Neural
Mechanisms
of Conditioning

Neural Mechanisms of Conditioning

Edited by
Daniel L. Alkon
National Institute of Neurological Communicative Diseases and Stroke
National Institutes of Health
at the Marine Biological Laboratory
Woods Hole, Massachusetts
and
Charles D. Woody
Mental Retardation Research Center
Brain Research Institute
University of California at Los Angeles
Los Angeles, California

Plenum Press • New York and London

Library of Congress Cataloging in Publication Data

Main entry under title:

Neural mechanisms of conditioning.

   Papers presented at a symposium held at the Marine Biological Laboratory in Woods
Hole, Mass., Nov. 1983.
   Includes bibliographical references and index.
   1. Neurophysiology — Congresses. 2. Conditioned response — Congresses. 3. Inver-
tebrates — Physiology — Congresses. 4. Vertebrates — Physiology — Congresses. I.
Alkon, Daniel L. II. Woody, C. D. (Charles D.).
QP356.N482   1985   591.1'88   85-19325
ISBN 0-306-42041-4

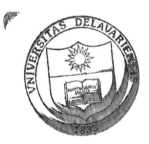

© 1986 Plenum Press, New York
A Division of Plenum Publishing Corporation
233 Spring Street, New York, N.Y. 10013

Printed in the United States of America

Contributors

WILLIAM B. ADAMS
Friedrich Miescher-Institut
CH-4002 Basel, Switzerland
Present address:
Biozentrum
University of Basel
CH-4056 Basel, Switzerland

DANIEL L. ALKON
Section on Neural Systems
Laboratory of Biophysics
IRP
National Institute of Neurological and
    Communicative Disorders and Stroke
National Institutes of Health at the Marine
    Biological Laboratory
Woods Hole, Massachusetts 02543

HIROSHI ASANUMA
The Rockefeller University
New York, NY 10021

H. L. ATWOOD
Department of Physiology
Faculty of Medicine
University of Toronto
Toronto, Ontario
Canada M5S 1AB

TAMAS BARTFAI
Department of Biochemistry
Arrhenius Laboratory
University of Stockholm
S-106 91 Stockholm, Sweden

G. BAUX
Laboratoire de Neurobiologie Cellulaire
Centre National de La Recherche Scientifique
F-91190 Gif sur Yvette, France

JACK A. BENSON
Friedrich Miescher-Institut
CH-4002 Basel, Switzerland
Present address:
Ciba-Geigy AG
Entomology Basic Research
CH-4002 Basel, Switzerland

NEIL E. BERTHIER
UCLA Medical Center
Mental Retardation Research Center
Brain Research Institute
Departments of Anatomy and Psychiatry
Los Angeles, California 90024
Present address:
University of Massachusetts
Amherst, Massachusetts 01003

LYNN J. BINDMAN
Department of Physiology
University College London
London WC1E 6BT, England

J. BRUNER
Laboratoire de Neurobiologie Cellulaire
C.N.R.S.
91190-Gif sur Yvette, France
Present address:
Laboratoire de Neurobiologie Cellulaire
Universite de Picardie
80039-Amiens, France

J. H. BYRNE
Department of Physiology and Cell Biology
University of Texas Medical School
Houston, Texas 77225

D. O. CARPENTER
Center for Laboratories and Research
New York State Department of Health
Albany, New York 12201

J. E. CHAD
Department of Biology and
  Ahmanson Laboratory of Neurobiology
University of California, Los Angeles
Los Angeles, California 90024

WAYNE E. CRILL
Department of Physiology and Biophysics
University of Washington
Seattle, Washington 98195

G. CZTERNASTY
Laboratoire de Neurobiologie Cellulaire
C.N.R.S.
91190-Gif sur Yvette, France
Present address:
Laboratoire de Neurobiologie Cellulaire
University de Picardie
80039-Amiens, France

W. JACKSON DAVIS
The Thimann Laboratories
University of California at Santa Cruz
Santa Cruz, California 95064

ROBERT J. DELORENZO
Department of Neurology
Yale University School of Medicine
New Haven, Connecticut 06510

JOHN F. DISTERHOFT
Department of Cell Biology and Anatomy
Northwestern University Medical School
Chicago, Illinois 60611

ROBERT W. DOTY
Center for Brain Research
University of Rochester
Rochester, New York 14642

R. ECKERT
Department of Biology and
  Ahmanson Laboratory of Neurobiology
University of California, Los Angeles
Los Angeles, California 90024

JOSEPH FARLEY
Department of Psychology
Princeton University
Princeton, New Jersey 08544

J. M. H. FFRENCH-MULLEN
Center for Laboratories and Research
New York State Department of Health
Albany, New York 12201

P. FOSSIER
Laboratoire de Neurobiologie Cellulaire
Centre National de La Recherche Scientifique
F-91190 Gif sur Yvette, France

JAMES R. GOLDENRING
Department of Neurology
Yale University School of Medicine
New Haven, Connecticut 06510

BRITTA HEDLUND
Department of Biochemistry
Arrhenius Laboratory
University of Stockholm
S-106 91 Stockholm, Sweden

N. HORI
Center for Laboratories and Research
New York State Department of Health
Albany, New York 12201
Present Address:
Department of Pharmacology
Kyushu University School of Dentistry
Fukuoka, Japan

GRAHAM HOYLE
Institute of Neuroscience
University of Oregon
Eugene, Oregon 97403

MASAO ITO
Department of Physiology
Faculty of Medicine
University of Tokyo
Bunkyo-ku, Tokyo 113
Japan

L. K. KACZMAREK
Departments of Pharmacology and
  Physiology
Yale University School of Medicine
New Haven, Connecticut 06510

ELLEN H.-J. KIM
UCLA Medical Center
Mental Retardation Research Center
Brain Research Institute
Departments of Anatomy and Psychiatry
Los Angeles, California 90024

K. KRNJEVIĆ
Departments of Anaesthesia Research
  and Physiology
McGill University
Montréal, Quebec H3G 1Y6
Canada

DENNIS M. D. LANDIS
Departments of Neurology, Developmental
  Genetics and Anatomy
Case Western Reserve University
Cleveland, Ohio 44106

JOSÉ LEMOS
Friedrich Miescher-Institut
CH-4002 Basel, Switzerland
Present Address:
Worcester Foundation for Experimental Biology
Shrewsbury, Massachusetts 01545

IRWIN B. LEVITAN
Friedrich Miescher-Institut
CH-4002 Basel, Switzerland
Present Address:
Graduate Department of Biochemistry
Brandeis University
Waltham, Massachusetts 02254

JEFFREY D. LEWINE
Center for Brain Research
University of Rochester
Rochester, New York 14642

R. MILES
Department of Physiology and Biophysics
University of Texas Medical Branch
Galveston, Texas 77550

JOHN W. MOORE
Department of Psychology
University of Massachusetts
Amherst, Massachusetts 01003

SHIGEMI MORI
Department of Physiology
Asahikawa Medical College
Asahikawa, Hokkaido
Japan 078-11

JOSEPH T. NEARY
Section on Neural Systems
Laboratory of Biophysics
National Institute of Neurological and
  Communicative Disorders and Stroke
National Institutes of Health at the Marine
  Biological Laboratory
Woods Hole, Massachusetts 02543

ILSE NOVAK-HOFER
Friedrich Miescher-Institut
CH-4002 Basel, Switzerland

R. E. NUMANN
Department of Physiology and Biophysics
University of Texas Medical Branch
Galveston, Texas 77550

K. O. OCORR
Department of Physiology and Cell Biology
University of Texas Medical School
Houston, Texas 77225

YOSHIHIRO OHTA
Department of Physiology
Asahikawa Medical College
Asahikawa, Hokkaido
Japan 078-11

C. A. PRINCE
Department of Physiology
University College London
London WC1E 6BT, England

JAMES L. RINGO
Center for Brain Research
University of Rochester
Rochester, New York 14642

STEVEN P. R. ROSE
Brain Research Group
The Open University
Milton Keynes, MK7 6AA
United Kingdom

TAKASHI SAKAMOTO
Department of Physiology
Asahikawa Medical College
Asahikawa, Hokkaido
Japan 078-11

PHILIP A. SCHWARTZKROIN
Department of Neurological Surgery
University of Washington
Seattle, Washington 98195

W. SHAIN
Center for Laboratories and Research
New York State Department of Health
Albany, New York 12201

VICTOR E. SHASHOUA
Mailman Research Center
McLean Hospital
Harvard Medical School
Belmont, Massachusetts 02178

T. SHIMAHARA
Laboratoire de Neurobiologie Cellulaire
C.N.R.S.
91190 Gif-sur Yvette
France

C. N. SINBACK
Center for Laboratories and Research
New York State Department of Health
Albany, New York 12201
Present Address:
Laboratory of Cell Biology
National Cancer Institute
National Institutes of Health
Bethesda, Maryland 20205

J. STINNAKRE
Laboratoire de Neurobiologie Cellulaire
C.N.R.S.
91190-Gif sur Yvette
France
Present address:
Laboratoire de Neurobiologie Cellulaire
Universite de Picardie
80039-Amiens, France

JEFFREY TAUBE
Departments of Physiology and Biophysics
University of Washington
Seattle, Washington 98195

L. TAUC
Laboratoire de Neurobiologie Cellulaire
Centre National de La Recherche Scientifique
F-91190 Gif sur Yvette, France

R. D. TRAUB
IBM T.J. Watson Research Center
Yorktown Heights, New York 10598
and

Neurological Institute
New York, New York 10032

NAKAAKIRA TSUKAHARA
Department of Biophysical Engineering
Faculty of Engineering Science
Osaka University, Toyonaka
and National Institute for Physiological Sciences
Okazaki, Japan

MARY LOU VALLANO
Department of Neurology
Yale University School of Medicine
New Haven, Connecticut 06510
Present address:
Department of Pharmacology
State University of New York
Upstate Medical Center
Syracuse, New York 13210

J. P. WALSH
Department of Physiology and Cell Biology
University of Texas Medical School
Houston, Texas 77225

E. T. WALTERS
Department of Physiology and Cell Biology
University of Texas Medical School
Houston, Texas 77225

CRAIG WEISS
Graduate Program in Neuroscience
Northwestern University Medical School
Chicago, Illinois 60611

R. K. S. WONG
Department of Physiology and Biophysics
University of Texas Medical Branch
Galveston, Texas 77550

CHARLES D. WOODY
UCLA Medical Center
Mental Retardation Research Center
Brain Research Institute
Departments of Anatomy and Psychiatry
Los Angeles, California 90024

Foreword

This is the second volume to be based on a series of symposia being held periodically on the neurobiology of conditioning. The first, entitled *Conditioning: Representation of Involved Neural Functions* was based on a symposium held in Asilomar, California, in October 1982 (Woody, 1982). The present volume is based on a symposium, organized by D. Alkon and C. Woody, held at the Marine Biological Laboratory in Woods Hole, Massachusetts in November 1983. This series of symposia and their publication are more than justified by the extraordinary progress being made during recent years in all branches of neuroscience and its application to our understanding of some of the basic neuronal mechanisms of conditioning and learning.

Invertebrate models of conditioning have been used by many in the attempt to obtain a more thoroughly controlled analysis at the single cellular and synaptic level of the mechanisms involved in elementary conditioning in a simple nervous system. Examples of this approach are presented in this volume and utilize insects (grasshopper), crustacea (crayfish), and particularly the relatively simple nervous systems of mollusks (*Aplysia* and *Hermissenda*). In such preparations it is possible to carry out precise electrophysiological and neurochemical studies of single identified cells and synapses involved in such simple processes as habituation and sensitization, as well as simple forms of "associative" conditioning, usually using simple aversive or withdrawal reflexes.

The question is raised by several contributors to this volume as to whether these precise studies of single cells and synaptic circuits in invertebrate models are actually pertinent to an understanding of mechanisms of conditioning and learning in higher vertebrates, such as cats, monkeys, and man. It is truly remarkable the degree to which the economy of nature has reproduced the same or very similar metabolic and biophysical mechanisms in nerve cells, in the electrical properties of their membranes, and even in the chemical substances used in the transmission across synaptic junctions in simple invertebrate nervous systems and in the most complex, including monkey and man. For example, the neuroactive amino acids, particularly glutamate, aspartate, and GABA play excitatory and inhibitory roles, respectively, in synaptic transmission in simple and complex forms, and they play the same role in neuromuscular transmission in crustacea.

Acetylcholine, which plays several important roles in the vertebrate nervous system, as a neurotransmitter at neuromuscular junctions, in sympathetic ganglia, and transmitter, as well as more a general neuroactivator or modulator in the vertebrate CNS, plays similar roles in invertebrate ganglia. The monamines, noradrenaline, dopamine, and serotonin, are also found to be either neurotransmitters or modulator substances in both invertebrates and the higher vertebrates. The same will probably be found to be true for many of the neuroactive peptides found to be of such importance in the regulation of synaptic excitability, even influencing the learning process in vertebrates. Ionic mechanisms, such as the effects of K^+, Na^+, Ca^{2+}, and Cl^- on synaptic transmission and upon intracellular metabolism is similar for all nerve cells. However, there are some important differences in the mode and location of action of these substances, differences that are particularly important when evaluating the degree to which invertebrate models of conditioning are valid for the far more complex processes in higher vertebrates.

In general, conditioning in vertebrates involves more highly specialized neuronal mechanisms and a centralization of mechanisms that may appear in simple, more peripheral, sensory motor reflex circuits in invertebrate ganglia. This is especially true for higher-order associative conditioning that may not be possible in lower invertebrate models and may even involve different mechanisms and specialized circuits such as the limbic system, the cerebellum, or the brain stem reticular system, which play special roles in higher vertebrate conditioning processes. Fortunately, with the improvement of microelectrode techniques for studying the properties of single brain cells in the intact vertebrate preparations, it is now possible to make a precise analysis of conditioning in higher forms at the cellular level. Some good examples are presented in this volume.

For example, in the experiments of Alkon and associates on the marine mollusk (*Hermissenda*), long-lasting changes in membrane conductance were found in the B-cell photoreceptor following a light-cued avoidance conditioning or in "associative" conditioning with light combined with rotation. Intracellular Ca^{2+} was elevated and K^+ currents reduced, with important changes in protein phosphorylation, which persisted even after removal of the photoreceptor. This may be a good model for some conditioning mechanisms at the postsynaptic cellular level, but such changes would probably not occur in vertebrate photoreceptors since they would have to preserve their normal function for non-conditioned responses. If such changes do occur in higher vertebrate preparations, they would probably be confined to central circuits or assemblies of neurones more widely distributed. Alkon himself presented a similar point of view at the previous symposium in Asilomar (Alkon, 1982).

There are many other important studies of basic biophysical and neurochemical mechanisms in single cells and synaptic circuits in invertebrates, for instance in *Aplysia*, showing the possible importance of serotonin in the modulation of Ca^{2+} flux in presynaptic or postsynaptic terminals with consequent changes in intracellular metabolism mediated by cyclic nucleotides, which may well be of great importance in our understanding of the ionic and molecular mechanisms of conditioning in general. The importance of specialized neuronal circuits and enduring changes in the biophysical properties of single cells in vertebrate preparations are also discussed in this volume, which covers a wide range of neurobiological studies of importance to our understanding of basic mechanisms of conditioning and learning.

Herbert H. Jasper

REFERENCES

Alkon, D. L., 1982, A biophysical basis for molluscan associative learning, in: *Conditioning: Representation of Involved Neural Functions*, C. D. Woody, ed., Plenum Press, New York, pp. 147-170.
Woody, C. D., 1982, Conditioning: Representation of Involved Neural Functions, Plenum Press, New York.

Contents

Contributors v

Foreword ix
Herbert H. Jasper

Part I—Invertebrate Models

1. Changes of Membrane Currents and Calcium-Dependent
   Phosphorylation during Associative Learning 3
   Daniel L. Alkon

2. Cellular Mechanisms of Causal Detection in a Mollusk 19
   Joseph Farley

3. Analysis of Associative and Nonassociative Neuronal Modifications
   in *Aplysia* Sensory Neurons 55
   J. H. Byrne, K. A. Ocorr, J. P. Walsh, and E. T. Walters

4. Mapping the Learning Engram in a "Model" System,
   the Mollusk *Pleurobranchaea californica* 75
   W. Jackson Davis

5. Recent Progress in Some Invertebrate Learning Systems 107
   Graham Hoyle

Part II—Vertebrate Models

6. Cellular Basis of Classical Conditioning Mediated
   by the Red Nucleus in the Cat 127
   Nakaakira Tsukahara

7. Dendritic Spine Structure and Function 141
   Dennis M. D. Landis

8. Rapid Conditioning of an Eye Blink Reflex in Cats 151
   Charles D. Woody, Neil E. Berthier, and Ellen H.-J. Kim

9. Neuronal Mechanisms Underlying Plastic Postural Changes
   in Decerebrate, Reflexively Standing Cats 167
   Shigemi Mori, Takashi Sakamoto, and Yoshihiro Ohta

10. Recovery of Motor Skill Following Deprivation of Direct Sensory Input
    to the Motor Cortex in the Monkey 187
    Hiroshi Asanuma

11. Motoneuronal Control of Eye Retraction/Nictitating
    Membrane Extension in Rabbit 197
    John F. Disterhoft and Craig Weiss

12. Two Model Systems 209
    John W. Moore

13. How Can the Cerebellar Neuronal Network Mediate
    a Classically Conditioned Reflex? 221
    Masao Ito

14. Mnemonic Interaction between and within Cerebral Hemispheres
    in Macaques 223
    Robert W. Doty, Jeffrey D. Lewine, and James L. Ringo

15. Passive Avoidance Training in the Chick: A Model for the Analysis
    of the Cell Biology of Memory Storage 233
    Steven P. R. Rose

    Part III—Membrane Physiology

16. Role of Calcium Ions in Learning 251
    K. Krnjević

17. Calcium-Dependent Regulation of Calcium Channel Inactivation 261
    R. Eckert and J. E. Chad

18. Calcium Action Potential Induction in a "Nonexcitable" Motor Neuron
    Cell Body: A Study with Arsenazo III. 283
    T. Shimahara, G. Czternasty, J. Stinnakre, and J. Bruner

19. Persistent Changes in Excitability and Input Resistance
    of Cortical Neurons in the Rat 291
    Lynn J. Bindman and C. A. Prince

20. A Critique of Modeling Population Responses for Mammalian
    Central Neurons 307
    Wayne E. Crill

21. Hippocampal Pyramidal Cells: Ionic Conductance and
    Synaptic Interactions 311
    R. K. S. Wong, R. E. Numann, R. Miles, and R. D. Traub

22. Mechanisms Underlying Long-Term Potentiation 319
    Philip A. Schwartzkroin and Jeffrey S. Taube

23. Modifiability of Single Identified Neurons in Crustaceans 331
    H. L. Atwood

24. Acetylcholinesterase and Synaptic Efficacy 341
   P. Fossier, G. Baux, and L. Tauc

25. Segregation of Synaptic Function on Excitable Cells 355
   D. O. Carpenter, J. M. H. ffrench-Mullen, N. Hori,
   C. N. Sinback, and W. Shain

   Part IV—Biochemistry

26. Phosphorylation of Membrane Proteins in Excitable Cells and Changes
   in Membrane Properties: Experimental Paradigms and Interpretations,
   a Biochemist's View 373
   Tamas Bartfai and Britta Hedlund

27. Calcium- and Calmodulin-Dependent Protein Kinase: Role
   in Memory 383
   Mary Lou Vallano, James R. Goldenring, and Robert J. DeLorenzo

28. Regulation of Neuronal Activity by Protein Phosphorylation 397
   José R. Lemos, William B. Adams, Ilse Novak-Hofer, Jack A. Benson,
   and Irwin B. Levitan

29. The Control of Long-Lasting Changes in Membrane Excitability by
   Protein Phosphorylation in Peptidergic Neurons 421
   L. K. Kaczmarek

30. Protein Phosphorylation, K^+ Conductances, and Associative Learning
   in *Hermissenda* 441
   Joseph T. Neary

31. The Role of Brain Extracellular Proteins in Learning and Memory 459
   Victor E. Shashoua

   Index 491

I

Invertebrate Models

Changes of Membrane Currents and Calcium–Dependent Phosphorylation during Associative Learning

DANIEL L. ALKON

1. INTRODUCTION

Much of what we learn concerns temporal relationships between stimuli or groups of stimuli. How does a system of neurons learn the temporal relationship between distinct sensory stimuli, as occurs, for instance, with Pavlovian conditioning? What are the biophysical and biochemical transformations that actually store the learned temporal relationship?

To address these questions in my laboratory we first developed a working blueprint of three separate sensory pathways (Alkon, 1973, 1974b, 1975, 1983) in a nudibranch mollusc called *Hermissenda crassicornis*. We then developed a model of Pavlovian conditioning by stimulating two of these pathways (Alkon, 1974a; Crow and Alkon, 1978) that had specific points of convergence; i.e., these pathways interacted in reproducible ways in every adult organism examined. Repeated pairings of light and rotation, which stimulate these separate sensory pathways beginning with the eye and statocyst, are followed by a long-lasting change in the animal's behavior. The nature of this change was most clearly manifest when light, the conditioned stimulus (CS) to which the animal is weakly attracted, elicits contraction of its caudal foot, an entirely new muscular response after training. This same contraction is reliably elicited, independent of training, as part of the animal's response to rotation, the unconditioned stimulus (UCS). As a result of training, the

DANIEL L. ALKON ● Section on Neural Systems, Laboratory of Biophysics, IRP, National Institute of Neurological and Communicative Disorders and Stroke, National Institutes of Health at the Marine Biological Laboratory, Woods Hole, Massachusetts 02543.

response to light has acquired some of the quantifiable features of the response to rotation (Lederhendler *et al.*, 1983). Also, as already described, this learned behavior has many of the hallmarks of Pavlovian conditioning of vertebrates. The learning is pairing specific and stimulus specific (Crow and Alkon, 1978). It increases as a function of practice and can be retained for several weeks. It shows extinction (Richards *et al.*, 1983), savings, and a requirement for contingency (Farley and Kern, 1984).

To find loci of neural changes that were causally related to the learning, we recorded intracellularly from many sites within the visual pathway, particularly from convergence sites, in conditioned and control animals. We accumulated evidence, with several different types of experiments, that the medial Type B photoreceptors play a causal role in the conditioning. The major findings that implicated these cells included:

1. *Extensive correlation* of Type B changes with learning of intact animals during acquisition, retention, and extinction (Crow and Alkon, 1980; West *et al.*, 1982; Farley and Alkon, 1982; Alkon *et al.*, 1982; Farley *et al.*, 1984; Alkon *et al.*, 1985).
2. *Intrinsic membrane changes* measured in Type B cells entirely isolated (i.e., in the absence of synaptic interactions with any other neuron) from conditioned, but not control, animals (Alkon *et al.*, 1982a; West *et al.*, 1982; Farley *et al.*, 1984; Alkon *et al.*, 1985).
3. *Prediction* of output changes (i.e., changes of motor impulse activity exiting from the central nervous system along nerves to muscle groups) by Type B changes based on known synaptic interactions, i.e., the flow of information through the visual pathway (Lederhendler *et al.*, 1982).
4. *Synthesis* of learned behavior by current injections (simulating depolarizing synaptic effect of rotation) paired with light (and not by injections alternating with light) in intact animals as well as isolated nervous systems (Farley *et al.*, 1983).

Given these sites of primary neural change during conditioning we could then ask, "What are the biophysical and biochemical transformations that lead to and actually store the learned information?" Based on our observations for *Hermissenda*, I would like to propose that the learning physiologist look at ionic channel properties within new temporal domains, extending from many minutes to hours to days. Within this new temporal domain, biophysical and ultimately biochemical mechanisms regulate ionic channels in ways that are not significant or appreciable within the milliseconds-to-seconds domain studied by most biophysicists during the last 40 years.

Briefly, the Type B cell soma membrane undergoes a conditioning-induced increase of excitability that can last for many days. The ionic channel changes that mediate this semipermanent increase of excitability, well within the learning temporal domain, arise first out of the electrical responses of the visual-vestibular network to light paired with rotation, i.e., within the millisecond-to-second temporal domain.

2. STIMULUS PAIRING

Light alone elicits a voltage-dependent depolarizing response from the Type B cell (Alkon and Grossman, 1978). The depolarization is sustained during the light and persists for many seconds after the light's cessation (Fig. 1). Rotation alone produces a synaptic hyperpolarization of the Type B cell followed by prolonged synaptic depolarization (Fig. 2; Tabata and Alkon, 1982). The temporal relationship of the two stimuli, light and rotation, strictly determines what happens to the Type B membrane potential (Figs. 2, 3, and 4). If light and rotation begin simultaneously or if rotation follows light by 1–2 sec, the depolarization of the Type B cell after the stimuli is substantially enhanced. This is due to two principal effects following stimulus pairing: (1) increased synaptic excitation of the Type B cell, and (2) increased input resistance of the Type B cell. In addition, these two effects of stimulus pairing are mutually enhancing. Stimulus pairing also enhances Type B depolarization relative to Type A depolarization during a light step. This is because inhibitory input from the hair cells during light is effective in blocking Type A impulses and not Type B impulses (Alkon, 1973; Tabata and Alkon, 1982). This biases the network in the eye in favor of Type B depolarization and against Type A depolarization.

When rotation onset follows the offset of light or when rotation offset precedes the onset of light, these two main effects are reversed (Fig. 3). The early hyperpolarization of the Type B cell produced by rotation does not occur during light because the input resistance of the Type B cell is low, thus shunting the synaptic input from the hair cells. The hyperpolarization produced by rotation will not be shunted if it occurs before the light and will actually be enhanced if it occurs after the light. The late depolarization of the Type B cell produced by rotation will be shunted if rotation precedes light and will be reduced if rotation onset follows light offset.

These features, then, of the network (Fig. 4) responses to different temporal

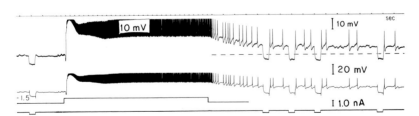

FIGURE 1. Effect of light on intact Type B photoreceptor. Cell was impaled simultaneously with two microelectrodes: one to measure voltage only, the other to measure voltage as well as to inject current (lower voltage traces). Depolarization during, and long-lasting depolarization associated with, decreased membrane conductance following a 30-sec light step (indicated by lowest trace and intensity expressed in −log units). Membrane conductance was measured by injection of negative current pulses (indicated by lowest trace). Dashed line indicates level of resting membrane potential. From Alkon and Grossman (1978).

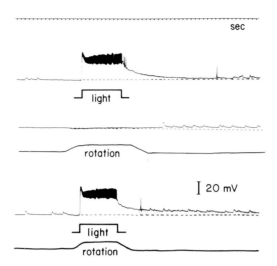

FIGURE 2. Responses of Type B photoreceptor to light and rotation. Rotation alone (middle panel) causes an initial synaptic hyperpolarization followed by prolonged depolarization and increased frequency of excitatory postsynaptic potentials (EPSPs). Light alone (upper panel) causes a depolarizing response as in Fig. 1, followed by a slight increase of EPSP frequency (some increase is typical). The light and rotation stimuli when presented alone were of somewhat longer duration than when presented together, i.e., paired (lower panel). Note that the paired presentation is followed by a larger depolarization and a greater EPSP frequency than following either stimulus presented alone.

relationships of the two stimuli will be expressed in terms of the net mean membrane potential of the Type B cell. Optimum pairing produces maximal mean depolarization (Fig. 5). The network responses, the resultant of an aggregate of neuron responses and their synaptic interaction within and between the visual and statocyst pathways, provide a basis for *temporal as well as stimulus specificity* of the learning process.

3. REPEATED STIMULUS PAIRING

When stimulus pairings are repeated, the residual membrane depolarization becomes progressively larger, reaching 10–15 mV after ten pairings (Fig. 5; Alkon, 1980). This progressive increase is really an accumulation of depolarization, since some depolarization after each pairing still remains when the next successive pairing occurs. Because of the voltage dependence of the depolarization following each light (Alkon, 1979), cumulative depolarization further enhances the depolarizing effects of each stimulus pairing. The effects (Fig. 6) of repeated stimulus pairing

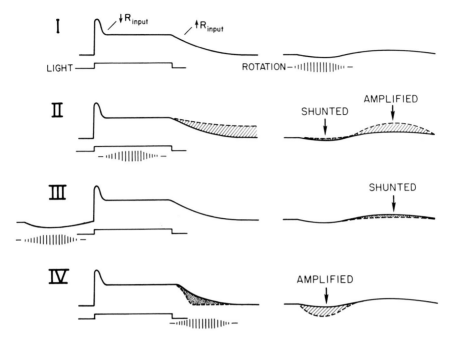

FIGURE 3. Effects of temporal relationship of light and rotation stimuli on Type B photoreceptor responses. Schematic responses to light stimuli (bars) are on left; responses to rotation stimuli (sequence of vertical lines) are on right. During light, input resistance (R_{input}) of Type B cell is low, thus shunting synaptic current due to activation of statocyst synaptic effects by rotation. Immediately after light, input resistance is two to three times higher than that prior to light, thereby amplifying rotation-induced synaptic input.

provide a basis for *acquisition* of the learned behavior. These effects include (1) cumulative membrane depolarization, (2) elevation of mean intracellular Ca_i^{2+} (Connor and Alkon, 1984), and (3) increased input resistance and excitability of the Type B cell.

4. PERSISTENT INCREASED EXCITABILITY

On days after acquisition, there is no residual depolarization nor is there evidence of elevated intracellular Ca_i^{2+}. The Type B cell remains, however, more excitable; i.e., in response to light or current injection, the Type B cell shows a greater depolarization. The medial Type B cells are not the only cells that change. Complementary changes also occur in the medial Type A photoreceptors (in each eye) that receive synaptic inhibition from the medial B cell (Richards *et al.*, 1983, 1984). Unlike the Type B cells, the medial Type A photoreceptors become less excitable as a result of training. What occurs, then, is a learning-induced bias in

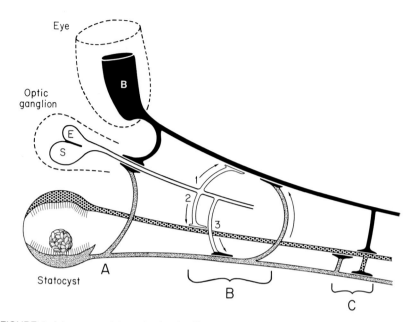

FIGURE 4. Intersensory integration by the *Hermissenda* nervous system. (A) Convergence of synaptic inhibition from Type B and caudal hair cells on S-E cell. (B) Positive synaptic feedback onto Type B photoreceptor. (1) Direct synaptic excitation. (2) Indirect excitation: E-S excites cephalic hair cell that inhibits caudal hair cell and thus disinhibits Type B cell. (3) Indirect excitation: E-S inhibits caudal hair cell and thus disinhibits Type B cell. (4) Indirect excitation: B cell inhibits C cell and thus disinhibits E cell; C-cell effects are not illustrated. (C) Intra- and intersensory inhibition. Cephalic and caudal hair cells are mutually inhibitory. Type B cell inhibits mainly the cephalic hair cell. All filled endings indicate inhibitory synapses; open endings indicate excitatory synapses. From Tabata and Alkon (1982).

the responsiveness of the neural system within each *Hermissenda* eye. It is a shift of the *relative* excitability of the sensory cells that encodes the learned temporal relationship of light with rotation. Stimulus pairing elicits responses from the visual-vestibular system, which selectively enhances the excitability of some cells while reducing that of others. Subsequent stimulation that is not selective, for example, presentations of light alone, will reduce the training-induced bias, i.e., will reduce the acquired difference in excitability of the Type B and A photoreceptors. The increased excitability, discussed above, which is intrinsic to the Type B soma membrane, provides a basis for *retention* of the learned behavior at least for many days. What changes of ionic channels account for this increased excitability and how do they arise?

5. LONG-TERM CHANGES OF IONIC CHANNELS

Voltage-clamp analysis reveals that there are four voltage-dependent currents that occur without light in response to depolarizations of 60 mV or less above the resting potential (Alkon *et al.*, 1984).

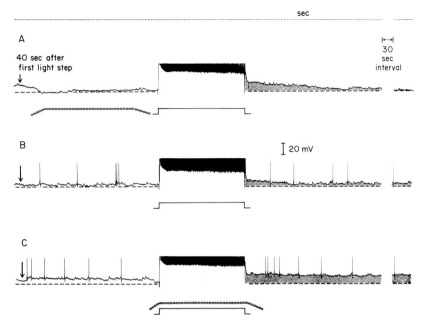

FIGURE 5. Intracellular voltage recordings of *Hermissenda* neurons during and after light and rotation stimuli. Responses of a Type B photoreceptor to the second of two succeeding 30-sec light steps (with a 90-sec interval intervening). The cell's initial resting potential, preceding the first of the two light steps in (A), (B), and (C), is indicated by the dashed lines. Depolarization above the resting level after the second of the two light steps is indicated by shaded areas. (A) Light steps ($\sim 10^4$ erg cm^{-2} sec^{-1}) alternating with rotation (caudal orientation) generating $\sim$ 1.0 g. The end of the rotation stimulus preceded each light step by 10 sec. (B) Light steps alone. (C) Light steps paired with rotation. By 60 sec after the first and second light steps, paired stimuli cause the greatest depolarization and unpaired stimuli the least. The minimal depolarization was in part attributable to the hyperpolarizing effect of rotation. Depolarization after the second presentation of paired stimuli was greater than that after the first. From Alkon (1980).

1. An early outward K$^+$ current known as I_A which shows rapid activation and inactivation.
2. A Ca^{2+}-dependent outward K$^+$ current with rapid activation and slow but substantial inactivation.
3. An inward Ca^{2+} current that is sustained, showing very little inactivation.
4. A late voltage-dependent K$^+$ current, the delayed rectifier, which is minimally activated at potentials $\leqslant 60$ mV.

In addition, there are two light-induced inward currents (Alkon, 1979): (1) an inward Na$^+$ current that inactivates within 2–3 sec, and (2) an outward Ca^{2+}-dependent K$^+$ current that arises from light-induced release of Ca^{2+} from intracellular stores.

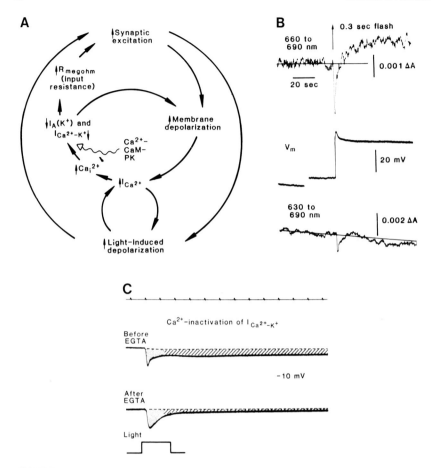

FIGURE 6. (A) Regenerative synaptic and light-induced excitation of the Type B photoreceptor. Light-induced depolarization facilitates synaptic excitation and vice versa in response to temporally associated light and rotation. Analyzed in biophysical terms, synaptic depolarization causes transient activation and then prolonged inactivation of I_A and $_{Ca^{2+}-K^+}$ and thereby enhancement of a voltage-dependent Ca^{2+} current. Increased intracellular Ca^{2+} causes further inactivation of I_A and $I_{Ca^{2+}-K^+}$ and thus a further increase of effective input resistance. These in turn cause more membrane depolarization. (B) Prolonged elevation of intracellular Ca^{2+} accompanies depolarizing response of isolated Type B cell to light. The cell was previously injected with arsenazo III. Absorbance changes at wavelength pairs of 660–690 and 630–690 nm (top and bottom records) and membrane voltage response (middle) following a 0.3-sec light flash. Differential absorbance changes at 660–690 nm measure changes of intracellular Ca^{2+}, while those at 630–690 nm measure changes of pH. (C) Ca^{2+}-inactivation of $I_{Ca^{2+}-K^+}$. Isolated type B cell soma is placed under voltage clamp at -60 mV in ASW. After 10 minutes' dark adaptation, the onset of command depolarizing step to -10 mV (15 seconds) is followed by brief light step ($10^{3.5}$ erg cm^{-2} sec^{-1}). Long-lasting apparent inward current following light step results from intracellularly released calcium causing inactivation of steady-state $I_{Ca^{2+}}-K^+$. With the same state of dark adaptation, the light induced decrease of $_{Ca^{2+}-K^+}$ is reduced after injection (under isopotential conditions) of EGTA (-2.0 nA, for 4 minutes). Calcium inactivation of $C_{Ca^{2+}-K^+}$ occurs in the absence of any activation of $I_{Ca^{2+}}$. (From Alkon, 1984.)

As mentioned above, several studies have shown that the isolated as well as the intact Type B cell depolarizes more in response to injection of positive current or light for conditioned as compared to control animals. This larger depolarizing response, which I previously described as an increased excitability, could arise from (1) a decrease in the voltage-dependent K^+ currents that act to hyperpolarize the membrane, and/or (2) an increase in the voltage-dependent Ca^{2+} current that acts to depolarize the membrane.

All available data (Alkon *et al.*, 1982, 1984) indicate that the first of these two possibilities, i.e., decreased K^+ currents (Alkon *et al.*, 1982b; Farley *et al.*, 1984; Forman *et al.*, 1984, Alkon *et al.*, 1985), largely accounts for conditioning-induced increase of the Type B excitability.

Blind voltage-clamp studies in fact revealed that the I_A and $I_{Ca^{2+}-K^+}$ are reduced across Type B soma membranes isolated from conditioned, but not control, animals (Fig. 7). The magnitude of this decreased I_A and $I_{Ca^{2+}-K^+}$ can account for most, if not all, of the Type B excitability increase. Although much of I_A and $I_{Ca^{2+}-K^+}$ inactivate, enough of these currents remain activated during a positive pulse to be responsible for a significant fraction of the total current flowing across the Type B soma membrane. Quantitative assessment of these currents is consistent with the effects of 1–3 mM external 4-aminopyridine (4-AP). 4-AP, which eliminates I_A without affecting the other Type B currents, causes the Type B input resistance (a measure of excitability) to increase during a light step (Acosta-Urquidi *et al.*, 1984). Substitution of Ba^{2+} for external calcium, which eliminates $I_{Ca^{2+}-K^+}$ without reducing the other Type B currents, causes a similar increase of input resistance and enhancement of the Type B depolarizing response to light.

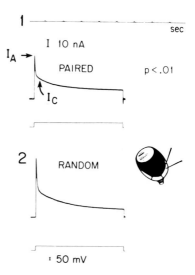

FIGURE 7. Membrane current changes with learning. Type B cell is isolated by axotomy after behavioral measurements are made preceding and following training. Cartoon depicts placement of two microelectrodes for voltage clamp. Ionic currents from holding potential of -60 mV: (1) paired I_A (early peak outward K^+ current) and $I_{Ca^{2+}-K^+}$ (late current, maximal at 300 msec after onset of command) are smaller than random (2) or naive values (not shown). From Alkon (1984).

6. BIOPHYSICAL STEPS IN CHANGING IONIC CHANNELS

How do these persistent reductions of K^+ currents arise? Again, how does a specific pattern of ionic fluxes elicited by stimulus pairing in one temporal domain, i.e., milliseconds to seconds, lead to a new balance of ionic fluxes in a much longer temporal domain, i.e., days to weeks? The process begins, we believe, with the cumulative depolarization of the Type B cell during repetitive stimulus pairing (Alkon, 1980). Intracellular Ca^{2+} is elevated during such pairing as measured with differential absorption spectrophotometry, and the mean Ca_i^{2+} (Connor and Alkon, 1984) remains elevated during the period of cumulative depolarization (Fig. 6). Elevation of intracellular Ca^{2+} can reduce most of the known Type B membrane currents, i.e., two of the voltage-dependent K^+ currents (I_A and $I_{Ca^{2+}-K^+}$), the voltage-dependent Ca^{2+} current and the light inward Na^+ and Ca^{2+} currents (Alkon et al., 1982b; Alkon et al., 1984; Alkon and Sakakibara, 1984). Ca^{2+}-mediated reduction of ionic flux was demonstrated with a number of experimental protocols. Using I_A as an example, we measured the I_A amplitude and level of Ca_i^{2+} before and after an abrupt rise of intracellular Ca^{2+} (Alkon et al., 1982a; Acosta-Urquidi et al., 1983). The reduction of I_A closely followed the level of Ca_i^{2+} as measured by differential spectrophotometry with arsenazo III. As I_A gradually increased (from its maximally reduced level) following the Ca^{2+} load, the level of intracellular Ca^{2+} gradually decreased. Any manipulation that reduced Ca_i^{2+} elevation, such as iontophoresis of EGTA, replacement of external Ca^{2+} with Ba^{2+} or block of Ca^{2+} currents with external Cd^{2+}, caused a corresponding decrease of the Ca^{2+}-mediated reduction of I_A. In other experiments Ca_i^{2+} was elevated by simulating the effect on the Type B soma of stimulus pairing (Alkon et al., 1982b). The isolated soma under voltage clamp was exposed to pairing of light with command depolarizing steps. The pairing (but not unpaired presentation) produced long-lasting depression of I_A. This depression did not occur when external Ca^{2+} (and thus the inward flux) was drastically reduced or replaced with Ba^{2+}. The same depression occurred when Ca^{2+} was iontophoresed with a third barrel under voltage-clamp control. Finally the magnitude of Ca^{2+}-mediated reduction of I_A was very dependent on the resting membrane potential of the Type B cell. As the cell becomes more depolarized, exactly as occurs during cumulative depolarization with stimulus pairing, the reduction becomes amplified and more prolonged.

Calcium-mediated decrease of $I_{Ca^{2+}-K^+}$ was first suggested by the observation that prior depolarization caused drastic reduction of $I_{Ca^{2+}-K^+}$ elicited by a depolarizing step under voltage clamp in the absence of any reduction of the calcium current (Alkon et al., 1984). This observation ruled out inactivation of $I_{Ca^{2+}-K^+}$ indirectly by calcium-mediated inactivation of $I_{Ca^{2+}}$ (which causes elevation of Ca_i^{2+} via voltage-dependent flux across the membrane) as described for other neurons (cf. Tillotson and Horn, 1978; Eckert and Lux, 1977; Eckert and Tillotson, 1978, 1981; Eckert and Ewald, 1981, 1983a,b; Eckert et al., 1981). In a series of other experiments, light was shown to cause intracellular release and thus elevation of calcium. Light was also shown to cause prolonged inactivation of of $I_{Ca^{2+}-K^+}$ via elevation of Ca_i^{2+} (Alkon and Sakakibara, 1984, 1985). The most direct demonstration of the latter was provided by the findings that intracellular iontophoresis of EGTA markedly reduced light-induced decrease of $I_{Ca^{2+}-K^+}$ (Fig. 6C) and that intracellular iontophoresis of Ca^{2+} reduces $I_{Ca^{2+}-K^+}$.

Different levels of Ca^{2+} are necessary to reduce Type B soma currents. Inactivation of I_A and $I_{Ca^{2+}-K^+}$ that remain decreased on retention days are results of elevation of Ca_i^{2+}, considerably below calcium levels necessary for inactivation of the delayed rectifying K^+ current and the voltage-dependent Ca^{2+} current. The voltage-dependent Ca^{2+} current shows, in fact, no inactivation unless external Ca^{2+} is substantially elevated (e.g., from 10 to 100 mM, thus elevating the voltage-dependent influx). This Ca^{2+}-dependent reduction of ionic fluxes not only requires different levels of Ca_i^{2+} to affect different ions. Differences between mechanisms for such inactivation of different channels were also suggested by iontophoresis of Mg^{2+} under voltage clamp instead of Ca^{2+}. Mg^{2+} elevation causes long-lasting reduction of the light-induced inward Na^+ current without affecting I_A (Alkon et al., 1982a,b).

During conditioning, as a function of elevated mean intracellular Ca^{2+}, many of the ionic currents are undergoing reduction. Because the voltage-dependent Ca^{2+} current itself shows no inactivation at normal levels of external Ca^{2+}, this current alone is sustained and can thus significantly determine the cumulative depolarization as well as the elevated Ca_i^{2+}. During acquisition of the conditioned behavior, reduction of I_A and I_C (the Ca^{2+}-dependent K^+ current) acts to depolarize the Type B membrane and increase resistance, i.e., increase excitability. Reduction of the inward light-induced Na^+ current acts to hyperpolarize the Type B membrane in response to successive light stimuli. With stimulus pairing, the effects of I_A and I_C reduction are greater than the effects of I_{Na^+} reduction. This is at least partly due to the fact that I_{Na} is more transient in nature; i.e., I_{Na^+} substantially inactivates during a Type B response to a single light step and thus does not greatly contribute to the steady-state depolarization of the cell during the light. Also, inactivation of I_{Na^+} apparently reverses more quickly than does inactivation of I_A and $I_{Ca^{2+}-K^+}$. The presence of I_{Na^+} inactivation, however, dampens the process of cumulative depolarization and increased excitability, preventing an explosive or unlimited increase. Cumulative depolarization, then, approximates an asymptote of membrane potential accompanied by increased input resistance; these effects are the resultant of Ca^{2+}-mediated current reductions in flux through at least three distinct channels, and these reductions, at least partially, have opposing effects.

During acquisition, the maximal depolarization achieved by each stimulus pair can be represented as the peak of an oscillating curve of membrane potential, while minimum depolarization reached just prior to each pair could correspond to the lower extreme of each wave (Fig. 8). Both maxima and minima increase during stimulus pairing and approach asymptotes, again as resultants of the opposing effects on membrane potential produced by waxing and waning of Ca^{2+}-mediated reduction of ionic currents.

The transition from electrical responses of a neural system to temporally related stimuli to prolonged changes of membrane potential, ionic flux, and excitability appears to be mediated by intracellular Ca^{2+}. The transition from these latter

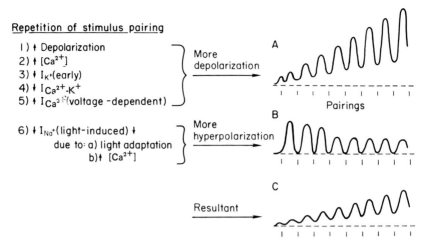

Repetition of stimulus pairing

1) ↑ Depolarization
2) ↑ [Ca²⁺]
3) ↓ I_K⁺(early)
4) ↓ I_Ca²⁺-K⁺
5) ↓ I_Ca²⁺(voltage -dependent)

More depolarization

6) ↓ I_Na⁺(light-induced) ↓
     due to: a) light adaptation
             b)↑ [Ca²⁺]

More hyperpolarization

Resultant

FIGURE 8. Summary of the effects of repeated stimulus pairing on Type B soma currents. On the right are schematic representations of progressive changes of Type B membrane potential with successive stimulus pairs.

changes to semipermanent (i.e., lasting for days) reduction of K^+ fluxes and the accompanying increased excitability is less clear-cut. A body of evidence now indicates that such a transition involves particular biochemical transformations.

7. BIOCHEMICAL STEPS FOR CHANGING IONIC CHANNELS

In an initial study using one-dimensional gel electrophoresis, phosphorylation of a low molecular weight protein (20,000) was found to change for eyes from conditioned when compared to naive animals or animals trained with randomized light and rotation (Neary *et al.*, 1981). Subsequently, it was shown that phosphorlyation of several low molecular weight proteins (20–25,000) was calcium-dependent. Exposure of *Hermissenda* neurons to high K^+ solutions (Neary and Alkon, 1983), effecting prolonged depolarization, caused phosphorylation differences of the same proteins (e.g., 25,000). Pharmacologic blockade of I_A, one of those K^+ channels which are changed after conditioning, also caused the same change in phosphorylation of the 25,000 mol. wt. protein. More recently, it was shown by Naito, *et al.*, 1985 that depolarization-induced changes of 25,000 mol. wt. protein phosphorylation persist long *after* the high K^+ solution is replaced with normal ASW.

Furthermore, intracellular manipulations which influence calcium-dependent phosphorylation cause persistent calcium-mediated reduction of $I_{Ca^{2+}-K^+}$ across the Type B soma membrane. Iontophoretic injection of a calcium–calmodulin-dependent kinase into the Type B soma (Fig. 9) produces a long-lasting calcium-dependent decrease of I_A and $I_{Ca^{2+}-K^+}$ (Acosta-Urquidi *et al.*, 1984). Iontophoretic

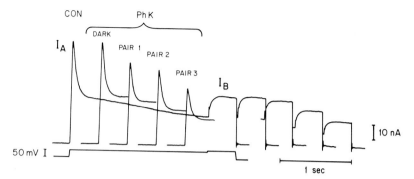

FIGURE 9. Effects of a single injection of phosphorylase kinase (60 nC) on axotomized Type B photoreceptor K$^+$ currents in normal Ca^{2+} - ASW. (Artificial Sea Water). From a V$_H$ of -60 mV, I$_A$ (left) was elicited by the first command step to -10 mV and decayed within approximately 1 sec to the steady state. A second superimposed step to 0 mV, applied 1.9 sec after the first step, elicited I$_B$. The family of K$^+$ currents (I$_A$ and corresponding I$_B$) show that phosphorylase kinase had no effect in I$_A$ or I$_B$ in darkness but reduced I$_A$ after a 20-sec pairing of light with depolarization to give a Ca^{2+} load (pair 1, to -10 mV). Further reduction of I$_A$ and also I$_B$ was evident after two additional pairings associated with increasing command steps (pair 2, to 0 mV; pair 3, to 15 mV). A full record is shown only for the control condition before the phosphorylase kinase injection. From Acosta-Urquidi *et al.* (1984).

injection of inositol triphosphate (but not inositol monophosphate) also produced a long-lasting reduction of I$_A$ and I$_{Ca^{2+}-K^+}$ (Sakakibara *et al.*, 1985). Exposure to activators of C-kinase enhanced and prolonged calcium-dependent decrease of I$_A$ and I$_{Ca^{2+}-K^+}$ (Alkon *et al.*, 1986). Finally, pharmacologic blockade of calcium-dependent phosphorylation (using calmidazolium or trifluoperazine) produced larger I$_A$ and I$_{Ca^{2+}-K^+}$ amplitudes and inhibited calcium-dependent reduction of these currents.

These observations, taken together, provide support for the conclusion that calcium-calmodulin-dependent protein phosphorylation is involved in the transition from short (minutes) to long (days or longer) term inactivation of those K$^+$ channels responsible for I$_A$ and I$_{Ca^{2+}-K^+}$.

8. CONCLUSION

Ca^{2+}–calmodulin-dependent protein phosphorylation could link the temporal domains of the acquisition phase of the learning to the temporal domain of retention. Repetitive pairing of light and rotation would cause cumulative depolarization and elevated Ca$_i^{2+}$. Elevated Ca$_i^{2+}$ in turn would stimulate Ca^{2+}-dependent phosphorylation of proteins that are part of or that regulate voltage-dependent K$^+$ channels. The consequent increased Type B excitability would decrease excitation of the medial Type A cell in response to light and thereby reduce interneuron and motor neuron excitation responsible for orienting the animal's movement toward a light source. This sequence of biophysical processes extends from a temporal domain of seconds (with a single stimulus pair) to one of hours for repetitive stimulus pairing to one of days for retained after-effects. These processes arise out of ionic channels and channel properties and protein transformations that have been remarkably conserved in the course of evolution from *Paramecia* to mammals and therefore could have relevance to our own learning and memory functions. This relevance has recently been supported by direct demonstration of conditioning-induced neuronal changes intrinsic to rabbit hippocampal slices (Disterhoft *et al.*, 1984, 1985). Comparison of intracellularly recorded afterhyperpolarizations of CNl cells from conditioned, pseudoconditioned, and naive animals showed a clear reduction on retention days only for the conditioned group. Thus, the Ca^{2+}-dependent K^+ current, $I_{Ca^{2+}-K^+}$, which is responsible for the afterhyperpolarization undergoes long-lasting reduction with rabbit conditioning exactly as has been observed with conditioned *Hermissenda*.

REFERENCES

Acosta-Urquidi, J., Alkon, D. L., Connor, J. A., and Neary, J. T., 1983, Intracellular injection of a Ca^{2+}-dependent protein kinase amplifies Ca^{2+}-mediated inactivation of a transient K^+ current (I_A) in *Hermissenda* giant neurons, *Soc. Neurosci. Abstr.* **9**:501.

Acosta-Urquidi, J., Alkon, D. L., and Neary, J. T., 1984, Ca^{2+}-dependent protein kinase injection in a photoreceptor mimics biophysical effects of associative learning, *Science* **224**:1254–1257.

Alkon, D. L., 1973, Intersensory interactions in *Hermissenda*, *J. Gen. Physiol.* **62**:185–202.

Alkon, D. L., 1974a, Associative training of *Hermissenda*, *J. Gen. Physiol.* **64**:70–84.

Alkon, D. L., 1974b, Sensory interactions in the nudibranch mollusc *Hermissenda crassicornis*, *Fed. Proc.* **33**:1083–1090.

Alkon, D. L., 1975, A dual synaptic effect on hair cells in *Hermissenda*, *J. Gen. Physiol.* **65**:385–397.

Alkon, D. L., 1979, Voltage-dependent calcium and potassium ion conductances: A contingency mechanism for an associative learning model, *Science* **205**:810–816.

Alkon, D. L., 1980, Membrane depolarization accumulates during acquisition of an associative behavioral change, *Science* **210**:1375–1376.

Alkon, D. L., 1983, Learning in a marine snail, *Sci. Am.* **249**:70–84.

Alkon, D. L., 1984, Calcium-inactivated potassium currents: A biophysical memory trace, *Science* **226**:1037–1045.

Alkon, D. L. and Grossman, Y., 1978, Long-lasting depolarization and hyperpolarization in eye of *Hermissenda*, *J. Neurophysiol.* **41**:1328–1342.

Alkon, D. L. and Sakakibara, M., 1984, Prolonged inactivation of a Ca^{2+}-dependent K^+ current but not Ca^{2+}-current by light-induced elevation of intracellular calcium, *Soc. Neurosci. Abstr.* **10**:10.

Alkon, D. L. and Sakakibara, M., 1985, Calcium activates and inactivates a photoreceptor soma K^+ current, *Biophys. J.* (in press).

Alkon, D. L., Lederhendler, I., and Shoukimas, J. J., 1982a, Primary changes of membrane currents during retention of associative learning, *Science* **215**:693–695.

Alkon, D. L., Shoukimas, J., and Heldman, E., 1982b, Calcium-mediated decrease of a voltage-dependent potassium current, *Biophys. J.* **40**:245–250.

Alkon, D. L., Farley, J., Sakakibara, M., and Hay, B., 1984, Voltage-dependent calcium and calcium-activated potassium currents of a molluscan photoreceptor, *Biophys. J.* **46**:605–614.

Alkon, D. L., Sakakibara, M., Harrigan, J., Lederhandler, I., and Farley, J., 1985, Reduction of two voltage-dependent K^+ currents mediates retention of a learned association, *Behav. Neural Biol.* (in press).

Alkon, D. L., Kubuta, M., Neary, J. T., Naito, S., Coulter, D., and Rasmussen, H., 1986, C-kinase activation prolongs Ca^{2+}-dependent inactivation of K^+ currents, *Proc. Natl. Acad. Sci. USA* (in press).

Connor, J. A. and Alkon, D. L., 1984, Light- and voltage-dependent increases of calcium ion concentration in molluscan photoreceptors, *J. Neurophysiol.* **51**:745–752.

Crow, T. J. and Alkon, D. L., 1978, Retention of an associative behavioral change in *Hermissenda crassicornis, Science* **201**:1239–1241.

Crow, T. J. and Alkon, D. L., 1980, Associative behavioral modification in *Hermissenda:* Cellular correlates, *Science* **209**:412–414.

Disterhoft, J., Coulter, D. A., and Alkon, D. L., 1984, Conditioning causes intrinsic membrane changes of rabbit hippocampal neurons *in vitro, Biol. Bull. Abstr.* **167**:526.

Disterhoft, J. F., Coulter, D. A., and Alkon, D. L., 1985, Conditioning-specific membrane changes of rabbit hippocampal neurons measured *in vitro, Proc. Nat. Acad. Sci. USA* (in press).

Eckert, R., and Ewald, D., 1981, Calcium-mediated calcium channel inactivation determined from tail current measurements, *Biophys. J.* **33**:145a.

Eckert, R., and Ewald, D., 1983a, Calcium tail currents in voltage-clamped intact nerve cell bodies of *Aplysia californica, J. Physiol. (Lond.)* **245**:533–548.

Eckert, R. and Ewald, D., 1983b, Inactivation of calcium conductance characterized by tail current measurements in neurons of *Aplysia californica, J. Physiol. (Lond.)* **245**:549–565.

Eckert, R., and Lux, H. D., 1977, Calcium-dependent depression of late outward current in snail neurons, *Science* **197**:472–475.

Eckert, R. and Tillotson, D., 1978, Potassium activation associated with intraneuronal free calcium, *Science* **200**:437–439.

Eckert, R. and Tillotson, D., 1981, Calcium mediated inactivation of the calcium conductance in caseium-loaded giant neurones of *Aplysia californica, J. Physiol. (Lond.)* **314**:265–280.

Eckert, R., Tillotson, D., and Brehm, P., 1981, Calcium mediated control of calcium and potassium currents, *Fed. Proc.* **40**:2226–2232.

Farley, J., 1985, Contingency learning and causal detection in *Hermissenda:* Behavioral and cellular mechanisms, *Behav. Neurosci.* (in press).

Farley, J. and Alkon, D. L., 1982, Associative neural and behavioral change in *Hermissenda* consequences of nervous system orientation for light- and pairing-specificity, *J. Neurophysiol.* **48**:785–807.

Farley, J., Richards, W. G., Ling, L. J., Liman, E., and Alkon, D. L., 1983, Membrane changes in a single photoreceptor cause associative learning in *Hermissenda, Science* **221**:1201–1203.

Farley, J., Sakakibara, M., and Alkon, D. L., 1984, Associative-training correlated changes in I_{Ca-K} in *Hermissenda* Type B photoreceptors, *Soc. Neurosci. Abstr.* **10**:270.

Forman, R., Alkon, D. L., Sakakibara, M., Harrigan, J., Lederhendler, I., and Farley, J., 1984, Changes in I_A and I_C but not I_{Na} accompany retention of conditioned behavior in *Hermissenda, Soc. Neurosci. Abstr.* **10**:121.

Lederhendler, I., Goh, Y., and Alkon, D. L., 1982, Type B photoreceptor changes predict modification of motorneuron responses to light during retention of *Hermissenda* associative conditioning, *Soc. Neurosci. Abstr.* **8**:824.

Lederhendler, I., Gart, S., and Alkon, D. L., 1983, Associative learning in *Hermissenda crassicornis* (Gastropoda): Evidence that light (the CS) takes on characteristics of rotation (the UCS), *Biol. Bull. Abstr.* **165**:528.

Naito, S., Neary, J. T., Sakakibara, M., and Alkon, D. L., 1985, Elevated external potassium causes persistent change of specific protein phosphorylation in *Hermissenda* nervous sytem, *Soc. Neurosci. Abstr.* (in press).

Neary, J. T., and Alkon, D. L., 1983, Protein phosphorylation/dephosphorylation and the transient, voltage-dependent potassium conductance in *Hermissenda crassicornis, J. Biol. Chem.* **258**:8979–8983.

Neary, J. T., Crow, T. J., and Alkon, D. L., 1981, Change in a specific phosphoprotein band following associative learning in *Hermissenda, Nature* **293**:658–660.

Richards, W., Farley, J., and Alkon, D. L., 1983, Extinction of associative learning in *Hermissenda:* Behavior and neural correlates, *Soc. Neurosci. Abstr.* **9**:916.

Richards, W. G., Farley, J., and Alkon, D. L., 1984, Extinction of associative learning in *Hermissenda:* Behavior and neural correlates, *Behav. Brain Res.* (in press).

Sakakibara, M., Alkon, D. L., Neary, J. T., DeLorenzo, R., Gould, R., and Heldman, E., 1985, Ca^{2+}-mediated reduction of K^+ currents is enhanced by injection of IP_3 or neuronal Ca^{2+}.calmodulin kinase type II, *Soc. Neurosci. Abstr.* (in press).

Tabata, M. and Alkon, D. L., 1982, Positive synaptic feedback in the visual system of the nudibranch mollusc *Hermissenda crassicornis*, *J. Neurophysiol.* **48:**174–191.

Tillotson, D. and Horn, R., 1978, Inactivation without facilitation of calcium conductance in caseium-loaded neurons of *Aplysia, Nature* **273:**312–314.

West, A., Barnes, E. S., and Alkon, D. L., 1982, Primary changes of voltage responses during retention of associative learning, *J. Neurophysiol.* **48:**1243–1255.

2

Cellular Mechanisms of Causal Detection in a Mollusk

JOSEPH FARLEY

1. INTRODUCTION

A primary function of associative learning and memory in the nudibranch mollusk *Hermissenda crassicornis* is to allow this animal to detect, anticipate, and to respond appropriately to *causal relations* within its environment. The cellular mechanisms by which this is accomplished reflect the integrated effects of the synaptic organization of the visual and vestibular systems, in conjunction with the intrinsic electrophysiological characteristics of the component neurons.

From the standpoint of efficiency, any biological system designed to detect causal relations should at minimum satisfy the following criteria. First, the system should be able to store information concerning those events that co-occur and those that do not in a rapid and enduring manner, days at minimum. Second, it should be able to distinguish between regularities that are merely coincidental and those likely to reflect causal structure inherent within the environment. That is, it should distinguish between mere contiguity and contingency. Third, the system should reflect the fidelity of the temporal relations implicit in environmental causal relations. Since perception often imitates logic and entails that causes typically precede effects, it is crucial that temporal sequence information be represented within associative memory if efficient adaptive use of the causal relation is to be made. Fourth, representations of causal relations within a system should be updateable. If the environmental regularity should cease or become ambiguous or degraded for any reason, then this should be reflected within the record of associative memory. Students of animal learning will recognize these generic features of causal detection systems as paralleling many of the salient empirical characteristics of Pavlovian conditioning: long-term retention, contingency sensitivity, the customary superiority

JOSEPH FARLEY ● Department of Psychology, Princeton University, Princeton, New Jersey 08544.

of forward vs. simultaneous and backward conditioning sequences, extinction, and partial reinforcement.

The associative suppression of phototaxic behavior in the nudibranch *Hermissenda* provides one interesting example of causal detection that is understood at the cellular level. Indeed, at present it is the sole preparation for which such an understanding exists. As will be shown, the parallels between training-produced behavioral changes in the intact animal and the neurophysiological characteristics of identified neurons, which mediate both the simple and more complex phenomenology of associative learning, encourage the view that relatively simple nervous systems may yield cellular insights into not only the phenomena of associative learning and memory but also more complex forms of behavioral adaptation as well.

2. SIMPLE AND COMPLEX CHARACTERISTICS OF ASSOCIATIVE LEARNING IN *HERMISSENDA*

2.1. Pairing- and Stimulus-Specific Behavioral Changes

Hermissenda typically locomotes towards a light source when tested during the daylight portion of its diurnal cycle (Alkon, 1974). Five pairings of light and rotation (Farley and Alkon, 1982b, 1985b) result in the suppression of phototaxic behavior for up to 25 min or so following training. Prolonged exposure to pairings of light and rotation (Crow and Alkon, 1978; Farley and Alkon, 1980b) results in a long-term suppression that persists for 3–4 days (Fig. 1) or longer (J. S. Harrigan and D. L. Alkon, in preparation), depending upon the extent of original training. This suppression of phototaxic behavior is specific to pairings of these two stimuli, and reflects neural changes in two of three Type B photoreceptors in each eye of the animal (Farley and Alkon, 1980b, 1982b; Alkon, 1980). Pairings of light and rotation consistently produce greater phototaxic suppression than equivalent numbers of random presentations of light and rotation (Crow and Alkon, 1978; Farley and Alkon, 1980a, 1982a; Farley, 1985), light-alone, rotation-alone, or explicitly unpaired presentations of the two stimuli (Crow and Alkon, 1978), when light and rotation intensities are equated for across-treatment conditions.

Suppression of phototaxic behavior in *Hermissenda* is also stimulus specific. The training-produced decreased movement towards light is not attributable to either generalized decreases in arousal or a diminished capacity for evoked locomotion of any sort, since pairings of light and rotation produce no consistent reduction of animals' locomotor behavior induced by gravitational stimulation (Farley and Alkon, 1982a). Moreover, posttraining tests of phototaxic behavior with light intensities substantially different from that customarily used in training generally fail to reveal significant effects of training (Vold *et al.*, 1985). This failure of conditioning to generalize along the dimension of light intensity is paralleled by diminished training-produced differences in light-induced impulse activities in Type B photoreceptors, when light intensities deviate too greatly from the standard training

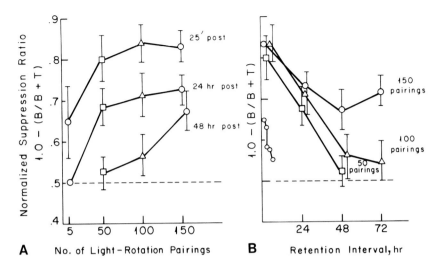

FIGURE 1. Acquisition and retention curves for associative suppression of phototaxic behavior in *Hermissenda*. Strength of conditioning is expressed in terms of the suppression ratio: B/B + T (B = baseline pretraining latency; T = retention test latency), normalized to 1.0 so that more positive values correspond to greater conditioning. (A) Conditioning strength expressed as a function of the number of light–rotation pairings. Each point along a curve represents the results of a separate group of animals [adapted from Farley and Alkon, 1980a; 1982a (150 pairings); Farley and Alkon, 1982b, 1985b (5 pairings); Richards *et al.*, 1983, 1984 (100 pairings); J. Farley and G. Kern, unpublished (50 pairings)]. Each curve depicts the results for the designated retention interval. (B) Persistence of associative suppression as a function of the number of pairings administered during training [same results and sources as in (A)].

level (Farley and Alkon, 1982a). In all probability, these effects do *not* reflect the capacity of the animal to exhibit associative discriminations among lights of varying intensities as in vertebrates. Although the experiment has not been done, discriminative conditioning between lights of differing intensities (e.g., dim light–rotation, bright light–no rotation, and vice versa) would be surprising, since the light intensities that are effective in producing training comprise a subset of those that elicit phototaxis (Farley and Alkon 1982a, 1985a). All other things being equal, training lights that are too bright or too dim fail to produce the associative training effect (see Section 3.4). The possibilities for additional tests of specificity within the visual modality are necessarily circumscribed. For example, the prerequisites for color vision appear to be lacking in *Hermissenda*, thereby precluding generalization tests along the dimension of hue.

Associative learning in *Hermissenda* occupies an apparently unique position within invertebrate—particularly gastropod—learning: nonassociative learning processes, such as habituation, sensitization, and pseudoconditioning, simply fail to play an appreciable role (see Richards *et al.*, 1983, 1984; Farley and Alkon, 1985a). Attempts to produce a persistent suppression of phototaxis by maximizing any nonassociative effects of light and/or rotation have been singularly unsuccessful. Distributing extra light- or rotation-alone presentations throughout a sequence of pairings fails to enhance the associative suppression and instead attenuates it (Farley, 1985). Pre-exposure of animals to large number of light- or rotation-alone presentations prior to pairings, which might be expected to either retard (latent inhibition) or alternatively enhance acquisition (latent facilitation), fails to affect subsequent conditioning (G. Means and J. Farley, in preparation). Moreover, increased intensities of light and rotation produce no suppression that exceeds durations of an hour or so, when efforts to simulate the associative effects of the customary stimulus intensities through nonassociative training protocols are undertaken (e.g., light-alone, rotation-alone, explicitly unpaired sequences; J. Farley, in preparation). Insofar as modifications of phototaxic behavior by prior experience with light and rotation are concerned, there seems to be primarily one way in which to produce suppressed phototaxis: by pairing light and rotation. These results imply that those cellular mechanisms (see Sections 3.3 and 3.6) that mediate phototaxic suppression are specialized for *associative learning*. They in no sense represent an elaboration upon a more primitive nonassociative process, such as sensitization, as has been argued for alpha-conditioning of the gill- and siphon-withdrawal reflexes of *Aplysia* (Kandel and Schwartz, 1982; Byrne *et al.*, Chapter 3, this volume).

2.2. Contiguity vs. Contingency

"Pairings" of stimuli represent one extreme case of environmental regularity to which traditional conceptions of animal learning have attached paramount importance. However, as originally noted by Prokasy (1965) and Rescorla (1968), both animals and humans are sensitive to other "correlations" between events, even in the relatively rarified and simplified experimental paradigms of classical conditioning. Organisms can learn that events consistently fail to co-occur, as in conditioned inhibition training (Pavlov, 1927; Konorski, 1967; Rescorla, 1975). Animals' learned behavior also often reflects the extent to which cues are reliable and consistent predictors of one another (Kamin, 1969; Mackintosh, 1975). In short, they are sensitive to both the sign and magnitude of the contingency between stimuli, with respect to the dimensions of both space (Testa, 1974) and time (Rescorla, 1972).

One of the more striking demonstrations of the sensitivity of vertebrates to stimulus contingencies, rather than stimulus contiguity, involves an apparent failure of animals to learn under what would otherwise appear to be favorable conditions. Consider the following classical conditioning experiment, one which has been repeated with a variety of vertebrate preparations. In one condition, subjects receive 50 CS–UCS pairings. Following training, the strength of conditioning is assessed and it is observed that a strong conditioned response (CR) has developed. A second group of subjects receives 50 UCSs interspersed among the 50 CS–UCS pairings. None of these extra UCSs is contiguous with a CS. They are delivered throughout training, either a long time before or after the CS–UCS pairings. Following training it is observed that conditioning is severely reduced. The dilemma that such results pose for views of learning that stress the number of contiguous pairings of CS and

UCS as crucial for learning is obvious: the extra UCSs attenuate conditioning despite the presence of an otherwise adequate number of CS–UCS pairings. It appears that the relation that most strongly controls the animal's behavior is that of CS–UCS contingency, rather than simply the number of pairings. A convenient descriptive metric that captures this intuition is the conditional probability difference: [P(UCS/CS) − P(UCS/no CS)]. Positive values of this statistic entail "excitatory" conditioning, viz., normal CR acquistion, while negative values correspond to conditioned inhibition procedures.

Contingency experiments with *Hermissenda* indicate that these animals behave in much the same fashion as vertebrates. A behavior demonstration of contingency (Farley, 1985) sensitivity was first arranged by comparing the extent of phototaxic suppression produced by consistent pairings of light and rotation [p(R/L) = 1.0; p(R/no L) = 0] with that resulting from a degraded contingency treatment in which either extra rotation-alone [p(R/no L) = .75] or light-alone [p(R/L) = .33] presentations were delivered between pairings of light and rotation. As Fig. 2 indicates, animals that received only pairings of light and rotation exhibited pronounced suppression of phototaxis during retention, while animals that experienced a degraded contingency exhibited little conditioning at all. These results demonstrate that the behavior of *Hermissenda* is sensitive not only to the number of light–rotation pairings (that is, the relation of temporal contiguity) but also to the degree to which light is a valid and reliable predictor of rotation (contingency).

Since the original demonstrations of contingency (Rescorla, 1968), at least two distinct theoretical conceptions of the phenomena have been suggested. One class of account regards animals as sensitive to the *correlation* between CS and UCS (Rescorla, 1972). According to this view, event correlations are dimensionless relations that characterize the degree to which events consistently occur—or fail to occur—together, and it is assumed that animals in some way are directly responsive to such relations. A second view of contingency-sensitivity derives the animal's apparent sensitivity to CS–UCS correlations from a more basic trial-by-trial conditioning process. According to one such model (Rescorla and Wagner, 1972), any and all CSs present on conditioning trials compete with one another for association with the UCS. Added UCS-alone presentations degrade conditioning because they allow for the possibility of "contextual conditioning," i.e., conditioning to static environmental cues, which then compete for control of behavior with the nominal CS. Added CS-alone trials allow for "extinction." Other accounts of contingency-sensitivity eschew the notion of "correlation" entirely and instead attempt to account for contingency effects by noting the unfavorable mixture of interstimulus interval (ISI) relations entailed by contingency schedules. For example, a UCS-delivered adjacent to a CS–UCS pairing may be viewed as constituting two pairing "trials," one with a favorable temporal relationship between CS and UCS and one with a long, variable, and presumably unfavorable delay (Millenson *et al.*, 1977).

A primary difference among these accounts is the degree to which they emphasize the importance of the local temporal context of reinforcement. According to the original correlational view, a conditioning protocol that entails strict CS–UCS pairings is one entailing a maximum positive correlation of CS and UCS, regardless of whether the time elapsing between such pairings (ITI) is particularly long or

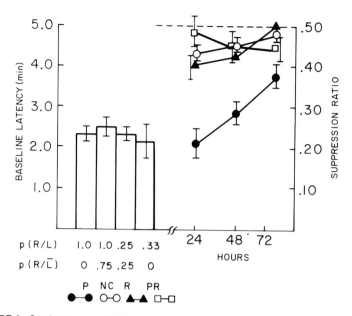

FIGURE 2. Contingency-sensitivity of phototaxic suppression in *Hermissenda*. Retention data (right ordinate) expressed as suppression ratio: B/B + T, where B = baseline pretraining latency, T = posttraining test latency. Group P, for whom a positive training contingency existed, received the standard three successive days of training, 50 trials/day, average ITI = 2.0 min [p(R/L) = 1.0]. Group NC (noncontingent training) received the same 50 pairing trials/day (ITI = 2.0 min), but in addition received 100 extra 30-sec rotation-alone presentations distributed throughout each training session [p(R/L) = 1.0; P(R/no L) = .75]. This entailed an average rotation ISI of 40″. Group PR received the same experience with paired light and rotation, but received 100 extra 30-sec light-alone presentations distributed throughout each training session [p(R/L) = .33]. Group R (random control) received 50 light and rotation presentations on each training day, delivered with an average ISIs of 2.0 min, randomly and independently of one another. Only group P, for which a substantial positive light-rotation contingency existed, exhibited retained phototaxic suppression. Note the absence of conditioning for groups NC and PR. (From Farley, 1985.)

short. Degrading a CS–UCS contingency through the addition of unpaired UCS-alone presentations to a sequence of CS–UCS pairings would be expected to depend little upon the precise temporal relation of unpaired UCSs and pairings of CS and UCS (i.e., the local temporal context of reinforcement). Yet local temporal context and trial-by-trial CS and UCS ISIs are potent determinants of learning. The effects of additional UCS-alone or CS-alone presentations clearly depend upon their temporal relationship to CS–UCS pairing (Farley, 1980; Ayres *et al.*, 1975; Jenkins and Shattuck, 1981; Kremer and Kamin, 1971). Indeed, whether CSs and UCS are regarded as "paired" or "unpaired" for an animal presumes an underlying temporal contiguity gradient to which the animal is sensitive. The relation of contingency depends in a fundamental way upon the temporal characteristics of sensory and

contiguity gradient to which the animal is sensitive. The relation of contingency depends in a fundamental way upon the temporal characteristics of sensory and more central systems: their ability to resolve near contiguous presentations of light and rotation into single vs. joint occurrences.

Figure 3 illustrates this dependence of contingency learning upon the capacity for temporal resolution of *Hermissenda*'s nervous system (Farley, 1985). Depicted in Fig. 3 are the retained changes in phototaxic suppression for each of four treatment conditions. One group (50 L–R) received the standard pairing treatment: fifty

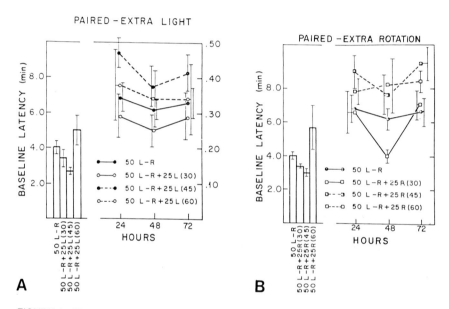

FIGURE 3. (A) Baseline and normalized test ratios for phototaxic behavior of *Hermissenda* exposed to either 50 or 75 pairings of light and rotation (results have been pooled and are designated by 50 L–R) or 50 pairings of light and rotation with added light-alone presentation presented either 30, 45, or 60 sec prior to a randomly selected 50% of pairings [groups 50 L–R + 25 L (30), (45), (60), respectively]. The left-hand portion depicts the mean locomotor latencies for animals prior to training. The right-hand portion (note change of ordinate) depicts the mean test ratios for animals during tests conducted 24, 48, and 72 hr after the conclusion of training. Response measure is a suppression ratio of the form B/(B + T), where B indicates baseline latency and T indicates test latency; numbers less than .50 indicate suppression. Error bars are standard deviations. Note attenuation of suppression for group 50 L–R + 25 L (45 sec) relative to group 50 L–R (Farley, 1985). (B) Baseline and normalized test ratios for phototaxic behavior of *Hermissenda* exposed to either 50 or 75 pairings of light and rotation (results have been pooled and are designated by 50 L–R; same as in (A), or 50 pairings of light and rotation with added rotation-alone presentations presented either 30, 45, or 60 sec prior to a randomly selected 50% of pairings. Note attenuation of suppression for groups 50 L–R + 25 R (30, 45) relative to group 50 L–R. (From Farley, 1985.)

light–rotation pairings on each of three successive training days. The remaining three groups received these same pairings but in addition received extra light-alone presentations that terminated either 30, 15, or 0 sec prior to a randomly selected half of the pairings. The major point is clear: the added light steps failed to attenuate associative conditioning when their offsets occurred either 0 or 30 sec prior to pairings. They appeared to be processed either as part of a joint occurrence of light and rotation [group 50 L–R and 25 L (30 sec)] or as an event with no significant effect upon the degree of suppression due to pairings [group 50 L–R and 25 L (60 sec)]. However, when terminating 15 sec prior to a pairing, the added light steps reduced conditioning. The results of a similar experiment substituting rotation-alone for light-alone presentations is also depicted in Fig. 3. Here, animals receiving extra rotation-alone steps which terminated either 15 or 30 sec prior to light-rotation pairings exhibited attenuated phototaxic suppression [groups 50 L–R and 25 R (45 sec, 60 sec)], while a group that received added rotation that terminated 0 sec before a pairing was no different from the standard pairing group. In general, the conditions under which the added light- and rotation-alone presentations will attenuate conditioning are predictable from our understanding of the neuronal organization of the visual and vestibular systems (cf. Section 3.4) and support the following conclusions: *The cellular machinery that provides for simple associative learning in Hermissenda also provides for contingency learning.*

Our contingency experiments also underscore the unique degree to which the behavioral changes resulting from the associative training procedure can be attributed to associative learning mechanisms in *Hermissenda*. Indeed, contingency experiments provide a general analytic means of distinguishing between whether *associative* or *nonassociative* processes account for the pairing-specific behavioral changes observed within other invertebrate conditioning paradigms (cf. Farley and Alkon, 1985a; Farley, 1985, for further discussion). If the greater behavioral change seen for paired vs. unpaired training paradigms reflects greater nonassociative learning process (such as greater sensitization of the gill and siphon withdrawal in *Aplysia*), then adding additional UCS-alone presentations would further enhance the effects of pairings, certainly not attenuate it. On the other hand, if the pairing-specific behavioral changes genuinely reflect an associative process, analogous to that of vertebrate conditioning, then the added UCS-alone presentations should attenuate conditioning due to pairings in these preparations as they do in *Hermissenda*.

2.3. Temporal Relations

In addition to the dimension of interevent correlations or contingency, the concept of a neural network as specialized for causal detection also implies that it is sensitive to particular orders of event occurrences. Although a number of examples of reliable associative learning occurring with simultaneous CS–UCS onsets (e.g., Heth and Rescorla, 1973) and "backward" UCS–CS sequences (Spetch *et al.*, 1981) have been provided in recents years, it remains true that forward CS–UCS sequences without question constitute the most favorable arrangement for producing a strong CR (Moore and Gormezano, 1977; Gormezano *et al.*, 1982).

For *Hermissenda,* the temporal order relation most commonly used is a "simultaneous" one, in which both the onsets and offsets of light and rotation occur together. However, this designation of the temporal arrangement as "simultaneous" is only approximately correct. Owing to the inertia of the turntable motor used to deliver rotational stimulation, maximum g is reached with a delay of 500–1000 msec. Hence, the arrangement more closely approximates a forward sequential arrangement. Recent experiments by Grover and Farley (1983) that explicitly compared the relative effectiveness of forward, simultaneous, and backward pairings indicate the nominal simultaneous procedure to be superior to backward conditioning, as well as to a forward delayed conditioning procedure in which 30 sec intervened between light and rotation onsets. Whether phototaxic suppression in *Hermissenda* exhibits the steep ISI functions characteristic of many vertebrate preparations remains to be determined.

2.4. Updating of Causal Relations

Perhaps the simplest means of changing the current status of the causal relation implied by CS–UCS pairings is to repeatedly present the CS without the UCS (extinction). If indeed it is adaptive for *Hermissenda* to learn to suppress its positive response to light when it is paired with rotation, since such learning may permit the animal to successfully negotiate the hazards of intertidal life, then it is also sensible to expect a cessation of phototaxic suppression once the circumstances (light-rotation pairings) that initially gave rise to suppression no longer obtain. It is precisely this feature of reversibility that serves to distinguish those forms of causality learning in which the relation may change rapidly and repeatedly during the life of an individual animal from those in which the structure within the environment is more static and hence presumably under greater developmental constraint. In *Hermissenda,* Richards *et al.* (1983, 1984) have recently demonstrated extinction of phototaxic suppression (see Section 3.1) for animals repeatedly exposed to nonreinforced light presentations following the conclusion of successful conditioning. Aside from the criterion of reversibility that this demonstration exemplifies, extinction in *Hermissenda* is interesting for an additional reason. It occurs in the absence of any demonstrable habituation to light and fails to exhibit the features of spontaneous recovery and disinhibition (Pavlov, 1927). All three characteristics generally accompany extinction of Pavlovian conditioning in vertebrate species and historically have been influential in suggesting to some that extinction is little more than the process of habituation to the CS, and, correspondingly, spontaneous recovery and disinhibition are little more than reflections of dishabituation or sensitization. However, their absence in *Hermissenda* implies that a major portion of the decline of phototaxic suppression following extinction is attributable to a reversal of the original process of acquisition rather than to a simple masking of the original learning due to habituation. Intracellular recordings from cells known to play a causal role in acquisition and retention confirm this notion (cf. Section 3.2).

In summary, the associative suppression of phototaxic behavior in *Hermissenda* is characterized by most, if not all, of the critical and defining features of associative learning for vertebrates. These features include pairing and stimulus specificity, well-behaved acquisition and retention functions, and a virtual absence of nonassociative processes. In addition, *Hermissenda*'s learning also shares some of the more interesting and complex characteristics of associative learning and causal detection for more evolved animals, viz., contingency learning, extinction, superior conditioning for distributed vs. massed training procedures (Section 3.4), and sensitivity to the temporal order of light and rotation. It has been particularly gratifying in our research with *Hermissenda* to discover that the same neural networks and cellular principles that govern the acquisition and retention of the basic associative behavioral change also play fundamental roles in generating much of the more complex and nonintuitive phenomenology of associative learning. We now turn to our understanding of these cellular mechanisms.

3. NEUROPHYSIOLOGY OF ASSOCIATIVE LEARNING AND CAUSAL DETECTION

Any serious attempt to understand learning, memory, and the detection and perception of causal relations at the cellular level must address four issues. The first is that of localization of function. Where do neural changes occur within the animal that are causally related to the learned behavioral change? Secondly, how are these changes propagated throughout the nervous system so as to affect behavior? How is knowledge expressed in performance? Third, what are the mechanisms for acquisition of knowledge? For *Hermissenda,* how is the association between light and rotation encoded? Fourth, what are the mechanisms of retention and retrieval? What is the basis for enduring neural changes, and how is stored information accessed?

3.1. Localization of Sites of Learning: Type B and A photoreceptors

Three lines of evidence converge to imply that the somas of Type B photoreceptors in *Hermissenda's* eyes are primary sites of neural change that mediate acquisition, retention, and retrieval of the learned suppression of phototaxis. This evidence includes demonstrations of striking correlations between the training-produced electrophysiological characteristics of Type B cells and the behavior of intact animals: (1) during acquisition and retention of learning, (2) following extinction, partial reinforcement, and degraded contingency training, (3) for comparisons of massed vs. distributed training trials, and (4) for a variety of light-rotation ISI conditions. Second, these training-produced changes are intrinsic to the Type B cells; they are not secondary consequences of changes elsewhere. These changes are well correlated with, and in many cases allow us to predict, the training-produced light-evoked differences in interneurons and motoneurons involved in phototaxis. Finally, and most importantly, artificial induction of membrane changes in the Type B cells of previously untrained, semi-intact, behaving animals is sufficient to produce long-term changes in phototactic behavior.

Intracellular recordings from Type B photoreceptors, immediately following three days of associative training, significantly differ in three respects from cells from comparable control animals: (1) The resting potentials of paired condition B cells are more positive; (2) the long-lasting depolarization response (LLD) of these same cells in response to brief flashes of light is greater; (3) input resistances are enhanced (Crow and Alkon, 1980).

Similar correlations between *long-term* electrophysiological changes in Type B cells and associative modifications of phototaxis are also obtained (Farley and Alkon 1981, 1982a,b; Farley, 1985; Farley *et al.*, 1982a,b, 1983a; Richards *et al.*, 1983, 1984; Fig. 4 and 5). Increased input resistances and enhanced peak, steady state, and LLD responses are apparent for paired vs. random conditioning treatments, one and two days following training. These differences reflect membrane changes intrinsic to the neurons, since axotomizing the B cells—which isolates them from all synaptic interactions—fails to abolish the training-produced differences. In addition, impulse frequency during light steps is also greater for B cells from the paired training condition (Farley and Alkon, 1982a). Unlike the case of recordings obtained immediately following training, no difference in cells' resting potentials for paired vs. random treatment conditions is apparent. Pairing-specific depolarization of B cells seems to be a relatively transient expression of the membrane changes undergone by B cells, confined to the first hour or so following training (Farley and Alkon, 1982a,b, 1985b).

In addition to playing a major role in mediating the effects of simple associative learning, a wealth of data suggests that these same cells also play a crucial role in

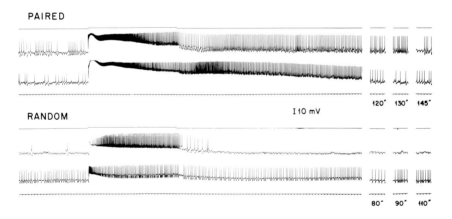

FIGURE 4. Training-produced differences in light-evoked impulse activities for two pairs of Type B photoreceptors in response to a moderate intensity light step. Top traces are for paired Type B cells; bottom traces are for random Type B cells. Recordings were obtained 24 hr after the conclusion of training. Note that paired B photoreceptors are more responsive during the light step than random Bs and more depolarized following light offset. Samples of impulse activities following light offset indicate the oscillatory patterns of B cell activity. Time scale is 1 sec. (From Farley and Alkon, 1982a.)

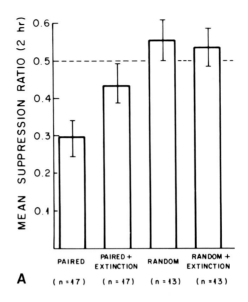

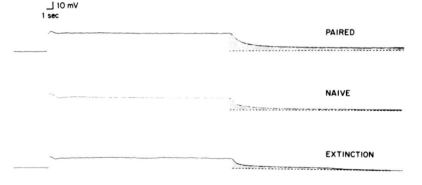

FIGURE 5. Behavioral (A) and neurophysiological (B) correlates of extinction training in *Hermissenda*. (A) Two-hour retention test data for animals exposed to the customary paired or random training protocols. Extinction animals received 25 nonreinforced presentations of light following the second day of 50 light–rotation pairings and exhibited no retention of phototaxic suppression. Additional results indicate that phototaxic suppression fails to spontaneously recover for these animals. (B) Examples of training-produced differences in isolated Type B photoreceptors. B cells from paired animals exhibited significantly greater peak and steady state-generator potentials, after depolarization, and enhanced input resistances when compared to extinction or control animals. (From Richards *et al.*, 1983, 1984.)

mediating some of the more complex phenomenology of associative learning as well. Following extinction training (Richards *et al.*, 1983, 1984), the light responses and input resistances of Type B cells are indistinguishable from that of naive or random control animals (Fig. 5), apparently reverting to an untrained state when light is no longer followed by rotation. Similarly, recordings obtained from animals exposed to degraded contingency conditions (see Table I) indicate that conditions that fail to produce substantial learning also fail to produce persistent changes in Type B cells. Similar correlations between the behavior of intact animals and B-cell membrane properties, as assessed shortly following recording and stimulation protocols that simulate the effects of training with natural stimuli, are obtained for massed vs. distributed training procedures, the effects of light intensity, and variations of the ISI relation between light and rotation (Section 3.3). Simply put, over a wide range of training conditions, the behavior of intact animals and the properties of the Type B cells parallel one another.

It would, of course, be simpleminded in the extreme to suggest that Type B cells are the *only* sites of change underlying associative learning. Recent evidence (Farley *et al.*, 1985; Richards *et al.*, 1983; Richards and Farley, 1984) indicates that the medial Type A cell is also changed by light–rotation pairings. Interestingly enough, whereas the B cell's light response is *enhanced* by light–rotation pairings, that of the A cell is *diminished* (Fig. 6). This complementary intrinsic change of the A cell combines with the increased synaptic inhibition from B cells following training (Farley and Alkon, 1982a) to produce further reductions in phototaxic behavior. The complementary nature of the Type B and A cell changes also underscores the point that learning is the response of a neural *system*, in this case one selected by evolution to detect consistent regularities in the temporal conjunction of light and rotation.

3.2. Knowledge and Performance: Increased Light Responses of B Cells Entails Reduced Visual Activation of Motoneurons by A Cells

The correlations between B-cell electrophysiology and behavior arise, at least in part, through well-characterized synaptic interactions involving Type B and A photoreceptors, interneurons, and motoneurons involved in phototaxis. Type B cells exert greater inhibition upon A cells following associative training (Farley and Alkon, 1982a). The A cells in turn are less effective in their excitation of identified interneurons and motoneruons which project to the pedal musculature (Goh and Alkon, 1982; Lederhendler *et al.*, 1982) (Fig. 7). No doubt, this particular pathway does not constitute a complete description of the neutral control of locomotion, and additional information is sorely needed.

3.3 Encoding Mechanisms: Cumulative Depolarization of Type B Cells

Since long-term storage of associative information occurs within the Type B photoreceptors, it is appropriate to inquire as to how these changes are brought

TABLE I. Degraded Contingency Training Conditions (A) and Neural Correlates in Type B Photoreceptors (B, C)[a]

A. Training conditions for behavior

Pairings	n's	Random	n's
50 L–R[b]	10	50 L/R	10
75 L–R	7	75 L/R	8
50 L–R + 25 L[b]	10	50 L/R + 25 L	9
50 L–R + 25 R[b]	11	50 L/R + 25 R	10

B. Contingency neural correlates during retention (means ± 1 S.E.M.)

	Paired (50 L – R)	Extra rotation (50 L – R + 25 R)	Extra light (50 L – R + 25 L)	Random (50 L/R)	$F_{(3, 20)}$	Scheffe confidence intervals ($P < .01$)	Significant comparisons
R input (MΩ)	95.67 ± 5.03	61.33 ± 4.29	67.33 ± 3.28	53.67 ± 4.85	6.48	29.20	50 L–R vs. 50 L/R, 50 L–R + 25 L, 50 L–R + 25 R
Impulse activity (per sec)	5.67 ± 0.68	3.80 ± 0.29	4.38 ± 0.29	3.88 ± 0.33	55.56	1.81	50 L–R vs. 50 L/R,

				50 L–R + 25 L, 50 L–R + 25 R	50 L–R vs. 50 L/R, 50 L–R + 25 L, 50 L–R + 25 R	50 L–R vs. 50 L/R, 50 L–R + 25 L, 50 L–R + 25 R
LLD duration (min)	6.45 ± 1.03	3.70 ± .97	4.50 ± 1.50	3.15 ± 1.12	21.10	2.30
Behavioral suppression ratio (24 hours)	0.24 ± .02	0.39 ± .01	0.36 ± .02	0.42 ± .03	9.25	.09

C. Cumulative depolarization (mV) for contingency simulations (means ± 1 S.E.M.)

	5 pairs	5 pairs + extra light	p^c	5 pairs	5 pairs + extra hair cell stimulation	p^c	5 random	p^d
30 sec	10.83 ± 0.80	7.77 ± 0.53	<.001	9.75 ± 0.79	8.92 ± 0.77	n.s.	5.25 ± 0.80	<.001
60 sec	9.80 ± 0.59	6.42 ± 0.62	<.001	7.42 ± 11.06	6.00 ± 1.12	<.01	3.11 ± 0.69	<.001
120 sec	9.75 ± 0.61	4.75 ± 0.70	<.001	7.42 ± 1.06	6.00 ± 1.12	<.01	2.05 ± 0.70	<.001

[a] Abbreviations: L, light; R, rotation.
[b] Also used for retention neural correlates study.
[c] Students t-test for matched samples.
[d] Students t-test comparing six cells from random condition, with pooled results (n = 12) of the two repetitions of pairings.

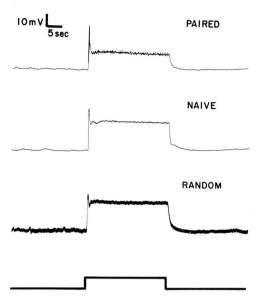

FIGURE 6. Training-produced differences in light response of Type A photoreceptor. Twenty-four hours following training, the A cell from a paired animal responds to light with a significantly smaller peak and steady state generator potential, but a greater afterhyperpolarization, than a cell from either a naive animal or an animal exposed to the random control treatment. (From Richards and Farley, 1984; Farley et al., 1985.)

about. It is now clear that a major role is played by a cumulative depolarization of the Type B cell, which occurs during the course of associative training and which derives from a pairing-specific synaptic facilitation of the B cells' long-lasting depolarizing (LLD) response to light. As a consequence of cumulative depolarization, intracellular levels of Ca^{2+} rise (Connor and Alkon, 1982), producing persistent changes in B-cell ionic conductances and hence excitability of B cells by light.

As is summarized in the schematic diagram of Fig. 8, the pairing-specific cumulative depolarization of Type B cells arises largely from two sources. First, both light and caudal hair cell stimulation produce inhibition of the S/E optic ganglion cell (Tabata and Alkon, 1982; Farley and Alkon, 1982b, 1985b) which responds to the termination of inhibition with a rebound-increase in depolarization and impulse activity. The S/E cell excites the B photoreceptor. Second, there is a pairing-specific disinhibition of Type B cells, which results from poststimulation hyperpolarization of caudal hair cells (Farley and Alkon, 1982b, 1985b).

The causal role of both these sources of synaptic facilitation has been documented through the development of *in vitro* conditioning techniques for the isolated nervous system of *Hermissenda* (Farley and Alkon, 1982b; 1985b). This simulation of the training that is received by intact animals entails intracellular stimulation and recording from three classes of neurons: the Type B photoreceptor, the S/E optic ganglion cell, and a caudal hair cell in the statocyst. Exposure of the isolated nervous system to five pairings of light and current-induced impulse activity of the caudal cell results in an average 10 mV depolarization of Type B cells, which is significantly greater than that produced by five random presentations of these two stimuli (Fig. 9). Cumulative depolarization of the B cell is substantially reduced

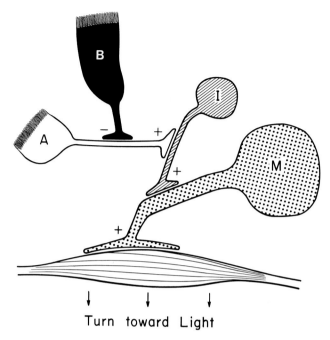

Turn toward Light

FIGURE 7. Schematic diagram of one identified pathway subserving phototaxic behavior in *Hermissenda*. The Type B photoreceptor (B) causes monosynaptic inhibition of the medial A photoreceptor (A). The medial A cell causes monosynaptic excitation of ipsilateral interneurons (I), which are also excited by caudal hair cells (not depicted here). These interneurons, in turn, produce both mono- and polysynaptic excitation of ipsilateral pedal motoneurons (M), which are responsible for the animal turning towards an ipsilateral source of illumination. Training-produced decreases in phototaxic behavior are thought to arise in part from the decreased response of the A cell, to light mediated in part by greater synaptic inhibition of the A cell by the B cells.

when the S/E cell is hyperpolarized throughout the course of pairings of light and caudal hair cell stimulation. Similarly, light paired with depolarizing current injections to the S/E cell are sufficient to produce large and prolonged cumulative depolarization in B cells. If pairings of light and current-induced caudal hair cell activity are carried out while the caudal hair cell is hyperpolarized during the intertrial interval—so as to preclude disinhibition—cumulative depolarization is also significantly attenuated. Thus, the S/E optic ganglion cell, which is a critical convergence point for visual and vestibular (statocyst hair cell) information, appears to be both necessary and sufficient to mediate the pairing effects of light and rotation upon the Type B photoreceptor (Farley and Alkon, 1982b, 1985b).

While the previously described results implicate cumulative depolarization and increased intracellular Ca^{2+} levels as major contributors to the persistent changes in Type B cell ionic conductances that occur with training, other mechanisms no doubt play a role as well. For example, accumulating evidence suggests a role for training-induced pharmacological modulation of B cell ionic currents, by serotonin (McElearney and Farley, 1983; Wu and Farley, 1984; Auerbach *et al.*, 1985).

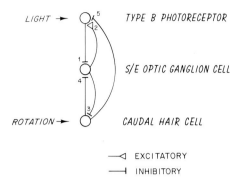

LIGHT → TYPE B PHOTORECEPTOR

S/E OPTIC GANGLION CELL

ROTATION → CAUDAL HAIR CELL

—◁ EXCITATORY
—┤ INHIBITORY

FIGURE 8. Schematic circuit of neurons involved in the production of cumulative depolarization in the Type B photoreceptors of *Hermissenda*, with pairings of light and rotation/electrical stimulation of caudal hair cells. Light results in long-lasting depolarization of the Type B cells, accompanied by an increase in the input resistance of these cells. Two important synaptic consequences of light are: (a) inhibition of the S/E optic ganglion cell (1) which results in cessation of EPSPs in the B cells (2) during light; (b) inhibition of the caudal hair cell (through a connection not illustrated here). Following the offset of light, EPSP frequency in the Type B cells increases (2) due to disinhibition of the S/E cell. In addition, there is a conductance-decreased enhancement of the EPSPs. Caudal hair cells respond to direct electrical or rotational stimulation with trains of impulse activity, which in turn result in inhibition of the S/E cell (4) and inhibition of the Type B photoreceptor (5). Following the termination of prolonged impulse activity, the caudal hair cell hyperpolarizes and becomes inactive. The S/E is disinhibited with a consequent increase in EPSP frequency in the Type B cell (4). In addition, the B cell is disinhibited (5) due to reduced impulse activity in the caudal hair cell. (From Farley and Alkon, 1982b, 1985b.)

We were first alerted to this possibility by the observation that *in vitro* conditioning of the isolated nervous system (cf. Fig. 9) was most effective if depolarization of the B cell was effected through *synaptic* means (i.e., either current stimulation of the hair cell or S/E optic ganglion cell), as opposed to direct depolarizing current stimulation of the B cell. This indicated to us that the cumulative depolarization and enhanced input resistances that B cells undergo during training could not be entirely reproduced by substituting electrophysiologically produced depolarization for synaptically produced depolarization. Perfusion of B cells with a crude optic ganglion cell homogenate (Fig. 10) confirmed the suspicion of the presence of a substance within the optic ganglion that resulted in depolarization and increased input resistance in the dark-adapted B cell. Recent evidence indicates the neuromodulator to be serotonin (Fig. 11): (1) bath application of serotonin reduces I_A, I_C and enhances I_{Ca} (Wu and Farley, 1984), (2) HPLC and immunocytochemistry analyses reveal that serotonin is found within the optic ganglia, is released during associative training, and serotonin fine processes extensively innervate the cerebropleural ganglia where photoreceptor axo-dendritic processes ramify (Auerbach *et al.*, 1985).

Nevertheless, cumulative depolarization of Type B cells represents the initial step in the production of long-term associative neural and behavioral changes in *Hermissenda*. Depolarization of B cells results in an initially *transient* suppression of K^+ (I_A and I_C) currents in Type B cells, through a voltage-dependent inactivation mechanism. Suppression of I_A and I_C in turn leads to sustained depolarization and results in an increase in intracellular Ca^{2+} levels throughout training (Connor and Alkon, 1982). Increased levels of intracellular Ca^{2+} may arise, in large part, from the depolarization enhancement of the inward light-induced Ca^{2+} current during light steps paired with rotation (Alkon *et al.*, 1983). Increased levels of intracellular Ca^{2+} may then, by biochemical mechanisms that may entail protein phosphorylation of specific K^+ ion channels (or regulatory proteins for these channels) produce *long-term* inactivation of the I_A current. Biochemical correlates of the associative training procedure (Neary, Chapter 30, this volume), biochemical correlates of I_A channel blockers (Neary and Alkon, 1982), and Ca^{2+}-dependent protein kinase regulation of K^+ currents (Acosta-Urquidi *et al.*, 1982) have now been demonstrated for *Hermissenda*, and it should prove interesting to determine the precise relevance of these correlates for the learned behavioral change.

3.4. Predictive Coding and Causal Detection within the Visual-Vestibular System: Contingency, Massed vs. Distributed Training Trials, and ISI Effects

In vitro simulation of the degraded contingency experiments (Figs. 2 and 3), by exposing preparations to either five pairings of light and caudal hair cell stimulation or pairings plus extra light or hair cell stimulation, results in a significant attenuation of cumulative depolarization in Type B cells. The disruptive effects of the extra light stimuli primarily arise from the introduction of temporary, nonassociative, light adaptation effects in B cells. Figure 12 indicates that the light-adapted B cell during such a treatment responds with less of a depolarizing generator potential than normally, and consequently the postpairing depolarization is less. Although each light-alone step results in some depolarization, this is insufficiently compensated for by its proactive interference with *pairing-produced depolarization*. A major role in the reduction of the light-induced generator potential is inactivation of the transient light-induced Na^+ current (see Fig. 13), mediated in part by residual intracellular Ca^{2+} (Alkon *et al.*, 1982; Farley, 1985). The attenuation of cumulative depolarization by the extra steps of unpaired caudal hair cell stimulation occurs for a different reason. Caudal hair cell impulse trains synaptically hyperpolarize Type B cells, thus reversing the depolarization produced by prior pairings (Fig. 14). Unlike the case of light-alone presentation, the effects of the added hair cell stimulation are primarily retroactive. In the absence of prior pairings, they exert little lasting effect upon the neural response of the B cell (or behavior of the intact animal). Once the cumulative depolarization of B cells has been initiated by the pairings of light and rotation, however, the added hair cell stimulation functions as a reset mechanism, acting to restore the original membrane potential of the cell and thus curtail increased intracellular Ca^{2+}. Thus, this demonstration that Type B cells both encode and store information concerning both contiguity and contingency relations strongly suggests that these two relations are encoded and stored through common biophysical mechanisms as well, viz., modulation of K^+ conductances, through regulation of cumulative depolarization and intracellular Ca^{2+}.

The neuronal organization of the visual and vestibular neural systems, which provides for simple associative and contingency learning also constrains, in predictable fashion, the conditions under which added rotation-alone and light-alone presentations will attenuate associative learning and those in which they will not.

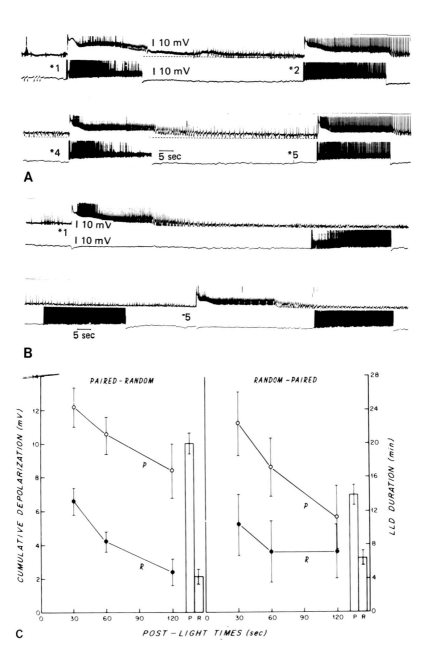

As indicated above, adding light very shortly before a light-rotation pairing fails to attenuate conditioning and may even slightly enhance it (Fig. 3). Under these conditions, the Type B photoreceptor fails to appreciably resolve the two presentations of light as distinct. The two light steps are responded to as one long step of illumination. This failure of the B photoreceptor to faithfully follow high-frequency light presentations is attributable in large part to activation of the sluggish voltage- and light-dependent Ca^{2+} current and prolonged inactivation of the I_A current, during the first light. Both conductance effects combine to maintain the cell's membrane potential at a depolarized level that diminishes slowly. At depolarized levels of membrane potential, a subsequent light gives rise to an additional steady Ca influx, serving to maintain the present level of membrane potential. In this range of membrane potentials the prior inactivation of I_{Na} (Fig. 13) has a negligible effect, since the Na current's role is largely limited to producing large and transient depolarization in the *dark-adapted* eye. Similarly, addition of extra rotation-alone presentations to the B cells at times substantially following a light-rotation pairing have correspondingly diminished effects in reversing cumulative depolarization and intracellular Ca^{2+} levels. Intracellular Ca^{2+} levels have already risen. Synaptic inhibition from the hair cells is reduced: the postlight enhancement of synaptic potentials due to the light-induced decreased conductance of the B cell has abated. It is a case of too little, too late.

Three further predictions concerning the behavior of intact animals can also be derived from the manner in which the characteristics of the intrinsic conductances of Type B photoreceptors interact with the synaptic circuitry. The first concerns the effects of light intensity. Cumulative depolarization of the B cell with light–rotation pairings builds upon the LLD response of the B cell to light alone and is extremely voltage dependent (Alkon, 1979). Hence, it is directly determined by the magnitude of the depolarizing generator potential. Therefore, dim lights would be expected to produce minimal cumulative depolarization and little suppression of phototaxic behavior (Fig. 15). Not so obvious is what the expected effect of very bright lights would be. Here, the *in vitro* simulated training procedure is a helpful guide. Lights

---

FIGURE 9. (A) Intracellular recordings from a medial Type B photoreceptor (top trace) and a caudal hair cell (bottom trace) during: successive pairings (trials #1, #2, #4, and #5) of light and current-induced impulse activity in the caudal hair cell. With pairings, the B cell progressively depolarized (dashed line indicates resting potential). Following the last light step, the B cell was 10 mV, 7.5 mV and 7.0 mV depolarized at .5-, 1.0-, and 3.0-min post-light intervals and remained depolarized for 30 min. (B) Intracellular recordings from the same cells as in (A) exposed to a conditioning sequence in which current-induced caudal hair cell activity occurred randomly with respect to light steps (light trials #1 and #5 are depicted). Following the last light step, the cell was 1, .5, and 1 mV hyperpolarized at .5-, 1.0-, and 3.0-min intervals. The order of training for this preparation was paired-random. (C) Summary statistics for the magnitude (left ordinate) and duration (right ordinate) of cumulative depolarization of type B photoreceptors from isolated nervous systems exposed to either five pairings of light and caudal-hair cell depolarization (p), or five random presentation of these two stimuli. The results of five preparations exposed to the reverse training order appear on the right. Error bar = ±1 S.E.M. For duration measures, 30-min score was the maximum possible. (From Farley and Alkon, 1982b, 1985b.)

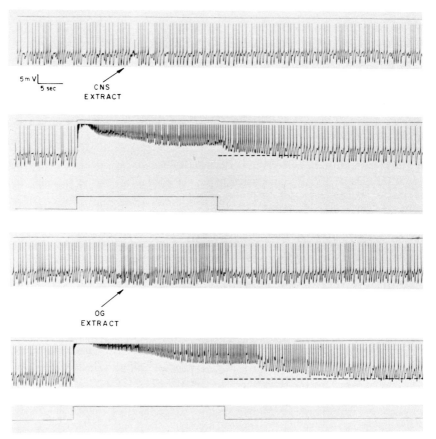

FIGURE 10. Addition of crude CNS (pedal ganglion) homogenate fails to affect B photorecep-tor's membrane potential (top) or its response to light. Addition of crude optic ganglion (OG) homogenate produces a transient depolarization and a pronounced enhancement of the B cell's light response (bottom). (From McElearney and Farley, 1983.)

which are too intense produce an initial cumulative depolarization, which thereafter declines to random control levels. Trial-by-trial analysis indicates that subsequent light steps actually give rise to a *hyperpolarizing* light response, presumably re-flecting a profound inactivation of I_{Na} and activation of the calcium-activated K^+ conductance (Farley and Alkon, 1982b, 1985b). Here, the effect of a rise in intra-cellular Ca^{2+} is one of too much too soon. The behavior of intact animals again parallels the cumulative depolarization results (Fig. 15). A similar mechanism underlies the effects of massed vs. distributed training trials. When delivered at frequencies exceeding 1/min, 30-sec pairings of light and rotation fail to produce either conditioning for intact animals or cumulative depolarization in the isolated nervous system (Farley and Alkon, 1982b, 1985b). Hyperpolarizing responses to light are often evident under these conditions. Conversely, extremely long intertrial

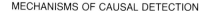
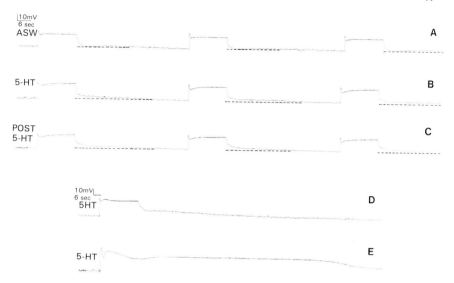

FIGURE 11. Effects of μM quantities of serotonin (5-HT) upon Type B photoreceptor light response. (A) Standard responses of B cell to an intermediate intensity light step of 3000 ergs. (B) Response of cell 1 min post-5-HT. Note enhancement of peak, steady state, and LLD components. (C) Persistence of serotonin's effects after washout (5 min). (D) Response of B photoreceptor in ASW to a bright (4500 ergs) light step. (E) Response of B cell to bright light following addition of 5-HT to bath. Note enhanced peak, steady state, and LLD components. (From McElearney and Farley, 1983.)

intervals also diminish cumulative depolarization of the Type B cell, as well as behavioral suppression in the intact animal. For this same reason—persistent light adaptation effects—we have been unable to simulate the effects of associative training by exposing animals to training schedules involving more frequent and/or brighter light-alone presentations. Perhaps we may eventuallly be able to do so, but light-alone presentations have so far proven to be an extremely ineffective means of producing long-term suppression of phototaxic behavior.

Cumulative depolarization of the B cell is also unique to vestibular stimulation of the *caudal* hair cells in the statocyst, since it is these that synaptically inhibit both the S/E cell and the Type B photoreceptor. Pairing light with *cephalad* hair cell stimulation fails to produce cumulative depolarization of B cells (Alkon, 1980; Farley and Alkon, 1980a), and training conditions that maximize this manner of vestibular stimulation also fail to produce persistent behavior suppression (Farley and Alkon, 1980b).

Finally, our understanding of the cellular interactions intrinsic to the visual-vestibular system has allowed the derivation of a set of predictions as to what the most effective temporal relation for pairings should be. It should be one in which light and rotation completely overlap; the onsets and particularly the *offsets* of stimulation should coincide. Synchronous offsets should maximize (1) S optic cell

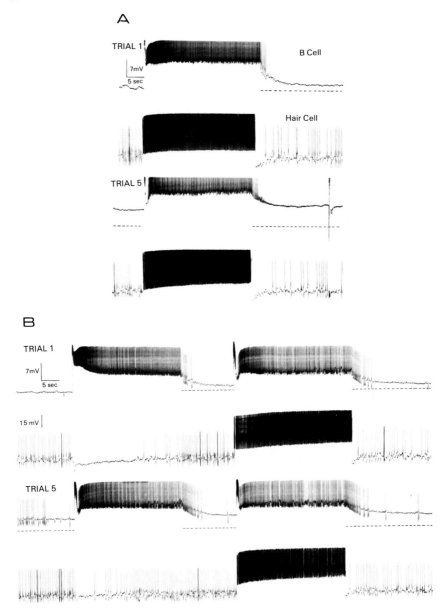

FIGURE 12. Simulation of the partial reinforcement degraded contingency effect in the isolated nervous system of *Hermissenda*. Light steps were 30 sec in duration and 3.0×10^4 ergs cm^{-2} sec^{-1} in intensity. Caudal hair cell depolarization consisted of 30 sec of depolarizing (20 mV) current steps injected through a balanced bridge circuit. Successive pairings were separated by 2.0 min, onset-to-onset. Adding light prior to each (B) pairing reduced the depolarizing generator potential and LLD response of the B cell (top trace of each record), during and following the subsequent pairing trial (depicted here are trials 1 and 5). Minutes after the conclusion of training, cells which received the extra light (B) were less depolarized than when the same cells

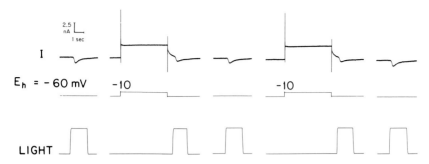

FIGURE 13. Voltage-clamp recordings from isolated Type B photoreceptor indicating reduction of a light-induced inward current (primarily carried by Na$^+$) by prior depolarization (and resulting concomitant increase in intracellular Ca^{2+}), comparable to that which would occur in the unclamped cell exposed to light. Outward K$^+$ current blockers have been added to the bath (TEA, 4-AP). From Farley (1985).

disinhibition (positive synaptic feedback), (2) disinhibition of the B cell by the hair cell, and (3) the intrinsic postlight conductance changes in the B cell (e.g., reduction of K$^+$ currents). Indeed, any substantial deviation from such a training procedure would be predicted to minimize the effects of pairings, as recent results confirm (Grover and Farley, 1983; Fig. 16).

Consider the effects of terminating light prior to the offset of rotation. Although Type B cells respond to the light with a depolarizing generator potential, the LLD response following light offset is reduced by synaptic inhibition from the hair cell. Although some synaptic depolarization would be expected following the termination of rotation, it is substantially reduced by not being paired with light. Its efficacy is further reduced because it is delayed. The decreased-conductance enhancement of EPSPs in the B cell has diminished. For similar reasons, initiating and terminating hair cell stimulation *before* light is a relatively ineffective means of producing cumulative depolarization. Any postrotation enhancement of EPSPs to the B cell is reduced by light-induced shunting of the synaptic currents. Membrane conductance increases by a factor of 10 or so during the initial few seconds of visual stimulation.

While the key relation for the visual-vestibular system is that of light-rotation offsets, I would nevertheless expect the relation of light-rotation onset to also play a modulatory role. Preceding the onset of rotation with the onset of light by 0.5–2.0

received only pairings (A). Three minutes after pairings, this cell was only 1 mv depolarized. One major contributing factor to the reduced depolarization by light alone vs. light paired with caudal hair cell stimulation is relatively less synaptic excitatory feedback to Type B cells following offset of light-alone steps. Pairings of light and caudal hair cell stimulation inhibit the S/E optic ganglion cell, which exhibits an anode-break excitation following the pairing. This occurs to a much lesser degree with light alone. In addition, the prior light steps inactivate the light-induced Na$^+$ current, leading to reduced depolarizing generator particles. The S/E cell is responsible for EPSPs in the B cell, which facilitates and prolongs the light-induced LLD. (From Farley, 1985.)

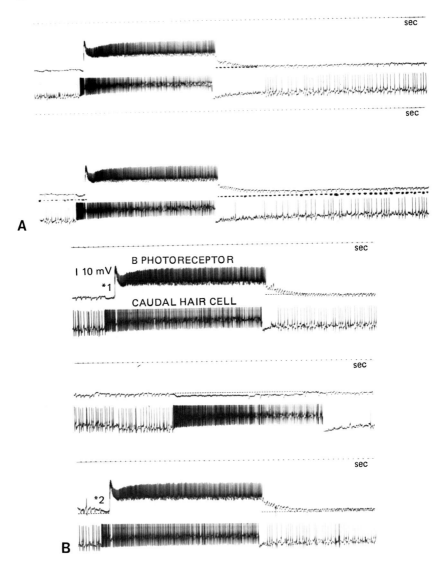

FIGURE 14. Simulation of the degraded contingency effects due to extra caudal hair cell stimulation. Adding hair cell stimulation (bottom trace each record) prior to each pairing resulted in synaptic hyperpolarization of the B cell (arrow, between trial 1 and 2), thereby partially reversing the prior depolarization. Minutes after the conclusion of training, cells which had received the extra hair cell stimulation were less depolarized then those same cells receiving only pairings. (From Farley, 1985.)

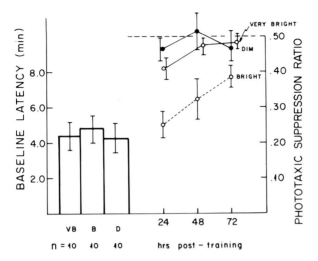

FIGURE 15. Behavioral results of dim, moderate, and bright lights used in standard conditioning protocols. Dim and very bright lights produce little retained suppression or cumulative depolarization. (From Farley and Alkon, 1982b, 1985b.)

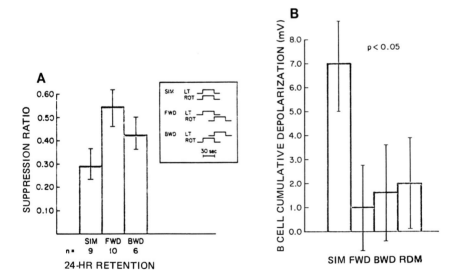

FIGURE 16. Behavioral and electrophysiological results of manipulating the light–rotation interstimulus interval. (A) Behavioral suppression 24-hr posttraining for forward-delayed, simultaneous, and backward-conditioned animals. Only the simultaneous animals, for whom light onset preceded peak rotation by .5 sec show retained suppression. (B) Summary data for simulation of ISI conditions in the isolated nervous system of untrained animals. Only simultaneous protocols (five pairings of light and caudal hair cell stimulation) result in pronounced cumulative depolarization. (From Grover and Farley, 1983.)

sec should exaggerate some of the cumulative depolarization due to simultaneous offsets. This would be expected to occur primarily because in the absence of simultaneous hair cell synaptic inhibition, the light-induced transient inward current should produce greater membrane depolarization of the B cell.

3.5. The Causal Role of B Photoreceptors in Associative Modification of Phototaxis

The preceding review of the research concerning neural correlates of associative learning in *Hermissenda* demonstrates striking correlations between the associatively produced behavioral changes in phototaxis and biophysical changes intrinsic to the Type B photoreceptors in the animal's eyes, during both acquisition and retention of associative learning. Despite the strength of these correlations, it is nonetheless important to recognize that they are only that—correlations. Indeed, it is important to realize that correlated neural changes, which occur with learning, are all that have been previously demonstrated for *any* simple system preparation, including those attempting to elucidate the mechanisms of habituation and sensitization. In no case has it proven possible to derive a quantitative estimate of the proportion of the learned behavioral change which is attributable to neural correlates. Recently, we have demonstrated a direct causal relationship between membrane changes, as they occur during acquisition, and long-term behavioral changes in phototaxis (Farley *et al.*, 1982, 1983b).

Our strategy in these experiments was to produce, through electrophysiological means, the acquistion-correlated membrane changes (cumulative depolarization and increased input resistance) in a single Type B cell in intact animals and to subsequently assess long-term changes in phototaxis. The experimental treatment designed to simulate the associative training procedure with natural stimuli involved exposing animals to five pairings of 30 sec of light and depolarizing current into Type B cells. These stimulation parameters were directly derived from our previous experience with *in vitro* conditioning (Section 3.3) of the isolated nervous system. We also examined two control conditions. One condition involved exposing animals to five *unpaired* presentations of light and depolarizing current, the general parameters of light and current being identical to those of the paired condition. The second simply involved microelectrode impalement of Type B cells, without administering any training stimulation. Animals were allowed to recover and were then tested, using "blind" observational procedures, for changes in phototaxic behavior.

Figure 17 summarizes the results of these experiments and illustrates that pairings of light and positive current produced a cumulative depolarization in Type B cells that was significantly greater than the negligible change that occurred for cells exposed to the unpaired treatment. The paired treatment cells also exhibited a significant 48% increase in input resistance, while the unpaired treatment yielded no change in this measure of cell conductance. In short, we successfully directly produced the membrane changes, which we had previously observed in the conditioning of isolated nervous systems, in Type B cells of intact animals.

One and two days following training, all animals exhibited longer phototaxic latencies (compared to initial baseline levels), but animals receiving paired presentations of light and depolarizing current exhibited significantly greater suppression of phototaxic behavior than either control group. Thus, pairings of light and membrane depolarization of Type B cells was *sufficient* to produce retained suppression of phototaxis. Furthermore, since the unpaired presentations of light and positive current produced no changes in phototaxis other than those attributable to the general suppressive effects of restraint and nervous system manipulation, these experiments also strongly imply that Type B cell membrane changes are *necessary* for long-term associative modification of phototaxis. Since these experiments were conducted with intact synaptic interactions between photoreceptors and other elements of the nervous system, our data speak only to the causal role of Type B cells during *acquisition* of learned suppression of phototaxic behavior. Current research is directed towards determining whether the same behavioral changes can be produced if Type B cells are "trained" under synaptic blockade, thereby directly demonstrating that they are sites for storage of memorial information which is causally related to long-term retention of phototaxic suppression.

3.6. Biophysical Mechanisms for Retention: Reduction of K^+ Conductances

Consistent with the likelihood that increased input resistances and enhanced light-induced depolarizing generator potentials of Type B cells from associatively trained animals reflected a decrease in one or more outward K^+ currents, Alkon *et al.* (1982) reported a 30% reduction in the peak amplitude and a more rapid inactivation of the fast, rapidly inactivating A current (Connor and Stevens, 1971) for associatively trained animals, one and two days following training. Subsequent research confirmed the suspicion that the A current could be suppressed for intermediate lengths of time (10–15 min) following introduction of Ca^{2+} loads into the cell (Alkon *et al.*, 1983a). Efforts to develop a Hodgkin–Huxley model of the voltage- and light-dependent currents in the B phototreceptor indicate that a 30% reduction in the A current can enhance the magnitude of the peak and steady-state components of the generator potential by 10–20% (Shoukimas and Alkon, 1983; in preparation), in a manner approximating the effects of training.

The question naturally arises as to whether the A current is the only current that is changed by associative training; if not, which other(s) change? Can changes in other currents be related to a training-produced rise in intracellular Ca^{2+}, as in the case of the A current? Or are additional mechanisms involved (e.g., cyclic nucleotides)? Preliminary evidence indicates that neither the transient inward light-induced Na^+ current (Alkon, 1979; West *et al.*, 1982) nor the delayed rectifier (I_K) (Alkon *et al.*, 1982) are affected by training. More recent results (Farley *et al.*, 1983a, 1984; Farley and Alkon, 1983) point to changes in the voltage-dependent calcium current (I_{Ca}) as well as the calcium-activated potassium current (I_{K-Ca}).

Reduction of training-produced differences in the contribution of I_A to Type B photoreceptor light responses seems to enhance, rather than attenuate, the associative differences. Following the conditioning of intact animals, light-induced peak and steady state generator potentials were greater for paired vs. random control animals, and these differences were further exaggerated when these same cells were

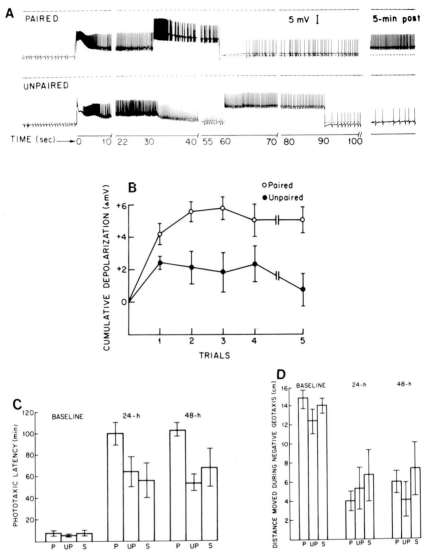

FIGURE 17. Membrane changes in Type B cells and behavioral changes in phototaxis produced by five paired presentations of light and depolarizing current administered to Type B cells in intact *Hermissenda*. (A) Illustration of training procedures of paired and unpaired treatment conditions. Preparations exposed to five paired presentations of light and depolarization (top) received light (time = 1 sec) followed immediately by positive current (time = 30 sec) injected through the balanced bridge circuit. Unpaired control preparations received depolarizing current 30 sec following the offset of the light (time = 60 sec). Five minutes following the conclusion of training, membrane potential (right) and input resistances were measured. The paired treatment condition resulted in a cumulative depolarization of 9 mV for this particular cell (top right), while the unpaired treatment resulted in a 2-mV hyperpolarization in this case (bottom right). (B) Cumulative depolarization of Type B cells, as a function of treatment condition (paired vs.

exposed to a 10 sec 40 mV depolarizing step just prior to light (so as to eliminate I_A for both groups; Fig. 18a; Farley et al., 1983a; Farley and Alkon, 1985c). Similarly, large training-produced differences in input resistances and generator potentials were observed when 4-aminopyridine (10 mM; 4-AP) was used to selectively block the A current (Farley and Alkon, 1983, 1985c; Fig. 18b). Direct measurement of the calcium-activated K^+ current (I_{K-Ca}) and the voltage-dependent Ca^{2+} current on retention days reveals that I_{K-Ca} is selectively reduced (Fig. 19) and I_{Ca} is selctively enhanced for paired animals (Farley et al., 1984; Farley and Alkon, 1985c; J. Farley, unpublished observations). Recent results (Alkon et al., 1983b) indicate that I_{K-Ca} can be inactivated by intracellular Ca^{2+} levels, without any detectable inactivation of I_{Ca} (cf. Eckert and Tillotson, 1981). Some of these effects may be mediated by calcium–calmodulin-dependent protein kinases (Acosta-Urquidi et al., 1982). However, both I_A and I_{K-Ca} are also reduced by activation of protein-kinase C in B cells (Farley and Auerbach, 1985; Fisher et al., 1985), an enzyme which is primarily phospholipid-sensitive. Serotonin has been reported to increase protein kinase C activity in several tissues (Berridge and Irvine, 1984). Elucidation of the interaction of Ca^{2+}, cyclic nucleotides, and phospholipid-metabolism in the production of long-term changes of membrane conductances is clearly a major goal of future research.

4. SUMMARY

A decade ago, the learning capacities of gastropods appeared rather impoverished, being limited to various forms of nonassociative behavioral modifications. The chief value of molluscan preparations, at that time, appeared to lie in their promise for revealing biophysical and biochemical bases of some rather primitive forms of behavioral plasticity. The relevance of such mechanisms for the more complex processes of learning and memory in vertebrates was, and continues to be, of uncertain import. As our work, with *Hermissenda* indicates, however, "simple" nervous systems are nevertheless capable of some rather sophisticated information processing. We are thus encouraged in our belief that fundamental insights into vertebrate learning and memory can be gleaned from simpler vervous systems by the general similarity of conditioning and learning processes across phylogeny implied by our demonstrations of contingency learning, extinction, and sensitivity to CS–UCS temporal order. Furthermore, we continue to be surprised by just how

---

unpaired) and number of training trials. Following the first trial, B cells exposed to light–depolarization pairings exhibited significantly greater depolarization than unpaired controls. For trials 1–4, depolarization was measured just prior to the onset of the subsequent ($n + 1$) trial (2 min after the beginning of the previous trial). For trial 5, the value was obtained 5 min following the final trial, once the cell had reached a steady state level of membrane potential. (C) Phototaxic behavior of *Hermissenda* before (left) and 24 and 48 hr after paired (P), unpaired (UP), or sham (S) treatment conditions. Bar: 1 S.E.M. Paired treatment animals were significantly less phototaxic than either control, both 24 and 48 hr following treatment. (D) Locomotor behavior of *Hermissenda,* in the dark, in response to a gravitational gradient. There were no significant differences among any of the groups either before or after treatment. (From Farley *et al.*, 1983b.)

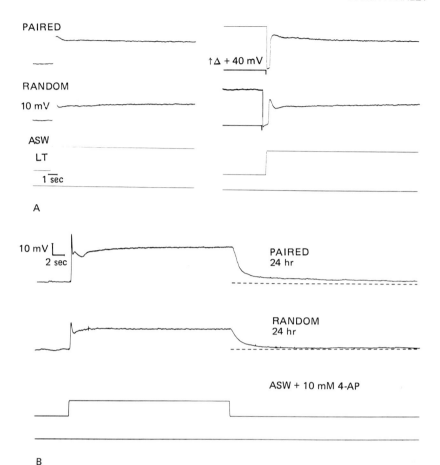

FIGURE 18. (A) Typical training-produced differences in peak and steady-state components of Type B photoreceptor's light-induced generator potential (left). Preceding the light step by a 10-sec, 40-mV depolarizing prepulse (right) *enhanced* the training-produced difference for paired vs. random B cells, by selectively enhancing the light response for the paired cell. Under voltage-clamp, prolonged depolarization selectively inactivates the I_A current (Farley *et al.*, 1983a). (B) Persistence of training-produced differences in peak and steady-state components of B cell's light-induced generator potential in presence of 10 mM 4-AP, which pharmacologically blocks I_A. Both results (A and B) indicate the presence of training-produced conductances other than I_A. (From Farley and Alkon, 1983.)

many of the more complex characteristics of associative learning for *Hermissenda* are implicit in the dynamic characteristics and neural organization of the visual-vestibular network. At the levels of ionic conductances in individual neurons, as well as in the network rules relating synaptic convergence to patterns of environmental stimulation by light and rotation and behavior in the intact animal, an impressive invariance holds. The combined effects of light and rotation are in a sense unique and are not predictable from the effects of either considered in isolation. The network is "tuned" to detect consistent regularities in the temporal patterning

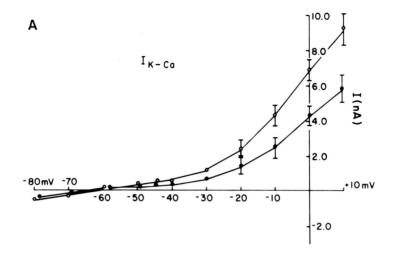

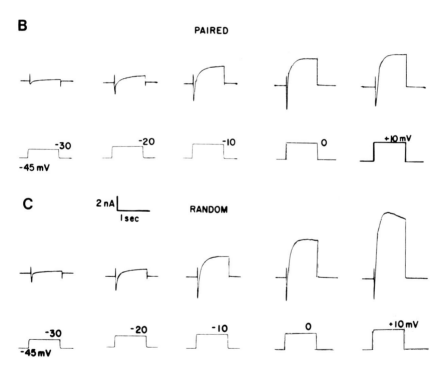

FIGURE 19. Associative training-produced reductions in I_{K-Ca}, measured in the absence of 4-AP but the presence of TEA (100 mM) and an elevated external calcium concentration (25 mM). B cells were voltage clamped at a holding potential of -45 mV, resulting in voltage-dependent inactivation of I_A. (A) Average results for paired ($n = 10$) vs. random control ($n = 9$) animals. Error bars = 1 S.E.M. (B) Typical records from a B cell from a paired animal. (C) Records from a random control animal.

of light and rotation, and this information is stored in a relatively permanent form. Finally, we have begun to appreciate how the combination of components that are characterized by associative memorial capacities (the Type B and A photoreceptors), when embedded within a network that resonates to the joint occurrence of two events, is sufficient to comprise a rudimentary causal detection system. The exciting possibility is thus raised that simple nervous systems may provide direct access to cellular mechanisms of at least some of the more complex, adaptive characteristics of cognition.

ACKNOWLEDGMENTS. I am grateful to William Richards and Lawrence Grover for their insightful discussion and comments upon this chapter, as to their contributions to the research described herein.

REFERENCES

Acosta-Urquidi, J., Neary, J. T., and Alkon, D. L., 1982, Ca^{2+}-dependent protein kinase regulation of K^+ (v)-currents: A possible biochemical step in associative learning of *Hermissenda, Soc. Neurosci. Abstr.* **8:**825.

Alkon, D. L., 1974, Associative training in *Hermissenda, J. Gen. Physiol.* **64:**70–84.

Alkon, D. L., 1979, Voltage-dependent calcium and potassium ion conductances: A contingency mechanism for an associative learning model, *Science* **205:**810–816.

Alkon, D. L, 1980, Membrane depolarization accumulates during acquisition of an associative behavioral change, *Science* **210:**1376–1378.

Alkon, D. L., Lederhendler, I., and Shoukimas, J. J., 1982, Primary changes of membrane currents during retention of associative learning, *Science* **215:**693–695.

Alkon, D. L., Shoukimas, J. J., and Heldman, E., 1983a, Calcium-mediated decrease of a voltage-dependent potassium current, *Biophys. J.* **40:**245.

Alkon, D. L., Farley, J., Hay, B., and Shoukimas, J. J., 1983b, Inactivation of Ca^{2+}- and Ca^{2+}-dependent K^+ current can occur without significant Ca^{2+}-current inactivation, *Soc. Neurosci. Abstr.* **9:**1188.

Auerbach, S., Grover, L., and Farley, J., 1985, HLPC and immunochemistry analyses of serotonin in *Hermissenda* central nervous systems, *Soc. Neurosci. Abstr.* (in press).

Ayres, J. J. B., Benedict, J. O., and Witcher, E. S., 1975, Systematic manipulation of individual events in a truly random control procedure in rats, *J. Comp. Physiol. Psychol.* **88:**97–103.

Benedict, J. O. and Ayres, J. J. B., 1972, Factors affecting conditioning in the truly random control procedure in the rat, *J. Comp. Physiol. Psychol.* **78:**323–330.

Berridge, M. J. and Irvine, R. F., 1984, Inositol triphosphate, a novel second messenger incellular signal transduction, *Nature* **312:**315–321.

Connor, J. and Alkon, D. L., 1982, Light-induced changes of intracellular Ca^{2+} in *Hermissenda* photoreceptors measured with Arsenazo III, *Soc. Neurosci. Abstr.* **8:**944.

Connor, J. and Stevens, C. F., 1971, Voltage-clamp studies of a transient outward current in gastropod neural somata, *J. Physiol. (London)* **213:**21–30.

Connor, J. A. and Alkon, D. L., 1984, Light- and voltage-dependent increases of calcium ion concentration in molluscan photoreceptors, *J. Neurophysiol.* **51:**745–752.

Crow, T. J. and Alkon, D. L., 1978, Retention of an associative behavioral change in *Hermissenda, Science* **201:**1239–1241.

Crow, T. J. and Alkon, D. L., 1980, Associative behavioral modification in *Hermissenda:* cellular correlates, *Science* **209:**412–414.

Eckert, R., and Tillotson, D., 1981, Calcium-mediated inactivation of the calcium conductance in caesium-loaded giant neurones of *Aplysia Californica, J. Physiol. (London)* **314:**265–280.

Farley, J., 1980, Automaintenance, contrast, and contingencies: effects of local vs. overall, and prior vs. impending reinforcement context, *Learn. Motiv.* **11:**19–48.

Farley, J., 1985, Contingency-learning and casual detection in *Hermissenda:* Behavior and cellular mechanisms, *Behavioral Neuroscience* (in press).

Farley, J. and Alkon, D. L., 1980a, Neural organization predicts stimulus specificity for a retained associative behavioral change, *Science* 210:1373–1375.

Farley, J. and Alkon, D. L., 1980b, Neural organization predicts stimulus specificity for a retained associative behavioral change, *Soc. Neurosci. Abstr.* 6:786.

Farley, J. and Alkon, D., 1981, Associative neural and behavioral change in *Hermissenda:* Consequences of nervous system orientation for light- and pairing-specificity, *Soc. Neurosci. Abstr.* 7:325.

Farley, J. and Alkon, D., 1982a, Associative and behavioral change in *Hermissenda:* Consequences of nervous system orientation for light- and pairing-specificity, *J. Neurophysiol.* 48:785–807.

Farley, J. and Alkon, D. L., 1982b, Cumulative cellular depolarization and short-term associative conditioning in *Hermissenda, Soc. Neurosci. Abstr.* 8: 825.

Farley, J. and Alkon, D. L., 1983, Changes in *Hermissenda* Type B photoreceptors involving a voltage-dependent Ca^{2+} current and a Ca^{2+}-dependent K^+ current during retention of associative learning, *Soc. Neurosci. Abstr.* 9:167.

Farley, J. and Alkon, D., 1985a, Cellular analysis of gastropod learning, in: *Cell Receptors and Cell Communication in Invertebrates* (A. J. Greenberg, ed.), Marcel-Dekker (in press).

Farley, J. and Alkon, D. L., 1985b, *In vitro* associative conditioning of *Hermissenda:* cumulative depolarization of Type B photoreceptors and short-term associative behavioral changes, *J. Neurophysiol.* (in press).

Farley, J. and Alkon, D. L., 1985c, Associative training results in persistent reductions in a calcium-activated potassium current in *Hermissenda* Type B photoreceptors. *J. Neurophysiol.* (in press).

Farley, J. and Auerbach, S., 1985, Phorbol esters reduce voltage-dependent and calcium-activated K^+ currents in *Hermissenda* Type B photoreceptors, *Biophys. J.* 47:386a.

Farley, J., Richards, W., Ling, L., Liman, E., and Alkon, D. L., 1982, Membrane changes in a single photoreceptor cause retained associative behavioral changes in *Hermissenda, Biol Bull.* 163:383.

Farley, J., Richards, W., Alkon, D. L., 1983a, Evidence for an increased voltage-dependent Ca^{2+} current in *Hermissenda* B photoreceptors during retention of associative learning, *Biophys. J.* 41:294a.

Farley, J., Richards, W., Ling, L., Liman, E., and Aldon, D. L., 1983b, Membrane changes in a single photoreceptor during acquisition cause associative learning in *Hermissenda, Science* 221:1201–1203.

Farley, J., Richards, W. G., Grover, L., 1985, Associative learning changes intrinsic to *Hermissenda* Type A photoreceptors, *Brain Res.* (in press).

Farley,, J., Sakakibara, M., Alkon, D. L., 1984, Associative-training correlated changes in I_C and I_{Ca} in *Hermissenda* Type B photoreceptors, *Soc. Neurosci. Abstr.* 10:270.

Fisher, D., Auerbach, S., and Farley, J., 1985, Protein kinase C reduces K^+ currents and enhances a Ca^{2+} current in *Hermissenda* Type B cells, *Soc. Neurosci. Abstr.* (in press).

Goh, Y. and Alkon, D. L., 1982, Convergence of visual and statocyst inputs on interneurons and motoneourons of *Hermissenda:* A network design for associative conditioning, *Soc. Neurosci. Abstr.* 8:825.

Gormezano, I., Kehoe, E. J., and Marshall, B. S., 1982, Twenty years of classical conditioning research with the rabbit, *Progress in Psychobiology and Physiological Psychology* 10:98–275.

Grover, L., and Farley, J., 1983, Temporal order sensitivity of associative learning in *Hermissenda, Soc. Neurosci. Abstr.* 9:915.

Heth, C. D. and Rescorla, R. A., 1973, Simultaneous and backward fear conditioning in the rat, *J. Comp. Physiol. Psychol.* 82:434–443.

Jenkins, H. M. and Shattuck, D., 1981, Contingency in fear conditioning: A reexamination, *Bull. Psychonomic Soc.* 17:159–162.

Kamin, L. J., 1969, Predictability, surprise, attention and conditioning, in: *Punishment and Aversive Behavior* (B. Campbell and R. Church, eds.), Appleton-Century-Crofts, New York, pp. 279–296.

Kandel, E. R. and Schwartz, H. J., 1982, Molecular biology of learning: Modulation of transmitter release, *Science* 217:433–443.

Konorski, J., 1967, *Integrative Activity of the Brain,* University of Chicago Press.

Kremer, E. F. and Kamin, L. J., 1971, The truly random control procedure: Associative or nonassociative effects in rats, *J. Comp. Physiol. Psychol.* **74**:203–210.

Kupfermann, I., 1979, Modulatory actions of neurotransmitters, *Ann. Rev. Neurosci.* **2**:447–465.

Lederhendler, I., Goh, Y., and Aldon, D. L., 1982, Type B photoreceptor changes predict modification of motoneuron responses to light during retention of *Hermissenda* associative conditioning, *Soc. Neurosci. Abstr.* **8**:825.

Mackintosh, N. J., 1974, *The Psychology of Animal Learning,* Academic Press, New York.

Mackintosh, N. J., 1975, A theory of attention: Variations in the associability of stimulus with reinforcement, *Psychol. Rev.* **82**:276–298.

McElearney, A. and Farley, J., 1983, Persistent changes in *Hermissenda* B photoreceptor membrane properties with associative training: A role for pharmacological modulation, *Soc. Neurosci. Abstr.* **9**:915.

Millenson, J. R., Kehoe, E. J., and Gormezano, I., 1977, Classical conditioning of the rabbits' nictitating membrane response under fixed and mixed CS–UCS intervals, *Learn. Motiv.* **8**:351–366.

Moore, J. W., and Gormezano, I., 1977, Classical conditioning, in: *Fundamentals and Applications of Learning* (M. H. Marx and M. E. Bunch, eds.), MacMillan Co., New York, pp. 87–120.

Neary, J. T. and Alkon, D. L., 1982, K^+ conductances of protein phosphorylation in *Hermissenda:* Decrease in ^{32}P incorporation in a 24,000 MW phosphoprotein band in the presence of 4-aminopyridine, *Soc. Neurosci. Abstr.* **8**:825.

Pavlov, I. P., 1927, *Conditioned Reflexes* (G.V. Anrep, trans.) Oxford University Press, London.

Prokasy, W. F., 1965, Classical eyelid conditioning: Experimenter operations, task demands, and response shaping, in: *Classical Conditioning: A Symposium* (W. F. Prokasy, ed.), Appleton-Century-Crofts, New York, pp. 208–225.

Rescorla, R. A., 1968, Probability of shock in the presence and abscence of CS in fear conditioning, *J. of Comp. and Physiol. Psych.* **66**:1–5.

Rescorla, R. A., 1972, Informational variables in Pavlovian conditioning, in: *The Psychology of Learning and Motivation,* Vol. 6 (G. Bower, ed.), Academic Press, New York.

Rescorla, R. A., 1975, Pavlovian excitatory and inhibitory conditioning, in: *Handbook of Learning and Cognitive Processes: Conditioning and Behavior Theory,* Vol. 2 (W. K. Estes, ed.), Lawrence Erlbaum Associates, Hillsdale, New Jersey, pp. 7–35.

Rescorla, R. A. and Wagner, A. R., 1972, A theory of Pavlovian conditioning: Variations in the effectiveness of reinforcement and non-reinforcement, in: *Classical Conditioning II: Current Theory and Research* (A.H. Black and W. F. Prokasy), Appleton-Century-Crofts, New York, pp. 64–99.

Richards, W. and Farley, J., 1984, Associative-learning changes intrinsic to *Hemissenda* Type A photoreceptors, *Soc. Neurosci. Abstr.* **10**:623.

Richards, W., Farley, J., and Alkon, D. L., 1983, Extinction of associative learning in *Hermissenda:* Behavior and neural correlates, *Soc. Neurosci. Abstr.* **9**:916.

Richards, W. G., Farley, J., and Alkon, D. L., 1984, Extinction of associative learning in *Hemissenda:* Behavior and neural correlates, *Behavioural Brain Research* **14**:161–170.

Shoukimas, J. J. and Alkon, D. L., 1980, Voltage-dependent, early outward current in a photoreceptor of *Hermissenda crassicornis, Soc. Neurosci. Abstr.* **6**:17.

Shoukimas, J. J. and Alkon, D. L., 1983, Effect of voltage-dependent K^+ conductances upon initial generator response in B-photoreceptors of *H. Crassicornis, Biophys. J.* **41**:37a.

Spetch, M. L., Wilkie, D. M., and Pinel, J. P. J., 1981, Backward conditioning: A reevaluation of the empirical evidence, *Psych. Bull.* **89**:163–175.

Tabata, M. and Alkon, D. L., 1982, Positive synaptic feedback in visual system of nudibranch mollusk *Hermissenda crassicornis, J. Neurophysiol.* **48**:174–191.

Testa, T. J., 1974, Causal relationship and the acquisition of avoidance responses, *Psychol Rev.* **81**:491–505.

Vold, L., Grover, L., and Farley, J., 1985, Training and testing determinants of phototaxic behavior in *Hermissenda, Soc. Neurosci. Abstr.* (in press).

West, A., Barnes, E., and Alkon, D. L., 1982, Primary changes of voltage responses during retention of associative learning, *J. Neurophysiol.* **48**:1243–1255.

Wu, R. and Farley, J., 1984, Serotonin reduces K^+ currents and enhances a Ca^{2+} current in *Hermissenda* Type B photoreceptors, *Soc. Neurosci. Abstr.* **10**:620.

3

Analysis of Associative and Nonassociative Neuronal Modifications in *Aplysia* Sensory Neurons

J. H. BYRNE, K. A. OCORR, J. P. WALSH, and E. T. WALTERS

1. INTRODUCTION

There is a growing interest among psychologists, neurobiologists, and adaptive system theorists in the mechanisms that underlie the capacity of the nervous system for associative and nonassociative information storage. In this chapter, we briefly review our attempts to examine this question utilizing the defensive tail withdrawal reflex in *Aplysia* as a simple test system. Because this system is a relatively new one, we first describe some of its features and characterize some of the underlying neurocircuitry. We then review electrophysiological, biochemical, and biophysical correlates of sensitization, a nonassociative form of learning exhibited by this reflex. An important extension of our work on sensitization was the demonstration of a cellular analog of associative learning. Some of these results and a possible mechanism for this associative information storage, termed activity-dependent neuromodulation, are discussed. Finally, we describe some recent biochemical correlates of associative cellular conditioning.

2. THE TAIL WITHDRAWAL REFLEX

Figure 1 illustrates a side view of *Aplysia californica*. When a mechanical or an electrical stimulus is applied to the tail, there is a brisk reflex withdrawal of the

J. H. BYRNE, K. A. OCORR, J. P. WALSH, and E. T. WALTERS ● Department of Physiology and Cell Biology, University of Texas Medical School, Houston, Texas 77225.

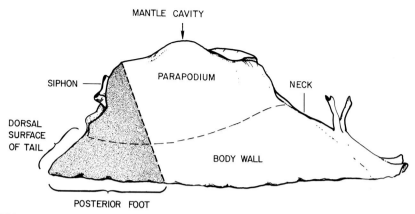

FIGURE 1. Side view of an intact *Aplysia*. The general tail region (stippled) also includes the posterior aspects of both the parapodia and the midbody. The tail itself extends to the left from the termination of the parapodia (which cover the mantle cavity). Stimulation of the skin in the general tail region elicits the short-latency tail withdrawal reflex. When maximally activated, this reflex produces contraction of all the stippled area, causing most of the tail region to retract into the body. (From Walters *et al.,* 1983a.)

tail, which presumably serves a defensive role, protecting the tail. Strong stimuli cause the entire stippled region to withdraw into the soft body cavity. Unlike the extensively examined siphon and gill withdrawal reflex, which is controlled by neurons in the abdominal ganglion (Koester and Kandel, 1977; Byrne, 1981; Hawkins *et al.,* 1981), the tail withdrawal reflex is mediated by neurons in the pleural and pedal ganglia (Walters *et al.,* 1983a).

The cell bodies of the sensory neurons that innervate the tail comprise a subset of a distinct cluster of about 200 sensory cells (the PLVC cluster) located in the pleural ganglion (Fig. 2). A tactile stimulus to the tail excites the afferent terminals of the tail sensory neurons and the resulting action potentials propagate through the pedal ganglion into the pleural ganglion. Before reaching the pleural ganglion, the sensory neurons make excitatory monosynaptic connections in the pedal ganglion with at least three identified tail motor neurons known as P5, P6, and P7. Sufficient activation of the sensory neurons causes activation of the tail motor neurons; the resulting action potentials propagate out the peripheral nerves, causing muscles in the tail to contract and withdraw the tail.

The experimental preparation we used is illustrated in Fig. 3. The animal was split almost in half, leaving only the tail intact. The pleural and pedal ganglia were placed in a small inner chamber so that the periphery and the ganglia could be perfused with separate solutions. Simultaneous intracellular recordings were made from both motor neurons and sensory neurons. Mechanical or electrical stimuli were delivered to the tail and the resultant reflex contractions were measured with a tension transducer.

Figure 4 illustrates typical recordings obtained when a mechanical stimulus was presented to the tail in this preparation. In Part A a brief pinch was delivered to the skin (indicated by the arrow), leading to a brisk discharge of action potentials

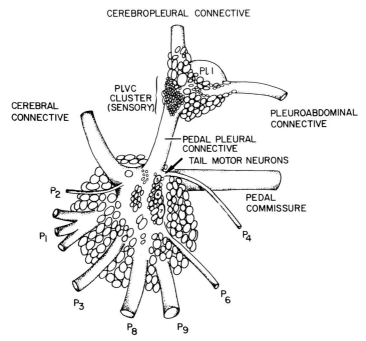

FIGURE 2. Schematic diagram of the left pleural and pedal ganglia. Symmetrical clusters are located in the right pleural and pedal ganglia. The pleural ventrocaudal (PLVC) cluster of mechano-afferent somata lies on the root of the pedal-pleural connective. Near the opposite root of the pedal-pleural connective is a cluster of presumptive motor neurons in the pedal ganglion containing identified cells P5, P6, and P7 that cause tail withdrawal. Electrophysiological (Walters *et al.*, 1983a) and morphological (Cleary and Byrne, 1984) observations indicate that both the sensory neurons and motor neurons send their axons out the peripheral nerves. (From Walters *et al.*, 1983a.)

in the sensory neuron, a discharge of action potentials in the motor neuron, and a reflex withdrawal of the tail. In order to assess the contribution of this sensory neuron to the reflex, the cell was artificially activated in an attempt to mimic roughly the firing produced by the mechanical stimulus to the tail. Firing the sensory neuron led to a burst of spikes in the motor neuron and a contraction of the tail that was about 30% of the magnitude of the tail withdrawal produced by actually stimulating the skin. This indicates that each sensory neuron makes a sizable contribution to the reflex withdrawal of the tail.

3. SENSITIZATION OF THE TAIL WITHDRAWAL REFLEX

Having analyzed some of the features of the tail withdrawal reflex and its neural circuit, we then examined various forms of plasticity in the connections between the sensory neurons and motor neurons.

Figure 5 shows an example of sensitization of this reflex and the correlates of

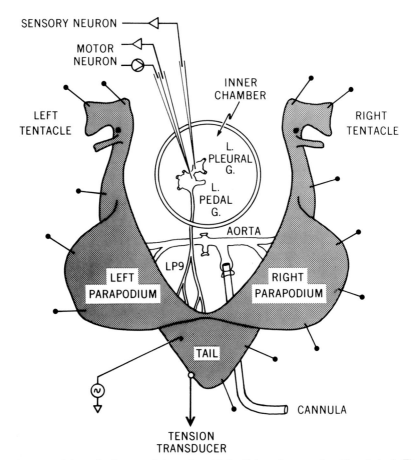

FIGURE 3. Schematic diagram of the reduced tail withdrawal preparation (dorsal view). The mantle organs, viscera, and all the ganglia except for the left pleural and pedal ganglia (shown enlarged) were removed, and the animal was completely bisected except for the tail, which was connected to a tension transducer. The preparation was restrained with pins inserted through the body except in the region innervated by the left posterior pedal nerve (LP9). All other nerves (not shown) were transected. The aorta was cannulated for perfusion of the body, and separate perfusion was used in the inner chamber for the CNS. A motor neuron was impaled in the pedal ganglion, while one or more tail sensory neurons were recorded from in the pleural ganglion. In most experiments mechanical or electrical stimuli were applied to the tail. (From Walters *et al.*, 1983a.)

sensitization in the sensory and motor neurons. In this experiment simultaneous recordings were made from a sensory neuron and a motor neuron, and the magnitude of the tail withdrawal was monitored with a tension transducer. Part A of Fig. 5 shows the tension and motor neuron recordings. Here very weak tail shocks were repeatedly delivered to the skin at 5-min test intervals. These weak test stimuli did not excite the particular sensory neuron being monitored (not shown). The test stimuli produced bursts of synaptic input to the motor neuron, but no tail withdrawal,

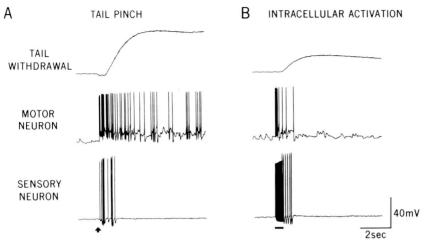

FIGURE 4. The tail withdrawal reflex. (A) Responses of the tail, a tail motor neuron (P5), and a tail sensory neuron to brief stimulation of the margin of the tail with fine forceps. (B) Intracellular activation (bar) of the sensory neuron produced 20 spikes (including an afterdischarge of 8 spikes), which resulted in activation of the motor neuron and a withdrawal of the tail that was 35% of the amplitude produced by the tail pinch. This suggests that the coactivation of the small number of VC sensory neurons may normally be sufficient to produce the tail withdrawal reflex. (From Walters *et al.*, 1983a.)

because the stimulus intensity was so weak. A sensitizing stimulus was then given to a part of the tail distant from the location where the test stimuli were applied and outside the receptive field of the sensory neuron being monitored. In response to the next test stimulus (trial 5), the tail withdrew briskly. One correlate of this sensitization was increased synaptic input and enhanced spike activity in the tail motor neuron in response to the test stimulus. Part B of Fig. 5 suggests that at least part of the increased synaptic input in the motor neuron is a result of heterosynaptic facilitation of the monosynaptic EPSP from the sensory neurons. Prior to the sensitizing stimulus, an action potential artificially produced in this sensory neuron resulted in the monosynaptic EPSP in the motor neuron shown to the left of Part B. Immediately after the sensitizing stimulus was delivered, the EPSP from the same sensory neuron was facilitated. Also note that in this example the sensory neuron triggered polysynaptic excitatory components that were not present prior to the sensitizing stimulus. Thus, enhancement of the sensory neuron connections may also increase the probability of recruiting interneuronal input to the motor neurons during sensitization.

4. ROLE OF SEROTONIN (5-HT)

The gill withdrawal reflex in *Aplysia* shows sensitization (Pinsker *et al.* 1970, 1973) similar to that described above for the tail withdrawal reflex. In addition, the siphon sensory neurons that trigger the gill withdrawal reflex also shows het-

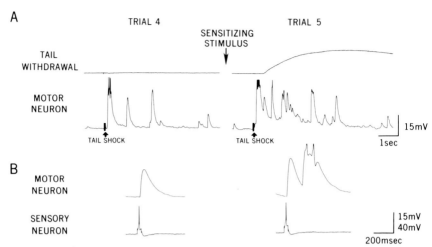

FIGURE 5. Sensitization and synaptic facilitation produced by a weak mechanical stimulus. (A) Test responses of the tail and a tail motor neuron 3 min before (trial 4) and 2 min after (trial 5) brief application of a 5-g von Frey hair (sensitizing stimulus) to the tail. The test stimuli were 70-msec shocks (approximately 1 mA) delivered at 5-min intervals through an electrode implanted in the tail. The sensitizing stimulus was applied after four tests in which neither a withdrawal response nor a change in the motor neuron response was observed. In order to reduce the likelihood of action potential initiation and observe the underlying synaptic input, the motor neuron was kept hyperpolarized 30 mV from resting potential throughout the experiment. (B) EPSPs produced by a single tail sensory neuron spike 30 sec before and 90 sec after the sensitizing stimulus. Test EPSPs were elicited every 60 sec by intracellular activation of single sensory neuron action potentials. The short-latency component is the monosynaptic EPSP. After sensitizing stimulation, the sensory neuron spike evoked a large monosynaptic EPSP and, in addition, longer-latency polysynaptic EPSPs. Spikes in the motor neuron are clipped by the pen recorder. (From Walters *et al.*, 1983b.)

erosynaptic facilitation (Castellucci *et al.*, 1970; Castellucci and Kandel, 1976). In the gill withdrawal reflex serotonin (5-HT) or a related neuromodulator appears to mediate these facilitatory effects (Brunelli *et al.*, 1976; Klein and Kandel, 1978, 1980). To explore the possibility that 5-HT might also be a modulatory transmitter for the tail withdrawal reflex, we conducted the experiment shown in Fig. 6. This experiment was very similar to the one illustrated in Fig. 5 but instead of delivering a sensitizing stimulus to the animal, we perfused 5-HT (5×10^{-5} M) into the inner chamber of the preparation. A weak test stimulus (tail shock) was delivered to a point outside the receptive field of the sensory neuron being monitored (see below). This initial tail shock caused a burst of spikes in the motor neuron and produced a small reflexive withdrawal of the tail (Fig. 6A$_1$). After 5-HT was perfused into the chamber, the same shock was again delivered. This shock produced a larger burst of spikes in the motor neuron and a larger tail withdrawal (Fig. 6A$_2$). In Part B, the motor neuron EPSP was dramatically enhanced, illustrating the facilitation of the connection between the sensory neuron and motor neuron produced by 5-HT. Thus, 5-HT application can mimic a sensitizing stimulus and may be a modulatory transmitter used in the tail withdrawal reflex.

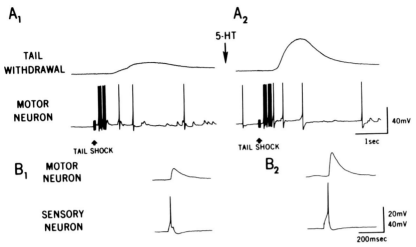

FIGURE 6. Sensitization of tail withdrawal reflex and heterosynaptic facilitation are mimicked by 5-HT. (A) Simultaneous recordings of the responses of the tail and a tail motor neuron to a weak tail shock (outside the excitatory receptive field of the sensory neuron, see part B) 4 min before and 1 min after superfusion of the ganglia with 5×10^{-5} M 5-HT. The 5-HT did not reach the peripheral tissues, which were separated from the inner chamber. (B) Facilitation of the monosynaptic EPSP from the sensory neuron to the motor neuron. The EPSP was tested 30 sec before each test shown in Part A. (From Walters *et al.*, 1983b.)

Serotonin has four distinct but related effects on the sensory neurons and their EPSPs (Fig. 7). First, it increases the size of the PSP produced in the motor neuron by an action potential in the sensory neuron. Second, it often produces a slow and long-lasting depolarization of the sensory neuron. Third, there is an increase in excitability of the sensory neuron. In Fig. 7 this increase in excitability is shown by the fact that the same constant current pulse that had produced only a single action potential in the absence of 5-HT produced a burst of action potentials in the presence of 5-HT. Fourth, although not visible in Fig. 7A, 5-HT also enhances the duration of the sensory neuron action potential. This can be more clearly seen when one perfuses the preparation with a low concentration of TEA or 4-AP to partially block repolarizing potassium currents (Klein and Kandel, 1978; Walters *et al.*, 1983b).

The depolarizing effects of serotonin on the sensory neurons were examined in greater detail in the experiment illustrated in Fig. 7B. In this experiment, the entire sensory neuron cluster was surgically removed from the ganglion to minimize the possible indirect effects from 5-HT-sensitive interneurons. In addition, input resistance of the sensory neuron was monitored by applying brief constant current hyperpolarizing pulses. Bath application of 5-HT led to a slow and long-lasting depolarization that was associated with an increase in input resistance. Additional voltage–clamp and ion substitution experiments indicate that the slow depolarization is, at least in part, due to a decrease in a resting K^+ conductance (Walsh and Byrne, 1983, 1984).

Similar depolarizations and conductance changes are associated with hetero-

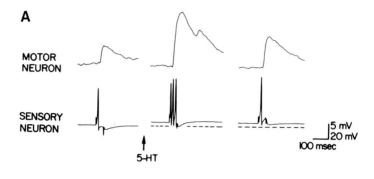

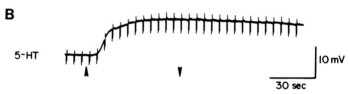

FIGURE 7. Effects of serotonin on the tail sensory neurons. (A) Effects of 5-HT on membrane potential and monosynaptic EPSP amplitude in the semi-intact preparation. Constant current suprathreshold depolarizing pulses (50 msec) were injected into the sensory neuron at 60-sec intervals. After 10^{-4} M 5-HT was perfused into the chamber (arrow), the brief depolarizing test pulse elicited multiple spikes. The stimulus current was then decreased so that only a single action potential was elicited (third panel). (B) Effects of 5-HT on membrane potential and input resistance in a nearly isolated sensory cell soma. In the absence of most (possibly all) synaptic input, 5-HT produced a depolarizing response accompanied by a 30% increase in input resistance, which was monitored by delivering constant current hyperpolarizing pulses through a second intracellular electrode. (From Walters *et al.*, 1983b.)

synaptic facilitation of the siphon sensory neurons in the gill withdrawal reflex (Klein and Kandel, 1978). In that system, 5-HT appears to be mediating its effects through cyclic AMP (Bernier *et al.*, 1982; for review, see Kandel and Schwartz, 1982). To determine whether cyclic AMP is used as a second messenger by the tail sensory neurons as well, we obtained simultaneous recordings from two tail sensory neurons (Fig. 8). Sensory neuron 1 was used to monitor voltage changes while sensory neuron 2 was voltage clamped at the resting potential. At the arrow, a 1-sec 10^{-5} M pulse of 5-HT was pressure ejected at a location approximately midway between the two sensory neurons. This produced a depolarization and increased resistance in sensory neuron 1 and a slow inward current associated with a decreased input conductance in sensory neuron 2. We next bath applied a relatively high concentration (10^{-4} M) of the cyclase activator forskolin (Seamon and Daley, 1981) as shown in Part B. Forskolin mimicked the 5-HT response, producing a depolarization and increase in input resistance in sensory neuron 1 and an inward current associated with a decrease in membrane conductance in sensory neuron 2. The same 5-HT pulse as in Part A was again applied in the continued presence of

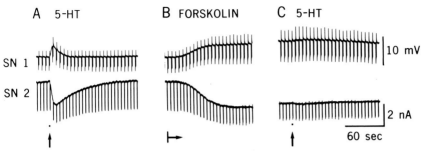

FIGURE 8. Forskolin effects on membrane properties and 5-HT response in an isolated sensory neuron cluster. (A) Responses of adjacent current-clamped (SN1) and voltage-clamped (SN2) sensory neurons to a 1-sec puff of 10^{-5} M 5-HT delivered between the two cells (arrow). Constant current and constant voltage hyperpolarizing pulses were applied in SN1 and SN2 respectively to monitor changes in input conductance. (B) Response of SN1 and SN2 to bath application of forskolin. Addition of 10^{-4} M forskolin mimicked the changes in membrane potential, current, and conductance produced by 5-HT. Forskolin was added at the arrow in (B) and remained present throughout (B) and (C). (C) Forskolin blocks subsequent responses to 5-HT. In the presence of 10^{-4} M forskolin a 1-sec puff of 5-HT identical to that applied in (A) produced no observable change in membrane properties in either SN1 or SN2. (From Walsh and Byrne, 1983, 1984.)

forskolin, but this time there was little or no change in membrane potential or membrane current in either of the two sensory neurons (Part C). Thus, forskolin is capable of mimicking the response of these cells to 5-HT and, furthermore, of blocking subsequent responses to 5-HT. These and other electrophysiological and pharmacological experiments indicate a role for cyclic AMP in the 5-HT response (see also Byrne and Walters, 1982; Pollock *et al.*, 1982).

More direct biochemical evidence for an involvement for cyclic AMP in this response is illustrated in Fig. 9. Here we directly measured cyclic AMP levels by radioimmunoassay techniques in surgically isolated clusters of sensory neurons (Ocorr *et al.*, 1983, 1985). Because there are two symmetrical clusters of sensory

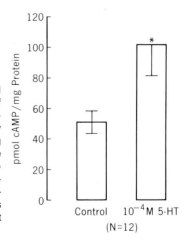

FIGURE 9. 5-HT elevates cAMP levels in isolated pleural sensory neuron clusters. Mean cyclic AMP levels of *Aplysia* tail sensory neurons are expressed as picomoles cyclic AMP/mg protein $\pm$ S.E.M. Isolated sensory neuron clusters were exposed either to ASW containing 10^{-4} M 5-HT or ASW alone (control) in the presence of RO 20-1724 for 5 min. Clusters were frozen immediately following the 5-HT or control treatment and assayed for cAMP content using standard radioimmunoassay techniques. Asterisk indicates difference is significant, $p < .005$, 1-tailed t-test for nonindependent groups. From Ocorr *et al.* (1983, 1985).

neurons, one in the left pleural ganglion and one in the right pleural ganglion, one cluster was used as a control for the other. Sensory neuron clusters exposed to 5-HT showed a significant enhancement in cyclic AMP content compared to their contralateral controls.

In summary, these results indicate that the tail withdrawal reflex can be sensitized and that the sensitization is mimicked by 5-HT. Furthermore, the 5-HT effects are associated with a decreased K^+ conductance, which appears to be produced by changes in cyclic AMP levels.

5. ASSOCIATIVE MODIFICATIONS OF SENSORY NEURONS

Because of its accessibility for detailed cellular analysis, we were interested in determining whether the tail withdrawal circuit displays associative modifications. Although simple, this system has some features that can be fit to some psychological theories of associative learning. For example, some psychologists have assumed that the formation of some associations depends largely upon the contiguous activation of sensory "analyzers" and modulatory "arousal centers" (Konorski, 1967; Mackintosh, 1974). We tested this general idea on the neuronal level by examining the associative interaction of electrophysiological activity in individual sensory neurons with neuromodulatory effects produced during defensive arousal or sensitization. Our results suggest a cellular mechanism for associative information storage that we call activity-dependent neuromodulation.

A cellular model of activity-dependent neuromodulation is illustrated in Fig. 10. Assume that two "sensory analyzers," here designated as sensory neuron 1 and sensory neuron 2, make weak subthreshold connections to a response system. Reinforcing stimuli have two effects. One is to directly activate the response system and produce an unconditioned response (UR). Second, reinforcing stimuli activate a diffuse modulatory or facilitatory system that nonspecifically enhances the connections of all the sensory neurons. Delivering a reinforcing stimulus alone would activate the response system and cause generalized sensitization or heterosynaptic facilitation of the sensory neurons by increasing their excitability and enhancing transmitter release. We propose that spike activity in one of the sensory neurons (indicated by the stippling) just prior to the modulatory stimulus causes a selective amplification of the modulatory effects in that specific sensory neuron (Walters and Byrne, 1983a). Unpaired activity or no activity (sensory neuron 2) would not modify the modulatory effects in the neuron. The amplification of the modulatory effects in the paired sensory neuron lead to an enhancement of the ability of that sensory neuron to activate the response system and produce the conditioned response (Part B).

The experimental preparation utilized to test this hypothesis is illustrated in Fig. 11. It is very similar to the preparation illustrated in Fig. 3. Simultaneous recordings were made from a single tail motor neuron and three tail sensory neurons. The reinforcing or unconditioned stimulus (US) was an electric shock delivered to the tail. Sensory neurons were selected that had receptive fields outside the region of the stimulating electrodes and thus were not activated by the US. The timing

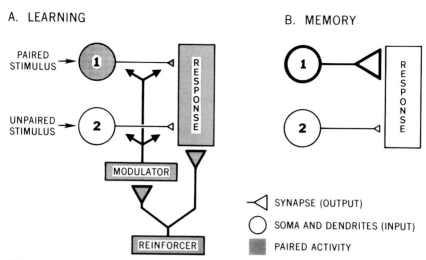

FIGURE 10. General model of associative information processing through the mechanism of activity-dependent neuromodulation. (A) Learning. Stippling indicates temporally contiguous activity. A motivationally potent reinforcing stimulus activates a neural response system and diffusely modulates (modulator) afferents to the response system. Increased spike activity in the paired afferent (1) immediately before the modulatory signal amplifies the degree and duration of the modulatory effects, perhaps through the Ca^{2+} sensitivity of the modulatory evoked second messenger. The unpaired afferent neuron (2) does not show an amplification of the modulatory effects. (B) Memory. The amplified modulatory effects cause increases in transmitter release and/or excitability of the paired neuron, which in turn strengthens the functional connection between the paired neuron (1) and the response system. (Modified from Walters and Byrne, 1983a.)

and number of spikes in the sensory neurons was artificially controlled with intracellular depolarizing current pulses. One sensory neuron was not activated at all and thus served as a monitor of changes in the EPSP that were produced by sensitization alone. A second cell (the CS +) received paired stimulation; it was artificially depolarized to produce a high-frequency burst of action potentials just prior to the tail shock. The third sensory neuron (CS −) received unpaired stimulation; it was also artificially fired (producing a similar burst of spikes), but this cell was fired 2 min after the tail shock was delivered.

Figure 12 illustrates details of the training and testing procedures and shows some of the raw data. The baseline EPSP amplitude was monitored in a single motor neuron that received input from each of the sensory neurons. Action potentials artificially induced in any one of these sensory neurons initially produced small monosynaptic EPSPs in the motor neuron (Fig. 12B). Each of these sensory neurons was assigned to receive the spike activity either paired with the modulatory stimulus (CS +), the unpaired activity, (CS −), or without high-frequency spike activity (SENS). The responses of the cell that received the paired spike activity (SN1) are shown in Fig. 12A. The high-frequency bursts of spikes was activated 600 msec before the tail shock (US), producing summating EPSPs in the motor neuron. The tail shock (note stimulus artifact in Fig. 12A) did not fire the sensory neuron in

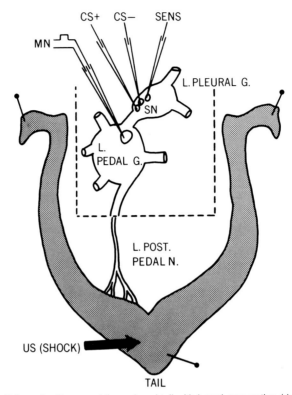

FIGURE 11. Schematic diagram of the reduced tail withdrawal preparation (dorsal view) used for associative conditioning procedures. Restraining and dissection procedures were identical to those described in Fig. 3. Three tail sensory neurons (SN) and a tail motor neuron (MN) were examined simultaneously. The CS + cell received depolarizing pulses that fired a burst of spikes in the sensory neuron and was paired with tail shock (US). The CS − cell received an identical burst of spikes specifically unpaired with the US (2 min after the US). The SENS cell received no CS and was used to monitor the nonspecific effects of heterosynaptic facilitation.

any of the three traces, but it produced EPSPs and spikes in the motor neuron. In the cell that received unpaired activity (SN2) the artificially induced spike activity followed the tail shock by 2 min (CS −). Finally, the sensitization control cell SN3 (SENS) received no high-frequency activation during the training procedure. Five training trials were given at 5-min intervals. Before, during, and after the training, the size of the EPSPs produced by individual spikes was tested at 5-min intervals to see if there were any differences in the amplitude of the EPSPs from the different cells. As shown in Part C, the EPSP from the sensory neuron that was paired was enhanced dramatically from its pretest levels. The EPSPs from the sensory neurons receiving the CS − training and SENS training were also enhanced, but to a lesser extent than the cell receiving the paired activity. The enhancement of the EPSP in SN3 is simply a reflection of the heterosynaptic facilitation produced by sensitization.

Figure 13 illustrates summary data from ten experiments and shows the size

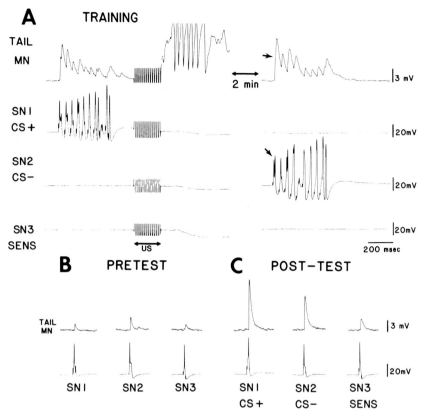

FIGURE 12. Associative conditioning of a sensory neuron. Three tail sensory neurons (SN) and a tail motor neuron (MN) were examined simultaneously. (A) Training procedure (illustrated by trial 3). Each CS consisted of nine intracellular suprathreshold depolarizing pulses. SN1 received the CS+ (which elicited 11 spikes on this trial) 600 msec before the US (tail shock artifacts are visible), and SN2 received the CS− (which elicited 12 spikes) 2 min later. The US was applied outside of the excitatory receptive fields of the sensory neurons examined. The resulting spikes in the motor neuron are clipped by the pen recorder. SN3 (SENS) received no CS, providing an index of nonspecific heterosynaptic facilitation. The first pulse during the CS− elicited a double spike in SN2 (arrow), causing summation of the resulting EPSPs in the motor neuron (arrow). (B) Monosynaptic test responses during the pretest. (C) Monosynaptic test responses during posttest (test 6, 10 min after training). The test response of SN1 (CS+) showed more facilitation (732% of baseline) than did SN2 (CS−, 254%) or SN3 (SENS, 214%) in this animal. (From Walters and Byrne, 1983a.)

of the EPSP in the pretest, in the training phase, and in the posttest phases. Initially the mean EPSP in each group was about 7 mV in amplitude. Three pretest trials were given to ensure stable responses. The tail shocks (US) during training are indicated by the arrows. During training there was an enhancement of the EPSPs in all the cells, but the EPSPs from the cells that received the paired training (CS+) showed a dramatic enhancement relative to the EPSPs from those cells that received the explicitly unpaired spike activity (CS−) or the cells that received no high-frequency burst of spikes at all (SENS).

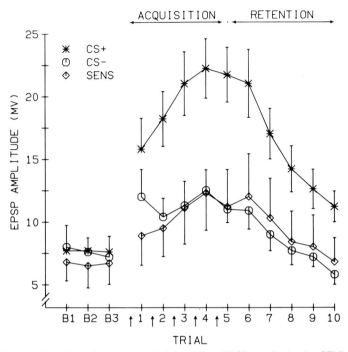

FIGURE 13. Activity-dependent neuromodulation. Mean EPSP amplitudes (± SEM) of CS+ group are greater than those of CS− and SENS groups. Arrows on abscissa indicate delivery of the US. B1 to B3 are baseline tests (pretest phase). The increase in SENS responses indicates the degree of nonspecific heterosynaptic facilitation. (From Walters and Byrne, 1983a.)

6. MECHANISM OF THE ASSOCIATIVE NEURONAL MODIFICATION

Given that there is a relatively long-term enhancement of synaptic transmission produced by activity-dependent neuromodulation, what are the mechanisms that might account for this associative phenomenon? Since activity seems to amplify the effects of sensitization, and since the effects of 5-HT and sensitization appear to be linked to increased levels of cyclic AMP, we predicted that pairing spike activity with a sensitizing stimulus would lead to an associatively specific enhancement of cyclic AMP levels. To begin to test this possibility, we utilized the isolated sensory neuron cluster and paired high K^+ depolarization (to mimic spike activity) with 5-HT application (to mimic the reinforcing US) and monitored changes in cyclic AMP levels in the sensory neurons.

For the paired procedure, sensory neurons were exposed for 5 sec to high K^+ saline followed immediately by a 15-sec application of 5-HT. For the unpaired procedure, the clusters were first exposed to a 5-sec application of high K^+ followed by a $2\frac{1}{2}$-min exposure to saline alone and then to the same application of 5-HT used in the paired procedure. The clusters were frozen after 5-HT application and subsequently assayed for cAMP content. Figure 14 illustrates the results. Sensory

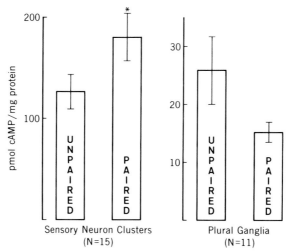

FIGURE 14. Effects of conditioning analog on cyclic AMP levels. Both sensory neuron clusters from single *Aplysia* were surgically isolated and the clusters, as well as the remaining portion of the pleural ganglia, were exposed to an analog of a differential conditioning paradigm. A 5-sec application of high K^+ ASW served as the conditioned stimulus (CS) and a 15-sec application of 5×10^{-6} M 5-HT served as the unconditioned stimulus (US). One cluster from each animal was exposed to a paired presentation of the CS and US. Exposure to high K^+ ASW immediately preceded exposure to 5-HT. The contralateral cluster was exposed to a specifically unpaired treatment (exposure to high K^+ ASW preceded the 5-HT application by 2.5 min). Identical manipulations were performed on the remainder of the pleural ganglia. Tissues were analyzed for cyclic AMP content using standard radioimmunoassay techniques. Mean cyclic AMP levels are shown (pmoles cAMP/mg protein $\pm$ S.E.M.); asterisk indicates difference is significant ($p < .01$, 1-tailed t-test for nonindependent groups). The difference observed for the pleural ganglia cAMP content was also significant ($p < .05$). In contrast to the results for the sensory neuron clusters, however, this difference was not replicable. (From Ocorr et al., 1983.)

neuron clusters exposed to the paired procedure showed a significant elevation of cyclic AMP levels compared to the contralateral control clusters that received the unpaired procedure. These results indicate that a single pairing of high K^+ depolarization with 5-HT leads to a specific enhancement of cyclic AMP levels. Figure 14B shows that this effect appears to be limited to the sensory neuron clusters; an identical pairing procedure applied to the remnants of the pleural ganglia (the portion remaining after removing the cluster of sensory neurons) produced no enhancement (and indeed a reduction) of cyclic AMP levels.

It is important to point out that these measurements of cyclic AMP levels were obtained with isolated sensory neuron clusters and thus the effects that we monitored presumably occurred in the cell body and not the synapses. This effect is interesting by itself because of the possibility that cyclic AMP may influence the synthetic capabilities of the cell soma (e.g., Severin and Nesterova, 1982). For example, changes in gene expression might be important for long-term retention of these associative changes (Walters and Byrne, 1985). If similar effects were also taking place at the terminal, a more immediate read-out of the memory might be an enhancement of transmitter release. A molecular model that attempts to explain the relationship between cAMP and transmitter release is shown schematically in Fig. 15. Neuromodulatory transmitters such as 5-HT, which activate the cAMP cascade, might initiate the phosphorylation of proteins associated with a resting potassium channel. If this phosphorylation resulted in the closure of these channels, a slow long-lasting depolarization would be produced in the cell. In addition, because of the reduction of repolarizing K^+ currents, subsequent action potentials would be broadened allowing additional calcium to enter the cell and, consequently, additional transmitter release. This is essentially the model proposed by Klein and Kandel (1980) for sensitization of the siphon withdrawal reflex in *Aplysia*. If, however, spike activity is paired with the modulating stimulus, the spike activity (in addition to directly causing transmitter release) might also enhance the subsequent activation of adenylate cyclase by the moldulatory transmitter. It is conceivable that calcium, which enters during the depolarization produced by spike activity (Walters and Byrne, 1983a,b; Hawkins *et al.*, 1983; Abrams *et al.*, 1983), can serve as an activator of adenylate cyclase (Brostrom *et al.*, 1978; Malnoe *et al.*, 1983). Thus Ca^{2+} could increase the response of the adenylate cyclase to 5-HT, causing an amplification of cAMP production. The enhanced cyclic AMP levels should in turn produce greater closure of potassium channels, increased spike broadening, and further transmitter release.

7. CONCLUSIONS

Our results indicate that activity-dependent neuromodulation can produce an associative enhancement of synaptic efficacy, and it is intriguing to think that such mechanisms may contribute to associative learning. Moreover, in light of the recent demonstration of differential classical conditioning of the tail withdrawal reflex (Ingram and Walters, 1984), it will be interesting to see if similar changes in the tail sensory neurons also underlie this form of conditioning. Hawkins *et al.* (1983)

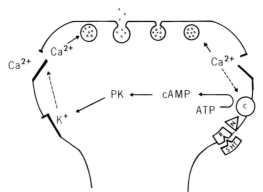

FIGURE 15. General model of molecular events underlying sensitization and activity-dependent neuromodulation. Neurotransmitter binding to receptor (R) activates adenylate cyclase (C) via a regulatory subunit (N). The cyclic AMP produced activates one or more protein kinases (PK) whose action(s) include closure of steady-state K^+ channels. Closing K^+ channels results, indirectly, in an increased Ca^{2+} influx and an increase in transmitter release during subsequent depolarizations. If Ca^{2+} entering during spike activity (CS) interacts synergistically with one or more of the components of the adenylate cyclase complex, subsequent activation by 5-HT (US) would result in an amplification of cyclic AMP levels. A consequence of the amplified cAMP levels would be an enhancement of transmitter release. (From Ocorr *et al.*, 1983, 1985.)

have shown similar activity-dependent neuromodulation in the siphon sensory neurons that mediate the gill and siphon withdrawal reflex, a system that also exhibits differential classical conditioning (Carew *et al.*, 1983).

The generality of activity-dependent neuromodulation remains to be established. It would be foolish to suggest that this is the only mechanism for associative learning, and other possibilities are discussed throughout this volume. It is interesting, however, that activity-dependent neuromodulation has been observed recently at the crayfish neuromuscular junction by Breen and Atwood (1983) and in hippocampal pyramidal cells by Hopkins and Johnston (1983). In addition, there is growing evidence from a number of vertebrate and invertebrate systems consistent with synergistic Ca^{2+} and cyclic nucleotide interactions (e.g., Woody *et al.*, 1978). Since Ca^{2+} and cyclic nucleotide tide control systems are so ubiquitous, it is attractive to think that their specific interactions are involved in general mechanisms of plasticity and learning.

Finally, there is a growing belief among developmental neurobiologists that both activity and neuromodulation are important for the formation and maintenance of synaptic connections (Changeux and Danchin, 1976; Kasamatsu *et al.*, 1981; Schmidt and Edwards, 1983). Models such as ours may help provide a mechanistic link between development and learning.

Clearly, much work remains. We need to examine the temporal constraints of the associative effects, the details of the interactions between spike activity (and presumably Ca^{2+}) and the cAMP system, and the relationship between the soma changes and changes in release at the synapse. Finally, we plan to examine the extent to which activity-dependent neuromodulation can account for associative modifications of behavior observed in the intact animal (Ingram and Walters, 1984).

ACKNOWLEDGMENTS. Supported by NIH grant NS19895 to J.H.B., fellowship MH09014 to K.A.O., and fellowship NS06455 to E.T.W.

REFERENCES

Abrams, T. W., Carew, T. J., Hawkins, R. D., and Kandel, E. R., 1983, Aspects of the cellular mechanism of temporal specificity in conditioning in *Aplysia:* Preliminary evidence for Ca^{2+} influx as a signal of activity, *Soc. Neurosci. Abstr.* **9:**168.

Bernier, L., Castellucci, V. F., Kandel, E. R., and Schwartz, J. H., 1982, Facilitatory transmitter causes a selective and prolonged increase in adenosine $3':5'$-monophosphate in sensory neurons mediating the gill and siphon withdrawal reflex in *Aplysia, J. Neurosci.* **2:**1682–1691.

Breen, C. A. and Atwood, H. L., 1983, Octopamine—a neurohormone with presynaptic activity-dependent effects at crayfish neuromuscular junctions, *Nature* **303:**716–718.

Brostrom, M. A., Brostrom, C. O., Breckenridge, B. M., and Wolff, D. J., 1978, Calcium-dependent regulation of brain adenylate cyclase, *Adv. Cyclic Nucleotide Res.* **9:**85–99.

Brunelli, M., Castellucci, V., and Kandel, E. R., 1976, Synaptic facilitation and behavioral sensitization in *Aplysia:* Possible role of serotonin and cyclic AMP, *Science* **194:**1178–1181.

Byrne, J. H., 1981, Comparative aspects of neural circuits for inking behavior and gill withdrawal in *Aplysia californica, J. Neurophysiol.* **45:**98–106.

Byrne, J. H. and Walters, E. T., 1982, Associative conditioning of single sensory neurons in *Aplysia.* II. Activity-dependent modulation of membrane responses, *Soc. Neurosci. Abstr.* **8:**38.

Carew, T. J., Hawkins, R. D., and Kandel, E. R., 1983, Differential classical conditioning of a defensive withdrawal reflex in *Aplysia californica, Science* **219:**397–400.

Castellucci, V. and Kandel, E. R., 1976, Presynaptic facilitation as a mechanism for behavioral sensitization in *Aplysia, Science* **194:**1176–1178.

Castellucci, V., Pinsker, H., Kupfermann, I., and Kandel, E. R., 1970, Neuronal mechanisms of habituation and dishabituation of the gill withdrawal reflex in *Aplysia, Science* **167:**1745–1748.

Changeux, J. P. and Danchin, A., 1976, Selective stabilization of developing synapses as a mechanism for the specification of neuronal networks, *Nature* **264:**705–712.

Cleary, L. and Byrne, J. H., 1984, Light and electron microscope examination of sensory neurons and motoneurons mediating the tail withdrawal reflex in *Aplysia, Soc. Neurosci. Abstr.* **10:**916.

Hawkins, R. D., Castellucci, V. F., and Kandel, E. R., 1981, Interneurons involved in mediation and modulation of gill-withdrawal reflex in *Aplysia*. I. Identification and characterization, *J. Neurophysiol.* **45:**304–314.

Hawkins, R. D., Abrams, T. W., Carew, T. J., and Kandel, E. R., 1983, A cellular mechanism of classical conditioning in *Aplysia:* Activity dependent amplification of presynaptic facilitation, *Science* **219:**400–405.

Hopkins, W. F. and Johnston, D., 1983, β-adrenergic receptor regulation of long-term potentiation in the hippocampus, *Soc. Neurosci. Abstr.* **9:**861.

Ingram, D. A. and Walters, E. T., 1984, Differential classical conditioning of tail and siphon withdrawal in *Aplysia, Soc. Neurosci. Abstr.* **10:**270.

Kandel, E. R. and Schwartz, J. H., 1982, Molecular biology of learning: Modulation of transmitter release, *Science* **218:**433–443.

Kasamatsu, T., Pettigrew, J. D., and Arg, M., 1981, Cortical recovery from effects of monocular deprivation: Acceleration with norepinepherine and suppression with 6-hydroxydopamine, *J. Neurophysiol.* **45:**254–266.

Klein, M. and Kandel, E. R., 1978, Presynaptic modulation of voltage-dependent Ca^{2+} current: Mechanism for behavioral sensitization in *Aplysia californica, Proc. Natl. Acad. Sci. USA* **75:**3512–3516.

Klein, M. and Kandel, E. R., 1980, Mechanism of calcium current modulation underlying presynaptic facilitation and behavioral sensitization in *Aplysia, Proc. Natl. Acad. Sci. USA* **77:**6912–6916.

Koester, J. and Kandel, E. R., 1977, Further identification of neurons in the abdominal ganglion of *Aplysia* using behavioral criteria, *Brain Res.* **121:**1–20.

Konorski, J., 1967, *Integrative Activity of the Brain,* University of Chicago Press, Chicago.

Mackintosh, N. J., 1974, *The Psychology of Animal Learning,* Academic Press, New York, pp. 70–124.

Malnoe, A., Stein, E. A., and Cox, J. A., 1983, Synergistic activation of bovine cerebellum adenylate cyclase by calmodulin and β-adrenergic agonists, *Neurochem. Int.* **5:**65–72.

Ocorr, K. A., Walters, E. T., and Byrne, J. H., 1983, Associative conditioning analog in *Aplysia* tail sensory neurons selectively increases cAMP content, *Soc. Neurosci. Abstr.* **9:**169.

Ocorr, K. A., Walters, E. T., and Byrne, J. H., 1985, Associative conditioning analog selectively increases cAMP levels of tail sensory neurons in *Aplysia, Proc. Natl. Acad. Sci. USA* **82:**2548–2552.

Pinsker, H. M., Kupfermann, I., Castellucci, V. F., and Kandel, E. R., 1970, Habituation and dishabituation of the gill-withdrawal reflex in *Aplysia, Science* **164:**1740–1742.

Pinsker, H. M., Hening, W. A., Carew, T. J., and Kandel, E. R., 1973, Long-term sensitization of a defensive withdrawal reflex in *Aplysia, Science* **182:**1039–1042.

Pollock, J. D., Camardo, J. S., Bernier, L., Schwartz, J. H., and Kandel, E. R., 1982, Pleural sensory neurons of *Aplysia:* A new preparation for studying the biochemistry and biophysics of serotonin modulation of K^+ currents, *Soc. Neurosci. Abstr.* **8:**523.

Seamon, K. B. and Daley, J. W., 1981, Forskolin, a unique diterpene activator of cAMP-generating systems, *J. Cyclic Nucleotide Res.* **7:**201–204.

Severin, E. S. and Nesterova, M. V., 1982, Effect of cAMP-dependent protein kinases on gene expression, *Adv. Enzyme Regulation* **20:**167–193.

Schmidt, J. T. and Edwards, D. L., 1983, Activity sharpens the map during the regeneration of the retinotectal projection in goldfish, *Brain Res.* **269:**29–39.

Walsh, J. P. and Byrne, J. H., 1983, Comparison of decreased conductance serotonergic responses in ink motor neurons and tail sensory neurons in *Aplysia, Soc. Neurosci. Abstr.* **9:**458.

Walsh, J. P. and Byrne, J. H., 1984, Forskolin mimics and blocks a serotonin-sensitive decreased K^+ conductance in tail sensory neurons of *Aplysia, Neurosci. Lett.* **52**:7–11.

Walters, E. T. and Byrne, J. H., 1983a, Associative conditioning of single sensory neurons suggests a cellular mechanism for learning, *Science* **219**:405–408.

Walters, E. T. and Byrne, J. H., 1983b, Slow depolarization produced by associative conditioning of *Aplysia* sensory neurons may enhance Ca^{2+} entry, *Brain Res.* **280**:165–168.

Walters, E. T. and Byrne, J. H., 1985, Long-term potentiation produced by activity-dependent modulation of *Aplysia* sensory neurons, *J. Neurosci.* **5**:662–672.

Walters, E. T., Byrne, J. H., Carew, T. J., and Kandel, E. R., 1983a, Mechano-afferent neurons innervating the tail of *Aplysia*. I. Response properties and synaptic connections, *J. Neurophysiol.* **50**:1522–1542.

Walters, E. T., Byrne, J. H., Carew, T. J., and Kandel, E. R., 1983b, Mechano-afferent neurons innervating the tail of *Aplysia*. II. Modulation by sensitizing stimulation, *J. Neurophysiol.* **50**:1543–1559.

Woody, C. D., Swartz, B. E., and Gruen, E., 1978, Effects of acetylcholine and cyclic GMP on input resistance of cortical neurons in awake cats, *Brain Res.* **158**:373–395

4

Mapping the Learning Engram in a "Model" System, the Mollusk *Pleurobranchaea californica*

W. JACKSON DAVIS

1. INTRODUCTION

In recent years, several laboratories have begun to employ relatively simple, invertebrate organisms for the study of the cellular basis of complex behavioral phenomena, in a paradigm that has become known as the "model systems" approach. The term is somewhat of a misnomer, since most experimental preparations, simple and complex, serve as models of fundamental biological principles that are presumed to apply more broadly. The term is nonetheless useful, in that it reflects two of the basic assumptions implicit in the model systems paradigm. The first of these assumptions is that evolution has been conservative in its solution to general biological problems, i.e., that "models" may in fact be useful tools toward a broader understanding. The second assumption is that complex behavioral phenomena are indeed accessible to reductionist analysis at the cellular level, i.e., that the formulation of feasible cellular models of behavior is possible.

Both assumptions of the model systems approach have received broad support in the last decades of experimental biology. Thus, it is widely acknowledged that studies of the fruit fly *Drosophila* have furnished general insights into the mechanisms of inheritance in all animals, including humans, although recent developments also suggest important differences. Similarly, the last decade has seen the elucidation of several complex behavioral phenomena at the cellular level through the use of the model systems approach, including forms of nonassociative learning such as habituation and sensitization (Castellucci *et al.*, 1978), motivation (Davis, 1984a,b,d; Davis *et al.*, 1983), and choice (Davis, 1979; Davis *et al.*, 1974a,b; Kovac and Davis, 1977, 1980). My purpose here is to review what has been

W. JACKSON DAVIS ● The Thimann Laboratories, University of California at Santa Cruz, Santa Cruz, California 95064.

discovered about the cellular mechanisms of associative learning in a particular model system, the mollusk *Pleurobranchaea californica.*

The practitioners of the model systems approach have adopted several different strategies for their individual quests. Thus Alkon and his colleagues (this volume), using the mollusk *Hermissenda,* are examining the cellular modifications that accompany a behavioral learning task at the level of the *sensory* neurons. In contrast, Carew, Kandel, and their associates have examined not a learned behavior in an intact organism but instead an *analog* of learning produced by electrical stimulation in a highly reduced preparation and pursued the analysis both at the level of sensory neurons and also central pathways (Carew *et al.,* 1983; Hawkins *et al.,* 1983). A third model system, the land slug *Limax,* has been studied by Gelperin and Sahley primarily from a behavioral perspective (Gelperin, 1975; Sahley *et al.,* 1981a; Sahley *et al.,* 1981b). *Limax* thus provides the best examples of higher-order learning phenomena of the kind seen also in vertebrates.

In contrast to all three of these approaches, our research on the cellular basis of associative learning in *Pleurobranchaea* seeks to understand the neural mechanisms of a complex and well-defined *real* learning task (as opposed to a learning analog) within the *central* pathways (as opposed to sensory neurons) that mediate the learned task. This diversity of approaches promises to reveal a rich variety of mechanisms; the challenge will be to extract the generalities, so that the promise of the model systems approach can be fully realized.

Regardless of the specific approach that is taken to learning, certain common areas of experimental analysis emerge as inevitable. The first step toward understanding learning at the cellular level is to establish that learning (or its analogs) occurs in a behaviorally meaningful context. Learning, like habituation or breathing or walking, is a *behavioral* term that applies to the actions of an intact, functioning organism; otherwise, a behavioral modification cannot be correctly termed learning, regardless of how it is induced. The second step toward an understanding of learning is to identify and untangle the neural pathways in which the underlying physiological modifications take place. The third step is to establish the cellular mechanisms—neural, biophysical, biochemical—by which the modifications underlying learning are brought about within these identified neural pathways. This general organizational approach characterizes our study of learning in *Pleurobranchaea* and is adopted for purposes of structuring the present paper.

2. BEHAVIORAL ASPECTS OF LEARNING IN *PLEUROBRANCHAEA*

2.1. The Food Avoidance Learning Paradigm

Associative learning in the mollusk *Pleurobranchaea* (Fig. 1) was first demonstrated by means of classical and avoidance conditioning of feeding behavior (Mpitsos and Davis, 1973). Subsequent research (Mpitsos and Collins, 1975; Mpitsos *et al.,* 1978) utilized comparable procedures to establish the paradigm that we are now investigating from a cellular viewpoint. In this paradigm, a food stimulus (the conditioned stimulus or CS) is conditionally paired with aversive electric shock (the unconditioned stimulus or US) in a conventional avoidance conditioning paradigm. As is typical of an avoidance learning paradigm, the animals are naive in the early conditioning trials and hence the CS and US are invariably presented together as in a classical aversive conditioning paradigm. Animals quickly learn to avoid the specific food stimulus with which food has been paired, however, as indicated by active withdrawal from the conditioned stimulus (active avoidance learning) and by simultaneous suppression of the feeding behavior (passive avoid-

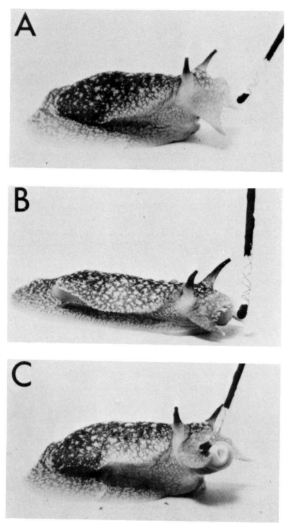

FIGURE 1. Different components of feeding behavior in the carnivorous marine gastropod *Pleurobranchaea californica*. (A) Orientation to a probe bearing a feeding stimulus; (B) extension of the feeding proboscis; (C) the consummatory bite-strike. (After Mpitsos and Davis, 1973.)

ance learning; Figs. 2–9). Thus, in later stages of conditioning the training protocol corresponds to an operant procedure.

Associative learning is generally considered as rigorously proven only after demonstration of several specific properties, including acquisition (i.e., the development of behavioral modifications during associative conditioning), long-term retention of the learned behavioral modification (i.e., for days or weeks), extinction of the learned behavioral modification (i.e., disappearance in absence of reinforcement), and savings of conditioning (i.e., accelerated acquisition as a consequence of previous conditioning and extinction). Moreover, numerous control procedures are essential in order to demonstrate that the learned behavioral modification is representative of associative learning. These control procedures include presentation of the CS and US alone, unpaired presentation of both the CS and US, random CS/US presentation, and backward conditioning. Finally, the case for associative learning is strengthened further by the demonstration of one-trial learning, stimulus selectivity, and differential conditioning. Each of these procedures has been performed successfully, repeatedly and independently in the case of food avoidance learning in *Pleurobranchaea,* as detailed in the remainder of this section (Figs. 2–9).

2.2. Acquisition Parameters

Acquisition parameters for the food avoidance learning task in *Pleurobranchaea* were first published nearly a decade ago (Mpitsos and Collins, 1975). Experimental animals (solid curves in Fig. 2) are associatively conditioned by presenting them with a food stimulus, homogenized squid (the CS), in ten sequential conditioning trials, each separated by 1 hr (the intertrial interval). If specimens either fail to withdraw from the CS or exhibit any component of the feeding response, they receive an aversive electric shock paired with continued CS delivery. Animals rapidly learn to associate food with shock and, as a result, withdraw increasingly from the food stimulus (Fig. 2A) and increasingly suppress the feeding responses, as expressed by increased response latencies of proboscis extension (Fig. 2B) and the bite-strike (Fig. 2C), and by an increase in the minimal concentration of food stimuli necessary to elicit these responses (the extension and bite-strike thresholds; Fig. 3). It has recently been reported that the acquisition of this food avoidance task is dependent upon feeding motivation (Gillette *et al.,* 1984), as seen also in vertebrate animals.

2.3. The Explicitly Unpaired CS/US Control Procedure

Modifications in the behavior of experimental animals cannot alone furnish evidence of learning, since nonassociative variables could in principle play a role in the observed changes. For example, repeated presentation of food or shock could alone increase withdrawal and/or suppress feeding. Alternatively, interaction between measures, nutritional history, general mechanical stimulation, or a host of other variables could modify the behavior of experimental (conditioned) animals. It is for these reasons that our experiments on learning in *Pleurobranchaea* have

FIGURE 2. Acquisition parameters for active (A) and passive (B and C) avoidance learning in *Pleurobranchaea* during simultaneous explicitly unpaired control procedures. The solid curve in (A) shows the percentage of experimental animals ($N = 25$; conditional pairing of food and aversive electric shock) that withdrew from the conditioned food stimulus (squid homogenate) during successive conditioning trials (intertrial interval, 1 hr). The dashed curve in (A) shows the percentage of control animals ($N = 24$; explicitly unpaired food and shock in the same absolute quantities as received by experimentals but separated in time by 0.5 hr) that withdrew from squid homogenate. Learning is indicated by significant differences between experimental and control percentages (asterisks; chi-square test, $p \le 0.01$). (B) and (C) show respectively the learned suppression of feeding behavior in the same animals as in (A), as expressed by increases in the latency from application of conditioned food stimuli to the first occurrence of the indicated feeding response, namely proboscis extension (B) or the bite-strike (C). Learning is indicated by significant differences between experimental and control means (asterisks; Mann-Whitney U tests, $p \le 0.01$). Vertical bars are standard errors. (From Mpitsos *et al.*, 1978.)

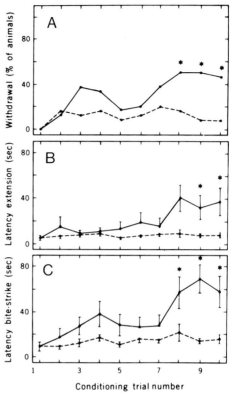

invariably entailed parallel control procedures aimed at eliminating the possible influence of nonassociative variables.

In our experiments, for example, prior to conditioning, each animal is always matched for size and responsiveness to food stimuli with a second specimen. Assignment of the two specimens to experimental and control categories is then accomplished using a random procedure. Control specimens subsequently receive exactly the same treatment as experimentals, in all respects but one, CS/US contingency. Thus, control animals have the same nutritive history; they receive the same absolute quantities of conditioned and unconditioned stimuli; measurements are made in the same way as on experimental animals, so that control animals receive the same amount and type of mechanical stimulation; their home cages are interspersed with those of experimental animals, so that they receive the same amount of light, noise, and other stimuli; and postconditioning measurements are made in the same way on experimental and control animals, without knowing the identity of specimens. Such a "blind" testing protocol guarantees lack of experimental and interpretative bias.

The only difference between experimental and control specimens is in the relative timing of CS and US. Thus, any difference in behavior between experimental and matched control animals constitutes evidence that the experimental animals are responding to this contingency with behavioral modifications; i.e., they are learning to associate two previously unassociated stimuli. In one type of control, for example, the CS and US are presented in the same amounts as received by the corresponding experimental specimen, but they are separated by a half hour. Using this "explicitly unpaired" control procedure, significant differences between mean behavioral measurements in experimental and control animals typically develop during acquisition (asterisks in Fig. 2). It is these differences in responsiveness to the CS between experimental and control animals that constitute evidence of associative learning.

2.4. Retention and Savings

Such significant differences between experimental and control groups are typically retained for at least 1 week (Fig. 3), at which time measurements are stopped. Individual specimens show retention for a month or more without reinforcement (not shown). Moreover, once extinction has been allowed to run its course, reconditioning of the same experimental animals (with parallel control procedures on the same control animals) reveals much more rapid acquisition than seen in the first conditioning trials. That is, significant differences between experimental and control groups develop earlier during training, typically by the second conditioning trial (Fig. 4). This phenomenon is known as "savings of conditioning" and is one of the requisite properties of associative learning as defined in vertebrate animals.

2.5. The Random CS/US Control Procedure

Although the explicitly unpaired control procedure described above and invariably employed in our conditioning experiments is considered sufficient by some learning psychologists, others believe that random presentation of the CS and US provides a theoretically sounder control procedure. Application of the random control to the food avoidance paradigm in *Pleurobranchaea* yielded little evidence of learning during acquisition (Fig. 5); but within 12 hr of the last conditioning trial, significant differences between experimentals and the random controls had developed (Fig. 6). These differences were retained for up to a week, at which time the experiment was terminated. Thus, within the above limits, the food avoidance learning in *Pleurobranchaea* also meets the stringent random CS/US control procedure.

2.6. Single Trial Learning and Backward Conditioning

Pleurobranchaea can even learn the food avoidance task in a single conditioning trial (Fig. 7), although the resultant behavioral modification can generally be observed only statistically in a large group of animals (total $N = 135$ in Fig. 7) and retention is predictably much shorter than in the case of repeated conditioning trials. In this same experiment (Fig. 7), several additional controls for nonassociative variables were performed, including the US (shock) alone, the CS (food) alone,

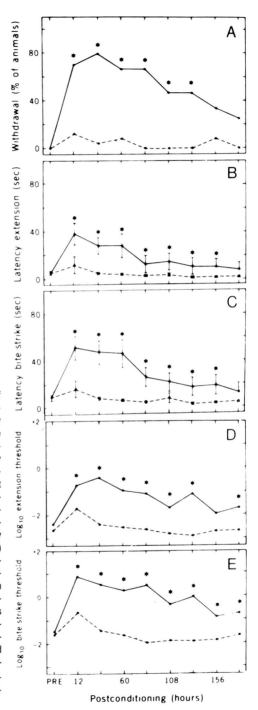

FIGURE 3. Retention and extinction of food avoidance learning in *Pleurobranchaea* following simultaneous explicitly unpaired control procedures. (A) Active avoidance learning (conditioned withdrawal from food stimuli), expressed by the percentage of animals that withdrew from the CS before (pre) and at various times after associative conditioning. Learning is indicated by the significant difference between experimental (solid curve) and control (explicitly unpaired food and shock; dashed curve) percentages (asterisks; $p \leq 0.01$; chi-square tests). (B–E) Passive avoidance learning (conditioned suppression of feeding), expressed by feeding response latencies (B, C) and thresholds (D, E). Learning is indicated by the significant difference between experimental (solid curve) and control (dashed curve) means ($p \leq 0.01$, Mann-Whitney U tests). Same animals as in Fig. 2. Vertical bars are standard errors. (From Mpitsos *et al.*, 1978.)

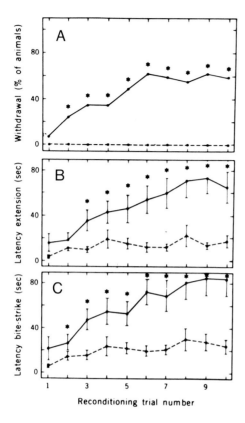

FIGURE 4. Saving of food avoidance learning, as indicated by more rapid acquisition of the learned task on reconditioning. Same animals and format as in Fig. 2. Note that significant differences between experimental and control animals occurred earlier than in the first conditioning sessions (cf. Fig. 2). Vertical bars are standard errors. (From Mpitsos et al., 1978.)

forward pairing (CS followed either 1 or 10 min later by the US) and backward conditioning (US followed either in 1 or 10 min by the CS). Neither the CS nor US alone causes the same modification seen in experimental animals, as demonstrated earlier (Davis et al., 1974a). In accord with learning laws as established in vertebrates, only forward conditioning resulted in a significant difference between experimental and control groups.

2.7. Selectivity in *Pleurobranchaea's* Food Avoidance Learning

Although the foregoing control procedures establish the conditioned behavioral modification in *Pleurobranchaea* as associative learning, the possibility remained that the behavioral modification was unselective, i.e., representative of a general suppression of responsiveness to any food stimulus. To test this hypothesis, animals were conditioned against squid and then tested not only with squid but also with an extract of sea anemone, an organism known to serve as a normal component of *Pleurobranchaea's* diet (Ottoway, 1977). Following conditioning, specimens exhibited suppressed feeding responses to squid, but normal responses to the sea

FIGURE 5. Acquisition parameters for active (A) and passive (B and C) food avoidance learning in *Pleurobranchaea* during simultaneous random control procedures. The solid curve in (A) shows the percentage of experimental animals (*N* = 24; conditional pairing of food and aversive electric shock) that withdrew from the conditioned food stimulus (squid homogenate) during successive conditioning trials (intertrial interval, 1 hr). The dashed curve in (A) shows the percentage of control animals (*N* = 25; *random* presentation of food and aversive electric shock in the same absolute quantities as received by experimentals) that withdrew from the squid

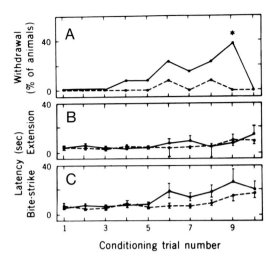

homogenate. Learning is indicated by the development of significant differences between experimental and control percentages (asterisk; $p \leqslant 0.01$; chi-square test). (B) and (C) show feeding responses of experimental (*N* = 24) and control (*N* = 25) animals, respectively. Significant differences indicative of learning do not appear until 12 hr postconditioning (see Fig. 6). Vertical bars are standard errors. (From Mpitsos *et al.*, 1978.)

anemone extract (Fig. 8). Therefore, this form of learning does not simply represent a generalized suppression of feeding responses but instead is selective to the food stimulus with which aversive shock is paired.

2.8. Differential Food Avoidance Conditioning in *Pleurobranchaea*

The discovery of selectivity in *Pleurobranchaea's* food avoidance learning made possible the application of a differential conditioning procedure (Davis *et al.*, 1980), considered the most powerful test for associative learning. In one set of experiments, squid homogenate was used as the CS$^+$, while homogenate of *Corynactis* served as the CS$^-$. In a second series of experiments on a different population of animals, the roles of squid and *Corynactis* were reversed; i.e., *Corynactis* became the CS$^+$, while squid was used as the CS$^-$. In both cases, training was accomplished by conditionally pairing the CS$^+$ with electric shock on the hour, while the CS$^-$ was presented alone on the half hour. In both cases, following training, the response to CS$^+$ was significantly less than to the CS$^-$, although statistical comparison of groups was necessary to demonstrate the small mean difference (Fig. 9).

2.9. The Case for Associative Learning in *Pleurobranchaea*

As illustrated by the data summarized above, the major conventional controls for learning have been performed numerous times for the food avoidance learning paradigm in *Pleurobranchaea*, on literally thousands of animals over a 10-year

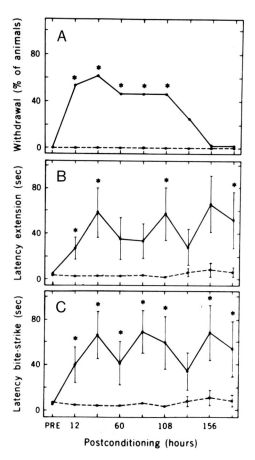

FIGURE 6. Retention and extinction of food avoidance learning in *Pleurobranchaea* following simultaneous random control procedures (random presentation of food and aversive electric shock). (A) Active avoidance learning (conditioned withdrawal from food stimuli, expressed by the percentage of animals that withdrew from the CS before (pre) and at various times after associative conditioning. Learning is indicated by the significant difference between experimental (solid curve) and control (random food and shock; dashed curve) percentages (asterisks; $p \leq 0.01$; chi-square tests). (B and C) Passive avoidance learning (conditioned suppression of feeding), expressed by proboscis extension latencies (B) and bite-strike latencies (C). Learning is indicated by significant differences between experimental (solid curves) and control (dashed curve) means ($p \leq 0.01$, Mann-Whitney U tests). Same animals as in Fig. 5. Vertical bars are standard errors. (From Mpitsos *et al.*, 1978.)

period. The same learning paradigm has been exhaustively tested and applied independently by a dozen investigators in at least three different laboratories (that of G. Mpitsos, R. Gillette, and our laboratory). The paradigm is extremely robust; in our experience more than 80% of experimental specimens show some evidence of learned behavioral modification, and more than two thirds of trained animals meet the stringent quantitative criteria for learning of a summed proboscis and bite-strike threshold elevation of four orders of magnitude following conditioning (Kovac *et al.*, 1985). Acquisition and retention parameters have been repeatedly published; controls for nutritional history and other nonassociative variables have been extensively performed and published; interactions between measurements have been excluded as a cause of behavioral modification in conditioned animals by a variety of control procedures; single trial learning has been demonstrated; selectivity in the food avoidance learning has been shown; and differential conditioning of the feeding behavior under the avoidance paradigm has been accomplished. On these grounds we believe that the case for an advanced form of associative learning in *Pleurobranchaea* has been adequately established, and attention is now properly turned toward the underlying neurophysiological mechanisms.

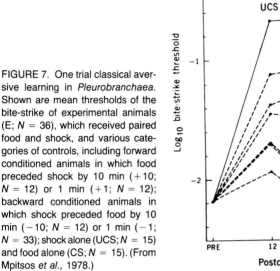

FIGURE 7. One trial classical aversive learning in *Pleurobranchaea*. Shown are mean thresholds of the bite-strike of experimental animals (E; $N = 36$), which received paired food and shock, and various categories of controls, including forward conditioned animals in which food preceded shock by 10 min ($+10$; $N = 12$) or 1 min ($+1$; $N = 12$); backward conditioned animals in which shock preceded food by 10 min (-10; $N = 12$) or 1 min (-1; $N = 33$); shock alone (UCS; $N = 15$) and food alone (CS; $N = 15$). (From Mpitsos *et al.*, 1978.)

3. CENTRAL NEURAL PATHWAYS MEDIATING LEARNED BEHAVIOR IN *PLEUROBRANCHAEA*

A decade ago we hypothesized that the neural modifications underlying the above associative learning in *Pleurobranchaea* would at least partially entail physiological changes within the neural circuitry mediating the learned behavior, i.e., within the withdrawal and feeding circuitry (Davis *et al.*, 1974c). To test this hypothesis, it was necessary to unravel the neural circuitry controlling these behaviors in order to permit experiments on learning at the level of the identified neuron. The task was far from simple; feeding in particular is a relatively complex behavior, involving distance and contact stimulus detection, selective stimulus recognition, appetitive consummatory behavioral components, rhythmic, goal-directed movements, and plastic modifications according to complicated motivational variables. Several years of research have now furnished a fairly comprehensive view of the participating neural circuitry, however, beginning with the sensory systems responsible for detecting food stimuli and terminating with the motoneurons and muscles that mediate the behavior.

3.1. Sensory Mediation of Feeding Behavior in Pleurobranchaea

On the anterior end of *Pleurobranchaea* are located the major sensory organs involved in food detection (Davis and Matera, 1982; Matera and Davis, 1982), namely the large oral veil with fused lateral tentacles, and the rhinophores (Fig.

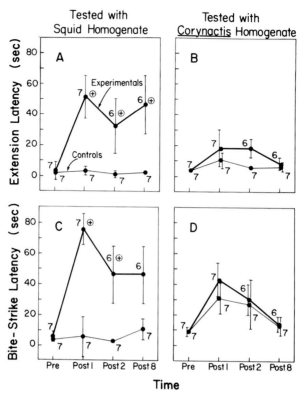

FIGURE 8. Selectivity in food avoidance learning of *Pleurobranchaea*, as manifest in the latencies of the proboscis extension (A and B) and the latencies of the bite-strike (C and D) following application of the indicated food stimulus, before (pre) and on various days after (post) conditioning. Squid homogenate served as the CS for food avoidance conditioning. Animals were then tested with squid homogenate (A and C) or extract of the sea anemone *Corynactis* (B and D). Dark curves are experimental animals, while light curves are explicitly unpaired controls. Numbers indicate sample sizes (numbers of specimens), while circled plusses indicate significant differences from control means at $p \leq 0.05$ or less (Wilcoxon test). Bars signify two standard errors. (From Davis *et al.*, 1980.)

10A). The oral veil is a broad, flat structure that bears numerous sensory papillae, while both the tentacles and rhinophores are tubular structures open to the outside, with sensory receptors lining the internal lumen. Scanning electron microscopy of these regions (Matera and Davis, 1982) has revealed a characteristic cell type comprising the sensory epithelium (Fig. 10B), consisting of a soma 10 μm in diameter bearing numerous cilia that project into the external medium (Fig. 10C). Each cilium is expanded at its distal tip into a flattened, discoid structure (Fig. 10C) and hence these receptors have been termed "discociliated." Transmission electron microscopy of the cilia (Fig. 10D) has shown that the discoid tips are composed of conventional bilamellar membrane that surrounds the looped tip of the cilium and therefore that the discs are genuine and presumably functional morphological

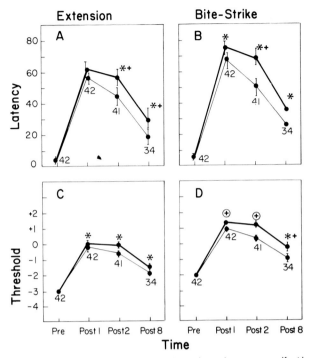

FIGURE 9. Differential food avoidance learning in *Pleurobranchaea,* as manifest in the latencies and thresholds of the indicated feeding responses following application of the CS, before (pre) and on various days after (post) conditioning. The dark curve shows means from CS$^+$ specimens, while the lighter curves show means of CS$^-$ specimens (*N* indicated by the number adjacent to means). Asterisks indicate significant differences in the means at $p \leq 0.05$ (Wilcoxon test). (From Davis *et al.,* 1980.)

entities. Electron microscopy has also revealed that the soma of each receptor sends a single axon centrifugally.

The anterior regions of *Pleurobranchaea* are the only areas of the exterior body surface that exhibit chemosensory capacity (Davis and Matera, 1982), and the disociliated receptors are the predominant, and in some areas exclusive, cell type located in these chemosensory regions (Matera and Davis, 1982). Therefore, the disociliated receptors are presumed to be the chemoreceptors known from electrophysiological studies to detect food stimuli (Bicker *et al.,* 1982a; Bicker *et al.,* 1982b). These same areas of the body, however, are sensitive to mechanical stimuli. Therefore, it is possible that the disociliated receptors are multimodal, transducing both chemical and mechanical stimuli.

3.2. Peripheral Processing of Food Stimuli

Centrifugal (i.e., toward the central nervous system) back-injection of the axons of the disociliated receptors with cobaltous chloride indicates that their axons

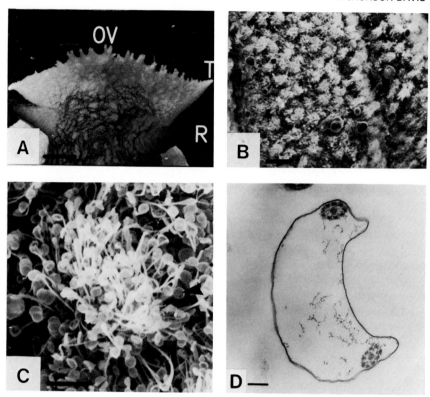

FIGURE 10. Sensory apparatus used in food detection. (A) Macrophotographs of the oral veil showing the sensory papillae. OV, oral veil; T, tentacle; R, rhinophore. Bar, 1 cm. (B) Scanning electron micrograph of the sensory epithelium of the rhinophore showing an overview of the discociliated receptors that characterize anterior sensory structures. Bar, 20 μm. (C) Scanning electron micrograph showing a closer view of the discocilia in a single receptor cell. Bar, 5 μm. (D) Transmission electron micrograph through the discoid tip of a discocilia. Bar, 0.2 μm. (From Matera and Davis, 1982.)

project without interruption to the peripheral ganglia located at the base of the tentacles and rhinophores, the tentacle and rhinophore ganglia (Bicker *et al.,* 1982b). These peripheral ganglia are elaborate neural structures, containing well-defined commissural tracts and highly articulated neuropilar regions. Each ganglion also contains the somata of a population of approximately 100 neurons that project directly to the central cerebropleural ganglion or brain, as revealed by centripetal cobaltous chloride back-injection of the nerve connecting the peripheral ganglion with the brain. The neurons stained by this procedure do not send peripheral processes beyond the tentacle and rhinophore ganglia, and therefore they have the structural properties of interneurons.

Intracellular recording from the somata of these interneurons has shown that they fall into three general categories: chemosensory, mechanosensory, and bimodal. Some show relatively simple responses, while others display a complex but consistent pattern of excitation to one stimulus mode, and inhibition to another (Bicker *et al.*, 1982b). The integrative capacities of the peripheral ganglia are evidently well developed. These studies have shown that the sensory interneurons located in the tentacle and rhinophore ganglia represent the first integrative station for the processing of incoming information about food stimuli. Peripheral ganglia in invertebrates were once believed to serve mainly as autonomous reflex centers for mediating simple movements (Bullock and Horridge, 1965). The peripheral ganglia of *Pleurobranchaea* may indeed serve such a role, but our studies show that they also serve as major peripheral integrative centers for complex stimuli associated with food detection.

3.3. Central Neural Machinery of the Feeding Motor System

Following the integration of food stimuli in the peripheral ganglia, the processed information is relayed to central ganglia that mediate the feeding behavior. These ganglia include the cerebropleural ganglion or brain, which is attached by connectives to the peripheral ganglia; the buccal ganglion, attached by the cerebrobuccal connectives to the brain; and the lateral pedal ganglia, attached to each other and the brain by the cerebropedal connectives (Fig. 11).

The neural circuitry that controls feeding behavior in this "simple" system is in reality astonishing in its complexity. Circuitry involved in the control of feeding is distributed in all of the above ganglia, but the buccal ganglion and brain have been investigated most intensively (Davis *et al.*, 1984; Davis *et al.*, 1974c; Davis *et al.*, 1973; Gillette and Davis, 1977; Gillette *et al.*, 1980, 1982a, 1982b; Gillette *et al.*, 1982c; Kovac *et al.*, 1983a,b; Kovac *et al.*, 1982; Siegler, 1977; Siegler *et al.*, 1974). The most important neurons, from the viewpoint of learning, are "command" interneurons in the brain that initiate feeding behavior. These neurons were first discovered by cobaltous chloride back-injection of the cerebrobuccal connectives (Davis *et al.*, 1974c). This procedure fills the somata of three classes of brain neurons: the paired metacerebral giant neurons; the opisthocerebral neurons; and the paracerebral neurons (Fig. 12). Little is known about the opisthocerebral neurons, and the metacerebral neurons, although well studied (Gillette and Davis, 1977), have but a weak effect on the feeding motor output.

In contrast, the paracerebral neurons (PCNs) play a major role in feeding behavior, and as will be detailed below, they are in addition critical components of the central neural pathway that is modified by associative conditioning of feeding behavior. Accordingly, these neurons have been analyzed extensively (Croll *et al.*, 1985b; Davis *et al.*, 1984; Gillette *et al.*, 1978, 1982c; Kovac *et al.*, 1983a,b; Kovac *et al.*, 1982). In behaving, whole animal preparations, intracellular stimulation of a single PCN induces feeding movements, i.e., rhythmic protraction and retraction of the feeding proboscis accompanied by ingestion of food (Gillette *et al.*, 1978, 1982c). Therefore, single PCNs are *sufficient* to cause feeding motor output. During such feeding behavior the PCNs are active cyclically in phase with the rhythmic feeding movements. Therefore, PCNs are also *appropriate* to the occurrence of feeding motor output. When one or two PCNs are silenced by hyperpolarization, however, feeding movements can still take place, although they

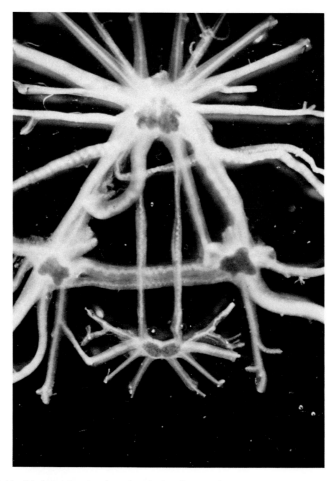

FIGURE 11. Photograph showing the isolated central nervous system of *Pleurobran-chaea*, including the cerebrobuccal ganglion or brain (top of picture), buccal ganglion (bottom), cerebrobuccal connectives (connecting the brain and buccal ganglion), lateral pedal ganglia and connectives, and various severed nerves.

appear weaker (Gillette *et al.*, 1982c). Therefore, single PCNs are not *necessary* to feeding movements, presumably because the role of initiating feeding is distributed redundantly over a large number of individual neurons. As a consequence of this redundancy, no individual member of the command population is indispensable to the behavior.

Studies on the technically more amenable isolated central nervous system (CNS) preparation have corroborated the command capacity of the PCNs. Intracellular stimulation of single PCNs causes rhythmic brain and buccal motor output (Croll *et al.*, 1985b; Davis *et al.*, 1984; Gillette *et al.*, 1978, 1982c), which is identifiable by several criteria as the ingestion or feeding motor program (Croll and

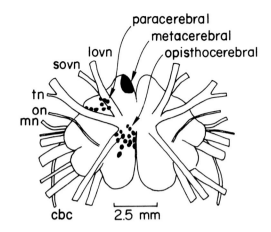

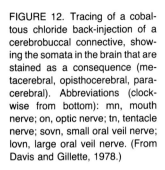

FIGURE 12. Tracing of a cobaltous chloride back-injection of a cerebrobuccal connective, showing the somata in the brain that are stained as a consequence (metacerebral, opisthocerebral, paracerebral). Abbreviations (clockwise from bottom): mn, mouth nerve; on, optic nerve; tn, tentacle nerve; sovn, small oral veil nerve; lovn, large oral veil nerve. (From Davis and Gillette, 1978.)

Davis, 1981, 1982; Croll *et al.*, 1985a,b). Experiments on the isolated CNS preparation have also revealed considerable specialization of function within the PCN population. The eight neurons on each side of the brain that were previously classified homogeneously as PCNs are now known to include both "tonic" PCNs (two neurons per hemiganglion) and phasic PCNs, or PC_ps (six neurons per hemiganglion), differentiated on both structural and functional grounds (Kovac *et al.*, 1982). The six PC_ps are in turn divided into two "standard" PC_ps, identified by their unique position and synaptic relation with the remaining PC_ps; two polysynaptic excitors (PSEs) of the standard PC_ps; and two type II electrotonically coupled (with the standard PC_ps) neurons (ET_{II}s). All of these subclasses of PCNs exhibit the capacity to cause feeding motor output when intracellularly stimulated, although their command efficacy increases in the order ET_{II}, standard PC_p, PSE (Davis *et al.*, 1984; Kovac *et al.*, 1983a).

In addition to excitatory influences on the standard PC_ps, a number of inhibitory influences have been identified, including monosynaptic inhibitors (MSIs) and several identified classes of polysynaptic inhibitors (PSIs). For each of these identified excitatory and inhibitory neurons, the morphology of the individual neurons has been established by repeated injection of Lucifer Yellow; the synaptic relationships with the standard PCNs has been determined by intracellular stimulation and recording and ion substitution experiments; and the normal discharge pattern of the neuron during the feeding motor program has been described (Kovac *et al.*, 1983a,b). Typical neuroanatomical and neurophysiological procedures used to identify and characterize each member of the command system are illustrated for a single neuron, an ET_{II}, in Fig. 13.

Among the most interesting and, from the viewpoint of learning, important inhibitory components of the command circuitry is the so-called "cyclic inhibitory network" (CIN), which impinges on all subclasses of PCNs. This network, known only from its inhibitory postsynaptic potentials (IPSPs) recorded intracellularly from feeding command interneurons, supplies cyclic bursts of inhibition to all PCNs at the frequency of the feeding rhythm (Gillette *et al.*, 1978, 1982c). By this mech-

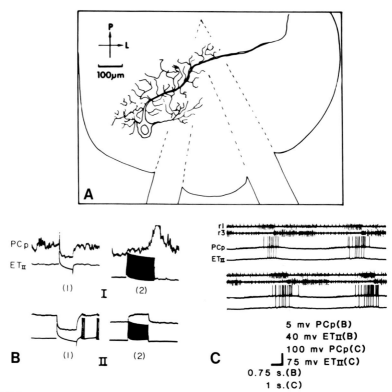

FIGURE 13. Tests performed, in this case on a type two electrotonic neuron or ET$_{II}$, to identify and characterize each interneuron in the feeding command system of *Pleurobranchaea*. (A) Lucifer Yellow injection of the neuron, seen in dorsal aspect in the left anterior lobe of the brain, with the midline on the left side of the picture and the tracts of the oral veil nerve and tentacle nerve shown. P, posterior; L, lateral. (B) Physiological effects of an ET$_{II}$ on a phasic paracerebral command interneuron (PC$_p$). I, hyperpolarization (1) and depolarization (2) of the ET$_{II}$ in normal sea water. Note short latency electrical and long latency chemical polysynaptic effect on PC$_p$. II, same experiment in zero Ca^{++} sea water. Note loss of chemical polysynaptic effect of PC$_p$. (C) Discharge pattern of ET$_{II}$ and a PC$_p$ during fictive feeding in the isolated CNS preparation. r1 and r3, extracellular recordings from buccal roots 1 and 3. (From Kovac *et al.*, 1983a.)

anism the CIN is presumed to be at least partially responsible for the bursting output of the paracerebral command neurons and, therefore, for setting the repetition period of the feeding rhythm. In addition, and as will be detailed below, the CIN is intimately involved in neurophysiological modifications that attend learning in this motor system.

This entire assembly of neurons is wired together to form the command system for feeding behavior in *Pleurobranchaea* (Fig. 14). The details of this command system are complex (Fig. 14A), but the underlying conceptual organization is more straightforward (Fig. 14B). The central organizational principles that operate in this system are: sensory inputs diverge both to the command elements and their excitatory and inhibitory synaptic inputs (although this interfacing remains to be explored in

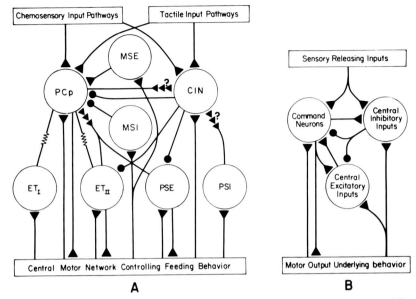

FIGURE 14. Wiring diagrams of the neural circuitry of the feeding command system of *Pleurobranchaea,* as established by experiments such as those illustrated in Fig. 13. (A) Details; (B) Organizational principles. (From Kovac et al., 1983b.)

detail); the standard PC_ps receive cyclic inhibition from the CIN; this same inhibition is routed to excitatory inputs to the standard PC_ps, including the $ET_{II}s$, and the PSEs; the command elements recurrently excite this inhibitory network; and all of the command elements are reciprocally connected with the motor network that mediates the feeding behavior (Fig. 14B).

Many additional details of the central feeding motor network have been elucidated, especially in the buccal ganglion, where numerous identified interneurons and motoneurons that participate in the control of feeding musculature are located. For purposes of learning, however, the critical central pathways appear to involve the command circuitry in the brain, as summarized above and in Fig. 14. The learned behaviors that follow associative conditioning are accompanied and presumably caused by neurophysiological modifications within this command network, as described next.

4. CELLULAR MECHANISMS OF ASSOCIATIVE LEARNING IN THE FEEDING COMMAND PATHWAY

4.1. The Whole Animal Preparation

Having elucidated the central pathways that mediate feeding behavior, we hypothesized that the neurophysiological processes underlying learning would be manifest, at least in part, in these pathways. Accordingly, we made intracellular recordings from the identified feeding command interneurons of avoidance conditioned preparations. In all of our work, parallel experiments are performed on control animals, including naive (untrained) specimens, explicitly unpaired CS/US controls, and food-satiated animals (a control for general motivational changes). The experimenter is generally unaware of the identity of the animal during the experiment in order to avoid experimental bias, and the resultant data are also analyzed blind, to avoid interpretative bias.

Figure 15 shows intracellular recordings from the feeding command interneurons of these four groups of animals, i.e., naive, experimental, control, and food satiated. These recordings were made from behaving, whole animal preparations to guarantee their relevance to associative learning (a *behavioral* concept). In naive specimens, food stimuli excite (depolarize) the command interneurons, leading to cyclic bursting that is phase-locked to rhythmic feeding movements (Fig. 15A), as described above. In contrast, the feeding command interneurons of avoidance-conditioned animals show an absence of excitation to food stimulation and are instead powerfully inhibited (hyperpolarized) by the conditioned food stimulus (Fig. 15B). The inhibition takes the form of a prolonged train of IPSPs that typically outlast the duration of the food stimulus. The responses of control animals (unpaired

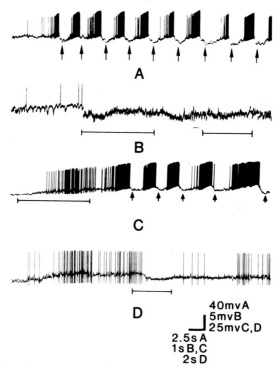

FIGURE 15. Intracellular responses of paracerebral command interneurons of whole animal preparations to food stimulation of the anterior chemosensory structures. (A) Naive (untrained, hungry) animal; (B) associatively conditioned animal; (C) control animal; (D) food-satiated animal. (From Davis and Gillette, 1978 and Gillette *et al.,* 1982c.)

food and shock) are the same as those of naive animals (Fig. 15C); i.e., food stimuli excite the feeding command interneurons. Therefore, the reduced excitation and increased inhibition seen in conditioned animals does not result either from food or from shock but rather from the temporal contiguity between these stimuli.

The responses of food-satiated animals, however, are indistinguishable from conditioned animals (Fig. 15D). That is, the feeding command interneurons show an absence of the usual excitatory response to food stimuli and are instead inhibited. This important result indicates that the decline in excitation and increase in inhibition seen in the feeding command interneurons of whole animal preparations cannot necessarily be ascribed to associative processes but instead represents a neurophysiological manifestation of *behavioral motivation,* regardless of its cause. These results furnish the first neurophysiological explanation of behavioral motivation; they illustrate that control experiments for motivational variables, which have generally not been performed in model systems research on learning, are advisable; and finally these results illustrate that physiological distinctions between associative and nonassociative processes cannot be made at the level of the command neurons. These neurons represent a central "final command pathway" for all experiential variables that affect feeding behavior. Instead, the physiological distinctions between associative and nonassociative processes must be sought at the level of neurons that are presynaptic to the command interneurons. These considerations led us to develop the technically more amenable isolated brain preparation to study learning, as described next.

4.2. The Isolated Brain Preparation

If the physical manifestation of learning is stable enough to remain within the animal and modify its behavior for several weeks, as indicated by retention studies, then we hypothesized that it would also be stable enough to survive the surgical isolation of the brain, so that it could be analyzed intracellularly at the level of identified neurons. Accordingly, brains were removed from animals that had been previously trained in the aforementioned food avoidance task, and intracellular recordings were made from various identified neurons in the command system. The anterior chemosensory structures, including the oral veil, tentacles, and rhinophores, were left attached to the brain by the appropriate nerves (Fig. 16) so that the normal afferent pathways involved in food detection could be stimulated as naturally as possible. Blind experiments were again performed on four classes of preparation, naive, conditioned, control, and food-satiated, and all data were again analyzed blind.

Figure 17 illustrates typical results from experiments on the isolated brain preparation. Application of food stimuli to the anterior chemosensory structures excites the feeding command interneurons of naive specimens (Fig. 17A), as seen in the whole animal preparations. In brains removed from animals trained 1–3 days earlier in the food avoidance task, however, the command neuron response to the conditioned food stimulus shows the same absence of excitation and presence of strong inhibition as seen in trained whole animal preparations (Fig. 17B). Therefore, the physiological manifestation of avoidance learning (the memory trace or "en-

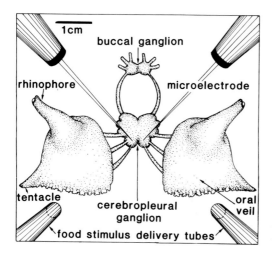

FIGURE 16. Drawing of the isolated central nervous system (CNS) preparation used to study the cellular mechanisms of associative learning in *Pleurobranchaea*, as seen from above and anterior. (From Kovac *et al.*, 1985.)

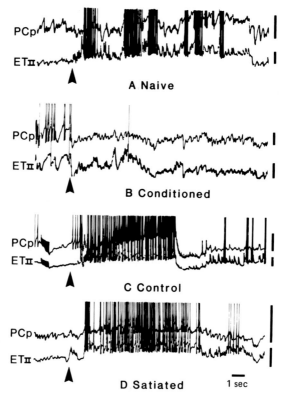

FIGURE 17. Intracellular responses of command interneurons to food stimuli in the isolated CNS preparation. (A) Brain taken from a naive (untrained, hungry) animal; (B) associatively conditioned animal; (C) control animal; (D) food-satiated animal. cf. Fig. 15. (From Kovac *et al.*, 1985.)

gram"), demonstrated previously in the behaving, whole animal preparation, persists even when the brain is removed for cellular analysis. The organism's "memories" of experiences obtained during its lifetime, represented by concrete, physical changes in central neural pathways, are so firmly embedded in the circuitry of the brain that they persist even following such a traumatic procedure as surgical isolation of the brain. This finding in turn opens the way to a detailed analysis of the engram at the cellular level in the technically amenable isolated brain preparation.

In brains removed from control specimens, food stimuli are excitatory to the feeding command interneurons (Fig. 17C), also as seen in whole animal preparations. In contrast to results in the whole animal, however, the feeding command interneurons in brains removed from food-satiated specimens are excited, rather than inhibited, by food stimuli (Fig. 17D). This result is not entirely unexpected, since isolation of the brain opens feedback pathways from gut stretch receptors that presumably normally provide the brain with signals that the gut is full. The result is nonetheless important, because it implies that the absence of excitation and presence of inhibition of feeding command interneurons in trained animals may be ascribed to a specific associative process, rather than to a more general motivational process. In other words, use of the isolated brain preparation enables the critical distinction between associative and nonassociative processes. Using the isolated brains of trained specimens, we can be confident that we are studying the specific cellular mechanisms of learning, rather than the more general neurophysiological mechanisms of motivation.

The isolated brain preparation has permitted the first analyses of the neural mechanisms of associative learning at the level of single, identified neurons within the central nervous system. Although this analysis has just begun, it has already furnished insights into the two critical cellular aspects of avoidance learning in *Pleurobranchaea:* the increase in synaptic inhibition of the feeding command interneurons seen in trained animals and the decrease in command neuron excitation.

4.2.1. Learning-Induced Increase in Command Neuron Inhibition

With respect to the increase in inhibition, two questions may be posed: Where does the inhibition originate? To what central loci is it distributed? Our answer to the first question is incomplete, but circumstantial evidence suggests that the source is, at least in part, the previously mentioned cyclic inhibitory network or CIN. This network produced IPSPs having their own, unique "signature," as expressed in their amplitude distributions and waveform. The IPSPs induced by food stimuli after associative training have the same signature, suggesting that they also originate from the CIN (Davis *et al.,* 1983). Moreover, and as detailed below, the distribution of CIN inhibition is identical to the distribution of learning-induced inhibition. On these grounds we propose that the CIN furnishes the command neuron inhibition seen following learning. Direct proof of this hypothesis will require locating the somata of the CIN neurons, which has not yet been accomplished.

Our answer to the second question, namely, where does the increased synaptic inhibition consequent to training go, is more complete. We have found that the same synaptic inhibition that affects the standard PC_ps is also routed to the other

PC_ps including the PSEs and the ET_{II}s (e.g., Fig. 17B; Kovac *et al.*, 1985). In other words, the command neuron inhibition that occurs following avoidance training exactly parallels in its distribution the inhibition furnished normally to the command neurons by the CIN.

4.2.2. Learning-Induced Decrease in Command Neuron Excitation

With respect to the decrease in command neuron excitation following training, the isolated brain preparation has also enabled progress to be made. Specifically, intracellular stimulation of a PSE in a naive (untrained) animal causes the characteristic polysynaptic excitatory response in a standard PC_p at a mean presynaptic spike threshold frequency of about 18 Hz ($N = 9$; Fig. 18A). Following training, however, the mean presynaptic spike threshold for a similar polysynaptic response in the PC_p is significantly elevated, to about 29 Hz ($N = 24$; Fig. 18B). In other words, associative training decreases the efficacy of the PSE on the standard PC_p, presumably accounting in part for the decline in food-induced excitation in the PC_ps seen following training. The mean PSE spike threshold frequencies for brains taken from control and satiated animals were respectively about 17 Hz ($N = 16$; Fig. 18C) and about 20 Hz ($N = 6$; Fig. 18D), neither of which is significantly different from the mean of naive animals (Kovac *et al.*, 1985).

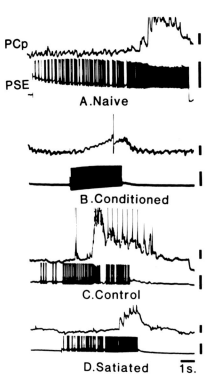

FIGURE 18. Effect of a polysynaptic excitor (PSE) on a standard PCN in isolated brain preparation taken from animals with different behavioral histories. (A) Brain taken from a naive (untrained, hungry) animal; (B) associatively conditioned animal; (C) control animal; and (D) food-satiated animal. (From Kovac *et al.*, 1985.)

This result indicates that somewhere in the central pathway between the PSE and the PC_ps, learning-induced physiological changes take place that reduce the functional efficacy of the pathway. In one respect this finding is puzzling, for it would not seem capable of explaining selectivity to specific conditioned food stimuli in the learned behavioral modification. Perhaps the decline in command neuron excitation is not in fact selective, but the increase in inhibition is. Further experiments are needed to resolve this question.

In another respect, however, the result is encouraging; namely, the pathway from the PSE to the PC_ps has now been fully elucidated. This pathway is known to include corollary discharge neurons in the buccal ganglion (Davis *et al.*, 1984), and the specific neurons involved have been identified and their synaptic connections with PSEs and PCNs fully established (M. P. Kovac, E. M. Matera, B. W. Volk, and W. J. Davis, in preparation). Therefore, the complete neural pathway in which this learning-induced modification occurs has been unraveled, promising a detailed cellular and subcellular understanding of the decline in command neuron excitation that is caused by associative conditioning.

5. CONCLUSIONS

The studies completed to date on the neural mechanisms of avoidance learning in *Pleurobranchaea* therefore indicate that the learned behavioral modification (suppression of feeding behavior) is caused by increased inhibition and reduced excitation of the command neurons that initiate feeding. The increase in inhibition appears to result from the enhancement of the activity of a pre-existing network of neurons, the cyclic inhibitory network, which normally serves as a "pacemaker" or "Zeitgeber" of the feeding rhythm. The inhibition is distributed not only to the standard phasic paracerebral command interneurons (PC_ps) but also to their identified excitatory inputs, including the other phasic paracerebral command interneurons (PSEs and $ET_{II}s$). The decrease in excitation results in part from increased inhibition of excitatory inputs and also from decreased efficacy of an identified excitatory pathway that begins with the PSE, ends with the standard PC_p, and includes identified buccal neurons in between.

Our studies to date permit formulation of a realistic and testable cellular model of associative learning in *Pleurobranchaea* (Davis *et al.*, 1983; Fig. 19). According to this model, the behavioral modifications that represent passive avoidance learning are caused by a training-induced change in the way that a pre-existing central neural network (the feeding command system) processes incoming information. Prior to conditioning, the sensory information that is associated with food detection is routed through predominantly excitatory pathways to the feeding command interneurons (Fig. 19A). The result is that these neurons are excited, and feeding behavior is accordingly initiated. As a consequence of associative training, identified elements of this central neural network are altered, such that incoming information is now routed to the command interneurons through predominantly inhibitory pathways (Fig. 19B). Specifically, excitatory pathways are reduced in potency (i.e., the PSE to PC_p pathway), and inhibitory pathways are facilitated (i.e., the CIN to PC_p

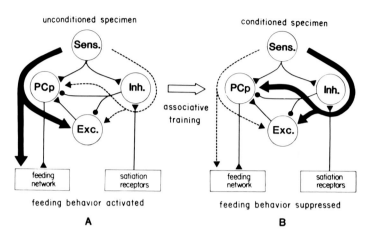

FIGURE 19. Cellular neurophysiological model of food avoidance learning in *Pleurobranchaea*. (A) and (B) schematically illustrate the activity of the feeding command circuitry before and after associative training. Before associative training (A), sensory information (sens) is routed to the feeding command interneurons (PC$_p$) through predominantly excitatory pathways (Exc), as indicated by the heavy arrows, causing feeding behavior. After associative training such information is routed through predominantly inhibitory pathways (Inh; heavy arrows), causing learned suppression of feeding. (From Davis *et al.*, 1983.)

pathway). As a consequence the feeding command neurons of trained animals are less excited and more inhibited than in naive animals, and feeding behavior is accordingly suppressed. This combination of mechanisms and wide distribution of cellular loci ensures powerful suppression of the feeding behavior in response to food stimuli in animals that have learned.

The cellular changes that have been shown to date to underlie food avoidance learning in *Pleurobranchaea* are summarized in the "engram map" of Fig. 20. This diagram shows the known wiring diagram of the feeding command system, including all of the identified synaptic junctions at which physiological changes underlying learning could in principal occur, with the locations that have been demonstrated to change as a function of associative learning superimposed. This map represents the first empirical representation of how a memory is stored within the central nervous system at the level of individual, identified neurons.

The engram mapped in Fig. 20 is certainly incomplete in its present form. At present, for example, we have not determined whether the neural changes that accompany learning result from synaptic modifications or from changes in the endogenous properties of single neurons and their membranes, or both. Of course, it is possible, indeed likely, that the cellular changes underlying food avoidance learning in *Pleurobranchaea* are more extensive than has been documented to date. For example, London and Gillette (1984) have recently reported physiological changes in identified inhibitory interneurons (PSIs) following associative training. It is possible that such neurons operate on the PC$_p$s through the CIN (Fig. 20). For the immediate future, our goal is to complete this engram map by determining as many as possible of the identified cellular loci at which the engram is stored and

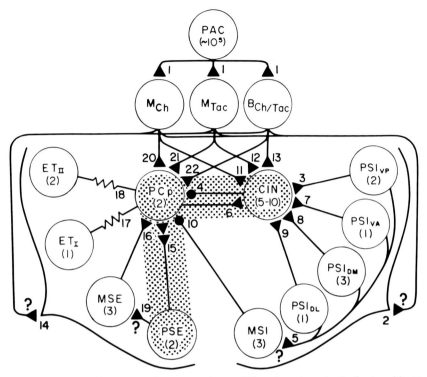

FIGURE 20. Map of the "engram," or memory trace, of *Pleurobranchaea* for the food-avoidance learning task. Question marks designate possible but undemonstrated connections. Shown is the central neural circuitry known to mediate feeding behavior. Superimposed shading designates that portion of the circuitry that is presently known to be functionally modified as a consequence of associative training. (From Kovac *et al.*, 1985.)

to test whether these physiological changes occur in the membranes of the participating neurons, at synapses between the neurons, or both. The long-term goal of our research is to determine how these neurophysiological changes are caused by the temporal contiguity of the CS and US, and how they are represented in terms of subcellular mechanisms, both biophysical and biochemical.

6. POSSIBLE GENERAL PRINCIPLES OF LEARNING DERIVED FROM THE MODEL SYSTEMS APPROACH

As indicated at the outset of this chapter, a central assumption of the model systems approach is that it can illuminate *general* biological principles. In the case of learning, several such principles appear already to be emerging from the numerous laboratories working on the problem, extending from the behavioral laws of learning to the underlying neurophysiological mechanisms. For example, several gastropod mollusks have now been shown capable of complex learning tasks seen also in vertebrates: classical conditioning, differential conditioning, and taste aversion learning; higher-order conditioning; effects of motivation on acquisition, and others (see Davis, 1984c, for a more detailed review). These many behavioral parallels encourage the view that the underlying cellular mechanisms will also have general relevance.

General principles are in fact already evident also at the level of cellular mechanisms. Work on several molluscan model systems, for example, suggests the principle that learning (or its analogs) entails functional modification of the neural circuitry that mediates the unconditioned/conditioned response. The details in support of this principle vary depending upon the preparation. Thus, in *Pleurobranchaea,* food avoidance learning entails functional modification of command and pattern-generating circuitry, while in *Aplysia* and *Hermissenda,* changes in sensory neurons have been implicated.

Similarly, work on several model systems suggests that learning (or its analogs) does not require the formation of new synaptic connections but rather can be explained in terms of functional modification of existing neurons and/or neuronal circuits. Our study of food avoidance learning in *Pleurobranchaea,* for example, supports the hypothesis that modifications in a pre-existing inhibitory network (the CIN) suppress feeding in conditioned animals. Similarly, Alkon and his colleagues (this volume) give evidence that endogenous changes in pre-existing sensory neurons are responsible for conditioned modifications of *Hermissenda*'s behavior. In *Aplysia,* a learning analog appears to involve broadening of action potentials in pre-existing neurons, rather than the *de novo* formation of new synapses. None of the studies on model systems disproves the possibility of *de novo* synapse formation as a cellular mechanism of learning, but neither do any available results require such a mechanism for their explanation.

Our study of food avoidance learning in *Pleurobranchaea* also suggests that learned modifications in behavior result from neurophysiological changes near the *input* side of the neural circuits that control the behavior, in this case at the command neuron level. The same principle is seen in more extreme form in *Hermissenda,* where the changes entail modification of sensory neurons. Similarly, in *Aplysia,* an analog of learning is explained in cellular terms by broadening of action potentials in sensory neurons. In view of the multifunctionality of motor systems (e.g., Ayers and Davis, 1977; Croll and Davis, 1981, 1982), such an arrangement makes good sense from a theoretical standpoint; it would ensure that the learning is selective to the particular behavior with which the conditioned stimulus is associated, rather than a different behavior that is nonetheless mediated by the same motoneurons. It must be admitted, however, that experimental approaches have concentrated attention on the input end of neural circuits, and hence the alternative of changes at the motor level have not been examined as thoroughly.

Finally, studies on gastropods have conclusively supported the general principle that the engram manifests in single, identifiable neurons. Prior to studies on model systems, it was possible to imagine that learning is a mass property of neural tissue, necessarily involving functionally affiliated events in hundreds or even millions of individual neurons. In this case the neural changes that cause learning might well be too small to detect at the level of single neurons. Studies on *Pleurobranchaea* and other model systems have permanently dispelled this gloomy scenario and shown that the engram may indeed be found and analyzed in the single, identified neuron (Fig. 20). The challenge now for model systems researchers is to dissect the engram into its component biophysical and biochemical components—a task that we may expect to see realized in the next decade of model systems work.

ACKNOWLEDGMENTS. The original research on which this article is based was supported by NIH Research Grant NS-09050 and NSF Grant BNS-8110235. This article was written during the tenure of a Senior Scientist Award from the Alexander von Humboldt Foundation, Federal Republic of Germany. I thank my German hosts, Dr. Hubert Markl (University of Konstanz) and Dr. Franz Huber (Max-Planck Institute, Seewiesen) for warm hospitality and excellent facilities during this time.

REFERENCES

Ayers, J. L. and Davis, W. J., 1977, Neuronal control of locomotion in the lobster *Homarus americanus*. I. Motor programs for forward and backward walking, *J. Comp. Physiol. A* **115**:29–46.

Bicker, G., Davis, W. J., Matera, E. M., Kovac, M. P., and Stormo-Gipson, J., 1982a, Mechano- and chemoreception in *Pleurobranchaea californica*. I. Extracellular analysis of afferent responses, *J. Comp. Physiol.* **149**:221–234.

Bicker, G., Davis, W. J., and Matera, E. M., 1982b, Mechano- and chemoreception in *Pleurobranchaea californica*. II. Neuroanatomical and intracellular analysis of centripetal pathways, *J. Comp. Physiol.* **149**:235–250.

Bullock, T., and Horridge, G. A., 1965, *Invertebrate Nervous Systems*, Freeman, San Francisco.

Carew, T. J., Hawkins, R. D., and Kandel, E. R., 1983, Differential classical conditioning of a defensive withdrawal reflex in *Aplysia californica, Science* **219**:397–400.

Castellucci, V. F., Carew, T. J., and Kandel, E. R., 1978, Cellular analysis of long-term habituation of the gill-withdrawal reflex of *Aplysia californica, Science* **202**:1306–1308.

Croll, R. P. and Davis, W. J., 1981, Motor program switching in *Pleurobranchaea*. I. Behavioural and electromyographic study of ingestion and egestion in intact specimens, *J. Comp. Physiol.* **145**:277–287.

Croll, R. P. and Davis, W. J., 1982, Motor program switching in *Pleurobranchaea*. II. Ingestion and egestion in the reduced preparation, *J. Comp. Physiol.* **147**:143–154.

Croll, R. P., Kovac, M. P., and Davis, W. J., 1985a, Neural mechanisms of motor program switching in the mollusc *Pleurobranchaea*. I. Central motor programs underlying ingestion, egestion and the "neutral" rhythm(s), *J. Neurosci.* **5(1)**:48–55.

Croll, R. P., Kovac, M. P., Davis, W. J., and Matera, E. M., 1985b, Neural mechanisms of motor program switching in the mollusc *Pleurobranchaea*. III. Role of the paracerebral neurons and other identified brain neurons, *J. Neurosci.* **5(1)**:64–71.

Davis, W. J., 1979, Behavioral hierarchies, *Trends Neurosci.* **2**:5–7.

Davis, W. J., 1984a, Neural consequences of experience in *Pleurobranchaea californica, J. Physiol. (Paris)* **78**:793–798.

Davis, W. J., 1984b, Neural mechanisms of behavioral plasticity in an invertebrate model system, in: *Model Neural Networks and Behavior* (A. I. Selverston, ed.), Plenum Press, New York (in press).

Davis, W. J., 1984c, Correlational aspects of memory: invertebrate model systems, in: *Learning and Memory: A Biological View* (J. L. Martinez and R. P. Kesner, eds.), Academic Press, New York (in press).

Davis, W. J., 1984d, Motivation and Learning: Neurophysiological Mechanisms in a model system, *Learn. Motiv.* **15**:377–393.

Davis, W. J. and Gillette, R., 1978, Neural correlate of behavioral plasticity in command neurons of *Pleurobranchaea*, *Science* **199**:801–804.

Davis, W. J. and Matera, E. M., 1982, Chemoreception in gastropod mollusks: Electron microscopy of putative receptor cells, *J. Neurobiol.* **13**:79–84.

Davis, W. J., Siegler, M. V. S., and Mpitsos, G. J., 1973, Distributed neuronal oscillators and efference copy in the feeding system of *Pleurobranchaea*, *J. Neurophysiol.* **36**:258–274.

Davis, W. J., Mpitsos, G. J., and Pinneo, J. M, 1974a, The behavioral hierarchy of the mollusk *Pleurobranchaea*. I. The dominant position of the feeding behavior, *J. Comp. Physiol.* **90**:207–224.

Davis, W. J., Mpitsos, G. J., and Pinneo, J. M., 1974b, The behavioral hierarchy of the mollusk *Pleurobranchaea*. II. Hormonal suppression of feeding associated with egg-laying, *J. Comp. Physiol.* **90**:225–243.

Davis, W. J., Mpitsos, G. J., Siegler, M. V. S., Pinneo, J. M., and Davis, K. B., 1974c, Neuronal substrates of behavioral hierarchies and associative learning in the mollusk *Pleurobranchaea*, *Am. Zool.* **14**:1037–1050.

Davis, W. J., Villet, J., Lee, D., Rigler, M., Gillette, R., and Prince, E., 1980, Selective and differential avoidance learning in the feeding and withdrawal behaviors of *Pleurobranchaea*, *J. Comp. Physiol.* A **138**:157–165.

Davis, W. J., Gillette, R., Kovac, M. P., Croll, R. P., and Matera, E. M., 1983, Organization of synaptic inputs to paracerebral feeding command interneurons of *Pleurobranchaea californica*. III. Modifications induced by experience, *J. Neurophysiol.* **49**:1557–1572.

Davis, W. J., Kovac, M. P., Croll, R. P., and Matera, E. M., 1984, Brain oscillator(s) underlying rhythmic cerebral and buccal motor output in the mollusc, *Pleurobranchaea californica*, *J. Exp. Biol.* **110**:1–15.

Gelperin, A., 1975, Rapid food-aversion learning by a terrestrial mollusk, *Science* **189**:567–570.

Gillette, M. U., London, J. A., and Gillette, R., 1984, Motivation to feed affects acquisition of food-avoidance conditioning in *Pleurobranchaea*, *Soc. Neurosci. Abstr.* **9**(Part 2): 914.

Gillette, R. and Davis, W. J., 1977, The role of the metacerebral giant neuron in the feeding behavior of *Pleurobranchaea*, *J. Comp. Physiol A* **116**:129–159.

Gillette, R., Kovac, M. P., and Davis, W. J., 1978, Command neurons in *Pleurobranchaea* receive synaptic feedback from the motor network they excite, *Science* **199**:798–801.

Gillette, R., Gillette, M. U., and Davis, W. J., 1980, Action potential broadening and endogenously sustained bursting are substrates of command ability in a feeding neuron of *Pleurobranchaea*, *J. Neurophysiol.* **43**:669–685.

Gillette, R., Gillette, M. U., and Davis, W. J., 1982a, Substrates of command ability in a buccal neuron of *Pleurobranchaea*. II. Potential role of cyclic AMP, *J. Comp. Physiol.* **146**:461–470.

Gillette, R., Gillette, M. U., and Davis, W. J., 1982b, Substrates of command ability in a buccal neuron of *Pleurobranchaea*. I. Mechanisms of action potential broadening, *J. Comp. Physiol.* **146**:449–459.

Gillette, R., Kovac, M. P., and Davis, W. J., 1982c, Control of feeding motor output by paracerebral neurons in the brain of *Pleurobranchaea californica*, *J. Neurophysiol.* **47**:885–908.

Hawkins, R. D., Abrams, T. W., Carew, T. J., and Kandel, E. R., 1983, A cellular mechanism of classical conditioning in *Aplysia:* Activity-dependent amplification of presynaptic facilitation, *Science* **219**:400–405.

Kovac, M. P. and Davis, W. J, 1977, Behavioral choice: Neurophysiological mechanism in *Pleurobranchaea*, *Science* **198**:632–634.

Kovac, M. P. and Davis, W. J., 1980, Neural mechanism underlying behavioral choice in *Pleurobranchaea*, *J. Neurophysiol.* **43**:469–487.

Kovac, M. P., Davis, W. J., Matera, E. M., and Gillette, R., 1982, Functional and structural correlates of cell size in paracerebral neurons of *Pleurobranchaea californica*, *J. Neurophysiol.* **47**:909–927.

Kovac, M. P., Davis, W. J., Matera, E. M., and Croll, R. P., 1983a, Organization of synaptic inputs of paracerebral feeding command interneurons of *Pleurobranchaea californica*. I. Excitatory inputs, *J. Neurophysiol.* **49**:1517–1538.

Kovac, M. P., Davis, W. J., Matera, E. M., and Croll, R. P., 1983b, Organization of synaptic inputs of paracerebral feeding command interneurons of *Pleurobranchaea californica*. II. Inhibitory inputs. *J. Neurophysiol.* **49**:1539–1556.

Kovac, M. P., Davis, W. J., Matera, E. M., Morielli, A., and Croll, R. P., 1985, Learning: Neural analysis in the isolated brain of a previously trained mollusc, *Pleurobranchaea californica, Brain Res.* **331**:275–284.

London, J. A. and Gillette, R., 1984, Changes in specific interneurons presynaptic to command neurons underlie associative learning in *Pleurobranchaea, Soc. Neurosci. Abstr.* **9**(Part 2):914.

Matera, E. M. and Davis, W. J., 1982, Paddle cilia (discocilia) in chemosensitive structures of the gastropod mollusc *Pleurobranchaea californica, Cell Tissue Res. 222:*25–40.

Mpitsos, G. J. and Collins, S. D., 1975, Learning: Rapid aversive conditioning in the gastropod mollusc *Pleurobranchaea, Science* **188**:954–957.

Mpitsos, G. J. and Davis, W. J., 1973, Learning: Classical and avoidance conditioning in the mollusk *Pleurobranchaea, Science* **180**:317–320.

Mpitsos, G. J., Collins, S. D., and McClellan, A. D., 1978, Learning: A model system for physiological studies, *Science* **199**:497–506.

Ottoway, J. R., 1977, *Pleurobranchaea novaezelandiae* preying on *Actinia tenebrosa, N.Z.J. Mar. Freshwater Res.* **11**:125–130.

Sahley, C. L., Gelperin, A., and Rudy, J., 1981a, One-trial associative learning modifies food odor preferences of a terrestrial mollusc, *Proc. Natl. Acad. Sci. USA* **78**:640–642.

Sahley, C. L., Rudy, J. W., and Gelperin, A., 1981b, An analysis of associative learning in a terrestrial mollusc: Higher-order conditioning, blocking and a transient US pre-exposure effect, *J. Comp. Physiol.* **144**:1–8.

Siegler, M. V. S., 1977, Motor neurone coordination and sensory modulation in the feeding system of the mollusc *Pleurobranchaea, J. Exp. Biol.* **71**:27–48.

Siegler, M. V. S., Mpitsos, G. J., and Davis, W. J., 1974, Motor organization and generation of rhythmic feeding output in the buccal ganglion of *Pleurobranchaea, J. Neurophysiol.* **37**:1173–1196.

5

Recent Progress in Some Invertebrate Learning Systems

GRAHAM HOYLE†

1. INTRODUCTION

The October 1983 *Discover* was dedicated to: MEMORY. Beneath these large letters on the cover page was the tantalizing statement "How it works." My first thought was that such a statement implied that we could "all go home because the party's over!" Inside the covers Dr. Eric Kandel was quoted: "we found that everyday molecular machinery is used for *mental* activity, but in novel ways. It helps de-mystify learning." Anything that can "de-mystify" learning must surely be approved by us all. But the extent to which any of us have regarded memory, or any other physiological process not yet intensely investigated as a mystery, is a highly in-dividual matter. Some will ask: "was there a mystery?" Others may be skeptical that the adaptive physiological phenomenon Dr. Kandel studies has anything to do with learning per se.

As nearly as I can determine, memory as a mystery is associated with the traditions of a professional group, composed of psychologists and philosophers, some of whom want "memory" to remain mysterious. Possibly though, this is no more than yet another example of semantic confusion. It is not the physiological bases of memory which, even potentially, are mysterious, but their association with the operations of the human mind, or minds (if the subconscious is to be separated from the conscious). All our mental activities are so heavily concerned with re-membered events and notations that the two seem inseparable. Our first task is to recognize that we must, as scientists, separate mind from memory. Mind may be nothing without memory, but memory, defined as an information store capable of being utilized to control specific reproducible behavior, has no need of mind. Possibly memory is the most valuable of all nervous system functions, but it is present in the lowliest of animal cells.

†GRAHAM HOYLE (deceased) ● Institute of Neuroscience, University of Oregon, Eugene, Oregon 97403.

The term *memory* is invariably used incorrectly. It derives from the Latin *memoria,* which was used to refer to remembered experiences *as they come into a conscious human mind.* It is entirely inappropriate to refer to the store of information in the nervous system of a female digger wasp, which it uses to ensure appropriate sequential feeding of its buried larvae, as memory, in the same context in which the term is used for humans, but it is too late to stop even involved scientists from doing so. The same is true of the bee dancing to express the directional message from its recent foraging experiences. Even worse, we use *to remember* as the common verb for "recall" of an information store, and for an event which prompts memory, we use an expression that forcefully indicates the price we must pay for our love of history in everyday language, namely a re*mind*er.

Only a totally new word to designate the cellular information stores that a nervous system acquires during experience and that can be called upon to guide a behavior (which includes a mental experience if the animal's brain is capable of one) could get us out of this dilemma. However, while we address this philosophically critical issue, it should be pointed out that neither of the two kinds of conditioning about which Dr. Eric Kandel's and Dr. Daniel Alkon's research groups have cellular knowledge, need be physiologically equivalent to the establishment of a majority of the addressable stores of information used by humans, or even insects, for which we use the term memory. This is true especially if the loose traditional meanings put upon the word memory by humans in their own everyday lives is under consideration. The simplest etymologically and scientifically correct designation for the altered cellular events responsible for any form of learning is to refer to them as *conditioned changes.* The multiguous term memory should be avoided at least until the term has been given a universally accepted and scientifically precise definition. Furthermore, the term learning also needs to be defined equally carefully. Unfortunately, achieving these desirable objectives seems to be beyond human capability! The issue is further complicated by the vastly different views of life mechanisms held by globally oriented zoophysiologists, like myself, and psychiatrico-physiologists. The only commonly used term in this field about which there is no ambiguity is "conditioning." Incidentally, conditioning is *not* to be equated with learning!

The best that can be said about any of the four experimental situations that have so far yielded information concerning the cellular events underlying a *conditioned* change is that they offer possible *candidate mechanisms* for learning and "memory". In chronological order these were as follows:

1. Woody and Black-Cleworth (1973): resistance change in cat cortical neurons.
2. Woollacott and Hoyle (1976): bidirectional resistance changes and associated change in soma/integrating region membrane potential, probably brought about by altered potassium conductance, in an identified locust retrainable tonic motor neuron.
3. Alkon (1979): increased input resistance following paired stimuli, in an identified *Hermissenda* sensory neuron.
4. Kandel and Schwartz (1982): resistance increase caused by potassium con-

ductance decrease, leading to prolonged action potential and transmitter release, in identified *Aplysia* sensory neurons following stimulus pairing.

The sites of 1, 2, and 3 are postsynaptic locales, whereas in 4 the site is presynaptic. What is perhaps the most remarkable feature of these four diverse preparations is that the cellular change which was found to underly the learned behavior was in each case a change in membrane potassium conductance.

There had long been a passionate desire on the part of many learning physiologists that a single common cellular event would turn out to be at the root of all *learned* changes. Great hopes were expressed for there being "memory molecule." Yet, in spite of the fact that there is a common feature in the four cases cited, I have yet to hear any widespread ringing of bells on behalf of the gK discoveries. Somehow, this was not the sort of process the early learning physiologists ever had in mind. There are some legitimate difficulties in the way of accepting the possibility that it is all done by controlling K^+ channels. To begin with, there are currently considered to be seven different types of potassium ion channels and at least four different potassium currents, and nobody believes that the list is complete. It should be comforting to think that a K^+ channel is responsible, if only because one of them must have been the first of all ion channels to evolve, initiating the bioelectric potential, which, by permitting a modulatable ionic current flow, launched animals on their path to behavioral complexity. Bear in mind though, that local ionic currents are as much a part of the lives of humble Protozoa as they are of higher mammals.

But it would be absurd to imagine that we now have *the* answer. During evolution nature will have used every trick at its disposal. Every ion channel is a candidate in principle, as is every modulator that can change one, for a learning mechanism in some cell or other. Add to all of these channels, of which some 20 are currently known, the emergent properties of neuronal circuits, the growth of new branches and synapses, alteration of the shapes of existing neuronal branches and spines, alterations in synaptic performance, altered genome readout, and other factors; and we have a formidable list of candidates for conditioning, learning, and memory events. It would neither surprise nor dismay me if it is eventually found that all the possibilities have been used somewhere or other. There will surely be many unsuspected surprises in store. The only surprise I currently feel is that anybody could have been so naive as to have ever thought otherwise!

2. A SURPRISE LOCATION AND MECHANISM OF LEARNED CHANGE IN A PRIMITIVE INSECT

Immediately following the First (Asilomar) Conference on Conditioning I went to New Zealand on sabbatical leave. New Zealand is now considered to have been the first part of Gondwanaland to split off, some 10^8 years ago. At this time the most advanced vertebrates were a few primitive lizards. There were some insects for them to feed on, including a family called the Stenopelmatidae. These insects found themselves the predominant species in a verdant land, where they have remained the dominant insect family to this day. Being interested in insect neurobiology, I was eager to determine the extent to which the neuroanatomy and physiology of these primitive insects resembles that of the present-day insects I am familiar with. In particular also, I wanted to know if they can "learn" by simple operant-conditioning of posture, as can some modern insect species (see Hoyle, 1982b).

I took with me microprocessor-controlled automatic training equipment and put it to work using simple aversive conditioning (Fig. 1 and Hoyle and Field, 1983a). The nocturnal insects, termed "wetas" (night devils) by the Maori natives, turned out to be remarkably good at detecting an experimentally set "window" position for the tibia of one joint, when this was coupled to a reinforcement. They learned, after a few self-generated experiences of the association between placing the free joint in the position window and the reinforcement, to have the joint occupy a site within the window (Table I). Most of the insects tested achieved a suitable learned position in less than 2 min.

Modern insects are also good at this; they do it by setting the rate of firing of a suitable tonic motor neuron to an appropriate fixed value, while at the same time suppressing antagonist activity (Hoyle, 1982a,b; Forman, 1984). A published example, for a locust, is shown in Fig. 2. But electromyograms obtained from trained wetas showed absolutely no electrical activity at all in the muscle generating force, following adoption of a position in the window, regardless of the window's location (Fig. 3). There was a lot of EMG activity during the exploratory movements and then one final burst in the agonist that terminated just before the final position was

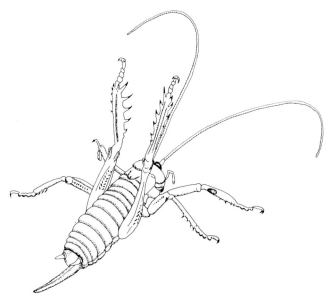

FIGURE 1. Drawing, from photograph, of a common New Zealand weta, *Hemideina femorata*, in raised-leg defense posture. The (presumed) threat was above and to the front of the head. (From Hoyle and Field, 1983a.)

TABLE I. Times to Adoption of a Position Window, Set Electronically at a Variety of Positions in Either Flexion or Extension, and With Various Window Sizes, Taken by the New Zealand Weta *Heemideina*[a,b].

Subject no.	Sex	Window size (approximate) (°)	Proximal window margin angle (°)	Learning criterion met?	Time from first experience to learning	Time from onset of learning to first error	Time from first error to relearning	Remarks
1	F	20	120	Yes	1 min 43 sec	2 hr 46 min	—	No relearning
2	M	20	120	Yes	1 min 19 sec	10 min	1 min 40 sec	
3	F	15	120	Yes	1 min 49 sec	44 min	1 min 36 sec	
4	F	15	120	Yes	54 sec	1 hr 40 min	No relearning	
5	M	15	140	No	—	—	—	No learning
6	F	10	140	Yes	47 sec	2 hr 0 min	1 min 32 sec	
7	M	10	160	No	—	—	—	No learning
8	M	10	40	Yes	1 min 34 sec	21 min	—	No relearning
9	M	10	40	No	—	—	—	No learning
10	F	5	Fully flexed	Yes	1 min 14 sec	1 hr 50 min	46 sec	
11	F	5	Fully flexed	Yes	1 min 2 sec	18 min	1 min 15 sec	
12	M	5	Fully flexed	No	—	—	—	No learning
13	F	10	40	No	—	—	—	No learning
14	F	10	30	Yes	42 sec	14 min	1 min 23 sec	
15	M	10	160	yes	1 min 59 sec	26 min	1 min 40 sec	
16	F	10	160	Yes	1 min 18 sec	48 min	1 min 4 sec	
				Mean	1 min 18 ± 26 sec	1 hr 2 ± 53 min	1 min 22 ± 19 sec	

[a] A loud 30-Hz sound was used as a negative reinforcement, coupled to the femoro-tibial joint angle (tibial position). The sound was off only when the preset window position was occupied by the tibia.

[b] From Hoyle and Field (1983a).

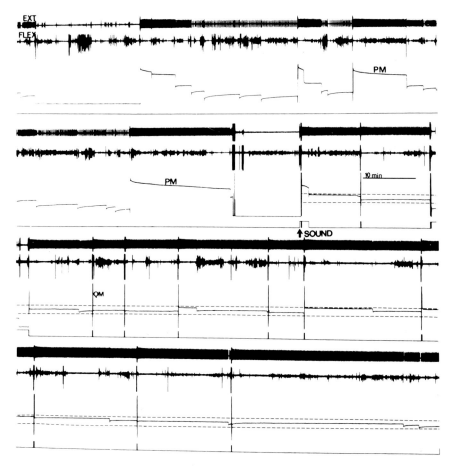

FIGURE 2. Continuous recording of a typical learning response of a grasshopper to the same paradigm used to train tibial position in weta (see Fig. 3). The preparation was lively and made many erratic movements before training started with the turning on of the aversive sound (arrow). Movements are registered on the third trace, extensor myogram (EXT) at top, flexor myogram (FLEX) second trace, sound on/off on bottom (fourth) trace. In addition to erratic flex/extend sequences, the preparation made regular plateau extension movements (PM). Within 2 min of the first experience of the relation between tibial position and sound the tibia was held steadily within the operational window, with progressively increasing intervals between errors. The position was attained by a combined steady discharge in the slow extensor motor neuron (SETi) with reduced flexion activity. Errors were entirely due to fast flexor activity causing a quick movement (QM). (From Hoyle, 1980.)

adopted. It was easy to determine the forces required to be developed to maintain each position, and these were of the order of a few grams.

Isolated nerve–muscle preparations did not show any persistent tonus, but some semi-intact preparations did (Hoyle and Field, 1983b). These preparations did not all start out by showing the ability to maintain tension following only a

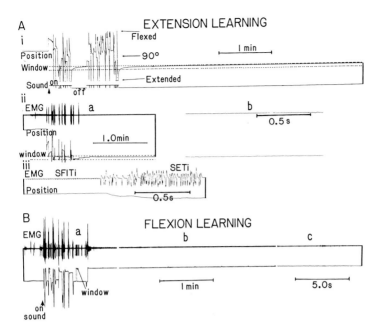

FIGURE 3. Postural shifts and electromyograms (EMGs) obtained during experiments (see Table I) in which the tibial position of a weta was conditioned by coupling femoro-tibial angle to an aversive loud sound. Learning to occupy a position in extension (A) and in flexion (B). A higher-speed excerpt made 10 min after occupation of the window is shown in each of the records in which electromyograms are displayed. In (A,i) the electronically set angular position window is indicated by a broken line, and moments of sound on and off by the marker below. In (A,ii) a different preparation is shown, accompanied by EMG from the whole femur. This includes both slow and intermediate flexor tibiae, and slow extensor tibiae (SETi) activity. A higher-speed excerpt is shown in (A,iii). In (B), a very narrow window was set in strong flexion. The window position was electronically tested automatically every 60 sec, as indicated by the small blips. (From Hoyle and Field, 1983a.)

burst of neural excitation, but gradually or even abruptly, they came to do so. This type of tension is commonly called "catch" (sperrung) or catchlike tension (CT). It was evident that a basic nerve–muscle system does not produce CT but that under a capricious influence emanating from the nervous system it may do so (Fig. 4).

Intracellular recordings of slow extensor tibiae (SETi) neuromuscular transmission in the CT state, compared with the normal, showed that a marked potentiation of excitatory junctional potentials and tension had occurred. It is known that potentiation is caused by the natural neuromodulator substance octopamine (O'Shea and Evans, 1979). This substance is synthesized by identified dorsal unpaired median (DUM) neurons (Hoyle and Barker, 1975; Evans, 1980), which make neurosecretory terminals in skeletal muscle cells in locusts (Hoyle et al., 1974, 1980). A close examination of weta ganglia quickly showed that they have DUM neurons that might be the homologues of those of locusts (Hoyle, 1978). The DUM neuron innervating the extensor tibiae (ETi), which is termed DUMETi in the weta, as

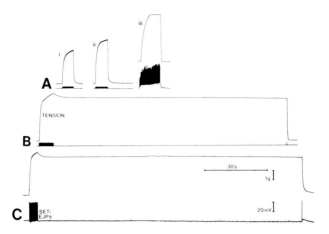

FIGURE 4. Results that afforded clues as to the mechanism of maintenance of a learned postural shift in wetas. (A, i–iii) Isometric tension development in semi-intact preparation of extensor of the tibia in response to the slow excitatory axon SETi. Intracellular recording of EJPs in (iii); stimulus artifacts only in (i), (ii). Progressive potentiation of the response occurred, associated with central events not under experimental control. (B) Response to SETi obtained later showed catchlike maintained tension remainder (CT). This was abruptly terminated by a single late excitation of the common inhibitory axon. (C) Still later response, with intracellular recording of EJPs. Note that these were potentiated to the point at which no facilitation occurred. In this example, CT was abruptly terminated following the tiny extra contraction caused by a single late EJP. Note that this EJP appears larger than preceding ones, due to posttetanic potentiation and elicitation of a small spike. It is believed that this muscle cell did not participate in producing CT. For participating muscle cells see Figs. 7 and 8. (From Hoyle and Field, 1983b.)

also in locusts/grasshoppers (Fig. 5), could be directly excited in preparations demanding position-setting of the tibia to a precise position in the extension range.

It was found that after a prior excitation of the weta DUMETi, a brief burst in its SETi led to a contraction that started out normally, but which was followed by some CT (Fig. 6). The strength of CT was proportional to the number and frequency of impulses in the SETi burst and also to the frequency and duration of the preceding DUMETi burst. Therefore, it was probable that it is octopamine released from DUMETi that determines the presence, or otherwise, of the CT.

Accordingly, octopamine (OCT) dissolved in insect saline in various concentrations was infused into the extensor muscle of isolated preparations not showing CT. Even high concentrations did not have any detectable direct effect on the muscle, but there was an immediate, marked potentiation of SETi EJPs (up to 10-fold) and contraction (up to 100-fold). Although absent at first, sooner or later, depending on the concentration of OCT, the relaxation rate slowed markedly, leaving a strong CT remainder. As little as 10^{-10} M OCT produced some CT, 10^{-8} M quite a lot, and 10^{-6} M a maximal amount.

Therefore, it was concluded that the weta produces a learned postural response by an unique peripheral mechanism that is not known elsewhere. A follow-up study

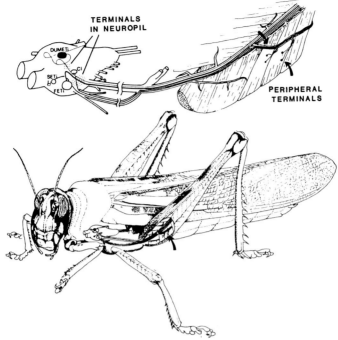

FIGURE 5. Diagram of the locations of the octopaminergic neuron DUMETi in the locust, and of its central and peripheral terminals. The homologous neuron of the weta has a similar morphology. (From Hoyle *et al.*, 1980.)

of events at neuromuscular junctions showed that at some of them a depolarization plateau, proportional in size to frequency and duration of the SETi burst, is developed following neural release, or infusion, of octopamine (Hoyle, 1984; Fig. 7).

The CT condition is abruptly relaxed by any of three neural events: a single common inhibitor impulse, a single fast extensor tibiae (FETi) excitor impulse, or a single late SETi impulse. The latter is the event that initiates CT in the presence of OCT in the first place, so this may seem surprising. However, at many of the synapses initially showing small excitatory junctional potentials (EJPs) even in the presence of OCT, there is a marked posttetanic potentiation (PTP). Thus, a late single EJP is markedly enhanced. An enhanced EJP elicits a graded action potential. Therefore, each of the events that can terminate CT abruptly has something in common with the others, i.e., activation of potassium conductance! The appearance of catch is associated with the development of the plateau of depolarization, which is probably due to a progressive loss of gK during the burst of SETi EJPs. Remarkably, the "learned" event in the weta, although it is peripheral in muscle cells, is probably (once again) altered gK. In the presence of OCT, the burst of EJPs evoked by SETi in some of the muscle fibers, which leads to initial depolarization

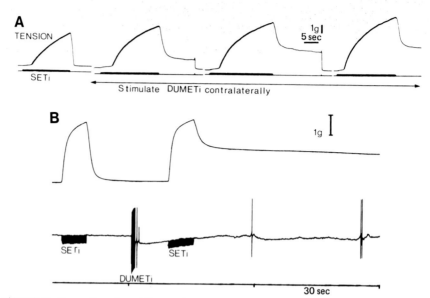

FIGURE 6. Generation of catchlike tension by tibial extensor muscle in weta, following SETi burst after stimulation of DUMETi. (A) DUMETi stimulated continually via its contralateral axon. (B) DUMETi soma stimulated intracellularly. (From Hoyle, 1984.)

of the cells, is followed by a persistent depolarization plateau (Fig. 8). Apparently the normal membrane potential restoration process following excitation, which is an activation of outward K^+ current, fails to occur, and the potential locks in to its new value.

There are several interesting questions arising out of these observations. One is whether there is any relation between the peripheral events in the weta and the central ones that occur during conditioning in the locust. There are central terminals of the octopaminergic neuron DUMETi in the vicinity of the tonic motor neurons that can be trained in the locust. Training alters the mean membrane potential of these neurons by altering gK in the soma and integrating regions. It is probable that OCT is required for the change to take place, although it is not automatic as is that occurring at the periphery in the weta. In the locust the correlation between the membrane potential, leg position, and reinforcement appear to be made within the motor neuron itself. In the weta the same correlation must be made, and it may be made in the motor neuron there also. But in the locust the final outcome is a central nervous, not a peripheral, membrane potential shift. Furthermore, the central shift in locust position training can last much longer. A trained weta has to refresh or reset its peripheral locking mechanism about every 20 min to maintain the posture constant. There may be some central "savings," i.e., retention of learned aspects of the correlations used in earlier successful adoption of the window position,

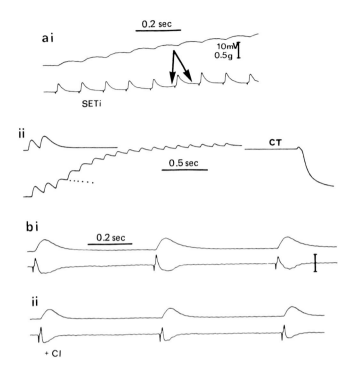

FIGURE 7. Catch evoked routinely in extensor tibae muscle by SETi burst in semi-isolated preparation following infusion of octopamine dissolved in saline into the muscle. Isometric tension above, intracellular record from sensitive muscle fiber below. 10^{-6} M OCT was infused 10 min before the tests, and then SETi was excited by a burst at progressively increasing frequency. A catchlike tension remainder followed each burst, and remained until terminated following a single, late EJP, which elicited a small spike. (From Hoyle, 1984.)

because far fewer error movements are made before the joint returns to the window after it has drifted out later. But the locking mechanism of CT is usually unlatched at each error and must be reset. While it may appear that the locust only needs to maintain the central nervous status quo, this too could require an equivalent resetting. Nevertheless, in the locust there does not appear to be an obligatory resetting requirement, for hours or even days can elapse between errors. It is fair to consider that the locust mechanism represents an evolutionary upgrade. But it involves the same neurons and may well use an identical cellular mechanism. Once again, this common mechanism is probably gK of a postsynaptic membrane. The major difference is that the peripheral mechanism lacks any capability for self-initiated perpetuation, which, incidentally, puts it in a similar category to the automatically-fading learned changes of both the *Aplysia* and the *Hermissenda* sensory cell learning.

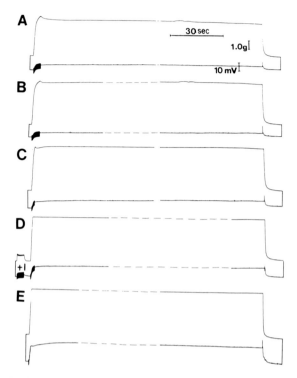

FIGURE 8. Basis of build-up of persistent depolarization in sensitive muscle fibers in response to a SETi burst in the presence of octopamine (OCT). There are two different types of EJPs, conventional, shown in (A,i), and biphasic, shown in (B). In the (A) type, late slow depolarizations occur in the presence of OCT (upper trace in Ai is tension). These are reflected in the tension as a marked slowing of relaxation (B,ii; broken line), leading to the build-up of catch like tension (CT). A single late EJP leads to a small twitch but also abolishes CT. In the (B) type there is a large undershoot which becomes reduced during repetition (B,i). Stimulation of the common inhibitor axon (CI) at the same time as SETi (B,ii) further enhances the undershoot, reduces the tension response, and prevents the build-up of CT. (From Hoyle, 1984.)

While the biochemical events that lead to the change in gK are already well characterized, at least in the *Aplysia* sensory neurons (Kandel and Schwartz, 1982), the question still remains paramount as to *why* a change occurs. In the *Aplysia* preparation, which is subjected to classical associative conditioning, the switch appears to be obligatory and sensitive only to the number of repetitions and the concentration of amine modulator, which in this case is 5-hydroxytryptamine. This change is necessarily unidirectional, returning to the baseline gradually with time following training, or more rapidly with noncontingent reinforcement.

In the insect preparations there is also an association between the reinforcement and motor output, but the latter is not directly driven, as it is when a UCS is used. In operant conditioning the animal makes its own moves voluntarily, and in the locust experiments there are both a qualitative directional component, flexion vs. extension, and two sensitive quantitative ones, the determinant of the mean positional requirement (center of the operational window) and the permitted error (determined by the size of the window, i.e., angular limits of the window in extension and flexion). The latter quantitative variant can be experimentally altered after the basic position has been learned, as a narrowing of the window (Hoyle, 1980). The preparation responds by reducing the variance in mean frequency of the motor neuron determining postion and/or with stronger inhibition of the antagonist. It responds to a shift in window position in extension by altered SETi frequency and to a shift in flexion, or from extension to flexion and vice versa, by altered frequency of one or more tonic flexor motor neurons.

The subtlety of the learned changes in the locust preparation are such as to suggest that a tonic motor neuron can assess the exact amount of altered gK required to occur within itself to achieve the desired mean frequency. This assessment is not done simply by a feedback onto a continually altering frequency, but rather as a stepwise decision after assessing the situation. The neuron appears to store within itself the results of experience. In the model I proposed earlier (Hoyle, 1982b), two principal specific short-term memory stores were invoked: *efference memory,* of recent motor outputs, and *afference memory,* of recent inputs, some of which are consequences of the recent motor output. In addition there is a general input indicative of goal-relatedness, which may be simply a sign of the "goodness" or "badness" of recent inputs for the animal's welfare. The preparation was shown some time ago to be able to function without specific afferent inputs (Hoyle, 1966). The least preparation that can learn is one quarter of an isolated ganglion. Such a quarter nevertheless contains the entire tonic motor neuron being trained.

I now consider it likely that each tonic motor neuron is "smart" and does its own associating of the inputs with the consequences of its own actions. It is probable that its efference memory is within itself and quite possible that a copy of the afference memory is kept within it also. It is virtually impossible to find a sensory stimulus of any modality that does not cause some synaptic input to occur onto one of the large tonic motor neurons. Their intensely multibranched dendritic trees fill more than an entire quarter of the ganglion. There are several thousand synaptic inputs onto them. There are few secrets within the nervous system, each tonic motor neuron being a party to all the incoming information.

The notion that individual neurons can be smart and have goals of their own is quite new (see Klopf, 1982). But why not? It may be that the adaptive capabilities of animals have arisen out of individual goals of their component neurons rather than the neural networks, as commonly presumed. Some Protozoa inherit "species memories" of instructions on how to build elaborate houses, of species-specific shape, from miniscule particles of silica. These single cells are aware if their house is damaged or has been removed and immediately set about seeking material with which to build a new one. This they "painstakingly" construct over many hours, using pseudopodia to test the suitability of each (there may be several hundred altogether) particle's shape. The pieces are cemented together, using two or three pseudopodia at a time, until a unit as neat as an Inca stone wall is completed.

Neurons are less mobile than these Protozoa after their initial growth period, but why should we assume that from the point of view of information storing and handling they are any less capable?

We must presume that although the tonic motor neuron appears to have a "mind of its own" in the locust, the biochemical events are basically just as stereotyped as they are in the *Aplysia* and *Hermissenda* sensory neurons. The differences are twofold. First, there must be antecedent intracellular events in the locust which cause the random movements which lead to the discovery of the relationship between the motor output and the reinforcement. All our attempts to drive the system to learn automatically by coupling the reinforcement of systematic frequency shifts caused by either synaptic input or directly applied membrane current failed. These failures suggest that the initiating shift is generated as part of a planned intrinsic self-testing mechanism in which the tonic motor neuron itself is involved.

This raises another important fundamental issue. Most neuroscientists still naively regard nervous systems as input → output information processors. Processing of input is only a secondary role of a nervous system, the primary function being to generate useful behavior spontaneously! Many, perhaps most, neurons are intrinsically active when not inhibited, especially in the presence of modulator(s). There may be several different intrinsic timing mechanisms in a single neuron, ranging from circannual through circadian to tonic rhythmic discharges, as well as a number that are aperiodic and governed by the immediate history of activity. In honest operant conditioning we are always dealing with the reinforcement of the latter, aperiodic randomly generated motor outputs. Neuroscientists have paid no attention to these extremely important events, so it is hardly surprising that they are almost always left out of consideration. However, it is clear that they must be responsible for the formidable facts of operant conditioning, the most important of all learning processes.

I suggest that it is an event within the spontaneous motor program generator networks that starts the ball rolling, by generating changes in output that result in the experience of the association between output and goal-related reinforcement. The second process, not present in simple associative-conditioning paradigms, is then set in motion. As long as the learned shift has produced a goal-related objective, there is no point in letting it slide back to normal. Unknown events are set in motion which stabilize the new condition. At least we can pinpoint their locale: once again, these are in the "smart" tonic motor neurons themselves (Woollacott and Hoyle, 1977; Hoyle, 1982a,b).

A simple diagram (Fig. 9) will suffice to illustrate the differences between the very elementary process of associative conditioning and the much more sophisticated one of operant conditioning. The two additional CNS mechanisms required for the latter are indicated. These are a neural mechanism for generating trial movements and a programmable memory. In higher mammals there is voluminous evidence for the involvement of "intelligence" in the unknown process of generating trial movements, or at least some of them. In higher invertebrates, the animal, or even a preparation, sooner or later makes any movement allowed it. It seems that no matter what this is, if it is associated with reinforcement, it will sooner or later become conditioned.

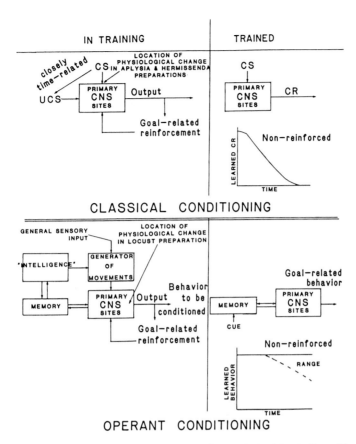

FIGURE 9. A comparison of the fundamental events in associative (classical) conditioning with those involved in the evolutionarily more advanced operant conditioning. There are at least two additional processes in operant conditioning. A true memory (store of experience of the relation between reinforcement and motor output) must operate in operant conditioning. In classical conditioning the cellular changes that occur themselves embody the learned changes. No memory process need be involved.

The important point that emerges from comparing the two forms of training is that there is a requirement for a memory process in operant conditioning, but not for classical conditioning. It is neither reasonable nor logical to use the term memory for the automatic physiological changes occurring in the CNS as a result of conditioning of either kind. Rather, these are adaptive mechanisms. However, the information store which holds the results of trial and error *experience* of the link between behavior and reinforcement in operant conditioning is equatable with memory no matter how this term is defined. This is the process we should try hard to unravel. The ion conductance shifts that are the consequences of its operation are trivial by comparison.

Concerning the models discussed herein and in previous chapters, we may wish to ask, "of what are they models?" Unfortunately, the term model has an extraordinary range of meanings. The most apt definition appears to be the following: a small copy of an existing object used as a toy. As scientists, we desire to pull our toys to pieces to find out how they work. Fortunately, we can all enjoy a feeling of common intensity, since each of these systems either already permits, or seems likely to permit, analysis of underlying events at the level of cellular mechanisms in identified neurons.

REFERENCES

Alkon, D. L., 1979, Voltage-dependent calcium and potassium ion conductances: A contingency mechanism for an associative learning model, *Science* **205**:810–816.

Alkon, D. L., 1980, Cellular analysis of a gastropod (*Hermissenda crassicornis*) model of associative learning, *Biol. Bull.* **159**:505–560.

Evans, P. D., 1980, Biogenic amines in the insect nervous system, *Adv. Insect Physiol.* **15**:317–473.

Forman, R., 1984, Leg position learning by an insect: a heat avoidance learning paradigm, *J. Neurobiol.* **15**:127–140.

Hoyle, G., 1966, An isolated ganglion-nerve-muscle preparation, *J. Exp. Biol.* **44**:413–427.

Hoyle, G., 1978, The dorsal, unpaired, median neurons of the locust metathoracic ganglion, *J. Neurobiol.* **9**:43–57.

Hoyle, G., 1980, Learning, using natural reinforcements, in insect preparations that permit cellular neuronal analysis, *J. Neurobiol.* **11**:323–354.

Hoyle, G., 1982a, Pacemaker change in a learning paradigm, in: *Cellular Pacemakers*, Vol. 2 (D. Carpenter, ed.), John Wiley and Sons, New York, pp. 3–25.

Hoyle, G., 1982b, Cellular basis of operant-conditioning, in: *Conditioning* (C. D. Woody, ed.), Raven Press, New York, pp. 197–211.

Hoyle, G., 1984, Neuromuscular transmission in a primitive insect: modulation by octopamine, and catch-like tension, *Comp. Biochem. Physiol.* **77C**:219–232.

Hoyle, G. and Barker, D. L., 1975, Synthesis of octopamine by insect dorsal median unpaired neurons, *J. Exp. Zool.* **193**:433–439.

Hoyle, G. and Field, L. H., 1983a, Defense posture and leg-position learning in a primitive insect utilize catchlike tension, *J. Neurobiol.* **14**:285–298.

Hoyle, G. and Field, L. H., 1983b, Elicitation and abrupt termination of behaviorally significant catchlike tension in a primitive insect. *J. Neurobiol.* **14**:299–312.

Hoyle, G., Dagan, D., Moberly, B., and Colquhoun, W., 1974, Dorsal unpaired median insect neurons make neurosecretory endings on skeletal muscle, *J. Exp. Zool.* **187**:159–165.

Hoyle, G., Colquhoun, W., and Williams, M., 1980, Fine structure of an octopaminergic neuron and its terminals, *J. Neurobiol.* **11**:103–126.

Kandel, E. R. and Schwartz, J. H., 1982, Molecular biology of learning. Modulation of transmitter release, *Science* **218**:433–443.

Klopf, A. H., 1982, *The Hedonistic Neuron*, Hemisphere, Washington.

O'Shea, M. and Evans, P. D., 1979, Potentiation of neuromuscular transmission by an octopaminergic neuron in the locust, *J. Exp. Biol.* **79**:169–190.

Woody, C. D. and Black-Cleworth, P., 1973, Differences in excitability of cortical neurons as a function of motor projection in conditioned cats, *J. Neurophysiol.* **36**:1104–1116.

Woollacott, M. and Hoyle, G., 1976, Membrane resistance changes associated with single, identified neuron learning, Abstr. 471, *6th Ann. Mtg. Soc. Neurosci.*

Woollacott, M. and Hoyle, G., 1977, Neural events underlying learning in insects: changes in pacemaker, *Proc. R. Soc. Lond. B* **195**:395–415.

II

Vertebrate Models

6

Cellular Basis of Classical Conditioning Mediated by the Red Nucleus in the Cat

NAKAAKIRA TSUKAHARA

1. SPROUTING IN RED NUCLEUS NEURONS

Synaptic plasticity is an important phenomenon because it provides a possible neuronal basis for learning and memory. The most remarkable long-term plasticity is sprouting and the formation of new synaptic connections. Sprouting has now been demonstrated in a variety of locations throughout the central nervous system using a variety of techniques (Cotman *et al.*, 1981; Tsukahara, 1981). The most common method to induce sprouting in the brain is to destroy some of the synaptic inputs to central neurons (lesion-induced sprouting). However, if sprouting and synapse formation in adult brain requires damage of the synaptic inputs, this phenomenon cannot be the neuronal basis of adaptive behaviors such as learning and memory. Recent studies in the red nucleus (Tsukahara and Fujito, 1976; Tsukahara *et al.*, 1982; Fujito *et al.*, 1982; Murakami *et al.*, 1984) have now revealed that a lesion is not essential and that it is possible to induce sprouting without any lesions of the brain. This finding (sprouting in the intact central neurons) appears to have reduced greatly the gap between sprouting and normal behavioral plasticity, such as learning and memory.

In order to test this view, we have attempted to reconstruct the learning behavior using the corticorubral synapses as the modifiable elements of the network for this behavior. Classical conditioning was used in this behavioral paradigm, because there is already evidence that midbrain structures are important for classical conditioned avoidance responses. The conditioned stimulus (CS) was delivered in the form of electric pulse train in a preparation in which the cerebral corticofugal outflow

NAKAAKIRA TSUKAHARA ● Department of Biophysical Engineering, Faculty of Engineering Science, Osaka University, Toyonaka, and National Institute for Physiological Sciences, Okazaki, Japan.

was largely restricted to the corticorubrospinal pathway by section of the cerebral peduncle caudal to the red nucleus. In this preparation we have found that after conditioning (by stimulating the cerebral peduncle as the CS and applying electric shock to the skin of the forelimb as the unconditioned stimulus; US), initially ineffective stimuli to the corticorubral fibers give rise to forelimb flexion. We performed several control experiments, that is, CS alone, US alone, or random pairing. In these stimuli, there was no acquisition of conditioned responses.

The primary site of conditioned change in this experimental paradigm was determined to be the corticorubral synapses for several reasons, and cellular correlates of conditioning were also observed by recording unit activities of the red nucleus in unanesthetized conditioned cats (Oda et al., 1981). Using intracellular recording techniques, we further analyzed the change of the postsynaptic potentials due to activation of corticorubral synapse after conditioning. We obtained some physiological evidence suggesting the sprouting of corticorubral synapses after establishment of conditioning (Tsukahara and Oda, 1981).

2. CLASSICAL CONDITIONING MEDIATED BY THE RED NUCLEUS

2.1. Behavioral Studies

During conditioning, cats were mounted on a frame, and the movement of the elbow joint was measured by a potentiometer attached to the joint. A series of stimuli was given daily during the training session. The CS was a train of five pulses with 2-msec intervals. The US was an electric shock and was preceded by CS from 60 to 200 msec, mostly 100 msec. CS–US pairing of 120 trials with an interval of 30 sec constituted the training of the day. After training, the score of performance (the ratio of positive responses above the predetermined elbow flexion) gradually increased and after about 1 week, the score attained a plateau. Figure 1C,D shows the mechanogram of elbow flexion at the first day and seventh day of training. The CS is delivered to the cerebral peduncle and the US to the forearm. On the first day, the CS alone produced no response. After the seventh day the CS produced elbow flexion. Figure 1E shows the time course of acquisition and extinction of the conditioned responses. The score of performance increased gradually attaining a plateau after about 1 week (Fig. 1E). In parallel with the increase in the score of performance, the minimum current intensity for producing 100 performances (100% performance current) decreased. After establishing the conditioned response by CS–US pairing, the backward pairing was used to extinguish the conditioned responses. Random control, as well as US alone and CS alone, produced no increase of score of performance. Therefore, it seems likely that this behavioral modification is an example of classical conditioning.

The primary site of the neuronal change in this pathway was tested. Red nucleus cells receive another excitatory input from the nucleus interpositus (IP) of the cerebellum. Thus, if the primary site of the neuronal change is below the red nucleus, we should produce a similar increase in the performance score by stimulating the

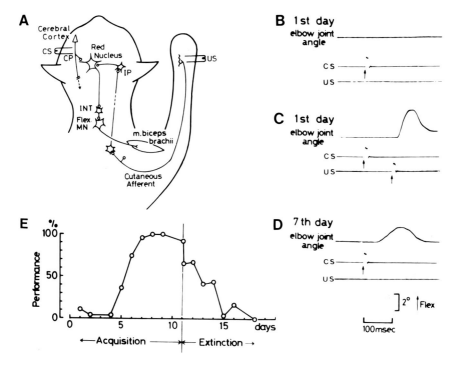

FIGURE 1. Classical conditioning mediated by the red nucleus in the cat. (A) Experimental design. CS, conditioned stimulus; US, unconditioned stimulus. (B–D) Specimen records of elbow flexion (uppermost traces) on 1st day and 7th day after training. Upwards arrows of middle and lowermost traces indicate the onset of the stimulus. (E) Change in performance (ordinate). Abscissa: day after onset of training, CS–US interval of 100 msec. After 11th day the stimulus sequence was reversed to US–CS with an interval of 900 msec. (Modified from Tsukahara *et al.*, 1981.)

nucleus interpositus or a decrease in the current intensity that gives the same performance score. This possibility was tested. There was no appreciable increase in the current intensities for eliciting the same score of performance by stimulating the nucleus interpositus, although the conditioned response was already established by stimulating the cerebral peduncle. This result indicates that the site of neuronal change is not below the red nucleus.

Furthermore, unit recording from the red nucleus before and after establishment of conditioning revealed that transmission through the corticorubral synapses was indeed facilitated after conditioning. Therefore, the most likely site is the corticorubral synapse.

2.2. Cellular Correlates of Conditioning

The next question is the possible mechanism for the increased efficacy of transmission of the corticorubral synapses. If the sprouting is the mechanism, one would expect to see changes in corticorubral EPSPs similar to that found after lesions of the nucleus interpositus (Fig. 2) or after cross-innervation. At least for these cases, electron microscopic studies have shown that they were due to sprouting at the proximal portion of the soma-dendritic membrane of red nucleus cells (Murakami *et al.*, 1982, 1984) (Fig. 3).

We tested this intracellular recording from red nucleus neurons in conditioned as well as in control cats. It was found that after establishment of the conditioned reflex, a new fast-rising component appeared in the corticorubral dendritic EPSPs.

Control cats had corticofugal lesions like the conditioned animals but were not subjected to any training regime. As shown in Fig.4A in conditioned animals, it was found that indeed a fast-rising component is superimposed on the slow-rising

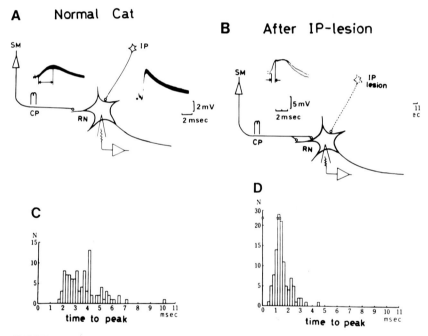

FIGURE 2. Lesion-induced sprouting in the adult feline red nucleus (RN). (A) Synaptic organization of the normal RN. Monosynaptic excitatory input from ipsilateral sensorimotor cortex (SM) through the cerebral peduncle (CP) impinges on the distal dendrites and that from the contralateral nucleus interpositus (IP) of the cerebellum on the soma. Stimulation of CP produces a slow-rising EPSP in an RN cell and stimulation of IP produces a fast-rising EPSP, as shown in the inset. (B) After IP lesion, a fast-rising component appears superimposed on the slow-rising CP EPSPs, as shown in the inset. (C) Frequency distribution of the time-to-peak of the CP EPSPs of normal cats measured as in the inset of (A). (D) Same as (C) but CP EPSPs of cats with chronic IP lesions measured as in the inset of (B). Modified from Tsukahara *et al.* (1975).

corticorubral dendritic EPSPs induced by stimulating CP. A similar fast-rising component is also evident in EPSPs induced by stimulating the sensorimotor cortex (Fig. 4B). In contrast, the cerebral peduncle EPSP from a control, nonstimulated cat shows only a slow-rising time course (Fig. 4C) like that in a normal nonlesioned cat (Fig. 4D). The time-to-peak of the cerebral pedunclar EPSPs was measured in both conditioned and control cats, and the frequency distribution of the time-to-peak of cerebral pedunclar EPSPs are illustrated in Figs. 4E–G. The data is from anesthetized cats. If dual peaks occurred, the first peak was measured to determine the time-to-peak of the EPSPs. The time-to-peak of cerebral pedunclar EPSPs in conditioned cats (Fig. 4E) appears shorter than that of control, nonstimulated cats (Fig. 4F), which was significant statistically ($p < 0.01$). In Fig. 4G, the frequency distribution of the cerebral peduncular EPSPs in normal nonlesioned cats from our previous experiments is illustrated. It should be noted that in some nonstimulated peduncular lesioned cats, the time-to-peak of the cerebral peduncular EPSPs is faster than that in the nonlesioned control cats.

The most attractive interpretation of these results seems to be that, by analogy with the previous experiments using nucleus interpositus lesions or cross-innervation, the corticorubral fibers sprout after conditioning to form new functional synapses on the proximal portion of the soma-dendritic membrane of red nucleus cells. At least for the case of interpositus lesions or cross-innervation, this interpretation of the physiological results was supported by subsequent electron microscopic studies (Murakami *et al.*, 1982, 1984).

However, other interpretations may also exist. One of the possible explanations is that the change of the synaptic potentials is due to morphological changes of dendritic spines. Crick (1982) has proposed that shortening of the spine stalk could possibly induce changes in the properties of the EPSPs, because spine shortening could decrease the electrotonic distance of synaptic currents propagating to the soma (Rall, 1970). Katsumaru *et al.* (1982) have indeed demonstrated by immunohistological techniques that the "actin" is present in the dendritic spine of the red nucleus neurons. The presence of actin in spines of other central neurons has also been reported (Matus *et al.*, 1982). In order to assess the possible role of spine shortening, Kawato and Tsukahara (1983) calculated the effects of morphological change in spines on the postsynaptic potentials using the Butz and Cowan Theorem (1974) and found that the effect of this morphological change on the EPSPs is very small. However, by introduction of a large synaptic conductance or some regenerative property of the spine membrane, it is possible to derive the change in synaptic potentials from the morphological changes in the spines (Koch and Poggio, 1983; Kawato and Tsukahara, 1984). However, Kawato *et al.* (1984) calculated the change of time course of the EPSPs of spine synapses produced by spine shortening in the neuron model based on the measurement of dendritic geometry of HRP-stained RN neurons.

They concluded that time-to-peak of the corticorubral EPSPs is not changed appreciably by the possible changes in the spine stalk, although the amplitude of the EPSPs may change depending upon the geometric parameters of the spine. Therefore, the possibility that the shortening of the time-to-peak of the corticorubral EPSPs is caused by the change of the morphology of the spine is remote.

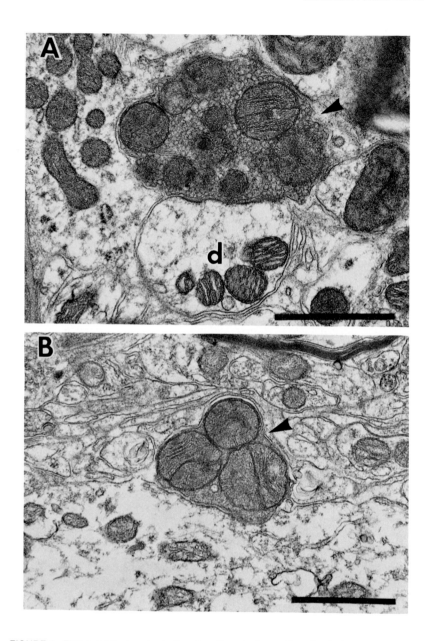

FIGURE 3. Electron-microscopic studies of corticorubral sprouting after lesions of the nucleus interpositus. (A) Degenerating corticorubral terminals in normal cat. An electron dense degeneration terminal (arrow) making synaptic contact with a dendrite (d) of small cross section. Synaptic vesicles are recognizable. (B) Cat with lesion of the nucleus interpositus (IP). A degenerating terminal in synaptic contact with a large dendritic profile. Scale: 1 μm. (C,D) Fre-

3. IN SEARCH OF THE INITIAL PROCESSES OF CONDITIONAL CHANGE

3.1. Long-Term Potentiation (LTP) of the Corticorubral Synaptic Transmission

In order to understand the initial events taking place in RN neurons when the CS was paired to the US, it is necessary to analyze the electrical activities of RN neurons after repetitive activation of the corticorubral input. Recently, we tested long-term effects in the corticorubral synaptic transmission using *in vitro* slice preparation or *in vivo* preparation.

Slice preparation has been used advantageously for the study of plasticity of synaptic transmission in several loci of the brain. Experiments were performed on a slice preparation of kitten midbrain containing the red nucleus. The stimulating electrodes were placed on the rostrolateral part of the red nucleus in order to stimulate the corticorubral fibers.

Tetanic stimulation of 50 Hz for 3 min induces potentiation lasting for an hour or so in the evoked EPSPs. The potentiation is prominent in the EPSPs with slow time-to-peak (Fig.5). This observation is in agreement with the LTP observed *in vivo* red nucleus for the corticorubral synaptic transmission (Kosar *et al.,* 1985). Furthermore, tetanic stimulation induced a later slow potential with a peak time of about 10–20 msec, which persisted several tens of minutes after tetanic stimulation

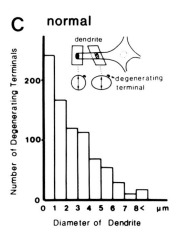
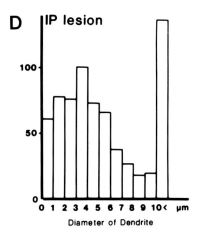

quency distribution of the dendritic diameters where degeneration terminals of corticorubral synapses were found. (C) Normal cat. (D) Cats with chronic destruction of the nucleus interpositus. Ordinates, number of degeneration presynaptic terminals; abscissa, minor diameters of dendrites on which the corticorubral degeneration terminals were found. (Modified from Murakami *et al.,* 1982.)

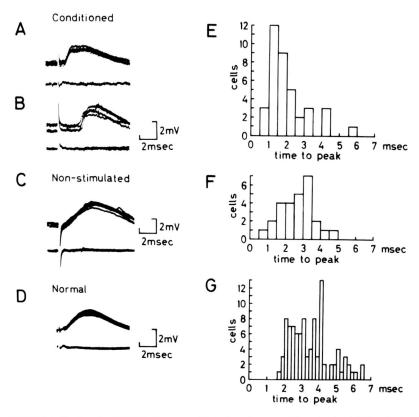

FIGURE 4. Corticorubral EPSPs from conditioned and nonconditioned cats. (A) Cerebral peduncle (CP) EPSPs induced in a red nucleus (RN) cell after the 8th day of conditioning, when conditioning is fully established. (B) Same as in (A), but an EPSP induced by stimulating the sensorimotor cortex (SM). (C) CP EPSPs induced in an RN cell in a nonconditioned control cat. (D) CP EPSPs induced in an RN cell in normal cat. Upper traces, intracellular potential. Lower traces, extracellular records corresponding to the upper traces. Time and voltage calibration of (B) also applied to (A). (E,F) Frequency distribution of the time-to-peak of CP EPSPs in the conditioned (E) and nonconditioned (F) cats. (G) The same histogram but taken from CP EPSPs of normal cats. The number of cells is shown on the ordinate, and the time-to-peak of CP EPSPs, recorded in milliseconds, on the abscissa. (From Tsukahara and Oda, 1981.)

(Fig. 5B). Interestingly, this slow depolarization is induced without tetanic stimulation but by applying dibutyryl cAMP extracelluarly as shown in Fig. 6B. Therefore, it is likely that the slow depolarization is associated with the increase of intracellular cAMP. Furthermore, during slow depolarization, which sometimes is produced without preceding fast EPSP under dibutyryl cAMP (Fig. 6C), the membrane resistance seems to be slightly increased for a short period of time, as shown by the increased amplitude of the electrotonic potentials produced by current pulse from the intracellular microelectrode (Figs. 6C,D). One possibility is that the slow depolarization is produced by the decrease in potassium conductance.

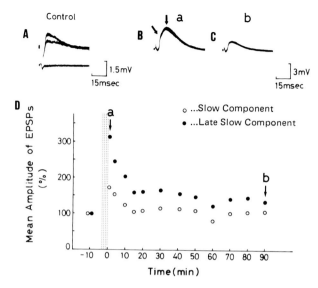

FIGURE 5. Long-term potentiation in the red nucleus neurons in slice preparation. (A, B, C) Specimen records before (A) and after tetanic stimulation of 50 HZ for 3 min (B, C) at the time indicated in (D). (D) Time course of potentiation of EPSPs. Ordinate: amplitudes of slow component (open circles) and late slow component (filled circles) of the EPSPs recorded in a RN cell. Abscissa: time in minutes. Dotted column: tetanic stimulation of 50 HZ for 3 min.

3.2. Ca^{2+}-Dependent Potentials in Red Nucleus Neurons

In order to understand the ionic basis of the slow depolarization, we analyzed the nature of ionic channels in the red nucleus cell membrane (Kubota *et al.*, 1984, 1985). Early electrophysiological study of red nucleus neurons indicated that an action potential of the RN neurons is characterized by an afterhyperpolarization (AHP), which is composed of an initial rapid phase followed by a prolonged slow phase. Addition of tetraethylammonium (TEA) to the perfusing solution increased the amplitude of the action potential, prolonged its falling phase, and abolished the fast AHP, leaving the slow AHP virtually unchanged. The slow AHP was reversibly abolished by perfusing with solutions containing Co^{2+} or Mn^{2+} but the fast AHP remained unchanged. Figure 7 shows an effect of Co^{2+} on the slow AHP. Addition of 2.5 mM Co^{2+} and lowering Ca^{2+} concentration to 1.2 mM abolished the slow AHP, but did not inhibit the fast AHP. When perfusing solution was changed to the normal one, the slow AHP appeared again. This result indicates that the slow AHP is Ca^{2+}-dependent. This hypothesis was further supported by experiments in which the extracellular K$^+$ concentration was changed. Figure 7B shows an effect of the extracellular K$^+$ concentration on the amplitude of the AHP. The amplitude of the slow (and also fast) AHP decreased when the extracellular K$^+$ concentration was raised from 6 mM to 12 mM. These results show that the slow AHP is dependent on both Ca^{2+} and K$^+$. Therefore , it is considered that the slow AHP is most probably produced by an increase in Ca^{2+}-dependent K$^+$ conductance.

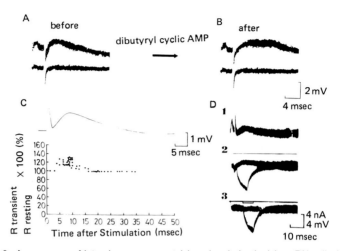

FIGURE 6. Appearance of late slow component (slow depolarization) in a RN cell after application of dibutyryl cAMP in the perfusing solution (A) before dibutyryl AMP and (B) after application of dibutyryl cAMP. Upper trace, intracellular records; lower trace, extracellular records
after withdrawal of the microelectrode. (C, D) Conductance decrease during slow depolarization.
(C) Ordinate: amplitudes of the electrotonic potentials produced by applying current pulses
through the microelectrode during slow depolarization (R transient) as the percentage of those
during resting membrane without slow depolarization (R resting). Abcissa; time after stimulation.
(D) Electrotonic potential produced by applying current pulses; D1, slow depolarization; D2,
slow depolarization and electrotonic potential; D3, electrotonic potential alone. Time and voltage
calibration in D3 also apply to D1, D2.

The existence of Ca^{2+}-dependent K^+ conductance raises a question whether
RN neurons, like other invertebrate and vertebrate neurons, have a voltage-dependent Ca^{2+} conductance. In order to answer this question, we abolished Na spikes
by adding tetrodotoxin (TTX) and inhibited the fast K^+ conductance by adding
TEA to the perfusing solution. As shown in Fig. 8, in a normal solution, a depolarizing current pulse evoked normal action potentials with a low threshold. Such
action potentials were abolished by the addition of TTX to the perfusing solution.
When TEA was further added, a long depolarizing current pulse evoked a regenerative depolarization that has a high theshold and a long duration. This regenerative
depolarization was TTX-resistant and evoked in an all-or none manner. This spike-
like depolarization was probably due to the activation of a voltage-dependent Ca^{2+}
conductance, because it was abolished in the solutions containing 0.6 mM Ca^{2+}
and 5 mM Mn^{2+} or 4 mM Co^{2+} only. Thus, it is likely that a voltage-dependent
Ca^{2+} conductance is also present in RN neurons. Furthermore, our preliminary
results indicate that dibutyryl cAMP reduced the Ca^{2+}-dependent K^+ conductance.
Therefore, our present hypothesis is that an increase of cAMP concentration in RN
neurons induces inhibition of Ca^{2+}-dependent K^+ conductance resulting in slow
depolarization with conductance decrease.

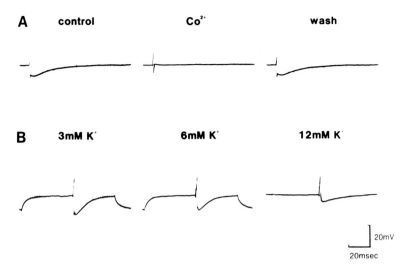

FIGURE 7. Effects of Co^{2+} and K^+ on the afterhyperpolarization in *in vitro* slice containing RN neurons. (A) (left) Action potential accompanied by the fast and the slow afterhyperpolarization (AHP) in the normal solution. (Middle) the slow AHP abolished 3 min after perfusing with the solution containing 1.2 mM Ca^{2+} and 2.5 mM Co^{2+}. Note that the fast AHP was not changed. The slow AHP recovered 8 min after perfusing with the normal solution. Action potentials are truncated. Resting membrane potential was -62 mV. Time and voltage calibration in (B) apply to (A). (B) (left) Action potential with the fast and the slow AHP in the normal solution (3 mM K^+). (middle) The amplitudes of the fast and the slow AHP decreased 30 min after perfusing with the solution containing 6 mM K^+. (Right) They decreased further 35 min after perfusing with the solution containing 12 mM K^+. The action potentials, which were elicitied by a 1-msec depolarizing current pulse, are truncated. Resting membrane potential in the normal solution (3mM K^+) was -63 mV. (From Kubota *et al.*, 1984.)

4. SUMMARY AND CONCLUSION

As for the long-term neuronal basis of conditioning, we believe that sprouting of the corticorubral fibers consitutes one of the long-lasting neuronal mechanisms of conditioning for the following reasons: (1) The site of the change is at the corticorubral synapses, where sprouting has been found. (2) Sprouting can in fact occur without lesions of the direct synaptic input, such as in the cross-innervation of peripheral flexor and extensor nerves (Tsukahara *et al.*, 1982; Fujito *et al.*, 1982; Murakami *et al.*, 1984). (3) The change of corticorubral EPSPs that occurs suggests sprouting at the proximal portion of the soma-dendritic membrane of red nucleus cells. (4) The time course of establishment of the conditioning is a slow process, requiring a week or so. At least for the acquisition process, the time course of conditioning is similar to that of sprouting, which takes place for about one week. However, the evidence is not sufficient and further experiments are required to substantiate this hypothesis.

normal   **TEA+TTX**   **TEA+TTX+Mn^{2+}**

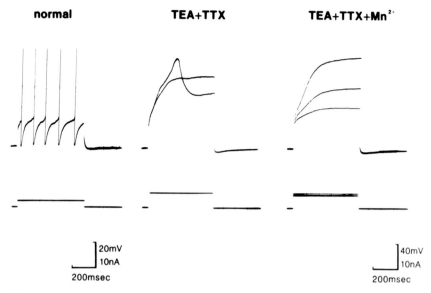

| 20mV |
| 10nA |

200msec

| 40mV |
| 10nA |

200msec

FIGURE 8. TTX-resistant regenerative depolarization. (left) Action potentials in the normal solution. They are retouched for clarity. (middle) In the solution containing 10 mM TEA and 0.4 μg/ml TTX, normal action potentials were abolished but an all-or-none regenerative depolarization was evoked by a long depolarizing current pulse. (right) Addition of 5 mM Mn^{2+} and lowering Ca^{2+} concentration to 0.6 mM abolished the regenerative depolarization. Upper traces are voltage records and lower ones current records. Resting membrane potential was −66 mV. (From Kubota et al., 1984.)

As for the inital events for triggering the long-term plasticity underlying conditioning changes, we found that corticorubral synaptic transmission is characterized by long-term potentiation. A slow depolarization, which is presumably due to a decrease of K$^+$ conductance, was also induced after tetanic stimulation of the corticorubral fibers. Since the slow depolarization could be induced by applying the dibutyryl cAMP, it is likely that an increase of intracellular cAMP is associated with the slow depolarization. To what extent these phenomena are related to the initial stage of conditioning is not known.

REFERENCES

Allen, G. I. and Tsukahara, N., 1974, Cerebrocerebellar communication system, *Physiol. Rev.* **54**:957–1006.

Butz, E. G. and Cowan, J. D., 1974, Transient potentials in dendritic system of arbitrary geometry, *Biophys. J.* **14**:661–689.

Cotman, C. W., Nieto-Sampedro, M., and Harris, E. W., 1981, Synaptic replacement in the nervous system of adult vertebrates, *Physiol Rev.* **61**:684–783.

Fujito, Y., Tsukahara, N., Oda, Y., and Yoshida, M., 1982, Formation of functional synapses in the adult cat red nucleus from the cerebrum following cross-innervation of forelimb flexor and extensor nerves. II. Analysis of newly-appeared synaptic potentials, *Exp. Brain Res.* **45**:13–18.

Katsumaru, H., Murakami, F., and Tsukahara, N., 1982, Actin filament in dendritic spines of red nucleus neurons demonstrated by immunoferritin localization and heavy meromyosin binding, *Biomed. Res.* **3**:337–340.

Kawato, M. and Tsukahara, N., 1983, Theoretical study on electrical properties of dendritic spines, *J. Theor. Biol.* **103**:507–522.

Kawato, M. and Tsukahara, N., 1984, Electrical properties of dendritic spines with bulbous end terminals, *Biophys. J.* **46**:155–166.

Kawato, M., Hamaguchi, T., Murakami, F., and Tsukahara, N., 1984, Quantitative analysis of electrical properties of dendritic spines, *Biol. Cybern.* **50**:447–454.

Koch, C. and Poggio, T., 1983, Electrical properties of dendritic spines, *Trends Neurosci.* **6**:80–83.

Kosar, E., Fujito, Y., Murakami, F., and Tsukahara, N., 1985, Morphological and electrophysiological study of sprouting of corticorubral fibers after lesions of the contralateral cerebrum in kitten, *Brain Res.* (in press).

Kubota, M., Nakamura, N., and Tsukahara, N., 1984, Calcium-dependent potentials in mammalian red nucleus neurons *in vitro*, *Neurosci. Res.* **1**:185–189.

Kubota, M., Nakamura, M., and Tsukahara, N., 1985, Ionic conductances associated with electrical activities of guinea-pig red nucleus neurons *in vitro*, *J. Physiol.* **362**:167–171.

Matus, A., Ackermann, M., Pehling, G., Byers, H. R., and Fujiwara, K., 1982, High actin concentrations in brain dendritic spines and postsynaptic densities, *Proc. Natn. Acad. Sci. USA* **79**:7590–7594.

Murakami, F., Katsumaru, H., Saito, K., and Tsukahara, N., 1982, A quantitative study of synaptic reorganization in red nucleus neurons after lesion of the nucleus interpositus of the cat: an electron microscopic study involving intracellular injection of horseradish peroxidase, *Brain Res.* **242**:41–53.

Murakami, F., Katsumaru, H., Maeda, J., and Tsukahara, N., 1984, Reorganization of corticorubral synapses following cross-innervation of flexor and extensor nerves of adult cat: A quantitative electron microscopic study, *Brain Res.* **306**:299–306.

Oda, Y., Kuwa, K., Miyasaka, S., and Tsukahara, N., 1981, Modification of rubral unit activities during classical conditioning in the cat, *Proc. Jpn. Acad. Ser. B* **57**:402–405.

Rall, W., 1970, Cable properties of dendrites and effects of synaptic location, in: *Excitatory Synaptic Mechanisms* (P. Anderson and J. K. S. Jansen, eds.), Oslo Universitesforlag, Oslo.

Tsukahara, N., 1981, Synaptic plasticity in the mammalian central nervous system, *Ann. Rev. Neurosci.* **4**:351–379.

Tsukahara, N. and Fujito, Y., 1976, Physiological evidence of formation of new synapses from cerebrum in the red nucleus following cross-union of forelimb nerves, *Brain Res.* **106**:184–188.

Tsukahara, N., Fujito, Y., Oda, Y., and Maeda, J., 1982, Formation of functional synapses in adult cat red nucleus from the cerebrum following cross-innervation of forelimb flexor and extensor nerves. I. Appearance of new synaptic potentials, *Exp. Brain Res.* **45**:1–12.

Tsukahara, N., Hultborn, H., Murakami, F., and Fujito, Y., 1975, Electrophysiological study of formation of new synapses and collateral sprouting in red nucleus neurons after partial denervation, *J. Neurophysiol.* **38**:1359–1379.

Tsukahara, N. and Oda, Y., 1981, Appearance of new synaptic potentials at corticorubral synapses after the establishment of classical conditioning, *Proc. Jpn. Acad. Ser. B* **57**:398–401.

Tsukahara, N., Oda, Y., and Notsu, T., 1981, Classical conditioning mediated by the red nucleus in the cat, *J. Neurosci.* **1**:72–79.

7

Dendritic Spine Structure and Function

DENNIS M. D. LANDIS

1. INTRODUCTION

While spines have long been considered a characteristic feature of neuronal architecture, the cellular mechanisms responsible for maintaining their peculiar shape have only recently come under detailed study. In this chapter, we review some recent studies of cytoskeletal structure in certain classes of dendritic spines, discuss the issue of heterogeneity of spine morphology in the hippocampus, and speculate about the capacity of spines for rapid shape change.

2. CYTOSKELETAL STRUCTURE IN SPINES

In tissue prepared for electron microscopic study by routine aldehyde fixation, it is exceedingly difficult to visualize more than a wispy background in spine cytoplasm. Fifkova and Delay (1982) accomplished a major advance in understanding spine structure by showing that spines in the hippocampus contain microfilaments that bind meromyosin fragments, and by that criterion suggested that spines contain actinlike molecules. Later, two other groups demonstrated the presence of actinlike immunoreactivity in spine cytoplasm (Matus *et al.*, 1982; Caceres *et al.*, 1983).

An alternative approach to tissue preservation has allowed us to recognize three distinct sets of filamentous structures in the cytoplasm of cerebellar Purkinje cell spines (Landis and Reese, 1983) (Figs. 1–5). Slices of cerebellar tissue were quickly excised from decapitated mice and frozen against a copper block cooled by liquid helium. The freezing in the superficial portion of the tissue slice is so

DENNIS M. D. LANDIS ● Departments of Neurology, Developmental Genetics and Anatomy, Case Western Reserve University, Cleveland, Ohio 44106.

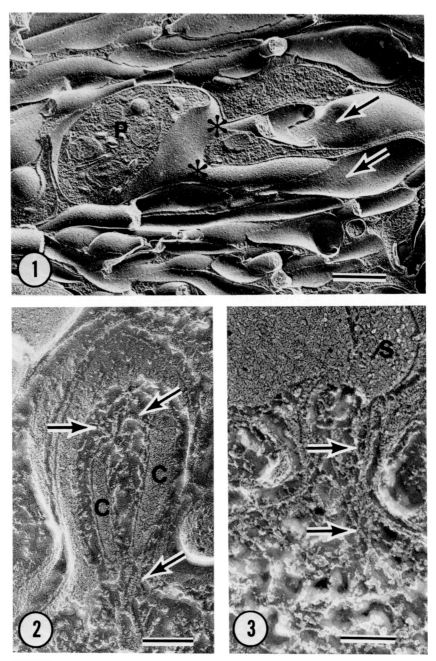

FIGURE 1. Purkinje cell spines in adult mouse cerebellar cortex. A cross-fractured Purkinje cell dendrite (P) gives rise to two spines (asterisks at spine origins), each of which synapses with a parallel fiber axon (oblique arrow). The upper oblique arrow indicates the cytoplasmic

rapid that ice crystals do not grow to a size that distorts cytoplasmic structure. The rapidly frozen tissue is then fractured in a Balzers freeze-fracture device, and water is allowed to sublime from the frozen surfaces, etching them to a depth of 20–40 nm. As cytoplasmic water sublimes, it exposes dissolved proteins, which may then be studied after platinum has been evaporated onto the surface of the specimen, replicating it. In the etched spines, there was a focal collection of short, anastomotic filaments 4–6 nm in apparent diameter, which was coextensive with the synaptic junction and which appeared to correspond to the electron-dense fuzz that characterizes postsynaptic cytoplasm in tissue fixed by more conventional means (Figs. 4, 5). In the core of the spine there is a second set of filaments, 8–9 nm in apparent diameter, which have a subtle periodicity and which resemble closely actin filaments as they are visualized in platinum-replicated preparations (Figs. 2, 4). These actinlike microfilaments were very close to the filaments of the postsynaptic web but did not appear to be continuous with them. Actinlike filaments extended through the body and neck of the spine, into the cytoplasm of the parent dendrite.

The most thought-provoking aspect of spine structure in this etched cerebellar tissue is a set of filaments 5–7 nm in diameter in the cortex of the spine cytoplasm (Figs. 2, 3, 4). These filaments insert on the true inner surface of the spine membrane and also intersect one another. The filaments are straight, and in the neck of the spine they can extend throughout the spine cytoplasm (Fig. 3). Similar, but much more sparse filaments lined the true inner surface of the dendritic membranes. We do not know the biochemical identity of these 5–7-nm filaments, but their location in the cortex of the spine and the spine neck led us to speculate that they might be involved in maintaining spine shape. If the points of insertion on the true inner surface of the membrane and the points of intersection with other filaments have mechanical strength, then this filament system could constitute a lattice that supports the inflection of the cell membrane at the spine neck. The filaments and their intersections are concentrated in the spine neck, where the mechanical requirements for maintaining membrane curvature are the greatest.

A time-honored approach to understanding structure is to examine the manner in which it is assembled during development. We have examined spine shape during normal postnatal synaptogenesis in mouse cerebellum, concentrating on Purkinje cell spines that contact parallel fibers (manuscript in preparation). We serially thin-

---

half of the fractured axonal membrane at the site of the active zone, and the lower oblique arrow indicates the extracellular half of the fractured axonal membrane and its active zone. (Aldehyde-fixed tissue; this and all the other freeze fracture micrographs has been photographically reversed, so that platinum appears light) (magnification 28,600×; calibration bar 0.5 μm).

FIGURE 2. Filaments in rapidly frozen, etched cerebellar Purkinje cell spine. The oblique arrows indicate larger (8–9 nm) actinlike filaments with a distinct periodicity. Horizontal arrows indicate smaller (5–7 nm) filaments in the periphery of the spine cytoplasm. Two cisterns (indicated by c) are present in the core of the spine (magnification 147,000×; calibration bar 0.1μm).

FIGURE 3. Fine filaments at the origin of a spine in rapidly frozen, etched cerebellar cortex. Horizontal arrows indicate the mesh of 5- to 7-nm filaments in the origin of the spine, extending downward into dendritic cytoplasm. The cytoplasmic half of the fractured spine membrane in the body of the spine is indicated by (s) (magnification 147,000×; calibration 0.1μm).

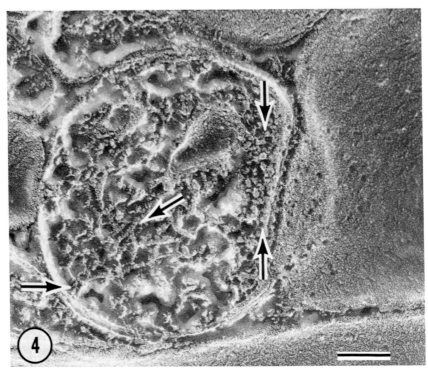

FIGURE 4. Cross-fractured Purkinje cell dendritic spine. The oblique arrows indicate actin-like, larger filaments toward the core of the spine. The 5- to 7-nm filaments are indicated by horizontal arrows. Between the apposed vertical arrows is the dense mesh of the postsynaptic fuzz (rapidly frozen, etched tissue; magnification 147,000 ×; calibration bar 0.1 μm).

sectioned developing tissue and found that spinous evaginations are present in distal portions of the arborization that have no synaptic junctions. These spinous evaginations resemble in shape, size, and content of membrane cisterns the dendritic spines of mature animals, but in mature animals, the dendritic spines are invariably part of a synaptic junction. Apparently, the cytoskeletal mechanisms which support spine formation and shape are independent of synaptic junctional specializations.

3. SPINES AND SYNAPTIC JUNCTIONS IN THE HIPPOCAMPUS

We would like to know whether the features of cytoskeletal structure are similar in spines arising from different types of neurons. In preparation for such an analysis, we have examined the dendritic arborization of pyramidal cells in the CA1 region of rat hippocampus, using fixed tissue prepared for electron microscopic study by freeze fracture techniques and by thin section techniques (Harris and Landis, 1983).

In freeze-fractured tissue, the spine membrane at the site of a synaptic junction is characterized by an aggregate of particles associated with the extracellular half

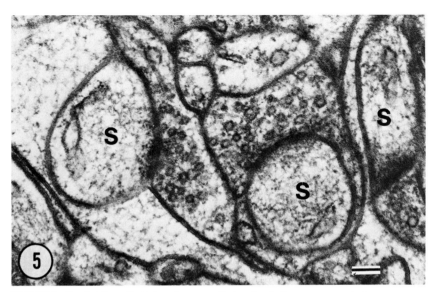

FIGURE 5. Parallel fiber: Purkinje spine synaptic junction in the mouse cerebellar cortex prepared by rapid freezing and freeze-substitution fixation. Within the cytoplasm of the cross-sectioned spines (s) there are filaments of at least two diameters (magnification 70,000 ×; calibration bar 1.0μm).

of the fractured membrane (Fig. 7). This aggregate is similar to those found at other synapses with an excitatory action in the mammalian central nervous system. The appearance of synaptic junctions on spines and on dendritic surfaces is remarkably similar. We compared the synaptic junctions of pyramidal cell spines with junctions formed by the same class of axon on interneuronal dendrites. The particle packing density and the appearance of the constitutent particles of the aggregates are similar in these junctions, though the range of junctional area is greater in spines.

In serially thin-sectioned tissue, the postsynaptic electron-dense fuzz in some of the larger pyramidal cell spines appears to be discontinuous. Such synaptic junctions have been variously described as perforated or complex. In freeze-fractured tissue, we have found particle aggregates in large spines that have particle-free zones within them. We presume that the particle-free zones correspond with the regions in which "fuzz" is absent in the postsynaptic specialization. Postsynaptic particle aggregates with particle-free zones have been described in other areas of the central nervous system and are not limited to spines. In general, the particle aggregates that are annular or have several particle free zones are large in area as compared to other synaptic junctions between the same types of neuronal processes. One might imagine that junctions have the capacity to grow within a range of surface area, but at the larger end of this range, the junction begins to break up. Perhaps this reflects some characteristic of the junctional materials, or perhaps it is a stage preceding subdivision to several synaptic junctions (Nieto-Sampedro *et al.*, 1982; Carlin and Siekevitz, 1983).

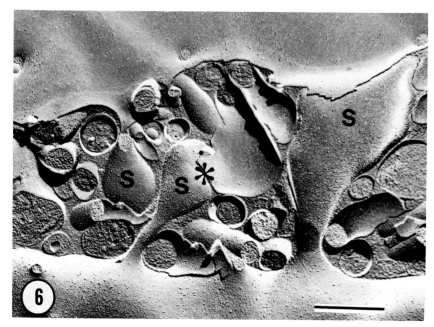

FIGURE 6. Spines arising from CA1 pyramidal cell dendrites in rat hippocampus. These spines in *S. radiatum* (s) exemplify the range of size and shape. The asterisk indicates the site of a synaptic junction (aldehyde-fixed tissue; magnification 38,000 ×; calibration bar 0.5μm).

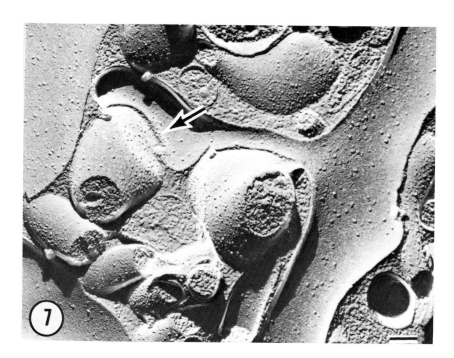

4. HETEROGENEITY OF SPINE STRUCTURE
IN THE HIPPOCAMPUS

We have been impressed by the heterogeneity of spine shape and size in area CA1 of the hippocampus, especially as it is apparent in serial thin sections. Variation in spine shape, size, and content of organelles has been noted in many studies (Westrum and Blackstad, 1962), but our attention was drawn to the issue by our freeze fracture preparations, in which neighboring spines can be seen to be very different at a glance (Fig. 6). In preliminary studies of serially thin-sectioned tissue, we have begun to measure various aspects of spines, and have found each to have a range of values. For example, the diameter of the spine origin, the diameter of the spine neck, the length of the neck, the volume of the spine head, the spine surface area, and the volume of membrane cisterns within the spine are all variable. Naturally, some of these aspects covary. Large volume spine heads tend to contain larger volumes of membrane cisterns. On the other hand, large volume heads may have long or short necks. We think that it will be necessary to serially section many spines and measure these parameters in them before patterns of covariation can be identified. Serial section analysis may also tell us whether neighboring spines influence one another, and whether position on the dendritic arbor is pertinent to spine shape.

Because neighboring spines arising from the same dendrite can be so different, the heterogeneity is unlikely to be simply a function of position on the dendritic arbor. We considered the possibility that spine shape would be regulated by the nature of the axon which contacted it. We used immunocytochemical methods to identify cells containing CCK-like immunoreactivity and found that immunoreactive axons do not contact spines in area CA1 (Harris et al., 1985). Other investigators have examined somatostatin and enkephalinlike immunoreactivity, and also have failed to identify axons contacting spines. For the present, it seems likely that a single population of axons—the Schaffer collaterals from area CA3—synapse with the vast majority of spines in stratum radiatum of CA1 and that these apparently similar axons contact spines with variable shapes.

Is it possible that synaptic activity has an influence on spine shape? In the hippocampus, the most florid example of the influence of activity on shape is the loss of spines that follows degeneration of the afferent axons. No activity somehow translates into no spine (e.g., Hoff et al., 1982). It is possible that differences in activity, such as firing rate of the afferent axon, also influence the spine. Repetitive or sustained transmitter release at a given synaptic junction might be reflected in the local inward currents of Na^+ and Ca^{2+} (Fifkova et al., 1982). It has been supposed that spine cisterns might be able to take up Ca^{2+}. If that is true, then spines synapsing with very active axons might require additional capacity for Ca^{2+} uptake and so a larger volume of spine cisterns is accumulated, with an incidental increase in the size of the spine.

FIGURE 7. Synaptic junction on a spine of a CA1 pyramidal cell. The synaptic junction has been cross-fractured. A portion of the particle aggregate on the extracellular half of the fractured postsynaptic spine membrane is indicated by an arrow (aldehyde-fixed tissue; magnification 70,000 × ; calibration bar 0.1 μm).

5. DO SPINES CHANGE SHAPE?

One of the most exciting concepts in neurobiology is that spine shape may be used by the cell to regulate the influence of a particular synapse upon it. Rall (1974) has argued that the diameter of the neck of a spine could be expected to influence the resistance to current flow through the spine to the parent dendrite. This inspired several efforts to identify changes in spine shape with morphological tools. Recently, Koch and Poggio (1983a,b) have lent support to Rall's ideas and point out that their models for spine function and shape correlate nicely with the shapes of spines seen in specific regions of Golgi-impregnated dendritic arborizations. On the other hand, Turner and Schwartzkroin (1983) have presented contrasting evidence, based on different assumptions and models, which seems to indicate that spine neck diameter is not a likely site for the regulation of synaptic efficacy.

Several efforts have been made to detect morphological changes associated with long-term synaptic potentiation in the hippocampus, but conflicting and confusing results have emerged (Van Harreveld and Fifkova, 1975; Fifkova and Van Harreveld, 1977; Moshkov et al., 1977; Lee et al., 1979, 1980; Moshkov et al., 1980; Fifkova and Anderson, 1981; Lynch and Baudry, 1982). All of these studies have failed to identify the particular potentiated synapses, and so are unable to directly compare potentiated and nonpotentiated synapses. Failing that, they rely on various samplings of the synaptic populations in which potentiation is presumed to have occurred. These samplings fail to fully consider the heterogeneity of spine shape and size in the hippocampus, and their results are of uncertain value. At present, we believe that one has to know much more about the range of spine variation in normal tissue before one can identify changes within that range which may correlate with long-term synaptic potentiation.

In our studies of spines arising form Purkinje cells, we wondered whether the spine cytoskeleton maintained shape permanently, or supported the capacity for change in spine shape. We do not believe that the morphological information available thus far has solved the issue. The presence of actinlike material in spines does not necessarily indicate that the actin participates in some contractile activity. In our studies, we did not identify cross-bridges between actin filaments or other branching structures resembling the interaction of actin and myosin in skeletal muscle. Furthermore, actinlike material is abundant in regions of cells which are known to be stable in shape. The role of the actin in spines is still unknown. It may have more to do with the synaptic junction than with the spine, since actin has invariably been found close to synaptic junctions, even when they occur on cell bodies or dendritic shafts.

ACKNOWLEDGMENTS. L. A. Weinstein, L. Cherkas, and D. M. Jackson provided valued assistance. This work supported in part by NS15573.

REFERENCES

Caceres, A., Payne, M. R., Binder, L. I., and Steward, O., 1983, Immunocytochemical localization of actin and microtubule-associated protein MAP2 in dendritic spines, *Proc. Natl. Acad. Sci. USA* **80:**1738–1742.

Carlin, R. K. and Siekevitz, P., 1983, Plasticity in the central nervous system: Do synapses divide? *Proc. Natl. Acad. Sci. USA* **80:**3517–3521.

Fifkova, E. and Anderson, C. L., 1981, Stimulation-induced changes in dimensions of stalks of dendritic spines in the dentate molecular layer, *Exp. Neurol.* **74:**621–627.

Fifkova, E. and Delay, R. J., 1982, Cytoplasmic actin in dendritic spines as a possible mediator of synaptic plasticity, *J. Cell Biol.* **95:**350–365.

Fifkova, E. and Van Harreveld, A., 1977, Long-lasting morphological changes in dendritic spines of dentate granular cells following stimulation of the entorhinal area, *J. Neurocytol.* **6:**211–230.

Fifkova, E., Markham, J. A., and Delay, R. J., 1982, Calcium in the spine apparatus of dendritic spines in the dentate molecular layer, *Brain Res.* **266:**163–168.

Harris, K. M. and Landis, D. M. D., 1983, Freeze-fracture study of membrane structure in the CA1 region of rat hippocampus. *Soc. Neurosci. Abstr.* **9:**1176.

Harris, K. M., Marshall, P. E., and Landis, D. M. D., 1985, Ultrastructural study of cholecystokinin-immunoreactive cells and processes in area CA1 of the rat hippocampus, *J. Comp. Neurol.* **233:**147–158.

Hoff, S. F., Scheff, S. W., Benardo, L. S., and Cotman, C. W., 1982, Lesion-induced synaptogenesis in the dentate gyrus of aged rats. I. Loss and reacquisition of normal synaptic density, *J. Comp. Neurol.* **205:**246–252.

Koch, C. and Poggio, T., 1983a, Electrical properties of dendritic spines, *Trends in Neurosci.* **6:**80–83.

Koch, C. and Poggio, T., 1983b, A theoretical analysis of electrical properties of spines, *Proc. R. Soc. London* **218:**455–477.

Landis, D. M. D. and Reese, T. S., 1983, Cytoplasmic organization in cerebellar dendritic spines, *J. Cell Biol.* **97:**1169–1178.

Lee, K. S., Oliver, M., Schottler, F., Creager, R., and Lynch, G., 1979, Ultrastructural effects of repetitive synaptic stimulation in the hippocampal slice preparation: A preliminary report, *Exp. Neurol.* **68:**478–480.

Lee, K. S., Schottler, F., Oliver, M., and Lynch, G., 1980, Brief bursts of high-frequency stimulation produce two types of structural changes in the rat hippocampus, *J. Neurophysiol.* **44:**247–258.

Lynch, G. and Baudry, M., 1982, Rapid structural modification in rat hippocampus—evidence for its occurrence and a hypothesis concerning how it is produced, in: *Changing Concepts of the Nervous System* (A. R. Morrison and P. L. Strick, eds.), Academic Press, New York, pp. 21–32.

Matus, A., Ackermann, M., Pehling, G., Byers, H. R., and Fujiwara, K., 1982, High actin concentrations in brain dendritic spines and postsynaptic densities, *Proc. Natl. Acad. Sci. USA* **79:**7590–7594.

Moshkov, D. A., Petrovskaia, L. L., and Bragin, A. G., 1977, Posttetanic changes in the ultrastructure of the giant spinous synapses in hippocampal field CA3, *Dokl. Akad. Nauk. USSR* **237:**1525–1528.

Moshkov, D. A., Petrovskaia, L. L., and Bragin, A. G., 1980, Ultrastructural study of the bases of postsynaptic potentiation in hippocampal sections by the freeze-substitution method, *Tsitologia* **22:**20–26.

Nieto-Sampedro, M., Hoff, S. F., and Cotman, C. W., 1982, Perforated postsynaptic densities: Probable intermediates in synapse turnover, *Proc. Natl. Acad. Sci. USA* **79:**5718–5722.

Rall, W., 1974, Dendritic spines, synaptic potency and neuronal plasticity, in: *Cellular Mechanisms Subserving Changes in Neuronal Activity* (C. Woody, K. Brown, T. Crow, J. Knipsel, eds.), Brain Information Service, UCLA, California.

Turner, D. A. and Schwartzkroin, P. A., 1983, Electrical characteristics of dendrites and dendritic spines in intracellularly stained CA3 and dentate hippocampal neurons, *J. Neurosci.* **3:**2381–2394.

Van Harreveld, A., and Fifkova, E., 1975, Swelling of dendritic spines in the fascia dentata after stimulation of the perforant fibers as a mechanism of post-tetanic potentiation, *Exp. Neurol.* **49:**736–749.

Westrum, L. E. and Blackstad, T. W., 1962, An electron microscopic study of stratum radiatum of the rat hippocampus (Regio superior, CA1) with particular emphasis on synaptology, *J. Comp. Neurol.* **119:**281–309.

8

Rapid Conditioning of an Eye Blink Reflex in Cats

CHARLES D. WOODY, NEIL E. BERTHIER, and ELLEN H.-J. KIM

1. INTRODUCTION

Associative conditioning may develop slowly, requiring many pairings, sometimes over many days (Woody, 1974), for acquisition of the conditioned motor response. Voronin and colleagues (Voronin, 1974; Voronin *et al.*, 1975) discovered that electrical stimulation of the hypothalamus could be used in combination with presentations of a CS and US to produce rapid development of an associatively conditioned startle response. Our studies evaluated whether acquisition of a conditioned eye blink movement could be accelerated by adding hypothalamic stimulation to pairing of a click and glabella tap. Earlier studies had shown that 700–1000 associative trace pairings of the same click CS and tap US were required for the development of a conditioned blink movement. The production of this associatively conditioned reflex depended on the integrity of neurons of the motor cortex and facial nucleus. Without the motor cortex, learning of the conditioned eye blink response was impaired, whereas performance of the unconditioned eye blink was not (Woody *et al.*, 1974). Application of 25% KCl to the motor cortex of eye blink-conditioned cats reversibly eliminated performance of the conditioned response, but not elicitation of the unconditioned eye blink response (Woody and Brozek, 1969).

Our earlier studies of conditioning of facial movements (Woody and Engel, 1972; Woody and Black-Cleworth, 1973; Brons and Woody, 1980; Woody, 1982a) showed that the patterns of activation of specific sets of units of the motor cortex determined the type of movement that was acquired, as well as the latency of the acquired response following presentations of the click CS. Consequently, the re-

CHARLES D. WOODY, NEIL E. BERTHIER, and ELLEN H.-J. KIM ● UCLA Medical Center, Mental Retardation Research Center, Brain Research Institute, Departments of Anatomy and Psychiatry, Los Angeles, California 90024. *Present address* for N.E.B.: University of Massachusetts, Amherst, Massachusetts 01003.

sponse of cortical units to the CS was investigated during accelerated conditioning using hypothalamic stimulation in combination with click CS and tap US. During training and testing, a hiss stimulus of comparable intensity to the click CS was presented as a discriminative stimulus.

2. METHODOLOGIES

All studies were made in conscious, unanesthetized cats. EMG activity was recorded bilaterally from the orbicularis oculi (eye) and levator oris (nose) muscles. Recordings were obtained from single units of the coronal pericruciate cortex during the training–testing paradigms described below. The technical procedures have been described in detail elsewhere (Woody and Black-Cleworth, 1973; Kim *et al.*, 1983; Woody *et al.*, 1983).

The hypothalamus was stimulated electrically with bipolar, concentric electrodes (four, 100-μsec rectangular pulses of 1–10 mA presented at 50 Hz). The electrodes were introduced into the hypothalamus via chronically implanted guide tubes.

2.1. Behavioral Training and Testing

Effects of the following paradigms of stimulus presentation were studied (see Fig. 1):

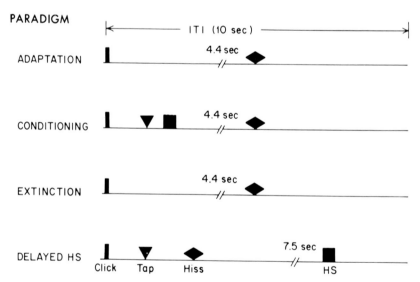

FIGURE 1. Temporal order and interval of presentations of click (CS), glabella tap (US), hypothalamic stimulation (HS), and hiss (DS) during different training paradigms. ISIs between clicks and immediately succeeding stimuli are specified in the text; those between clicks and stimuli succeeding the interrupted baseline are as indicated in the figure. (From Kim *et al.*, 1983.)

Adaptation: presentations of click and hiss alone.

Conditioning: presentations of click CS followed (340 msec) by glabella tap US followed (240 msec) by hypothalamic stimulation. Hiss DS given 3.8 sec after HS.

Extinction: presentations of click and hiss alone.

Backward (Delayed) HS: HS followed (2.5 sec) by click CS followed (340 msec) by tap US followed (240 msec) by hiss DS.

CS–US–DS paradigm: conditioning with omission of HS.

Each of the above paradigms used an intertrial interval of 10 sec.

3. BEHAVIORAL RESULTS

3.1. Adaptation

The physical characteristics of the click CS and hiss DS (75 db) used during adaptation and subsequent conditioning are shown in Fig. 2. During adaptation, some animals failed to respond to either stimulus, whereas other animals showed small blink responses that decreased and then disappeared during the adaptation period. When unconditioned eye blink responses to click and hiss were seen during the adaptation period, the responses evoked by hisses were bigger than those evoked by clicks. When present initially, blink responses to these stimuli appeared bilaterally as a consensual reflex response.

3.2. Conditioning

Given a satisfactory locus of hypothalamic stimulation, conditioning developed very rapidly, often within 20 pairings or less (see Fig. 3). During the initial paired presentations of CS, US, HS and DS, sensitized blink responses were elicited by the click and the hiss shown in the lower portion of Fig. 2. Soon thereafter (Fig. 3), the responses to the hiss DS diminished and a discriminative conditioned reflex emerged.* Averaged results from a group of cats conditioned to blink their eyes in this manner are shown in Fig. 3. The onset latencies of the major blink responses to the click CS, measured electromyographically, ranged between 80 and 320 msec. The unconditioned response to HS involved a broader spectrum of movements. Unconditioned motor responses elicited by HS included jaw opening, vocalization, and body movement. Those other movements were not part of the unconditioned response to the tap US. That response was an eye blink resembling the CR.

3.3. Extinction

Extinction was accomplished by giving presentations of clicks and hisses alone. The results showed learning savings of a discriminatively elicited conditioned eye

*In Voronin's studies discriminative conditioning could not be obtained within the same sensory modality.

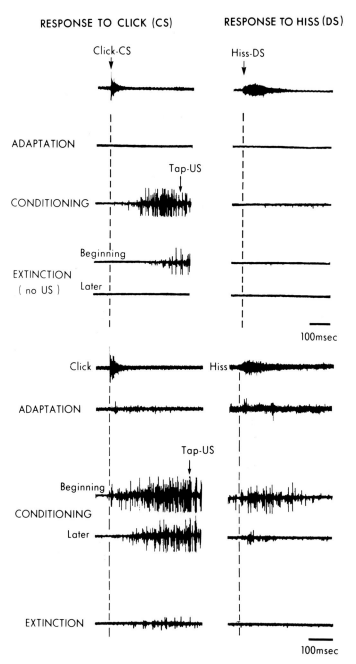

FIGURE 2. Superimposed traces (five each) of bipolar EMG recordings from the orbicularis oculi muscles (ipsilateral to HS) of two cats (above and below) demonstrating acquisition of selective eye blink CRs to the click CS during conditioning. The top traces show the physical characteristics of the two auditory stimuli, the click CS and hiss DS, converted into electric

blink response. Early during extinction, conditioned eye blink responses were elicited selectively by the click CS as opposed to the hiss DS (see Figs. 2 and 3). With repeated presentations of the CS and DS alone, the conditioned response was extinguished.

3.4. Backward HS Presentation

Explicitly unpaired presentations of stimuli (i.e., backwards conditioning wherein presentations of the HS preceded presentation of the click and tap) were used to assess the associative aspect of conditioning. Explicitly unpaired presentations provide a more precise assessment of associative variables than do so-called "random" stimulus presentations (see Woody, 1982b). Whereas presentations of HSs immediately after CS–US presentation resulted in rapid development of discriminative CRs, delivery of HSs 2.5 sec before each CS–US pairing did not. Presentations of the US and HS prior to presentations of the CS also failed to result in conditioning (cf. Kim et al., 1983).

Backward HS pairing resulted in the production of sensitized eye blink responses (Fig. 3). However, the numbers of such responses to the CS were fewer than those observed during forward associative conditioning. When extinction followed backward HS presentations, a few, small eye blink responses to *both* CS and DS occurred and then rapidly disappeared. These responses reflected some savings of sensitization.

3.5. CS–HS–DS Paradigm

Using a paradigm in which clicks, hypothalamic stimulation, and hisses were presented (without glabella tap), more than 100 pairings were required before any discriminative blink CRs emerged. This was consistent with the results of other investigators (cf. Sakurai and Hirano, 1983) and with the numbers of pairings of CSs and USs needed to produce conditioned nictitating membrane responses in rabbits (Gormezano, 1972).

After rapid production of eye blink conditioning using click CS, tap US, and HS, introduction of the CS–HS–CS paradigm (without US) resulted in maintenance of discriminatively conditioned responding to the click and augmentation of the magnitude of the conditioned eye blink response. In contrast, after rapid eye blink

---

signals via a microphone placed near the ear of the cat and then photographed from an oscilloscope after amplification. Arrows and dashed vertical lines indicate onsets of the auditory stimuli. A separate arrow indicates the time when the tap US was delivered. The time calibration (lower right) applied to both left and right traces. In the early adaptation period when clicks and hisses were first presented, small eye blinks were elicited by both stimuli in the animal shown below. The hiss-evoked responses were bigger than those evoked by clicks. During conditioning, the magnitude of the click-evoked eyeblinks was visibly larger than that of the hiss-evoked responses. Later, after repeated conditioning trials, the eyeblinks elicited by the DS diminished in size and were less frequently elicited than the CS-evoked responses. During the early extinction period after conditioning, eyeblinks were elicited selectively by the CS and not by the DS. (From Kim et al., 1983.)

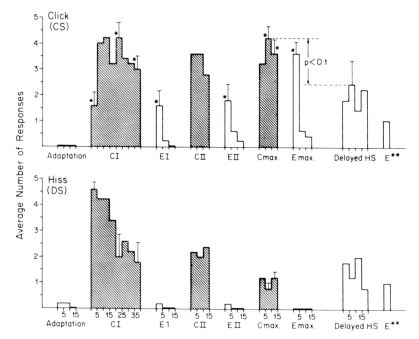

FIGURE 3. Establishment of discriminative response to the click CS over repeated conditioning sessions. Each bar represents the mean frequency of eyeblinks in the corresponding five-trial block averaged over five cats. Any EMG activity that was observed during the 580-msec period (equivalent to the CS–HS interval) following the two auditory stimuli that was distinguishably above the prestimulus baseline EMG activity was counted as "a response." CI and CII correspond, respectively, to the first and second conditioning sessions. The data shown in C_{max} were obtained from that later conditioning session in which the maximum frequency of eye blink CRs was noted. EI, EII, and E_{max} correspond to the extinction sessions given follwing the CI, CII, and C_{max} sessions, respectively. E** was the extinction session given after the "backward-delayed HS" session. Asterisks indicate the trial blocks in which the average number of eye blinks evoked by the click CS differed significantly from the average number of those elicited by the hiss DS (*t*-test, $p < .05$). Thin bars on the top represent standard error of the mean number of responses in these blocks. (From Kim *et al.,* 1983.)

conditioning, presentations of click CS and tap US (without HS) resulted in extinction of the blink responses conditioned by addition of HS.

Presentations of click, tap, and hiss (without associated HS) required many more pairings for the development of discriminative CRs than did pairings with associated HS presentations. Several days of training (totalling 700–1000 CS–US pairings) were required to reach 80% levels of CR performance (see Brons and Woody, 1980; Woody *et al.,* 1974).

Hypothalamic stimulation produced a facilitation of unconditioned eye blink response to glabella tap ipsilateral to the side of hypothalamic stimulation that was effective in accelerating conditioning. This is in agreement with earlier results of Murphy and Gellhorn (1945), which showed that hypothalamic stimulation could facilitate the production of limb movements elicited by electrical stimulation of the motor cortex in an "enduring" manner, as does repeated electrical stimulation of the motor cortex itself (Graham-Brown and Sherrington, 1912).

4. ELECTROPHYSIOLOGICAL RESULTS

4.1. Effects of Hypothalamic Stimulation on Cortical Unit Activity

Examples of the characteristic patterns of cortical unit discharge elicited by hypothalamic stimulation are shown in Fig. 4. Of 116 neurons studied, 26 responded with pattern A, 64 with pattern B, 13 with pattern C, and 13 with pattern D. Pattern A was characterized by short latency excitation followed by inhibition. Pattern B was characterized by short latency excitation followed by a sustained discharge. Pattern C was characterized by the late sustained discharge and pattern D by inhibition. Of the 26 neurons showing pattern A, 18 also showed long latency activation. Our results are in close agreement with those of Kita and Oomura (1981), who found that 71% of the neurons of the frontal cortex of rats responded to lateral hypothalamic stimulation with a short latency EPSP, as well as with earlier findings of Markevich and Voronin (1979), which indicated that the most typical short latency cortical response to stimulating the lateral hypothalamus was an EPSP–IPSP sequence. However, while the IPSP activity was conspicuous in intracellular recordings, the functional effect of the inhibition was not very pronounced, being of sufficient magnitude to produce conspicuous cessation of spike activity in but 11% of the neurons studied (cf. Woody et al., 1983; Kita and Oomura, 1981).

The pattern of cortical unit response to hypothalamic stimulation was predictive of loci of hypothalamic stimulation that were effective in producing enhanced rates of conditioned blinking. Different patterns of cortical unit activation were compared with hypothalamic stimulation that was (I) ineffective in producing CRs or sensitized responses, (II) effective in produced sensitized response, or (III) effective in producing conditioned and sensitized responses. As shown in Table I, there was a significant correlation between short latency activation of cortical units and rapid conditioning of an eye blink response. (For further analysis see Woody et al., 1983.) Many effective loci of stimulation were in or near the lateral hypothalamus (see Fig. 5). Electrodes placed in the internal capsule or the optic chiasm were ineffective in producing rapid conditioning even though they elicited unconditioned eye blinks.

4.2. Cortical Unit Activity during Rapid Conditioning

Recordings were made from neurons of the motor cortex during rapid eye blink conditioning and then during extinction and reconditioning of the blink CR. The patterns of activity of these neurons were found to be isomophic with the development, extinction, and reacquisition of the CR. Unit activity evoked by the click CS increased during conditioning, whereas activity evoked by the hiss DS did not. Averages are shown in Fig. 6. The increase in CS-evoked activity appeared shortly before or just at the time of behavioral acquisition of the CR. The latency

TABLE I. Different Patterns of
Response Elicited by Hypothalamic
Stimulation (HS) in Neurons of the
Coronal Pericruciate Cortex in Relation
to Different Behavioral Results
Observed during Conditioning[a,b]

Pattern	Group			
	I	II	III	Total
A	12	15	73	100
B	9	16	75	100
C	77	0	23	100
D	31	15	54	100

[a] For patterns A, B, C, D, see Fig. 4. See text (Section 4.1) for groups I, II, III. The values given are the percent of neurons that fell into that behavioral group out of the total number of cells showing that type of response pattern (A, B, C, or D).
[b] From Woody *et al.* (1983).

of activation of cortical units was comparable to that of production of the CR. Backward conditioning did not produce these effects (cf. Woody *et al.*, 1983).

5. DISCUSSION

5.1. Rapid Conditioning

It is interesting that eye blink conditioning that normally takes 1000 pairings of a click CS and glabella tap US can be accomplished in less than 20 pairings by adding electrical stimulation of the hypothalamus to paired presentations of the same CS and US. Given the complexity of the postulated underlying cellular mechanisms (Woody, 1982b), it is surprising that the conditioned reflex that develops so rapidly is discriminative within the same sensory modality, specific in that a highly selective motor response is acquired, and associative in its development. Forward pairings of the CS with both the US and HS are necessary for this rapid conditioning to occur.

Worth consideration is whether this phenomenon represents an acceleration of the normal conditioning process or, instead, a substitution of a different type of conditioned motor response from that produced by pairings of click CS and tap US alone. The possibility that a different motor response is conditioned arises because the latency (of response to the CS) of the rapidly conditioned eye blink response is longer than that of the response produced by conditioning with click and tap alone. If the rapidly acquired CR represents a different form of eye blink CR, there is still no clue as to how the type of motor response appropriate for substitution (an eye blink) would be selected from the entire repertoire of motor performance available to the organism. The CR that is acquired is the homolog of the uncon-

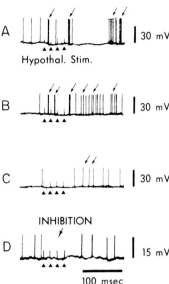

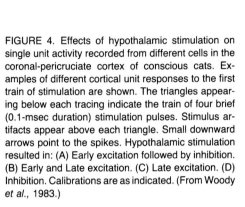

FIGURE 4. Effects of hypothalamic stimulation on single unit activity recorded from different cells in the coronal-pericruciate cortex of conscious cats. Examples of different cortical unit responses to the first train of stimulation are shown. The triangles appearing below each tracing indicate the train of four brief (0.1-msec duration) stimulation pulses. Stimulus artifacts appear above each triangle. Small downward arrows point to the spikes. Hypothalamic stimulation resulted in: (A) Early excitation followed by inhibition. (B) Early and Late excitation. (C) Late excitation. (D) Inhibition. Calibrations are as indicated. (From Woody et al., 1983.)

ditioned response to the tap US and not the homolog of the unconditioned response to HS. The fact that the ISIs between CS, US, *and* HS (340 and 240 msec) are comparable to those found optimal for many other forms of Pavlovian conditioning (cf. Table 3.1 in Woody, 1982b) and the failure of backwards presentation of HS to produce conditioned blinking suggest an acceleration of at least some part of the normal conditioning process.

Because hypothalamic stimulation produced a pronounced unconditioned eye blink, one might have assumed that strong activation of the eye blink musculature was the important factor for the rapid development of eye blink CRs. One notes, however, that stimulation of the internal capsule or the optic chiasm (which produced even larger unconditioned eye blink responses) did not lead to the production of conditioned eye blinks after 250 pairing trials (Kim *et al.*, 1983). In fact, contraction of peripheral muscles is not necessary for the acquisition of conventional eye blink conditioning (Beck and Doty, 1957; Crow and Woody, 1973). Evidently, muscle contraction is also not the crucial factor for accelerating the rates of acquisition of conditioned blinking by addings HS to click and glabella tap.

Previous studies have shown that some hypothalamic areas are positively reinforcing or rewarding when stimulated electrically, while others are negatively reinforcing or punishing. Reports of Voronin and colleagues (Voronin, 1974; Voronin *et al.*, 1975) of rapid conditioning using HS (though of conditioning that was not discriminative within the same sensory modality as the CS) indicated that their HS was rewarding since their animals would self-stimulate to receive the HS. One might therefore attribute the enhanced rapidity of acquisition of conditioning to a motivational effect of HS (cf., Voronin, 1974) or to an increased alertness or arousal.

Neither need be so. In our experiments the animals did not appear to find the

★ Most effective

• Effective

▲ Ineffective

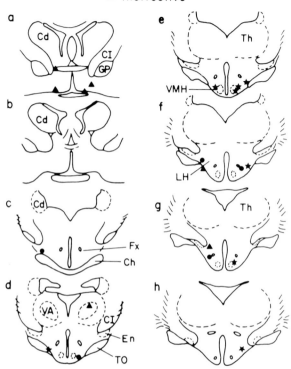

FIGURE 5. Loci of brain stimulation used in the present study. Filled stars represent hypothalamic sites, stimulation of which produced rapid acquisition of discriminative eye blink CRs at
over 90% performance level. The sites of stimulation that resulted in discriminative CRs being
performed less consistently are represented by filled circles. Behaviorally ineffective sites of
stimulation are indicated by filled triangles. Loci were determined from postmortem examination
of electrolytic lesions made at the locus of stimulation. Abbreviations: Cd, caudate nucleus; Ch,
optic chiasm; CI, interal capsule; FX, fornix; GP, globus pallidus; LH, lateral hypothalamus; Th,
thalamus; TO, optic tract; VMH, ventromedial hypothalamic nucleus. (From Woody *et al.,* 1983.)

HS noxious, but when tested in a shuttle box (Berthier *et al.,* 1982), instead of
seeking self-stimulation, they performed in such a way as to avoid receiving the
kinds of hypothalamic stimulation that produced rapid, discriminative conditioning.
Thus, a neurochemical effect not "motivational" in the rewarding sense, nor necessarily even in the punishing sense, may provide a basis for the processes underlying
rapid conditioning.

Arousal would not have been expected to facilitate discriminative elicitation
of an associatively conditioned response, nor to produce associative development
of a predominantly unilateral conditioned motor response. If the CRs were acquired
rapidly due to an increase in alertness, the blink responses should have been observed

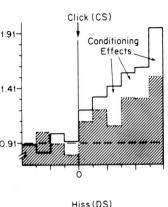

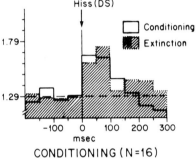

FIGURE 6. Averaged responses to click CS and hiss DS in 16 single units recorded from the coronal pericruciate cortex of four awake cats. The results from conditioning and extinction sessions are superimposed in the figure, with those from extinction denoted by shading. The auditory stimuli were given at time 0. The height of each bin represents the mean frequency of firing per each 50 msec time block. During conditioning and extinction, the mean prestimulus baseline activity (per 50 msec) was determined for the 200-msec period preceding the onset of each stimulus and that for conditioning is indicated by the dashed horizontal lines. For purposes of comparison, the extinction data were normalized relative to the same baseline activities (and ordinate scale increments) as the data from conditioning. (The ordinate shows the baseline for conditioning.) The mean pre-CS and pre-HS baseline activities during extinction were 0.93 and 0.91 impulses per 50 msec, respectively. Data were analyzed for a period of 300 msec after the click. (During conditioning, the US and HS were delivered 340 and 580 msec, respectively, after CS onset.) (From Woody et al., 1983.)

equally on both sides. In addition, a mechanism depending simply on increased alertness should have facilitated conditioning during the backward HS paradigm. With that paradigm, however, discriminative CRs failed to develop. Increased alertness may have contributed to the sensitization that appeared early during conditioning and during the backward HS paradigm. As shown in Fig. 3, this sensitization was readily distinguished from discriminative conditioning.

Effects of HS may have been expressed through activation of fibers *en passage* rather than through activation of local hypothalamic circuitry. Stimulation of several other hypothalamic regions besides the lateral hypothalamus was shown to be effective in producing rapid conditioning (Fig. 5).

The predictive value of short latency cortical activation by HS in determining loci of HS that would be effective in accelerating conditioning suggested that neurotransmission properties at the terminations of axons on these cortical cells might be an important factor in mechanisms supporting rapid conditioning.

5.2. Neural Mechanisms of Conditioning

5.2.1. Classical Eye Blink Conditioning

Earlier evidence (see Brons and Woody, 1980; Woody and Black-Cleworth, 1973; Woody et al., 1976) indicates that neural mechanisms supporting classical Pavlovian eye blink conditioning may be separated into at least two different types:

one found to support learned motor performance, the other found to support discrimination of the CS from the DS. Nonassociatively induced increases in postsynaptic neural excitability in cells of the motor cortex and facial nucleus appear to support the acquisition of the learned motor response (Brons and Woody, 1980; Matsumura and Woody, 1982). An increased input resistance resulting from a decreased potassium conductance may underlie the increased excitability to injected current that is found in neurons of these regions after conditioning and after presentations of US alone (Brons and Woody, 1980; Woody and Black-Cleworth, 1973; Woody and Wong, 1981). An increased excitability of neurons of the motor cortex and facial nucleus may produce a latent facilitation of subsequently conditioned eyeblink responses (Matsumura and Woody, 1982; Woody, 1982a), as well as the motor component of the enduring response produced by CS–US conditioning. Further details are given elsewhere (Brons and Woody, 1980; Brons *et al.,* 1982; Woody, 1982b; Woody, 1982c; Woody, 1984).

Other neuronal changes in more caudal cortical sensory association areas and other sensory receptive areas of the brain will help the central nervous system distinguish those incoming stimuli that should evoke the conditioned response from those that should not. Changes in neural excitability of this type facilitate spike production in response to the CS, but not to the DS, and are induced associatively (see Woody *et al.,* 1976; Woody, 1984). Given two different mechanisms supporting different features of conditioning, one mechanism might be expected to act more rapidly than the other. Accelerating the development of conditioning may simply require increasing the rate of the slower mechanism. It remains to be determined if the cellular mechanism governing the rate of acquisition of latent facilitation of motor performance can be accelerated by hypothalamic stimulation and if this can result in accelerated acquisition of discriminative conditioning.

5.3. Mechanisms of Rapid Conditioning

Our current attempts to identify the cellular mechanism(s) involved in enhancing the speed of conditioning are based on the postulate that HS potentiates the change in excitability in cells of the motor cortex and facial nucleus that underlies latent facilitation of the eye blink reflex. The responses to L-glutamate and acetylcholine are being studied in cortical cells that respond to hypothalamic stimulation with short latency discharge. In some cells, extracellularly applied L-glutamic acid diethylester suppresses this response to hypothalamic stimulation as well as the response to glutamate (Cooper and Woody, 1983). It is possible that glutamate, aspartate, or one of their related compounds is the agent released by stimulating fibers within the hypothalamus that project (probably polysynaptically) to these cortical cells. The release of glutamate at the synaptic terminals of cholinoceptive cortical neurons may potentiate the mechanism underlying latent facilitation.

A number of investigators have shown that cortical pyramidal tract (PT) cells are cholinoceptive (Crawford and Curtis, 1966; Krnjevic and Phillis, 1963). In the cat all PT cells of the motor cortex with somas identified by injection of HRP have been found to be layer V pyramidal neurons (Sakai and Woody, 1980). These cells are preferentially activated at short latencies by click stimuli similar to those used as CSs for short-latency eye blink conditioning (cf. Engel and Woody, 1972; Sakai and Woody, 1980), and regions of cortex containing the layer V PT cells are necessary for development of the classically conditioned eye blink response by pairing click CS with glabella tap US (Woody et al., 1974).

We have shown that long-lasting increases in input resistance can be produced in these cells by applying acetylcholine (ACh) extracellularly, while simultaneously delivering sufficient depolarizing current intracellularly to produce a sustained spike discharge (Woody et al., 1978). This increase in resistance persists for as long as the internal recording can be maintained. Its development can be blocked by extracellular application of atropine prior to administering ACh (Swartz and Woody, 1979). Comparable increases in resistance can be produced by substituting intracellular application of cyclic GMP for extracellular application of ACh.

Depolarization-induced discharge also plays a critical role in the development of associatively induced photophobic responses in *Hermissenda* (See Alkon, Chapter 1, this volume). There, a membrane phosphorylation, which appears to control changes in potassium conductance (an A current), can be related to the action of calcium entry on a calcium–calmodulin–dependent protein kinase. The calcium entry is induced by depolarization (Alkon et al., 1982; Connor and Alkon, 1982; Acosta-Urquidi et al., 1983).

Hori, Carpenter, and colleagues (Hori et al., 1981) have recently shown that effects of glutamate and acetylcholine on postsynaptic membrane properties can be mutually potentiating. This has been demonstrated in pyramidal neurons of the prepyriform cortex. Perhaps a comparable potentiation can occur in the pyramidal cells of the motor cortex. If so, an acceleration of the change in membrane property thought to underlie latent facilitation might be produced.

6. SUMMARY

We recently found that the number of pairings of click (CS) and glabella tap (US) needed to produce eye blink conditioning could be reduced from 1000 (Woody et al., 1974) to less than 20 by adding electrical stimulation of the hypothalamus (HS) 580 msec after the CS (Kim et al., 1983). The CRs were produced discriminatively to the CS and not to a hiss DS of comparable intensity. The CRs were produced associatively, their emergence depending on the order of CS, US, and HS presentations. The onset latencies of the major blink responses to the CS, measured electromyographically, ranged between 80 and 320 msec. The CRs were extinguished when click CSs and hiss DSs were presented alone.

The effect of HS was location dependent within the hypothalamus. Not every locus of hypothalamic stimulation produced accelerated rates of conditioning. Acceleration of conditioning was not seen with stimulation of the internal capsule or the optic chiasm, which produced a pronounced unconditioned eye blink response.

Patterns of unit activity recorded from the motor cortex were isomorphic with the development and extinction of the conditioned blink response. Intracellular recordings obtained from awake cats during these procedures indicated that the major effects of HS on the activity of cells in the motor cortex were 1) early excitation, 2) inhibition, and 3) late excitation. Short latency activation of layer V cortical pyramidal cells by HS was predictive of loci of hypothalamic stimulation that would accelerate conditioning (Woody *et al.*, 1983).

These findings are discussed in the context of current knowledge of cellular mechanisms of conditioning. The rapidly acquired eye blink CR affords a useful model for studying such mechanisms, intracellularly, in mammals during the development of associative conditioning.

ACKNOWLEDGMENTS. Supported by AFOSR F49620-85-C-0100, NINCDS HD 05958, and NSF BNS 78-24146.

REFERENCES

Acosta-Urquidi, J., Alkon, D.L., Connor, J.A., and Neary, J.T. 1983, Intracellular injection of a Ca^{++}-dependent protein kinase amplifies Ca^{++}-mediated inactivation of a transient K^+ current (I_A) in *Hermissenda* giant neurons, *Soc. Neurosci. Abstr.* **9**:501.

Alkon, D.L., Shoukimas, J., and Heldman, E., 1982, Calcium-mediated decrease of a voltage-dependent potassium current, *Biophys. J.* **40**:245–250.

Beck, E.C. and Doty, R.W., 1957, Conditioned flexion reflexes acquired during combined catalepsy and de-efferentation, *J. Comp. Physiol. Psychol.* **20**:211–216.

Berthier, N.E., Betts, B., and Woody, C.D., 1982, Discriminative conditioning of eyeblink with aversive brain stimulation, *Soc. Neurosci. Abstr.* **8**:1014.

Brons, J.F. and Woody, C.D., 1980, Long-term changes in excitability of cortical neurons after Pavlovian conditioning and extinction, *J. Neurophysiol.* **44**:605–615.

Brons, J., Woody, C.D., and Allon, N., 1982, Changes in the excitability to weak intensity electrical stimulation of units of the pericruciate cortex in cats, *J. Neurophysiol.* **47**:377–388.

Connor, J.A. and Alkon, D.L., 1982, Light-induced changes of intracellular Ca^{++} in *Hermissenda* photoreceptors measured with Arsenazo III, *Soc. Neurosci. Abstr.* **8**:944.

Cooper, P.H. and Woody, C.D., 1983, Effects of L-glutamate and L-glutamic acid diethyl ester (GDEE) on the response of cortical units to hypothalamic stimulation, *Soc. Neurosci. Abstr.* **9**:330.

Crawford, J.M. and Curtis, D.R., 1966, Pharmacological studies on feline Betz cells, *J. Physiol. (London)* **186**:121–138.

Crow, T.J. and Woody, C.D. 1973, Acquisition of a conditioned eyeblink response during reversible denervation of orbicularis oculi muscles in the cat, *Brain Res.* **64**:414–418.

Engel, J., Jr. and Woody, C.D., 1972, Effects of character and significance of stimulus on unit activity at coronal-pericruciate cortex of cat during performance of conditioned motor responses, *J. Neurophysiol.* **35**:220–229.

Gormezano, I., 1972, Investigations of defense and reward conditioning in the rabbit, in: *Classical Conditioning II. Current Research and Theory* (A.H. Black and W.F. Prokasy, eds.), Appleton-Century-Crofts, New York, pp. 151–181.

Graham-Brown, T. and Sherrington, C.S., 1912, On the instability of a cortical point, *Proc. R. Soc. B* **85**:250–277.

Hori, N., Auker, C.R., Braitman, D.T., and Carpenter, D.O., 1981, Lateral olfactory tract transmitter: glutamate, asparate, or neither?, *Cell. Molec. Neurobiol.* **1**:115–120.

Kim, E.H.-J., Woody, C.D., and Berthier, N.E., 1983, Rapid acquisition of conditioned eye-blink responses in cats following pairing of an auditory CS with a glabella-tap US and hypothalamic stimulation, *J. Neurophysiol.* **49**:767–779.

Kita, H. and Oomura, Y., 1981, Reciprocal connections between the lateral hypothalamus and the frontal cortex in the rat: Electrophysiological and anatomical observations, *Brain Res.* **213**:1–16.

Krnjevic, K. and Phillis, J.W., 1963, Acetylcholine-sensitive cells in the cerebral cortex, *J. Physiol. (London)* **166**:296–327.

Markevich, V.A. and Voronin, L.L., 1979, Synaptic responses of sensomotor cortical neurons to stimulation of emotionally significant brain structures, *Zhurnal Vysshei Nervnoi Deyatal' nosti* **29**:1248–1257 (*Neurosci. Behav. Physiol.* **12**:29–37, 1982).

Matsumura, M. and Woody, C.D., 1982, Excitability changes of facial motoneurons of cats related to conditioned and unconditioned facial motor responses, in: *Conditioning: Representation of Involved Neural Functions* (C.D. Woody, ed.), Plenum Press, New York, pp. 451–458.

Murphy, J.P. and Gellhorn, E., 1945, The influence of hypothalamic stimulation on cortically induced movements and on action potentials of the cortex, *J. Neurophysiol.* **8**:341–364.

Sakai, H. and Woody, C.D., 1980, Identification of auditory responsive cells in coronal-pericruciate cortex of awake cats, *J. Neurophysiol.* **44**:223–231.

Sakurai, Y., and Hirano, T., 1983, Multiple unit response in reward areas during operant conditioning reinforced by lateral hypothalamic stimulation in the rat, *Behav. Brain Res.* **8**:33–48.

Swartz, B.E., and Woody, C.D., 1979, Correlated effects of acetylcholine and cyclic guanosine monophosphate on membrane properties of mammalian neocortical neurons, *J. Neurobiol.* **10**:465–468.

Voronin, L.L., 1974, A study of neurophysiological mechanisms of learning on a simple behavioral model, *Proc. Int. Union Physiolog. Sci.* **10**:79–80.

Voronin, L.L., Gerstein, G., Kudriashov, I.E., and Ioffe, S.V., 1975, Elaboration of a conditioned reflex in a single experiment with simultaneous recording of neural activity, *Brain Res.* **92**:385–403.

Woody, C.D., 1974, Aspects of the electrophysiology of cortical processes related to the development and performance of learned motor performance, *Physiologist* **17**:49–69.

Woody, C.D., 1982a, Acquisition of conditioned facial reflexes in the cat: cortical control of different facial movements, *Fed. Proc.* **41**:2160–2168

Woody, C.D., 1982b, *Memory, Learning, and Higher Function: A Cellular View,* 1st ed., Springer-Verlag, New York.

Woody, C.D., 1982c, Neurophysiologic correlates of latent facilitation, in: *Conditioning: Representation of Involved Functions* (C.D. Woody, ed.), Plenum Press, New York, pp. 233–248.

Woody, C.D., 1984, The electrical excitability of nerve cells as an index of learned behavior, in: *Primary Neural Substrates of Learning and Behavioral Change* (D. Alkon and J. Farley, eds.), Cambridge University Press, Cambridge, pp. 101–127.

Woody, C.D. and Black-Cleworth, F., 1973, Differences in excitability of cortical neurons as a function of motor projection in conditioned cats, *J. Neurophysiol.* **36**:1104–1116.

Woody, C.D. and Brozek, G., 1969, Changes in evoked responses from facial nucleus of cat with conditioning and extinction of an eye blink, *J. Neurophysiol.* **37**:717–726.

Woody, C.D. and Engel, J., Jr., 1972, Changes in unit activity and thresholds to electrical microstimulation at coronal-pericruciate cortex of cat with classical conditioning of different facial movements, *J. Neurophysiol.* **35**:230–241.

Woody, C.D. and Wong, B., 1981, Intracellular recording of potassium in neurons of the motor cortex of awake cats following extracellular applications of acetylcholine, in: *Ion-Selective Microelectrodes and Their Use in Excitable Tissues* (E. Sykova, P. Hnik, and L. Vyklicky, eds.), Plenum Press, New York, pp. 125–131.

Woody, C., Yarowsky, P., Owens, J., Black-Cleworth, P., and Crow, T., 1974, Effect of lesions of cortical motor areas on acquisition of conditioned eye blink in the cat, *J. Neurophysiol.* **37**:385–394.

Woody, C.D., Knispel, J.D., Crow, T.J., and Black-Cleworth, P.A, 1976, Activity and excitability to electrical current of cortical auditory receptive neurons of awake cats as affected by stimulus association, *J. Neurophysiol.* **39**:1045–1061.

Woody, C.D., Swartz, B.E., and Gruen, E., 1978, Effects of acetylcholine and cyclic GMP on input resistance of cortical neurons in awake cats, *Brain Res.* **158**:373–395.

Woody, C.D., Kim, E.H.-J., and Berthier, N.E., 1983, Effects of hypothalamic stimulation on conditioned and unconditioned unit responses recorded from neurons of the sensorimotor cortex of awake cats. *J. Neurophysiol.* **49**:780–791.

9

Neuronal Mechanisms Underlying Plastic Postural Changes in Decerebrate, Reflexively Standing Cats

SHIGEMI MORI, TAKASHI SAKAMOTO, and YOSHIHIRO OHTA

1. INTRODUCTION

Our previous studies (Mori *et al.*, 1980a, 1982) have demonstrated brain stem areas subserving "setting" and "resetting" of the extensor muscle tone related to the reflex standing posture in acute precollicular-postmammillary decerebrate (mesencephalic) cats. Stimulation of the dorsal part of the caudal tegmental field (DTF) along the midline (Horsley-Clarke coordinates P3 to P7, H-4.5 to H-6) decreased the tone of the hindlimb muscles, with the force through the hindlimb and the tonic discharge of extensor muscles decreasing. Stimulation of the ventral part of the caudal tegmental field (VTF) along the midline area (P3 to P7, H-7.5 to H-9.5) increased the tone of the hindlimb muscles, with the force through the hindlimb and the tonic discharge of extensor muscles increasing.

In this chapter, the neuronal mechanisms for setting and resetting of extensor tone related to standing posture are discussed. We demonstrate that graded and long-lasting suppression of extensor muscle tone manifests itself in a long-lasting excitability suppression of alpha motoneurons (MNs) innervating hindlimb extensor muscles. We will also present evidence suggesting that DTF activation produces two types of inhibitory action upon alpha MNs innervating the soleus muscle. During DTF stimulation, postsynaptic inhibition plays a major role in terminating the tonic discharge of the cells along with the hyperpolarization of membrane potential, and

---

SHIGEMI MORI, TAKASHI SAKAMOTO, and YOSHIHIRO OHTA ● Department of Physiology, Asahikawa Medical College, Asahikawa, Hokkaido, Japan 078-11.

withdrawal of excitatory bombardment upon the cells by way of group Ia fibers, that is, disfacilitation, plays a major role in the subsequent suppression of moto-neuronal excitability that outlasts stimulation. This evidence was obtained from recent experimental studies (Atsuta *et al.*, 1985; Sakamoto *et al.*, in press).

2. METHODS

Experimental procedures were similar to those described previously (Mori *et al.*, 1980a,b, 1982). After surgical decerebration, the head of the animal was fixed in a stereotaxic instrument and the limbs placed on force transducers, the body being supported by a rubber hammock (see Fig. 1A). During such standing, the force exerted by each of the hindlimbs was measured by a force transducer placed underneath the foot. The force thus recorded was considered to represent the degree of hindlimb muscle tone (Mori *et al.*, 1982). In many of these decerebrate animals, extensor rigidity in the hindlimb was so well developed that when the animal was kept in a standing position, the hindlimbs could support the body weight almost without the aid of the rubber hammock (Mori *et al.*, 1983).

Glass microelectrodes filled with Woods metal, of which the tip was plated with platinum (Gesteland *et al.*, 1959), were used for stimulation of the DTF and the VTF areas. The stimuli consisted of 10- to 60-μA pulses of 0.2 msec duration and 50 pulses/sec rate that lasted 5–10 sec. The locations of electrode tips were confirmed by later histological examination and defined with reference to the stereotaxic atlases of Berman (1968) and Snider and Niemer (1961).

In a different group of animals, neuronal elements contributing to stretch reflexes such as alpha MNs, Renshaw cells, and group Ia and group Ib fibers were identified, and their activities were analysed in relation to the level of extensor muscle tone developed in the hindlimbs. To do this, the head and the vertebrae of the thoracic and lumbar segments were fixed in a stereotaxic instrument (Fig. 1D). In order to identify the spinal neuronal elements innervating the soleus muscle, bipolar electrodes made of thin (50 μm) stainless steel wires were implanted both for recording the electromyogram (EMG) and for stimulating the nerve endings within this muscle while maintaining the dorsal and the ventral roots intact (Atsuta *et al.*, 1985). The recording of neuronal activities was performed by means of bevelled micropipettes filled with 2 M potassium citrate. Alpha MNs were identified intracellularly by the conventional criteria (Brock *et al.*, 1953; Lipski, 1981). Renshaw cells were recorded extracellularly (Eccles *et al.*, 1954, 1961b; Renshaw, 1941, 1946). Group Ia and Ib fibers were impaled at the entry zone of L7 to S1 dorsal roots and were also identified according to the conventional criteria (Cameron *et al.*, 1981; Houk and Henneman, 1967; Houk and Rymer, 1981; Matthews, 1981).

In the last group of animals, attempts were made to study the cells of origin that projected their axons to the DTF area (Ohta *et al.*, 1984). To do this, double-barreled microelectrodes were employed, one made of a stimulating electrode filled with Woods metal, and the other made of a HRP-filled injecting micropipette. The HRP micropipette was filled with a mixture of 0.2 M NaCl and 10% HRP (Toyobo Grade I-C) in 0.1 M phosphate buffer at pH 7.6. The diameter of each micropipette

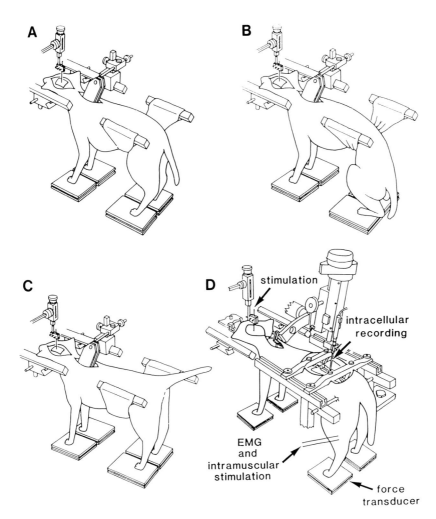

FIGURE 1. Decerebrate, reflexively standing posture. (A) Before stimulation; (B) after DTF stimulation (stimulus site, P5.5, LR0, H-4.5; stimulus strength, 40 μA); (C) after VTF stimulation (stimulus site, P5.5, LR0, H-9.5; stimulus strength, 40 μA);(D) experimental set-up for intra- and extracellular recording from spinal neuronal elements and for stimulating nerve endings within the soleus muscle.

was approximately 10 μm and the resistance was 0.3 and 10 MΩ for the stimulating electrode and for the injecting micropipette, respectively, HRP was passed from the injecting micropipette to a micro-lesioned site within the DTF area, by applying depolarizing current pulses of 5–10 μA for 400 msec of every 500 msec for 30 min. Following a survival time of 2 days, the animals were killed by cardiac perfusion, under pentobartital anesthesia, with a fixative containing 2% paraformaldehyde/0.5% glutaraldehyde in 0.1 M phosphate buffer at pH 7.4.

3. RESULTS

3.1. Plastic Postural Changes

Stimulation of the DTF area resulted in a decrease in the level of extensor muscle tone not only during the period of this stimulation but also during the period in which this stimulation was terminated. Behaviorally, the activity of extensor muscle tone was not strong enough to counteract the weight of the body, and the animal maintained a standing posture only passively with the aid of the rubber hammock (Fig. 1B). In contrast, stimulation of the VTF area resulted in an increase in the level of extensor muscle tone not only during the period of this stimulation but also during the period in which this stimulation was terminated. Behaviorally, the animal started to stand up with the beginning of this stimulation and maintained a standing posture without the aid of the rubber hammock during the period of increased force level (Fig. 1C).

The results in Fig. 2 represent a typical experiment in which the force and the EMG changes were elicited by a series of stimuli delivered to effective midline structures of the pons. Initially, periods of stimulation were delivered successively to the effective DTF area, resulting in a graded decrease of bilateral force levels. Then, the effective VTF area was stimulated successively. Following each stimulation period the force level increased in a staircase manner. After restoring the force to the original level the effective DTF and VTF areas were again stimulated alternately with a high intensity, which resulted in a "setting" and "resetting" of the force to the minimum and the maximum of the preceding levels. The discharges of extensor muscles were suppressed or augmented in parallel with the force changes (Mori *et al.*, 1982, 1983).

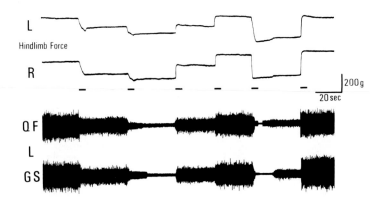

FIGURE 2. Setting and resetting of levels of hindlimb force. EMGs were recorded simultaneously with the force changes. Initial prestimulus levels of hindlimb forces were 0.43 kg for the left (L) and 0.45 kg for the right (R). DTF and VTF stimulations were delivered during periods indicated by bars under the force records (5.0 sec). Stimulus parameters: 30 μA for the first four sequences and 60 μA for the last two sequences. GS, gastrocnemius-soleus muscle; QF, quadriceps femoris muscle. Stimulus sites of inhibitory and facilitatory areas were P6.0, LR0, H-5.0, and P6.0, LR0, H-8.0. (From Mori *et al.*, 1982).

As will be found from such force records, the postural changes induced by stimulating the DTF and the VTF areas outlasted the periods of stimulation. Furthermore, the degree of decrease and increase in force levels changed depending on the stimulus intensity employed. All these results seemed to indicate that there existed neuronal structures within the brain stem that were capable of eliciting "plastic postural changes" in decerebrate, reflexively standing cats.

3.2. Neural Substrates of the Effective DTF and VTF Areas

The locations of the electrolytic lesions made in the DTF and the VTF areas were plotted on schematic drawings of the pontine brain stem (Fig. 3).

Careful histological examination of these electrolytic lesions indicated that the effective DTF area corresponded to the caudal portion of the nucleus centralis superior, where there were few cell bodies (Mori *et al.*, 1982). Therefore, it is possible that the effect was mediated by the fibers that cross at the level of the

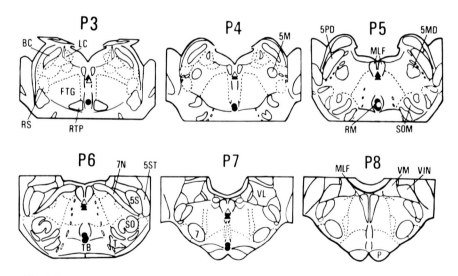

FIGURE 3. Representative locations of electrode tips identified by lesions made during experiments. Electrolytic lesions obtained from 20 animals were pooled. In a few animals, several lesions were made in a single experiment both in the effective DTF and the VTF regions. Triangles represent the effective DTF sites and each filled triangle is based on a single experiment. Open triangles represent eletrolytic lesions made sequentially in one animal. Circles represent effective VTF regions and each filled circle is based on a single experiment. The open triangles and the open circles were obtained from the same experiment. 5M, motor trigeminal nucleus; 5MD, motor trigeminal nucleus, dorsal division; 5PD, principal sensory trigeminal nucleus; 5ST, spinal trigeminal tract; 7, facial nucleus; 7N, facial nerve; 5S, sensory trigeminal nucleus; BC, brachium conjunctivum; FTG, gigantocellular tegmental field; LC, locus coeruleus; MLF, medial longitudinal fasciculus; P, pyramis; RM, nucleus raphe magnus; RS, rubrospinal tract; RTP, nucleus reticularis tegmenti pontis; SO, superior olive; SOM, medial nucleus of superior olive; T, nucleus of the trapezoid body; TB, trapezoid body; VIN, inferior vestibular nucleus; VM, medial vestibular nucleus; VL, lateral vestibular nucleus. (From Mori *et al.*, 1982).

nucleus centralis superior (Sakai *et al.*, 1977, 1979; Walberg, 1974). These fibers may activate the nucleus locus coeruleus, which could influence the spinal cord through its projections to the "medullary inhibitory" center of Magoun (Magoun and Rhines, 1946; Sakai *et al.*, 1984) or through its direct projection to the spinal cord via the coerulospinal pathway (Holstege and Kuypers, 1982; Kuypers and Maisky, 1975). It is also possible that we activated the bilateral tegmento reticular inhibitory tract (Sakai *et al.*, 1979, 1984).

The effective VTF area corresponded to the rostral portion of the nucleus raphe magnus (Mori *et al.*, 1982). This nucleus has been shown to send axons to the spinal cord (Kuypers and Maisky, 1975).

In order to study the possibility that we were stimulating passing fibers at the levels of the nucleus centralis superior, we injected HRP into the effective DTF area after making a microlesion there (Ohta *et al.*, 1984). With this method, we found that many cells in the dorsolateral tegmental area, including those with nucleus locus coeruleus (1 and 2 in Fig. 4A), in the pontine reticular formation, (4 in Fig. 4A), and in the medullary reticular formation (6 in Fig. 4A), were labeled. Searching for the putative descending pathways mediating DTF stimulus effects to the spinal cord, we also attempted to test whether cells activated by a single DTF stimulation could be activated or not by stimulating the spinal cord at the level of T12.

A representative result is shown in Fig. 4B. This neuron in the medial pontine reticular formation (P3, L1, H-6.6) was activated by stimulating the DTF area (P5, LR0, H-5.5), and it was also activated antidromically by stimulating the spinal cord. In contrast to the fixed latency from the spinal cord stimulation to the onset of antidromic spike potential, there was a jitter in the spike potential when the DTF area was stimulated. Such results suggest that either axon collaterals of this cell or the dendrites of this cell were activated by this stimulation. Conduction velocities of presumed axon collaterals and the descending axons were estimated to be about 5.6 m/sec and 101.9 m/sec, respectively.

We also made lesions at the level of T12 to interrupt descending pathways. Dorsal hemisection of the spinal cord did not abolish the DTF stimulus effects, but

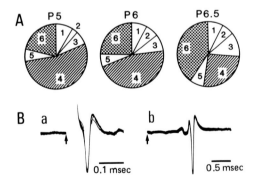

FIGURE 4. (A) Relative distributions of HRP-labeled neurons in the brain stem in three preparations (HRP-injected sites, P5, P6, and P6.5). 1, LC complex; 2, dorsolateral pontine tegmentum excluding LC complex; 3, central grey area; 4, pontin reticular formation (RF); 5, raphe complex; 6, medullary RF. Total numbers of labeled neurons: 188, 872, and 213 for the three preparations; in them, microlesions were made at the levels of P5, P6, and P6.5, respectively. (B) Orthodromic (a) and antidromic (b) activation of a pontine reticular neuron. Ten sweeps were superimposed. Stimulus site: P5.0, LR0, H-5.5 for the DTF, and T12 for the spinal cord. Stimulus frequency was 1 Hz. Recording site: P3.0, L1.0, H-6.6. Arrows represent the onsets of DTF and spinal cord stimulation.

additional lesion of the ventrolateral funiculus was effective in reducing the stimulus effects considerably. It has been shown that the ventral reticulospinal tract and the coerulospinal tract descend via the ventrolateral funiculus (Holstege and Kuypers, 1982; Jankowska *et al.*, 1968). It has also been shown that the ventral reticulospinal tract inhibits transmission from primary afferents to primary afferent terminals at an interneuronal level (Engberg *et al.*, 1968a,b) and that projections from the nucleus locus coeruleus exert inhibitory effects upon target cells (Amaral and Sinnamon, 1977; Foote *et al.*, 1983; Moore and Bloom, 1979). It is therefore plausible that the inhibitory effects are mediated by the ventral reticulospinal tract and the coerulospinal tract, but such a proposition does not necessarily rule out participation of other descending inhibitory pathways.

3.3. DTF-Elicited Suppression of Excitabilities in Alpha MNs, Renshaw Cells, and Group Ia and Group Ib Fibers

3.3.1. Alpha MNs

The records illustrated in Fig. 5A compare the time course of the changes in the soleus EMG with that of the intracellular activity of alpha MNs innervating the same muscle. The beginning of DTF stimulation was indicated by an upward arrow. During the prestimulus period, the force level was about 0.42 kg and vigorous EMG activity was recorded. Simultaneously recorded intracellular activity showed that this cell discharged tonically with a firing frequency of about 15 spikes/sec. With the beginning of DTF stimulation, interspike intervals of this cell gradually became more prolonged, and within about 1.1 sec after the onset of DTF stimulation, this cell ceased to fire. At this moment, the force level decreased to about 0.38 kg. Tonic activity of the soleus muscle was gradually suppressed during the period of DTF stimulation and was terminated within about 4.0 sec after the onset of DTF stimulation. The change in the firing frequencies of this cell in relation to various force levels is plotted in Fig. 5C (closed triangles).

The records illustrated in Fig. 5B were obtained from the same animal. Prestimulus force level was about 0.18 kg, and tonic discharges of three identifiable motor units were simultaneously recorded. Careful comparison of each intracellularly recorded spike with each motor unit activation showed that the activity of the motor unit with the smallest aplitude was phase-locked with that of the impaled cell. During the prestimulus period this cell discharged with a firing frequency of about 14 spikes/sec, and during the initial period of DTF stimulation it continued to fire for another 3.5 sec with almost the same firing frequency. After this period, however, the cell had gradually prolonged interspike intervals and finally ceased to fire about 7.0 sec after the onset of DTF stimulation. At this moment, the force level approached 0.12 kg. The change in the firing frequencies of this cell is plotted in Fig. 5C (closed circles).

It will also be seen that the motor unit with the largest amplitude was the first unit to terminate its tonic discharge after the onset of DTF stimulation. As shown in the records in Fig. 5B, it was sometimes possible to record tonic discharges of identifiable motor units. Therefore, we plotted the changes in the firing frequencies

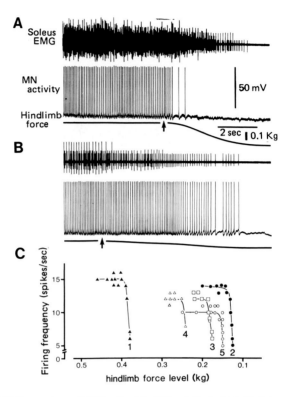

FIGURE 5. (A,B) Comparison of EMG with alpha MN activity. Left hindlimb force was recorded simultaneously with EMG and alpha MN activity. Arrows indicate the beginning of DTF stimulations. Stimulus parameters: 30 μA for (A), 10 μA for (B). (C) Relations between the firing frequencies of five alpha MNs and hindlimb force. Results were obtained from a single animal. Closed symbols represent intracellular MN activities. Open symbols represent motor unit activities. Unit 3 represents the larget amplitude motor unit in (B).

of identifiable motor units in relation to the various levels of hindlimb forces in Fig. 5C (open symbols). From such plots, it will be seen that each cell and each motor unit maintained tonic discharge with a relatively constant firing frequency when the level of hindlimb forces were within certain ranges. The critical level of hindlimb force at which each unit ceased to fire differed depending on the unit. Such results indicate that setting of extensor muscle tone is accomplished by a decrease in the firing frequency of individual alpha MNs and by derecruitment.

3.3.2. Renshaw Cells

Extracellularly recorded activity of Renshaw cells was correlated with the levels of hindlimb force in a similar manner as in alpha MNs. It was found that Renshaw cells discharge tonically with various frequencies depending on the level of hindlimb force. The smaller the prestimulus force level, the lower the firing frequency. As is shown in Fig. 6A, the firing frequency of Renshaw cells tended to be suppressed

FIGURE 6. (A) Setting of levels of hindlimb force and changes in the firing frequency of a Renshaw cell. Renshaw cell activity was recorded simultaneously with the force changes in the left hindlimb. Initial prestimulus level of hindlimb force was 0.37 kg (a). DTF stimulations were delivered during the periods indicated by bars under the force record (10 sec). Poststimulus force levels in (b) and (c) were 0.27 kg and 0.10 kg, respectively. The changes in the firing frequency of a Renshaw cell were represented by peristimulus frequency histogram, bin width being 0.5 sec. Dashed line represents the minimum force level. (B) Setting of levels of hindlimb force and changes in the activity of a group Ia fiber innervating soleus muscle. Format of (B) is the same as that of (A). Initial prestimulus force levels were 0.23 kg (a). Poststimulus levels in (b) and (c) were 0.17 kg and 0.10 kg, respectively. Conduction velocity of this fiber was 85.4 m/sec. (C) Setting of levels of hindlimb force and changes in the activity of a group Ib fiber innervating soleus muscle. Format of (C) is the same as that of (A). Initial prestimulus levels were 0.43 kg (a). Poststimulus levels in (b) and (c) were 0.34 kg and 0.24 kg, respectively. Firing frequencies of individual afferents were measured after termination of DTF stimulation, when the force showed a plateau level. Conduction velocity of this fiber was 77.4 m/sec.

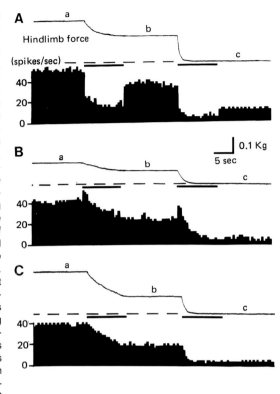

during the period of DTF stimulation. However, after the termination of stimulation, the Renshaw cell discharged with a higher frequency than during DTF stimulation. Renewed firing frequency was smaller than that of the prestimulus period. The changes in the firing frequency in this Renshaw cell were studied in repetitions throughout the range in which the level of hindlimb force was varied from a maximum level of about 0.50 kg to a minimum level of about 0.10 kg. It will be found from the results plotted in Fig. 7B that firing frequencies of Renshaw cells decreased almost linearly with decreases in the hindlimb force and that they continued to discharge with firing frequencies from 5–10 spikes/sec even when the hindlimb force was at the minimum level.

3.3.3. Group Ia and Ib Fibers

Most of these muscle afferents discharged tonically with various firing frequencies related to various levels of hindlimb force. In general, the smaller the

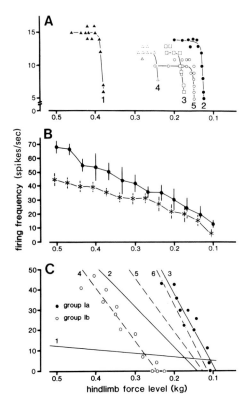

FIGURE 7. Discharge characteristics of alpha MNs, Renshaw cells, and group Ia and group Ib fibers. (A) Relations between the firing frequencies of five alpha MNs and hindlimb force (see Fig. 5C). (B) Relations between the firing frequencies of two Renshaw cells and hindlimb force. The mean and standard deviation of firing frequencies were plotted at a force level of X kg. Such values were calculated from the plotted samples (n = 5 to 10), which fell within the range $X \pm 0.016$ kg. Firing frequencies of individual cells were measured after termination of DTF stimulation. (C) Relations between the firing frequencies of three group Ia and three group Ib muscle afferents and and hindlimb force. Regression lines were drawn for each group Ia afferent fiber (solid line) and group Ib afferent fiber (dashed line). Filled and open circles represent the actual data for representative group Ia and group Ib afferents. Correlation coefficients (and conduction velocities) of each group Ia and each group Ib are as follows. Group Ia: 1, 0.47 (85.3 m/sec); 2, 0.89 (100.7 m/sec); 3, 0.80 (85.4 m/sec). Group Ib: 4, 0.94 (77.4 m/sec); 5, 0.96 (90.6 m/sec); 6, 0.94 (91.5 m/sec).

force level, the lower the firing frequency of individual muscle afferents tended to become. The examples illustrated in Figs. 6B and 6C were obtained from representative group Ia and Ib fibers, respectively. Periods of stimuli to the DTF area were delivered sequentially for two repetitions, and the changes in the firing frequencies of these fibers were correlated with those in the force levels.

For group Ia fibers, it was found that their firing frequencies tended to increase transiently at the initial declining phase of the force. The steeper and faster the decline of force, the larger the transient increase of firing frequency tended to become (Fig. 7C). However, group Ib fibers seldom exhibited such a clear transient increase (Fig. 7C). During the period of decreased force levels, after repetitions of DTF stimulation, individual group Ia fibers maintained stable and tonic discharges, but their firing frequency decreased to smaller values than that of the prestimulus period in each stimulus trial. The firing frequencies of group Ib fibers also decreased gradedly, corresponding to the graded decreases in the force levels. Furthermore, it was found that the time course of the decrease in firing frequency followed the trajectory of force decrease during DTF stimulation. The steeper the decline of force, the greater and faster the decrease in the firing frequencies of group Ib fibers tended to become.

The results summarized in Fig. 7C illustrate the relation between the firing frequencies of three representative group Ia and Ib muscle afferents each and the levels of hindlimb force. For each fiber, the correlation coefficient between firing frequency and hindlimb force was calculated. Correlation coefficients obtained from individual group Ia fibers ($n = 24$) varied between -0.06 and 0.91. For group Ib fibers ($n = 13$), they varied in the range between 0.88 and 0.98. Such a difference in correlation coefficients between group Ia and Ib fibers is reflected in the distribution of regression lines.

3.4. Long-Lasting Hyperpolarization of Membrane Potential Observed in Alpha MNs

DTF stimulation terminates tonic discharge of soleus alpha MNs along with hyperpolarization of membrane potential that outlasts the period of this stimulation (Atsuta *et al.*, 1985; Sakamoto *et al.*, 1983). A representative example is illustrated in record a of Fig. 8A. Before DTF stimulation, this cell discharged with a firing frequency of 4–6 spikes/sec with a mean membrane potential of about -54 mV. With the beginning of DTF stimulation, tonic discharge of this cell was terminated with a succeeding membrane hyperpolarization of about 4 mV. The hyperpolarized state outlasted this stimulation. In this cell, a direct hyperpolarizing current of 40 nA was passed through the 3 M KCl filled microelectrode to inject Cl⁻ intracellularly for 2 min.

Though the negative shift of membrane potential was small, synaptic noise became marked (record b in Fig. 8A). At such a membrane level, DTF stimulation

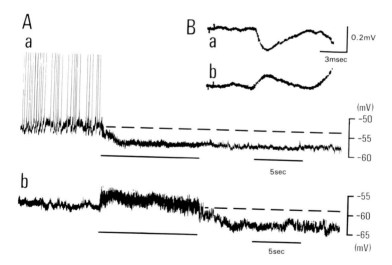

FIGURE 8. Comparison of the DTF-induced effects upon intracellular activity of an alpha MN before and after Cl⁻ injection. (A) Intracellular recordings from a single cell before (a) and after (b) Cl⁻ injection. The period of DTF stimulation is indicated by a solid line under the recordings. Broken lines were drawn to facilitate visualizing of membrane potential changes. (B) Antagonistic Ia IPSP before (a) and after (b) Cl⁻ injection. (From Sakamoto *et al.*, in press).

with the same stimulus strength as before Cl⁻ injection was delivered and resulted in a positive shift of membrane potential with further augmentation of synaptic noise. With an increase in the duration of DTF stimulation, which lasted 10 sec, the positive shift of membrane potential tended to decrease. Immediately after termination of DTF stimulation, membrane potential began to hyperpolarize below the prestimulus level and approached a steady level of -63 mV.

Along with the study of membrane potential changes induced by DTF stimulation, IPSPs were recorded from the same cell by stimulating the nerve endings within the tibialis anterior muscle, and they were averaged for 20 consecutive stimulus trials. Before Cl⁻ injection, an averaged IPSP had a latency of about 4.5 msec from the onset of intramuscular stimulation (see record a in Fig. 8A). This latency was 0.7 msec longer than that of EPSPs recorded in the same cell by stimulating the nerve endings within the soleus muscle. Immediately after Cl⁻ injection, the tibialis anterior muscle was again stimulated with the same stimulus strength that evoked ordinary IPSPs. Under such a condition, it was found that intramuscular stimulation evoked a positive deflection in potential (record b in Fig. 8B), the latencies from the onset of stimulation to the initial positive deflection and to the peak being almost the same as those of the averaged IPSP in record a in Fig. 8B.

These results suggested that the diffusion of Cl⁻ out of the intracellular recording electrode was sufficient to invert antagonistic Ia IPSPs. Accordingly, the injection of Cl⁻ seems to have inverted a DTF elicited hyperpolarizing response to a depolarizing response. From this series of studies, it can be concluded that different inhibitory mechanisms are acting during, vs. after, DTF stimulation, though membrane hyperpolarization is similarly evoked, and that the ionic mechanisms of this postsynaptic inhibitory process, during DTF stimulation, are similar to those of direct inhibition which is mediated by Cl⁻ ions (Llinas and Terzuolo, 1964).

To study further the difference in the inhibitory mechanisms during vs. after DTF stimulation, changes in membrane resistance were analysed along with membrane hyperpolarization. Motoneuron input resistance was determined by delivering repetitive depolarizing and hyperpolarizing current pulses (3–20 nA, 20 to 100 msec in duration) through the impaling microelectrode and dividing the voltage deflections by the amount of injected current (Llinas and Terzuolo, 1964; Morales and Chase, 1981). In measuring input resistance, we confirmed that the microelectrode resistance did not change during the measurement (Frank and Fuortes, 1956; Nelson and Frank, 1967) and that the artifact produced by the current flowing through the microelectrode was effectively compensated by the bridge circuit. When proper compensation was achieved, the voltage deflection was due solely to the input resistance of the MNs (Morales and Chase, 1981).

Representative results obtained from two different cells are illustrated in Fig. 9. The prestimulus membrane potential of the cell in Fig. 9A was -62 mV, and the DTF-induced hyperpolarization was about 4 mV. The amplitudes of induced voltage deflections were diminished during the period of DTF stimulation, indicating a decreased input resistance. It was found that input resistance decreased in parallel with the negative shift of membrane potential, attaining a minimum level at the end of 10 sec DTF stimulation. In the initial period of this stimulation, the changes

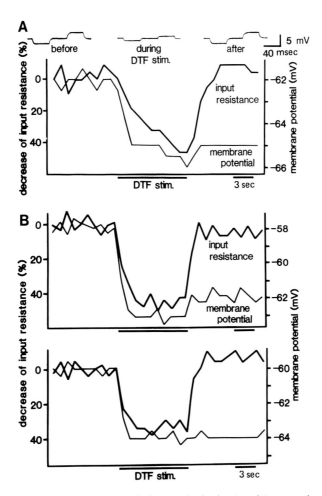

FIGURE 9. Representative time course of changes in the input resistance and membrane potential of two alpha MNs (A and B). Four nA anodal and cathodal pair pulses of 40-msec duration each were applied at a frequency of 1 Hz. Induced voltage deflections are illustrated at the top of record (A). It was confirmed that input resistance calculated by the injected anodal pulse and by the cathodal pulse was the same. The decrease of input resistance relative to that estimated during prestimulus stage was plotted along the ordinate. Input resistance and membrane potential are plotted by a thick and a thin line, respectively. (From Sakamoto et al., in press.)

in input resistance lagged slightly behind those in membrane potential. After termination of this stimulation, input resistance returned close to the prestimulus level, while the membrane potential remained hyperpolarized.

In the other cell, DTF stimulus trials were performed twice to evaluate the replicability of the stimulus effects that were induced. The second trial was performed after restoring the membrane potential close to the prestimulus level (Sakamoto *et al.*, in press). As illustrated in Fig. 9B, input resistance changed in parallel with a change in membrane potential in each trial. Induced changes in the membrane potential in the first and second trials were -6 mV and -5 mV, respectively. Reflecting such a difference, the change in input resistance in the first trial was larger than that in the second trial. There was again a clear dissociation between the changes in input resistance and the membrane hyperpolarization after termination of DTF stimulation.

All these results reinforce our proposition that different neuronal mechanisms are acting during, vs. after, termination of DTF stimulation, inducing graded and long-lasting membrane hyperpolarization of soleus alpha MNs. Possible neuronal mechanisms will be discussed below, together with the results obtained from different series of studies from our laboratory.

4. DISCUSSION

One of the most important features of our observations was that the graded and long-lasting decrease in the level of extensor muscle tone manifested itself in a graded and long-lasting membrane hyperpolarization of alpha MNs innervating extensor muscles in the hindlimb (Atsuta *et al.*, 1985; Sakamoto *et al.*, 1984). The mechanism responsible for such a tonic hyperpolarization could either be disfacilitation, presynaptic inhibition of ongoing group Ia excitatory input, postsynaptic inhibition, or a combination of all these factors.

As to the activities of spinal neuronal elements contributing to the stretch reflex, our analysis demonstrated that Renshaw cells discharge tonically, and the smaller the extensor muscle tone, the lower the firing frequency. There was a quasi-linear relation between the level of extensor muscle tone and the firing frequency of single Renshaw cells. It was interesting to note that Renshaw cell activity was greatly depressed during the period of DTF stimulation compared to the activity following DTF stimulation, even though motor output was relatively similar. Such findings suggest that the activity of Renshaw cells can be suppressed not only by a decreased output from alpha MNs but also by additional inhibitory input to the Renshaw cells (Engberg *et al.*, 1968b).

Primary spindle afferents project to homonymous alpha MNs, and there is little doubt that monosynaptic Ia projection is an important source of excitation (Burke and Rudomin, 1977; Matthews, 1981). In this study, about half of the sampled group Ia fibers ($n = 14$) exhibited a high correlation between the level of extensor muscle tone and their firing frequencies, but the rest of them ($n = 10$) did not exhibit such a clear tendency. A transient increase in the firing frequency of group Ia fibers seemed to be due to a transient and passive extension of intrafusal muscle fibers, because the degree of increases was related to the changes elicited in the force levels. It should be noticed that in spite of a transient increase in the excitatory feedback input to alpha MNs, there was no remarkable increase in the excitability of alpha MNs.

Tendon organ afferents project to homonymous alpha MNs and inhibit them through intervening interneurons (Eccles *et al.*, 1957). The important role of the tendon organ lies in integrating the responses of synergists and antagonists, rather than in homonymous regulation, and there is no significant force feedback in the decerebrate preparation (Houk and Rymer, 1981). Our results have demonstrated very clearly that the smaller the level of extensor muscle tone, the lower the firing frequencies of group Ib fibers. Furthermore, the slope of the decrease in the individual group Ib firing frequencies correlates well with that of the force decrease elicited during DTF stimulation.

Comparison of the discharge characteristics of Renshaw cells and group Ia and Ib muscle afferents, in relation to those of alpha MNs (Fig. 7), has demonstrated that DTF-elicited excitability suppression of alpha MNs is not due to either Renshaw inhibition (Eccles *et al.*, 1954; Renshaw, 1946) or group Ib inhibition (Eccles *et al.*, 1957; Houk and Rymer, 1981) but is possibly due to other postsynaptic inhibition. Withdrawal of group Ia facilitation seems to be one of the main sources of the long-lasting suppression that outlasted DTF stimulation.

Such a proposition has been extensively studied in this laboratory (Sakamoto *et al.*, in press) along the following three lines. First, Ia EPSPs and antidromic spike potentials have been recorded from alpha MNs innervating the soleus muscle, and the effects induced by DTF stimulation analysed. Second, Cl^- was injected into cells to test whether or not the induced membrane hyperpolarization could be reversed during DTF stimulation and after termination of it. Third, changes in the input resistance of MNs were studied before, during, and after termination of DTF stimulation. Such analyses disclose the relative contribution not only of postsynaptic inhibition (Llinas and Terzuolo, 1964; Morales and Chase, 1981; Morrison and Pompeiano, 1965) and disfacilitation (Llinas, 1964; Terzuolo, 1959) but also of presynaptic inhibition (Eccles *et al.*, 1961a, 1962a,b) induced by the DTF stimulation upon impaled cells.

The decrease in spike peak potential that occurs when an antidromic action potential is conditioned by an inhibitory input has been considered to reflect conductance change occurring across the motoneuron membrane (Coombs *et al.*, 1955a; Llinas and Terzuolo, 1964). The changes in the characteristics of the IS spike are indicative of an increase in membrane conductance (Brock *et al.*, 1953; Chandler *et al.*, 1980). During DTF stimulation we observed a decrease in the antidromic spike summit level, which was independent of the decrease of membrane hyperpolarization that occurred. In other cells, IS–SD block was even observed. In addition, we observed a depression in the peak amplitude of the averaged Ia EPSP and a reduction in the time-to-peak (TTP) and half width (HW) during DTF stimulation as compared to the prestimulus state. These results are indicative of an increase in the postsynaptic input to the MNs (Burke, 1967; Cook and Cangiano, 1972; Rall *et al.*, 1965). All these data seem to converge on one main conclusion: the hyperpolarization of soleus MNs during DTF stimulation is a result of postsynaptic inhibition. This, of course, does not exclude the possibility that disfacilitation may also be present.

A second piece of evidence for postsynaptic inhibition was obtained by injecting Cl^- into the cell. When enough Cl^- was injected from the microelectrode to tonically increase the intracellular concentration of Cl^- ions, it would be expected that membrane hyperpolarization induced during DTF stimulation would change its polarity (Coombs *et al.*, 1955b,c; Eccles, 1964). We observed that the membrane potential was depolarized with the generation of action potentials and with increased synaptic noise during DTF stimulation. It can therefore be concluded that a sustained synaptic inhibitory impingement upon soleus alpha MN is an IPSP-generating mechanism that selectively increases the permeability of the synaptic membrane to Cl⁻ ions during DTF stimulation.

The third line of evidence is the changes in the input resistance associated with membrane hyperpolarization. It was found that input resistance diminished by 30% during DTF stimulation (Sakamoto *et al.*, 1984). This change in background could be enough to increase membrane conductance sufficiently to decrease the peak summit level. The diminished input resistance means that membrane resistance dropped in the vicinity of the microelectrode (Glenn and Dement, 1981). Under the reasonable assumption that the microelectrode tip was lodged in the soma, it follows that the hyperpolarization is the result of an asynchronous increase in the activity of inhibitory synapses on the motoneuron soma (Glenn and Dement, 1981; Morrison and Pompeiano, 1965).

The mechanisms responsible for the membrane hyperpolarization that outlasted stimulation could involve mostly disfacilitation. After termination of DTF stimulation, we observed that the spike summit level of antidromic action potentials did not change or increased slightly, and that the peak amplitude of monosynaptic EPSPs increased with the prolongation of its decay phase (Sakamoto *et al.*, in press). Such phenomena would be a result of the net increase in the cell's input resistance that would be produced by disfacilitation (Llinas, 1964; Terzuolo, 1959). In fact, input resistance was found to increase close to that of the prestimulus stage after termination of stimulation (Sakamoto *et al.*, 1984).

All these results suggest that different inhibitory neuronal mechanisms are acting at the level of the final common path during plastic postural changes in a decerebrate, reflexively standing cat. However, at this stage of study, the questions "what are the neuronal structures activated by the DTF stimulation?" and "how are the stimulus effects relayed to each of the neuronal elements participating in the stretch reflex?" have remained unsolved. It would be interesting to analyse the activity of the coerulospinal tract in relation to the sustained membrane hyperpolarization, because activation of efferent pathways of the nucleus locus coeruleus has been shown to produce a hyperpolarizing response of target cells accompanied by an increased membrane resistance (Moore and Bloom, 1979).

5. SUMMARY

We studied brain stem areas subserving "setting" and "resetting" of the extensor muscle tone related to the standing posture in precollicular-postmammillary decerebrate cats. Stimulation of the dorsal part and the ventral part of the pons along the midline decreased and increased the tone of the hindlimb muscles, respectively. Such a decrease and increase in the extensor muscle tone continued for more than 5 min. The degree of the changes in extensor muscle tone depended on the stimulus strength. Thus, it was possible to evoke plastic postural changes in decerebrate, reflexively standing cats by selecting the stimulus strength in relation to the site of stimulation.

To study neuronal mechanisms underlying such plastic postural changes evoked by stimulating the dorsal part of the pons along the midline, activities of alpha MNs, Renshaw cells, and group Ia and Ib muscle afferents innervating the soleus muscle were analysed along with the postural changes. It was found that the long-lasting decrease in the level of extensor muscle tone was accompanied by a long-lasting hyperpolarization of membrane potential in the alpha MNs. Neither Renshaw inhibition nor group Ib inhibition could account for the hyperpolarization induced during dorsal tegmental stimulation. Analyses of intracellular Cl⁻ injection and neuronal input resistance disclosed that different neuronal mechanisms were acting during, vs. after, termination of dorsal tegmental stimulation. During this stimulation, postsynaptic inhibition played a major role in producing hyperpolarization; after stimulation, withdrawal of ongoing group Ia excitatory bombardment, that is disfacilitation, played a major role in inducing membrane hyperpolarization. Possible descending neuronal mechanisms in mediating postsynaptic inhibitory effects upon alpha MNs were discussed.

ACKNOWLEDGMENT. We express our sincere thanks to S. Nonaka, K. Matsuyama, and K. Takakusaki for their generous assistance, to M. Nogami for typing the manuscript, and to K. Takehara for histological examination. This study was supported by Ministry of Education and Culture of Japan Grant-in-Aid for Scientific Research (B) 57480107, Developmental Scientific Research (2) 58870008, and Special Project Research 56121001, 57114001, and 58106001 to S. Mori.

REFERENCES

Amaral, D. G. and Sinnamon, H. M., 1977, The locus coeruleus: Neurobiology of a central noradrenergic nucleus, *Prog. Neurobiol.* **9**:147–196.

Atsuta, Y., Sakamoto, T., and Mori, S., 1985, Dynamic behavior of stretch reflex loop in the acute decerebrate, standing cat, *Electroenceph. Clin. Neurophysiol.* **6**: 11p.

Berman, A.L., 1968, *The Brain Stem of the Cat. A Cytoarchitectonic Atlas with Stereotaxic Coordinates,* University of Wisconsin Press, Madison.

Brock, L.G., Coombs, J.S., and Eccles, J.C., 1953, Intracellular recording from antidromically activated motoneurons, *J. Physiol. (London)* **122**:429–461.

Burke, R.E., 1967, Composite nature of the monosynaptic excitatory postsynaptic potential, *J. Neurophysiol.* **30**:1114–1137.

Burke, R.E. and Rudomin, P., 1977, Spinal neurons and synapses, in: *Handbook of Physiology,* Section 1, *The Nervous System,* Volume 2, *Motor Control* (J.M. Brookhart, V.B. Mountcastle, and V.B. Brooks, eds.), American Physiological Society, Bethesda, Maryland, pp. 877–944.

Cameron, W.E., Binder, M.D., Botterman, B.R., Reinking, R.M., and Stuart, D.G., 1981, "Sensory Partitioning" of cat medial gastrocnemius muscle by its muscle spindles and tendon organs, *J. Neurophysiol.* **46**:32–47.

Chandler, S.H., Chase, M.H., and Nakamura, Y., 1980, Intracellular analysis of synaptic mechanisms controlling trigeminal motoneuron activity during sleep and wakefulness, *J. Neurophysiol.* **44**:359–371.

Cook, W.A., Jr. and Cangiano, A., 1972, Presynaptic and postsynaptic inhibition of spinal motoneurons, *J. Neurophysiol.* **35**:389–403.

Coombs, J.S., Eccles, J.C., and Fatt, P., 1955a, The electrical properties of the motoneurone membrane, *J. Physiol. (London)* **130**:291–325.

Coombs, J.S., Eccles, J.C., and Fatt, P., 1955b, The specific ionic conductances and the ionic movements across the motoneuronal membrane that produce the inhibitory post-synaptic potential, *J. Physiol. (London)* **130**:326–373.

Coombs, J.S., Eccles, J.C., and Fatt, P., 1955c, The inhibitory suppression of reflex discharges from motoneurones, *J. Physiol. (London)* **130**:396–413.

Eccles, J.C., 1964, *The Physiology of Synapses*, Springer-Verlag, Berlin.

Eccles, J.C., Fatt, P., and Koketsu, K., 1954, Cholinergic and inhibitory synapses in a pathway from motor-axon collaterals to motoneurons, *J. Physiol. (London)* **126**:524–562.

Eccles, J.C., Eccles, R.M., and Lundberg, A., 1957, Synaptic actions on motoneurones caused by impulses in Golgi tendon organ afferents, *J. Physiol. (London)* **138**:227–252.

Eccles, J.C., Eccles, R.M., and Magni, F., 1961a, Central inhibitory action attributable to presynaptic depolarization produced by muscle afferent volleys, *J. Physiol. (London)* **159**:147–166.

Eccles, J.C., Rosamond, M., Eccles, A., Iggo, A., and Lundberg, A., 1961b, Electrophysiological investigations on Renshaw cells, *J. Physiol. (London)* **157**:461–478.

Eccles, J.C., Magni, F., and Willis, W.D., 1962a, Depolarization of central terminals of group I afferent fibres from muscle, *J. Physiol. (London)* **160**:62–93.

Eccles, J.C., Schmidt, R.F., and Willis, W.D., 1962b, Presynaptic inhibition of the spinal monosynaptic reflex pathway, *J. Physiol. (London)* **161**:282–297.

Engberg, I., Lundberg, A., and Ryall, R.W., 1968a, Reticulospinal inhibition of transmission in reflex pathways, *J. Physiol. (London)* **194**:201–223.

Engberg, I., Lundberg, A., and Ryall, R.W., 1968b, Reticulospinal inhibition of interneurons, *J. Physiol. (London)* **194**:225–236.

Foote, S.L., Bloom, F.E., and Aston-Jones, G., 1983, Nucleus locus ceruleus: New evidence of anatomical and physiological specificity, *Physiol. Rev.* **64**:844–914.

Frank, K. and Fuortes, M.G.F., 1956, Stimulation of spinal motoneurons with intracellular electrodes, *J. Physiol. (London)* **134**:451–470.

Gesteland, R.C., Howland, B., Lettwins, J.Y., and Pitts, W.H., 1959, Comments on microelectrodes, *Proc. IRE* **47**:1856–1862.

Glenn, L.L. and Dement, W.C., 1981, Membrane resistance and rheobase of hindlimb motoneurons during wakefulness and sleep, *J. Neurophysiol.* **46**:1076–1088.

Holstege, G. and Kuypers, H.G.J.M., 1982, The anatomy of brain stem pathways to the spinal cord in cat. A labeled amino acid tracing study, *Prog. Brain Res.* **57**:145–176.

Houk, J.C. and Henneman, E., 1967, Responses of Golgi tendon organs to active contractions of the soleus muscle of the cat, *J. Neurophysiol.* **30**:466–481.

Houk, J.C. and Rymer, W.Z., 1981, Neural control of muscle length and tension, in: *Handbook of Physiology*, Section 1, *The Nervous System*, Volume 2, *Motor Control* (J.M. Brookhart, V.B. Mountcastle, and V.B. Brooks, eds.), American Physiological Society, Bethesda, Maryland, pp. 257–324.

Jankowska, E., Lund, S., Lundberg, A., and Pompeiano, O., 1968, Inhibitory effects evoked through ventral reticulospinal pathways, *Arch. Ital. Biol.* **106**:124–140.

Kuypers, H.G.J.M. and Maisky, V.A., 1975, Retrograde axonal transport of horseradish peroxidase from spinal cord to brain stem cell groups in the cat. *Neurosci. Lett.* **1**:9–14.

Lipski, J., 1981, Antidromic activation of neurones as an analytic tool in the study of the central nervous system, *J. Neurosci. Methods* **4**:1–32.

Llinas, R., 1964, Mechanisms of supraspinal actions upon spinal cord activities. Differences between reticular and cerebellar inhibitory actions upon alpha extensor motoneurons, *J. Neurophysiol.* **27**:1117–1126.

Llinas, R. and Terzuolo, C.A., 1964, Mechanisms of supraspinal actions upon spinal cord activities. Reticular inhibitory mechanisms on alpha-extensor motoneurons, *J. Neurophysiol.* **27**:579–591.

Magoun, H.W. and Rhines, R., 1946, An inhibitory mechanism in the bulbar reticular formation, *J. Neurophysiol.* **9**:165–171.

Matthews, P.B.C., 1981, Muscle spindles: Their messages and their fusimotor supply, in: *Handbook of Physiology*, Section 1, *The Nervous System*, Volume 2, *Motor Control* (J.M. Brookhart, V.B. Mountcastle, and V.B. Brooks, eds.), American Physiological Society, Bethesda, Maryland, pp. 189–228.

Moore, R.Y. and Bloom, F.E., 1979, Central catecholamine neuron systems: anatomy and physiology of the norepinephrine and epinephrine system, *Ann. Rev. Neurosci.* **2**:113–168.

Morales, F. and Chase, M.H., 1981, Postsynaptic control of lumber motoneuron excitability during active sleep in the chronic cat, *Brain Res.* **225**:279–295.

Mori, S., Kawahara, K., and Sakamoto, T., 1983, Supraspinal aspects of locomotion in the mesencephalic cat, in: *Neural Origin of Rhythmic Movements,* (A. Roberts and B.L. Roberts, eds.), Cambridge University Press, Cambridge, pp. 445–468.

Mori, S., Nishimura, H., and Aoki, M., 1980a, Brain stem activation of the spinal stepping generator, in: *Reticular Formation Revisited,* Int. Brain Res. Monogr. Volume 6 (J.A. Hobson and M.A.B. Brazier, eds.), Raven Press, New York, pp. 241–259.

Mori, S., Aoki, M., Kawahara, K., and Sakamoto, T., 1980b, Level setting of postural muscle tonus and inhibition of locomotion by MLR stimulation, *Adv. Physiol. Sci.* **1**:179–182.

Mori, S., Kawahara, K., Sakamoto, T., Aoki, M., and Tomiyama, T., 1982, Setting and resetting of level of postural muscle tone in decerebrate cat by stimulation of brain stem, *J. Neurophysiol.* **48**:737–748.

Morrison, A.R. and Pompeiano, O., 1965, An analysis of the supraspinal influences acting on motoneurons during sleep in unrestrained cat. Responses of the alpha motoneurons to direct electrical stimulation during sleep, *Arch. Ital. Biol.* **103**:497–516.

Nelson, P.G. and Frank, K., 1967, Anomalous rectification in cat spinal motoneurons and effect of polarizing current on excitatory postsynaptic potentials, *J. Neurophysiol.* **30**:1097–1113.

Ohta, Y., Sakamoto, T., and Mori, S., 1984, The cells of origin projecting their axons to the dorsal part of the central tegmental field in the pons, *J. Physiol. Soc. Jpn.* **46**:377

Renshaw, B., 1941, Influence of discharge of motoneurons upon excitation of neighboring motoneurons, *J. Neurophysiol.* **4**:167–183.

Renshaw, B., 1946, Central effects of centripetal impulses in axons of spinal ventral roots, *J. Neurophysiol.* **9**:191–204.

Rall, W., Burke, R.E., Smith, T.G., Nelson, P.G., and Frank, K., 1967, Dendritic location of synapses and possible mechanisms for the monosynaptic EPSP in motoneurons, *J. Neurophysiol.* **30**:1169–1193.

Sakai, K., Touret, N., Salvert, D., Leger, L., and Jouvet, M., 1977, Afferent projections to the cat locus coeruleus as visualized by the horseradish peroxidase technique, *Brain Res.* 119:21–41.

Sakai D., Sastre, J.P. Salvert, D., Touret, M., Tohyama, M., and Jouvet, M., 1979, Tegmentoreticular projections with special reference to the muscular atonia during paradoxical sleep in the cat: An HRP study, *Brain Res.* **176**:233–254.

Sakai, D., Sastre, J.P., Kanamori, N., and Jouvet, M., 1984, State specific neurons in the pontomedullary reticular formation with special reference to the postural atonia during paradoxical sleep in the cat, in: *Brain Mechanisms of Perceptual Awareness and Purposeful Behavior* (C. Ajmone Marsan and O. Pompeiano, eds.), Raven Press, New York, in press.

Sakamoto, T., Atsuta, Y., and Mori, S., 1984, Long-lasting excitability changes of soleus alphamotoneuron induced by the midpontine stimulation in decerebrate, standing cat, *J. Neurophysiol.,* in press.

Sakamoto, T., Atsuta, Y., and Mori, S., 1983, Effects elicited by the stimulation to the dorsal part of tegmental field upon soleus alpha motoneurons in the decerebrate standing animal, *Neurosci. Lett.* suppl. **13**:s74.

Snider, R.S. and Niemer, W.T.A., 1961, *Stereotaxic Atlas of the Cat Brain,* University of Chicago Press, Chicago.

Terzuolo, C.A., 1959, Cerebellar inhibitory and excitatory action upon spinal extensor motoneurons, *Arch. Ital. Biol.* **97**:316–339.

Walberg, F., 1974, Crossed reticulo-reticular projections in the medulla, pons and mesencephalon, *Z. Anat. Entwicklungsgesch.* **143**:127–134.

10

Recovery of Motor Skill Following Deprivation of Direct Sensory Input to the Motor Cortex in the Monkey

HIROSHI ASANUMA

1. INTRODUCTION

Recovery of function following partial destruction of the central nervous system has been observed for a long time. It is well known that the motor deficit following a stroke is severest immediately after the attack but that the symptoms become less severe as time passes. The genesis of this functional recovery has been an intriguing question among neurologists and neurophysiologists. It has been known for a long time that section of a peripheral nerve produces loss of control of the body area previously innervated by the nerve but that as time passes the sectioned nerve sprouts from the proximal end and eventually reinnervates the same territory to restore the function. Whether the same process takes place when a part of the central nervous system is destroyed has been a challenging problem. Since it is well established that mitotic division of neurons does not occur after birth, the recovery of function must occur by rearrangement of remaining neurons. Ramón y Cajal (1928) studied this problem extensively. He transsected the spinal cord of young cats and dogs and examined the sprouting of nerve fibers following the lesion. He observed that large numbers of the severed intraspinal fibers sprouted new processes with cones of growth similar to those observed in the peripheral nerves. However, after 4 or 5 weeks, the number of sprouting fibers diminished and eventually the new fibers disappeared. He concluded that the processes of regeneration were followed by atrophy and absorption. Similar observations were made by other investigators and it was generally agreed that nerve fibers in the CNS commenced

HIROSHI ASANUMA ● The Rockefeller University, New York, New York 10021.

to regenerate but that, for some reason, the newly formed sprouts would not cross the transsection to make functional connections in the opposite side of the stump (Clemente, 1964).

In the meantime, various efforts were made to reexamine whether regeneration of nerve fibers in the central nervous system was possible. Sugar and Gerald (1940) transsected the thoracic cord of young rats with special care to preserve the blood supply below the transsection, and, in some animals, they were able to observe recovery of sensory and motor functions in the hindlimb. Stimulation of the brain stem produced hindlimb movements, and silver stain showed a complete scar bridged by bundles of new axons passing through the scar. This observation was confirmed by Freeman (1952), who further demonstrated that functional regeneration could occur in young rats, kittens, and puppies. Thus, the recovery of function, in some cases, could occur by regeneration of nerve fibers, as is the case in peripheral nerves.

A breakthrough in the study of the genesis of functional recovery was made by Liu and Chambers in 1958. In 1954, Nauta and Gygax introduced a new method that was capable of staining not only myelinated but also nonmyelinated portions of degenerating fibers in the central nervous system. Using this method, they examined the reaction of intact spinal fibers following a lesion in the central nervous system. They partially denervated the spinal cord of adult cats by sectioning the pyramidal tract or the dorsal roots, and, following the disappearance of the degeneration products, the remaining intact dorsal roots or the pyramidal tracts were severed. After 4–5 days survival, the animal was sacrificed, and the distrbution of degenerating fibers was examined. They found marked increase of degenerating fibers on the chronically denervated side, clearly indicating that by elimination of one input to a part of the central nervous system, the remaining fibers proliferated and increased their number. These results suggested that functional recovery following partial lesion of the CNS is not achieved by the regeneration of the severed fibers but by the sprouting of the remaining fibers. This observation was further supported by Raisman (1969) and Raisman and Field (1973), using the electron microscope. They eliminated the fimbrial or hypothalamic input to the rat septal nucleus, and, after disappearance of degeneration products, they made a second lesion to the remaining input. They then examined the distribution of regenerating terminals produced by the second lesion. They found a marked increase of degenerating terminals, strongly suggesting that new synapses were formed by the sprouting of the remaining fibers. Physiological experiments also supported this interpretation. Tsukahara et al. (1975) demonstrated in the cat that elimination of cerebellar input to the red nucleus changed the shape of postsynatic potentials in red nucleus neurons elicited by stimulation of the motor cortex. Based on the cable theory (Rall et al., 1967), they concluded that the vacancy created by elimination of cerebellar input was replaced by new synapses formed by sprouting of the fibers from the cerebral cortex. Thus, it is now firmly established that at least part of the functional recovery observed following CNS lesions is due to the formation of new synapses by the remaining fibers.

Recently we have shown in cats (Asanuma et al., 1979a) and monkeys (Asanuma et al., 1979b) that the motor cortex receives peripheral input directly from the thalamus, in addition to that coming through the sensory cortex. This direct input to the motor cortex ascends through the dorsal columns; i.e., the dorsal columns send input directly to both the motor and the sensory cortices (Asanuma *et al.*, 1980). The sensory cortex receives additional input through the spinothalamic tract. The results indicated that the section of the dorsal columns or ablation of the sensory cortex alone does not eliminate the peripheral input to the motor cortex. It is shown in the present study that total elimination of the sensory input produces severe motor deficit but that partial elimination produces a deficit that can be compensated for within a short period probably due to the reorganization of the remaining input system.

2. MATERIALS AND METHODS

Experiments were carried out using four cynomolgus monkeys (*Maccaca fascicularis*) of either sex weighing between 3 and 4 kg. The monkeys were trained to sit in a primate chair and to pick up a food pellet from a hole in a food board. The hole had slits on both sides so that the monkey could insert the thumb and the index finger to pick up food. The board was rotated at various speeds while the monkey attempted to pick up the food. The movement of the hand was recorded on video tape for later analysis. The monkeys were quickly accustomed to this situation and within a few days reached a stable state of performance. Then the first operations were carried out under inhalation anesthesia (50% oxygen, 50% nitrous oxide, plus 1.5% halothane). In two monkeys, the sensory cortex was removed, and in the others the dorsal columns were cut bilaterally at the level of C-3. The funtional deficit and the recovery following the operations were observed for 4–5 weeks. The monkeys were then operated on again, and the remaining intact cortex or the dorsal column was lesioned to observe the functional deficit produced by the combined lesions. At the end of the experiments, the monkeys were deeply anesthetized with Nembutal (40 mg/kg) and perfused with saline followed by 10% formaline. The brain and the cervical cord were removed and frozen sections were cut to examine the extent of the lesions.

3. RESULTS

3.1. Effect of Sensory Cortex Ablation

In two monkeys, the sensory cortex was removed first. The later histological examination revealed that in both monkeys the ablation extended to areas 1, 2, 3b, 5, and caudal part of area 3a, but not to areas 4 and 7. The mediolateral extent was from the neck to hindlimb areas, as judged by the distribution of evoked potentials in the same species (Asanuma *et al.*, 1980). It has been shown repeatedly that ablation of the postcentral cortex produces very little motor deficit (Travis and Woolsey, 1956; Denny-Brown, 1966; Tatton *et al.*, 1975). Our results were similar to those reported by previous investigators.

Immediately after recovery from the anesthesia, the monkeys tended to look

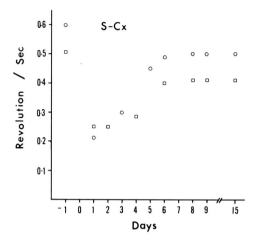

FIGURE 1. Recovery of hand skill following removal of the sensory cortex in two monkeys. Ordinate shows speed of the food board. At 0.5 rev/sec, the experimenter starts having a difficulty in putting the food correctly into the hole. Abscissa shows days before and after the operation.

at the hand contralateral to the ablated cortex, giving an impression that they were experiencing abnormal sensations. When given a peanut, they used the ipsilateral hand. However, both monkeys quickly adapted to the new situation, and, after a few hours, they started using the contralateral hand in much the same manner as the normal hand. The tactile placing reaction was lost during the entire period of observation, which lasted more than 2 months. Although the behavior of the monkeys in the cage looked nearly normal from 2 or 3 hr after the operation, further examination of the hand skill using the rotating food board revealed some clumsiness in the usage of the contralateral hand. On the day following the operation, the monkeys could bring the affected hand to the hole without difficulty, but could not use the proper fingers to pick up the food from the hole. Instead, both monkeys tried to use all fingers to pick up the morsel. This deficit in finger manipulation is reflected in the decrease in the ability of picking up food from the rotating table, as shown in Fig. 1. This clumsiness, however, diminished rapidly, and the monkeys started to use the proper fingers within a few days and regained nearly normal dexterity after a week, although the usage of the thumb and index finger was a little clumsier than normal during the period of observation, which lasted a month.

3.2. Effect of Dorsal Column Section

In two monkeys, the dorsal columns were sectioned first. Later histological examination revealed that in both cases the right dorsal column was cut completely. The observation of the motor skill was made using the right hand in both monkeys. The effect of dorsal column section as judged by simple observation was remarkably small. The monkeys could stand and walk normally even immediately after recovery from the anesthesia. Given a food pellet, they picked it up and ate without difficulty. Examination of hand skill with the rotating food board, however, revealed some deficit in motor function. Although the monkeys could bring the hand to a stationary hole, they could not always bring the fingers to the target hole when the board was

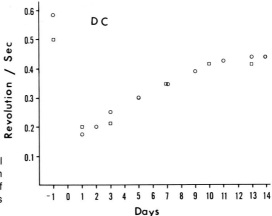

FIGURE 2. Recovery of hand skill
following dorsal column section in
two monkeys. Ordinate: speed of
food board rotation. Abscissa: days
before and after section.

rotated. When they tried to pick up the food from the hole, they could not coordinate
the thumb and the index finger and used all fingers in concert until accidental
insertion of one finger into the hole enabled them to pick up the food. The loss of
orientation and coordination recovered gradually, as shown in Fig. 2, and it took
2 weeks before the monkeys regained the ability of near-normal hand manipulation.
Thus, section of the dorsal columns produced motor deficit that was somewhat
severer than that produced by sensory cortex ablation, but the deficit was not
permanent and could be compensated for within 2 weeks.

3.3. Effect of Combined Lesions

After 4 or 5 weeks of observation, the monkeys were reanesthetized, and the
dorsal columns or the sensory cortex were ablated in addition to the previous lesions.
Later histological examination revealed that the lesions from the second operations
were as complete as those from the first operations. The results obtained with both
procedures were similar. When the monkeys recovered from the anesthesia, they
could stand in the cage cautiously but tended to fall when they tried to walk. The
hand contralateral to the cortical lesion was paralyzed, and they did not attempt to
use it at all. Several days after the operation, they tried to use the contralateral
hand occasionally, but the movement was disoriented, and the hand could not reach
the target. The ability to manipulate individual fingers was lost in spite of intact
visual guidance. When seated in the chair in front of the food board with the
ipsilateral hand restrained, they could occasionally pick up the food using all fingers
in concert when the food was placed on the smooth surface of the board, but not
in the hole. When the board was rotated with very slow speed (0.01 cycle/sec),
they could not pick up the food, even from the surface, and tended to abandon
attempts to pick it up. When a food pellet (such as a peanut) was brought in front
of the monkeys, they tried to grab the food using all fingers, but, in many trials,
the hand could not reach the target. Occasional success in grabbing the food en-

couraged the monkeys to continue their trials. When they picked up the food, they looked at the hand and brought the food cautiously to the mouth, but tended to drop the food when they tried to eat. This severe disturbance of motor function did not recover during the period of observation, which lasted 4–5 weeks following the second operation.

4. DISCUSSION

The importance of sensory input in motor performance has been known for a long time. In 1858, Claude Bernard reported that section of the dorsal roots produced impairment of movement in the frog and puppy. Mott and Sherrington (1895) reported that section of the dorsal roots in the monkey practically abolished the movement of hand and foot, although the movement of proximal joints was less impaired. Later study, however, demonstrated that by careful training, the deafferented monkey can learn to use the affected arm and leg but that the movements are abrupt and exaggerated (Knapp et al., 1963). A recent study on a deafferented patient (Rothwell et al., 1982) reported that the subject could learn to move then hand accurately as instructed, but, in daily life, the hands were useless. He was unable to fasten his shirt buttons or to hold a cup in one hand. The above results seem to suggest that interruption of dorsal root input produces impairment of fine movements primarily of distal limb muscles, a deficit resembling that observed following pyramidal section (Tower, 1940; Lawrence and Kuypers, 1968). However, since dorsal rhizotomy eliminates afferent input not only to the higher central nervous system but also to the spinal cord, the effect cannot exclusively be attributed to the elimination of the input to the motor cortex.

Concerning the functional role of the sensory input to the motor cortex, various hypotheses have already been proposed. Welt et al. (1967) proposed that the peripheral input might constitute the basis of postural reflexes such as tactile placing reaction. Rosén and Asanuma (1972) suggested that the input function as the neuronal basis for instinctive grasping reaction. Phillips (1969) proposed that input functions as a transcortical servo-loop that could dominate the segmental reflexes. The transcortical servo-loop theory was further advanced by various investigators (Marsden et al., 1972; Tatton et al., 1975; Evarts and Tanji, 1976). They proposed that these loops function to counteract unexpected loads during voluntary movements. All of these hypotheses, however, were based on the assumption that the motor cortex receives peripheral input through the sensory cortex. If this is the case, the functional role of the input must be minute because it has been shown repeatedly that removal of the sensory cortex produces very little motor deficit (Travis and Woolsey, 1956; Denny-Brown, 1966; Tatton et al., 1975). However, since it has been shown recently that the motor cortex receives peripheral input not only through the sensory cortex but also directly from the thalamus (Asanuma et al., 1979a,b; Lemon and van der Burg, 1979; Horne and Tracey, 1979) and since the direct input ascends through the dorsal columns (Asanuma et al., 1980), section of the dorsal columns, in addition to ablation of the sensory cortex, was necessary to examine the functional role of the sensory input. The functions explored by the combined lesions were control of orientation of the hand in space and control of fine movements, especially of distal extremities.

How are these functions, then, fitted to the known organization of the motor cortex? It has been shown that there are cortical efferent zones within the depth of the motor cortex that, when stimulated, can produce contraction of individual muscles in the cat (Asanuma and Sakata, 1967) and the monkey (Asanuma and Rosén, 1972) and that the effects are mediated primarily through the pyramidal tract (Asanuma and Sakata, 1968). These results suggested that there are connections from individual efferent zones to respective motoneuron pools through the pyramidal tract and that these connections constitute the basis of cortical motor function, i.e., control of fine movements of distal extremities. This interpretation may appear to be obscured by later electro-anatomical findings (Shinoda *et al.*, 1979, 1981) that each pyramidal tract fiber branches extensively in the spinal cord and innervates various interneurons and motoneurons. However, a further electro-anatomical study has shown that although each pyramidal tract fiber branches extensively, a group of PT neurons located in a small area of the cortex has a common target nucleus in the spinal cord (Asanuma *et al.*, 1979c). Furthermore a recent (C-14)-2-deoxy-glucose study has shown that microstimulation at a given efferent zone primarily activates a particular motor nucleus in the spinal cord, in addition to diffuse activation of the neighboring structures (Kosar and Asanuma, 1984). Since it is known that each efferent zone receives peripheral information related to the contraction of the target muscle (Rosen and Asanuma, 1972; Murphy *et al.*, 1975), it may be concluded that activity of a given efferent zone produces contraction of a particular muscle and that the same zone receives peripheral information related to the contraction of the target muscle, constituting a closed loop circuit. The present experiments revealed that the interruption of this loop circuit produced impairment in the orientation of the hand in space and control of fine movements. How, then, do the loop circuits participate in the execution of cortically induced movements?

One of the major differences between cortically induced movements and spinal reflexes is that the former are not automatic. In many cases, such movements necessitates long-term training. To become a musician, for example, years of training are necessary to play an instrument. After training, he is able to learn to contract only those specific muscles related to the manipulation of the instrument. When an animal is trained for a conditioned reflex, the response becomes restricted to these muscles necessary to acquire the desired behaviour as training procedes. Recent experiments revealed that when the training was completed, the excitability of cortical neurons projecting to these particular muscles was increased (Woody and Engel, 1972; Brons and Woody, 1980). There must be many neuronal mechanims subserving this increase of excitability, but one of the possible mechanisms is that this is achieved by reinforcing specific corticoperipheral loops.

This mechanism may function in the following way. When a subject is trained to pursue a specific movement, the repeated practice produces vigorous circulation of impulses in particular cortico-peripheral loops related to that movement. Continuous circulation of impulses in specific loops results in an increased efficiency of synaptic transmission in these loops. This may result in the increase of excitability of the related cortical neurons. It is a common experience that most neurons in the central nervous system show sustained discharges even when the animal is at rest, suggesting that neurons are always circulating impulses through various loop circuits, including the cortico-peripheral loop. Training of an animal might have increased the efficiency of synaptic transmission within these circuits, resulting in the increase of excitability of related neurons. The loss of learned skilled movements, such as picking up food pellets from a rotating table following interruption of the cortico-peripheral loop, suggests that this loop also plays an important role in the increased excitability of related cortical neurons.

5. RECOVERY OF MOTOR FUNCTION

As shown by the results, partial interruption of sensory input produced some motor deficits, but the function recovered within a week or two. It is unlikely that the deficit was caused by traumatic shocks produced by the surgery because the deficit could be detected only by a specific examination of hand skills. Without this test, the monkeys appeared normal even immediately after the operation. Therefore, it is more likely that the recovery was due to reorganization of remaining systems, which compensated for the lost function. In the case of dorsal column section, it is known that the sensory cortex still receives peripheral input (Brinkman et al., 1978), which is mediated by the spinothalamic pathway (Asanuma et al., 1980). It is most likely that recovery of function is the result of reorganization of connections between the sensory and the motor cortices, since the recovered function disappeared upon removal of the sensory cortex.

It has been shown that area 2 of the sensory cortex projects to the motor cortex (Jones et al., 1978). In normal monkeys, neurons in this area receive input primarily from receptors of deep tissues of the body (Powell and Mountcastle, 1959). It might be interesting to examine how the peripheral input to this area changes after dorsal column section and also whether the characteristics of the remaining input changes in relation to the recovery of motor function.

6. SUMMARY

The functional role of sensory input to the motor cortex was examined by observing hand skills following interruption of sensory pathways in the monkey. Section of the dorsal columns that send peripheral input directly to the motor cortex through the thalamus produced some disturbances in the orientation of the hand in the space, as well as in manipulation of fingers. However, function recovered within 2 weeks provided the sensory cortex was intact. Additional removal of the sensory cortex eliminated recovered function and produced severe motor deficit that did not recover during the period of observation, which lasted 4–5 weeks. It is concluded that the direct sensory input from the thalamus to the motor cortex plays an important role in the execution of learned movements but that loss of this input can be compensated for by the input from the sensory cortex. Possible neuronal mechanisms for the observed deficit and the recovery of function are discussed, and it is proposed that the sensory input functions by changing excitability of specific cortical efferent zones projecting to particular muscles related to the learned movement.

REFERENCES

Asanuma, H. and Rosén, I., 1972, Topograhical organization of cortical efferent zones projecting to distal forelimb muscles in the monkey, *Exp. Brain Res.* **14**:243–256.

Asanuma, H. and Sakata, H., 1967, Functional organization of a cortical efferent system examined with focal depth stimulation in cats, *J. Neurophysiol.* **30**:35–54.

Asanuma, H., Larsen, K. D., and Yumiya, H., 1979a, Receptive fields of thalamic neurons projecting to the motor cortex in the cat, *Brain Res.* **172**:217–228.

Asanuma, H., Larsen, K. D., and Yumiya, H., 1979b, Direct sensory pathways to the motor cortex in the monkey: A basis of cortical reflexes, in: *Integration in the Nervous System* (H. Asanuma and V. J. Wilson, eds.), Igaku-shoin, Toyko, pp. 223–238.

Asanuma, H., Zarzecki, P., Jankowska, E., Hongo, T., and Marcus, S., 1979c, Projection of individual pyramidal tract neurons to lumbar motoneuron pools of the monkey, *Exp. Brain Res.* **34**:73–89.

Asanuma, H., Larsen, K. D., and Yumiya, H., 1980, Peripheral input pathways to the monkey motor cortex, *Exp. Brain Res.* **38**:349–355.

Bernard, C., 1858, *Leçons sur la Physiologie et la Pathologie du Systeme Nerveux,* J. B. Bailliere et Fils, Paris, pp. 246–266.

Brinkman, J., Bush, B. M., and Porter, R., 1978, Deficient influences of peripheral stimuli on precentral neurones in monkeys with dorsal column lesions, *J. Physiol. (London)* **276**:27–48.

Brons, J. F. and Woody, C. D., 1980, Long-term changes in excitability of cortical neurons after Pavlovian conditioning and extinction, *J. Neurophysiol.* **44**:605–615.

Clemente, C. D., 1964, Regeneration in the vertebrate central nervous system, *Int. Rev. Neurobiol.* **6**:257–293.

Denny-Brown, D., 1966, *The Cerebral Control of Movement,* Charles C Thomas, Springfield, Illinois.

Evarts, E. V. and Tanji, J., 1976, Reflex and intended responses in motor cortex pyramidal tract neurons of monkey, *J. Neurophysiol.* **39**:1069–1080.

Freeman, L. W., 1952, Return of function after complete transection of the spinal cord of the rat, cat and dog, *Ann. Surg.* **136**: 193–205.

Horne, M. K. and Tracey, D. J., 1979, The afferents and projections of the ventroposterolateral thalamus in the monkey, *Exp. Brain Res.* **36**:129–141.

Jones, E. G., Coulter, J. D., and Hendry, S. H. C., 1978, Intracortical connectivity of architectonic fields in the somatic sensory, motor and parietal cortex of monkeys. *J. Comp. Neurol.* **181**:291–348.

Knapp, H. D., Taub, E., and Berman, A. J., 1963, Movements in monkeys with deafferented forelimbs, *Exp. Neurol.* **70**:305–315.

Kosar, E. and Asanuma, H., 1984, Focal and diffuse metabolic changes in the spinal cord elicited by microstimulation of differing motor cortical foci in the monkey, *Brain Res.* **310**:43–54.

Lawrence, D. G. and Kuypers, H. G. J. M., 1968, The functional organization of the motor system in the monkey. I. The effects of bilateral pyramidal lesions, *Brain* **91**:1–14.

Lemon, R. N. and Burg, van der J., 1979, Short-latency peripheral inputs to thalamic neurons projecting to the motor cortex in the monkey, *Exp. Brain Res.* **36**:445–462.

Liu, C. N. and Chambers, W. W., 1958, Intraspinal sprouting of dorsal root axons, *Arch. Neurol.* **79**:46–61.

Marsden, C. D., Merton, P. A., and Morton, H. B., 1972, Servo action in human voluntary movement, *Nature (London)* **238**:140–143.

Mott, F. W. and Sherrington, C. S., 1895, Experiments upon the influence of sensory nerves upon movement and nutrition of the limb, *Proc. R. Soc. Lond.* **57**:481–488.

Murphy, J. T., Wong, Y. C., and Kwan, H. C., 1975, Afferent-efferent linkages in motor cortex for single forelimb muscles, *J. Neurophysiol.* **38**:990–1014.

Nauta, W. H. J. and Gygax, P. A., 1954, Silver impregnation of degenerating axons in the central nervous system: A modified technique, *Stain Tech.* **29**:91–93.

Phillips, C. G., 1969, Motor apparatus of the baboon's hand, *Proc. R. Soc. Lond. B.* **173**:141–174.

Powell, P. S. and Mountcastle, B., 1959, The cytoarchitecture of the postcentral gyrus of the monkey *Macaca Mulatta, Bull. Johns Hopkins Hospital.* **105**:108–131.

Raisman, G., 1969, Neuronal plasticity in the septal nuclei of the adult rat, *Brain Res.* **14**:25–48.

Raisman, G. and Field, P. M., 1973, A quantitative investigation of the development of collateral reinnervation after partial deafferentation of the septal nuclei, *Brain Res.* **50**:241–264.

Rall, W., Burke, R. E., Smith, T. G., Nelson, P. G., and Frank, K., 1967, Dendritic location of synapses and possible mechanisms for the monosynaptic EPSP in motoneurons, *J. Neurophysiol.* **30**:1169–1193.

Ramón y Cajal, S., 1928, *Degeneration and Regeneration of the Nervous System* (R. M. May, ed. and translator), Oxford University Press, London.

Rosén, I. and Asanuma, H., 1972, Peripheral afferent inputs to the forelimb area of the monkey motor cortex: Input-output relations, *Exp. Brain Res.* **14**:257–273.

Rothwell, J. C., Traub, M. M., Day, B. L., Obeso, J. A., Thomas, P. K., and Marsden, C. D., 1982, Manual motor performance in a deafferenated man, *Brain* **105**:515–542.

Shinoda, Y., Zarzecki, P., and Asanuma, H., 1979, Spinal branching of pyramidal tract neurons in the monkey, *Exp. Brain Res.* **34**:59–72.

Shinoda, Y., Yokota, J., and Funtami, T., 1981, Divergent projection of individual corticospinal axons to motoneurons of multiple muscles in the monkey, *Neurosci. Lett.* **23**:7–12.

Sugar, O. and Gerard, R. W., 1940, Spinal cord regeneration in the rat, *J. Neurophysiol.* **3**:1–19.

Tatton, W. G., Former, S. D., Gerstein, G. L., and Chambers, W. W., 1975, The effect of postcentral cortical lesions on motor reponses to sudden upper limb displacements in monkeys, *Brain Res.* **96**:108–113.

Tower, S. S., 1940, Pyramidal lesion in the monkey, *Brain* **63**:36–90.

Travis, A. M. and Woolsey, C. N., 1956, Motor performance of monkeys after bilateral partial and total cerebral decortications, *Am. J. Phys. Med.* **35**:273–289.

Tsukahara, N., Hultborn, H., Murakami, F., and Fujito, Y., 1975, Electrophysiological study of formation of new synapses and collateral sprouting in red nucleus neurons after partial denervation, *J. Neurophysiol.* **38**:1359–1372.

Welt, C., Aschoff, J., Kameda, K., and Brooks, V. B., 1967, Intracortical organization of cat's sensory motor neurons, in: *Symposium on Neurophysiological basis of Normal and Abnormal Motor Activities* (D. P. Purpura and M. D. Yahr, eds.), Raven Press, Hewlett, N.Y., pp. 255–293.

Woody, C. D. and Engel, J., Jr., 1972, Changes in unit activity and thresholds to electric microstimulation at coronal-pericruciate cortex of cat with classical conditioning of different facial movements, *J. Neurophysiol.* **35**:230–241.

11

Motoneuronal Control of Eye Retraction/Nictitating Membrane Extension in Rabbit

JOHN F. DISTERHOFT and CRAIG WEISS

1. INTRODUCTION

The rabbit nictitating membane conditioning preparation, which was initially developed by Gormezano *et al.* (1962), has begun to be widely used as a model mammalian system in which to analyze the neurobiological substrates of learning. The preparation offers many technical advantages for this use (Thompson, 1976; Disterhoft *et al.*, 1977). Since conditioning occurs rapidly, even when the rabbit's head is fixed, the activity of single neurons may be related to behavioral response acquisition (Kraus and Disterhoft, 1982); auditory conditioned stimuli may be well controlled (Kraus and Disterhoft, 1981); and behavioral measurement is facilitated (Quinn *et al.*, 1984).

Our recent studies have concentrated on the final motor output pathway in this preparation (Disterhoft *et al.*, 1985). We have utilized neurophysiological, neuroanatomical, lesion, and stimulation techniques in these studies. Our goal has been to delineate the motoneuron pool(s) controlling the conditioned response (CR) output portion of the nictitating membrane (NM) reflex arc.

2. ANATOMICAL TRACING

Nictitating membrane extension in the rabbit occurs as a result of retraction of the eyeball into the orbit, which forces the NM out and across the cornea from the medial side in a passive fashion (Cegavske *et al.*, 1976). The retractor bulbi

JOHN F. DISTERHOFT ● Department of Cell Biology and Anatomy, Northwestern University Medical School, Chicago, Illinois 60611.   CRAIG WEISS ● Graduate Program in Neuroscience, Northwestern University Medical School, Chicago, Illinois 60611.

muscle, with slips which surround the optic nerve and insert onto the orbit medial and posterior to the other extraocular muscles, is ideally situated to retract the eyeball. Cegavske *et al.* (1976) reported that fibers in the VIth cranial nerve, the abducens, primarily controlled eye retraction and thus NM extension. They also found that multiple units in the principal abducens nucleus (ABD) fired with a very high correlation to both conditioned and unconditioned NM extension (Cegavske *et al.*, 1979).

We hypothesized that ABD might have subpopulations of neurons that control both lateral rectus and retractor bulbi muscles. To test this hypothesis, we injected horseradish peroxidase (HRP) into the retractor bulbi (Disterhoft and Shipley, 1980). However, we found that neurons in accessory abducens (ACC ABD), not ABD, were most heavily and reliably labeled after such injections (see Fig. 1). This accessory nucleus is a concentrated group of large cells ventral and slightly caudal to ABD and just dorsal to lateral superior olive. Axons from it course dorsal and rostrally through the principal abducens nucleus to exit the brain stem with the VIth nerve.

The ABD neurons may have been labeled as a result of leakage of HRP to lateral rectus within the orbit. To test this hypothesis, we made retractor bulbi injections after cauterizing the branch of the abducens nerve that goes to lateral rectus. We found normal uptake of HRP in ACC ABD and almost no transport to ABD. Thus, our anatomical experiments suggested that ACC ABD was the major source of motoneurons to retractor bulbi. Our conclusion regarding the dominant role of ACC ABD as the source of retractor bulbi motoneurons agreed with that of Cegavske and Moore and their colleagues on the basis of their anatomical experiments (Berthier and Moore, 1980; Cegavske *et al.*, 1984).

3. SINGLE NEURON RECORDING

In order to explore the role of ACC ABD motoneurons further, we recorded well-isolated single ACC ABD neurons in the conditioned and unconditioned rabbit (Quinn *et al.*, 1982). We found that neurons in ACC ABD had little or no background firing rate, that single unit activity always occurred during spontaneous or elicited NM sweeps, and that ACC ABD neurons were extremely responsive to corneal and periorbital somatosensory stimulation. Furthermore microstimulation in ACC ABD elicited NM sweeps at currents as low as 10 μA.

All of the ACC ABD cells showed an increase in firing associated with the beginning of the NM sweep, with some variation in response pattern during the remainder of the sweep. Figure 2 shows an example of three such cells. Some of these cells were recorded during the acquisition of the conditioned NM response. In these cases, the trial on which unit activity first appeared before US onset (in the CR period) was the first trial on which a CR appeared behaviorally.

Our single unit observations in the conscious rabbit have expanded upon those of Berthier and Moore (1983) in the anesthetized rabbit and on the observations that have been made in anesthetized cat (Grant *et al.*, 1979; Baker *et al.*, 1980).

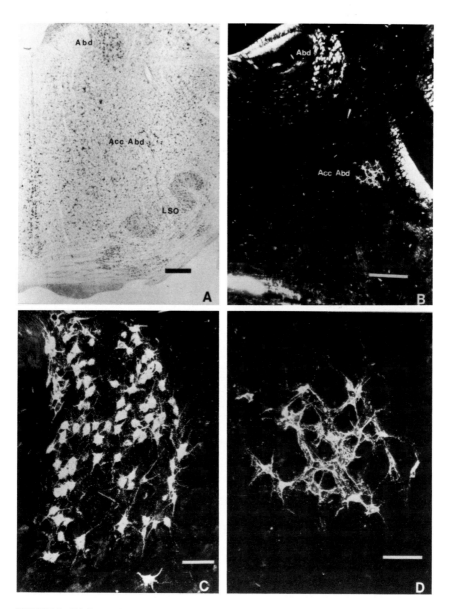

FIGURE 1. (A) Coronal section through rabbit brain stem. Abducens nucleus (Abd), accessory abducens nucleus (Acc Abd), and lateral superior olive (LSO) are indicated. Fascicles of nerve VI may be seen exiting toward the base of the brainstem. Bar = 0.5 mm. (B) Polarized light photomicrograph at same level as section in (A). HRP was injected into the retractor bulbi muscles. Cells in ACC ABD nucleus are heavily labeled. Bar = 0.5 mm. (C) Higher-power view of ABD shown in (B). Bar = 0.1 mm. (D) Higher-power view of ACC ABD shown in (B). Bar = 0.1 mm.

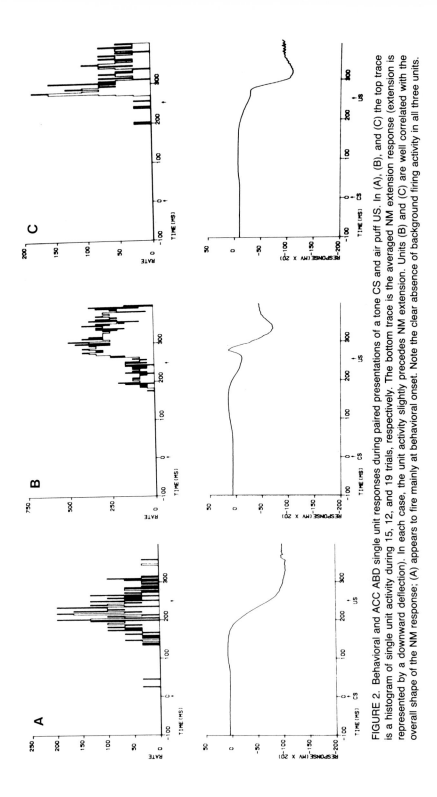

FIGURE 2. Behavioral and ACC ABD single unit responses during paired presentations of a tone CS and air puff US. In (A), (B), and (C) the top trace is a histogram of single unit activity during 15, 12, and 19 trials, respectively. The bottom trace is the averaged NM extension response (extension is represented by a downward deflection). In each case, the unit activity slightly precedes NM extension. Units (B) and (C) are well correlated with the overall shape of the NM response; (A) appears to fire mainly at behavioral onset. Note the clear absence of background firing activity in all three units.

The heavy corneal trigeminal input exists in both species (Grant and Horcholle-Bossavit, 1983). Our demonstration that single ACC ABD neurons are highly correlated with both unconditioned and conditioned NM extensions was anticipated on the basis of our anatomically demonstrated connections between ACC ABD motoneurons and the retractor bulbi muscles discussed above.

4. EYE RETRACTION MEASURED DIRECTLY

Nictitating membrane extension is an indirect consequence of eyeball retraction in the rabbit (Cegavske et al., 1976). We wished to measure the behavioral response directly to be able to evaluate lesion effects precisely. So we designed a method for doing accurate, repeatable measurements of eyeball retraction in the rabbit (Quinn et al., 1984). A film strip on which a light intensity grating has been exposed is attached to a contact lens. The lens is placed on the cornea and the intensity grating is placed between an LED and a photodiode. The contact lens film strip moves freely when the eyeball is retracted, and the photodiode gives a linear output with eyeball movement.

We have made some behavioral measurements with this device that are relevant to delineating the nictitating membrane, or perhaps more properly, eye retraction, conditioned response pathway. The average eye retraction latency to periorbital shock was 9.3 msec. This latency is about 8 msec shorter than values of NM extension latency that have previously been reported (Cegavske et al., 1976; Disterhoft et al., 1977; Moore and Desmond, 1982). It takes about 0.3–0.4 msec for the onset of the antidromic field potential at ACC ABD from a VIth nerve electric stimulus (Quinn et al., 1982). Berthier and Moore (1983) reported a 4-msec latency for ACC ABD neurons to respond to periorbital shock. The average eye retraction latency to VI nerve stimulation was 5.3 msec. The sum of these three values is 9.7 msec., a value very close to the 9.3-msec average latency for eye retraction produced by periorbital shock that we measured (see Fig. 3). Thus we would predict that premotor neurons that control ACC ABD (and probably the other motoneuron pools as well) should fire about 6–7 msec before the eye retraction behavioral response.

5. LESIONS

Both our anatomical and physiological experiments led us to conclude that ACC ABD was the principal source of retractor bulbi motoneurons. We reasoned that this muscle was the primary controller of eye retraction in rabbit because of its unique position in the orbit and because of the sensitivity of its neurons to corneal and periorbital stimuli, the major stimuli producing eye retaction. But there were two sources of conflicting data. First, Gray et al. (1981) had reported that both ACC ABD and 72% of ABD neurons sent axons to retractor bulbi. Second, activity of ABD multiple units had been demonstrated to be highly correlated with NM extension (Cegavske et al., 1979). We felt that if our dual hypothesis was correct, i.e., that retractor bulbi received its axons from ACC ABD and was the primary

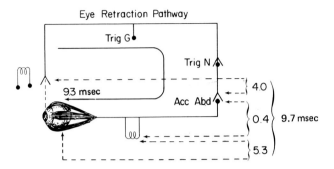

FIGURE 3. A schematic diagram of the unconditioned eye retraction response circuit. The average response latency to 10 mA periorbital shock trains was 9.3 msec. Berthier and Moore (1982) reported unit latencies of 4 msec to periorbital shock. We found onset latencies of the antidromic field potential to VI nerve stimulation of 0.3–0.4 msec (Quinn et al., 1984). Average eye retraction latency to VI nerve stimulation was 5.3 msec. The predicted latency value of 9.7 msec, obtained by adding the latencies obtained separately from three portions of the eye retraction unconditioned response arc, agrees with our measured value of 9.3 msec quite nicely.

cause of eye retraction, ACC ABD lesions should markedly reduce or eliminate eye retractions. Therefore, we performed a series of ACC ABD lesions to clarify the conflicting data.

We found that electrolytic lesions, which destroyed all or most of ACC ABD, immediately reduced the size of conditioned and unconditioned NM extensions in 8 of 10 cases. However, the responses generally returned to, or exceeded, prelesion amplitudes within 3 days (see Fig. 4). This result caused us to reexamine the report by Berthier and Moore (1980) that the extraocular muscles can mediate a NM response that is only reduced 50% from normal after VIth nerve section. Paradoxically, they found that extraocular muscle detachment alone had no effect on NM extension. In addition, Lorente de No (1933a) had shown many years ago, in quite a different context, that retractor bulbi and the other six extraocular muscles responded to corneal stimulation in rabbit.

In order to resolve the above paradox, we detached the recti and oblique extraocular muscles from the eyeball to get a more accurate estimate of reduction in retractor bulbi contraction strength after ACC ABD lesion. We found that the eye retraction response was reduced after extraocular muscle section, especially at high shock levels (see Fig. 5). In addition, qualitative behavioral observations indicated that the eyes were much less responsive to light puffs of air and corneal taps after extraocular muscle section. These data support the idea that the remaining extraocular muscles play a role in normal eye retraction in rabbit. In the two experiments in which we lesioned ACC ABD after extraocular muscle section, we found virtually complete and permanent elimination of eye retraction to periocular shock (see Fig. 6). That small retraction remaining was attributable to the small population of ABD and oculomotor neurons that send their axons to retractor bulbi (Spencer et al., 1980).

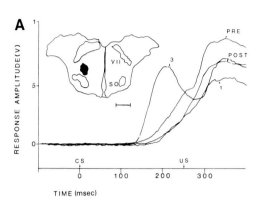

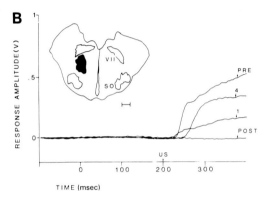

FIGURE 4. ACC ABD lesion effects on eyeball retraction response. (A) A lesion largely confined to ACC ABD caused an immediate reduction in conditioned and unconditioned response amplitude (Pre vs. Post). The postlesion effect on the conditioned response had disappeared by 3 days after the lesion, although in this case the unconditioned response remained reduced. (B) A large lesion caused a large postlesion unconditioned response reduction, which was still reduced 4 days after the lesion. The CS in (A) was white noise; the US in (A) and (B) was periorbital air puff. The eyeball retraction responses are 15 (A) and 10 (B) trial averages. The insets show outline drawings of sections through ACC ABD with largest lesion (VII, facial nerve; SO, superior olivary complex).

The most parsimonious interpretation of our lesion results is that ACC ABD is the major controller of retractor bulbi and therefore of eye retraction in the normal situation. When the extraocular muscles other than retractor bulbi are detached, eye retraction is relatively normal at low stimulus levels (see Fig. 5). The major effect is that the rise time of the retraction is slowed, indicating that the extraocular muscles contribute even at these low stimulus levels. As the stimulus intensity is increased, asymptotic retractor bulbi controlled eye retraction is reached, and the contribution of the remaining extraocular muscles becomes more apparent. When we lesioned ACC ABD and left the extraocular muscles attached, they soon increased their responsivity to periorbital stimuli. Thus, the initial reduction in NM response size soon disappeared. Of course, after the extraocular muscles had been sectioned, ACC ABD lesions eliminated the eye retraction response completely. Parenthetically, if 72% of ABD neurons send their axons to retractor bulbi (Gray *et al.*, 1981), the response should have been much less severely affected by ACC ABD lesions. Thus, our lesion data give strong support to our anatomical data, from which we concluded that ACC ABD is the main source of retractor bulbi motoneurons.

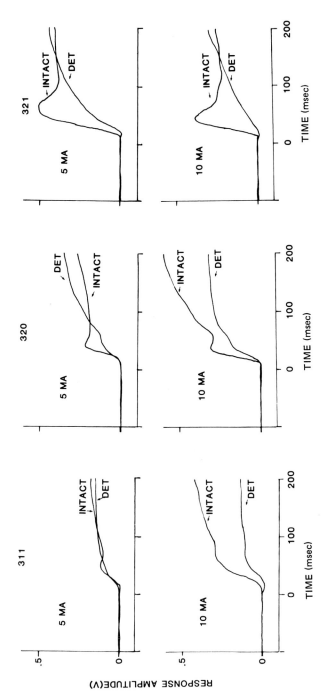

FIGURE 5. Extraocular muscle detachment effect on eye retraction. Average responses are shown for three rabbits (311,320,321) to 5 and 10 mA periorbital shock trains. The extraocular muscles other than retractor bulbi were detached from one orbit (DET); the other eye served as the unoperated control (INTACT). Detachment caused a clear reduction at the higher shock level. At the lower shock level, the effect was primarily to slow the rise time of the retraction; the asymptotic response was not affected.

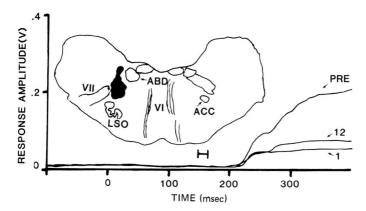

FIGURE 6. ACC ABD lesion plus extraocular muscle detachment effects on eyeball retraction response. Responses to periorbital shock (which began at 200 msec) are shown before (Pre), the day after (1), and 12 days after the ACC ABD lesion. All measurements were taken after extraocular muscle section, explaining why the Pre retraction is reduced from what would be expected in the intact situation (see Fig. 5). The bar represents 0.5 mm.

Apparently, Harvey *et al.* (1983) do not agree with our lesion results. They report that lesions of ACC ABD, leaving ABD intact, almost entirely eliminates NM extension. Extraocular muscle section was not necessary for their result. Since their lesions were done with knife cuts within the brain stem, designed to cut ACC ABD axons before they joined the sixth nerve, it is possible that the trigeminal afferents to the other extraocular muscles may have been cut as well. Our lesions were done electrolytically under physiological control. This is the only apparent explanation for our discrepant results. It should be noted that their current lesion result is at variance with their earlier report that 72% of ABD motoneurons send axons to retractor bulbi (Gray *et al.*, 1981), which were presumably not severed by their knife cuts.

We have multiple unit recording data from ABD which is in agreement with that of Cegavske *et al.* (1979), i.e., ABD multiple unit firing is highly correlated with NM extension. The recording data, with our ACC ABD lesion data, have led us to conclude that ABD nucleus can serve as one of the final output pathways for eyeball retraction in the rabbit. This, of course, is in agreement with the original report of Cegavske *et al.* (1976), although it is now obvious that the effect of cutting nerve VI was to immobilize both lateral rectus and retractor bulbi. When they stimulated nerve VI, they produced a coordinated eye retraction/NM extension because of the action of retractor bulbi. Had they stimulated axons to lateral rectus alone, the eye would have rotated laterally and retracted very little, if at all.

Oculomotor neurons also play a role in normal eyeball retraction, as was mentioned above. Lorente de No (1933a) showed by direct observation that the recti and obliques, in addition to retractor bulbi, contract after corneal stimulation. Harrison *et al.* (1978) have shown that oculomotor multiple units fire in correlation with NM extension. We have found that extraocular muscle section, other than retractor bulbi, reduced eye retraction. Thus, oculomotor neurons are involved in the normal rabbit eyeball retraction, since contraction of the recti and obliques can cause a substantial NM extension. The same considerations presumably apply to trochlear nucleus, which sends its axons to superior oblique. It is interesting to note that in their original experiments, Cegavske *et al.* (1976) found that stimulation of the oculomotor nerve caused correlated movement of the eye and NM, but not a coordinated retraction. This effect, due to the fact that lateral rectus and inferior oblique were not acting in concert with the other extraocular muscles, was reported but not weighted as heavily as the more dramatic VIth nerve effect (M. M. Patterson, personal communication).

6. CONCLUSIONS

Our conclusion is that two separate groups of motoneurons exist for controlling eyeball retraction: the ACC ABD forms one group; ABD, oculomotor, and trochlear nuclei form the other. Either ACC ABD or the other nuclei together may be sufficient but not necessary output pathways through which conditioned and unconditioned eyeball retraction may occur. Of course, in the intact rabbit, both groups act simultaneously to cooperatively produce eye retractions. We have not systematically tested the proposition, but it seems likely that all the extraocular muscles must contract synchronously in order to produce an effective eye retraction, as was discussed above. Thus, the three cranial motor nuclei that control the extraocular muscles other than retractor bulbi can be considered as one group, functionally, with regard to eye retraction.

Thompson has also shown that conditioned eye blink, controlled by the facial nucleus, is highly correlated with conditioned NM extension (McCormick *et al.*, 1982). This is understandable, since eye blink and NM extension are parts of the same defensive reflex in the rabbit's natural behavioral repertoire. The facial nucleus motoneurons that control orbicularis oculi are in the dorsomedial portion of the facial nucleus in rabbit (Disterhoft and Shipley, 1980). These facial motoneurons should also be under control of the premotor elements that govern ACC ABD, ABD oculomotor, and trochlear neurons in conditioned NM extension, given their close correlation.

The fact that there are apparently two groups of final output motoneurons controlling NM extension offers a unique experimental advantage for the next stage in retrogradely tracing the NM reflex arc. At some point, there should be a common premotor area that controls the two groups of output motoneurons, since all are highly correlated with NM extension. This common premotor interneuronal region should not be too many synapses upstream from the output motoneurons, given their close correlation. It is presumably between dentate-interpositus and the final output motoneurons since dentate-interpositus lesions eliminate conditioned, but not unconditioned, NM extensions (Lincoln *et al.*, 1982; McCormick and Thompson, 1984). We have begun retrograde tracing experiments at the final output motoneuron level by making physiologically controlled injections of wheat germ agglutinin-conjugated HRP (Weiss and Disterhoft, 1984). The most interesting premotor regions we have demonstrated, in regard to the eye retraction pathway, are from the perihypoglossal nuclei and reticular formation. We have not yet made injections into ACC ABD, oculomotor, or trochlear nuclei.

Our experiments, and those which other groups have been doing on rabbit NM/eyeball retraction conditioning, have sensitized us to the elegant complexity of the neuroanatomical and neurophysiological substrates that must underly this apparently simple, Pavlovian conditioning paradigm. This is certainly true even at the level of the final output motoneurons, as the experiments that we have described here demonstrate. The parallel loops and reciprocal connections that are known to exist in the brain stem regions through which information relevant to NM conditioning flows (Lorente de No, 1933b) offer several candidate loci for plastic change in addition to hippocampus (Thompson, 1980), neocortex (Kraus and Disterhoft, 1982), and cerebellum (Thompson et al., 1983). Matsumura and Woody (1982) have demonstrated excitability changes in cat facial nucleus motoneurons after blink conditioning. Their experiments strongly suggest that plastic change may be occurring even at the level of the final output motoneuron pools that we have discussed here. Systematic application of available extracellular techniques that relate the activity of single neurons to behavior, as well as further development and application of intracellular biophysical techniques to this conditioning preparation, should allow us to determine whether the "engram" for NM/eye retraction conditioning is localized or forms a distributed network within several levels of the neuraxis.

Acknowledgments. The research reported here was supported by NSF BNS 83 02488 and NIH 2 S07 RR05370.

REFERENCES

Baker, R., McCrea, R. A., and Spencer, R. F., 1980, Synaptic organization of cat accessory abducens nucleus, J. Neurophysiol. 43:771–791.

Berthier, N. E. and Moore, J. W., 1980, Role of extraocular muscles in the rabbit (Oryctolagus cuniculus) nictitating membrane response, Physiol. Behav. 24:931–937.

Berthier, N. E., and Moore, J. W., 1983, The nictitative membrane response: an electrophysiological study of the abducens nucleus in rabbit, Brain Res. 258:201–210.

Bienfang, D. C., 1978, The course of direct projections from the abducens nucleus to the contralateral medial rectus subdivision of the oculomotor nucleus in the cat, Brain Res. 145:277–289.

Cegavske, C. F., Harrison, T. A., and Torigoe, Y., 1984, Identification of the substrates of the unconditioned response in the classically conditioned, rabbit nictitating membrane preparation, in: Classical Conditioning (I. Gormezano, W. F. Prokasy, and R. F. Thompson, eds.), Lawrence Erlbaum Associates, Hillsdale, New Jersey.

Cegavske, C. F., Patterson, M. M., and Thompson, R. F., 1979, Neuronal unit activity in the abducens nucleus during classical conditioning of the nictitating membrane response in the rabbit (Oryctolagus cuniculus), J. Comp. Physiol. Psychol. 93:595–609.

Cegavske, C. F., Thompson, R. F., Patterson, M. M., and Gormezano, I., 1976, Mechanisms of efferent neuronal control of the reflex nictitating membrane response in rabbit (Oryctolagus cuniculus), J. Comp. Neurol. 90:411–423.

Disterhoft, J. F. and Shipley, M. T., 1980, Accessory abducens nucleus innervation of rabbit retractor bulbi motoneurons localized with HRP retrograde transport, Neurosci. Abstr. 6:478.

Disterhoft, J. F., Quinn, K. J., Weiss, C., and Shipley, M. T., 1985, Accessory abducens nucleus and conditioned eye retraction/nictitating membrane extension in rabbit, *J. Neuroscience* **5**:941–950.

Disterhoft, J. F., Kwan, H. H., and Lo, W. D., 1977, Nictitating membrane conditioning to tone in the immobilized albino rabbit, *Brain Res.* **137**:127–143.

Gormezano, I., Schneiderman, N., Deaux, E. B., and Fuentes, I., 1962, Nictitating membrane: Classical conditioning and extinction in the albino rabbit, *Science* **138**:33–34.

Grant, K., Gueritaud, J. P., Horcholle-Bossavit, G., and Tyc-Dumont, S., 1979, Anatomical and electrophysiological identification of motoneurons supplying the cat retractor bulbi muscle, *Exp. Brain Res.* **34**:541–550.

Grant, K. and Horcholle-Bossavit, G., 1983, Convergence of trigeminal afferents on retractor bulbi motoneurones in the anesthetized cat, *J. Physiol. (London)* **339**:41–60.

Gray, T. S., McMaster, S. E., Harvey, J. A., and Gormezano, I., 1981, Localization of retractor bulbi motoneurons in the rabbit, *Brain Res.* **226**:93–106.

Harrison, T. A., Cegavske, C. F., and Thompson, R. F., 1978, Neuronal activity recorded in the abducens and oculomotor nuclei during nictitating membrane conditioning in the rabbit, *Neurosci. Abstr.* **4**:259.

Harvey, J. A., Marek, G. J., Johannsen, A. M., McMaster, S. E., Land, T., and Gormezano, I., 1983, Role of the accessory abducens nucleus in the nictitating membrane response of the rabbit, *Neurosci. Abstr.* **9**:330.

Kraus, N. and Disterhoft, J. F., 1981, Location of rabbit auditory cortex and description of single unit activity, *Brain Res.* **214**:275–286.

Kraus, N. and Disterhoft, J. F., 1982, Response plasticity of single neurons in rabbit auditory association cortex during tone-signalled learning, *Brain Res.* **246**:205–215.

Lincoln, J. S., McCormick, D. A., and Thompson, R. F., 1982, Ipsilateral cerebellar lesions prevent learning of the clasically conditioned nictitating membrane/eyelid response, *Brain Res.* **242**:190–193.

Lorente de No, R., 1933a, The interaction of the corneal reflex and vestibular nystagmus, *Am. J. Physiol.* **103**:704–711.

Lorente de No, R., 1933b, Vestibulo-ocular reflex arc, *Arch. Neurol. Psychiatr.* **30**:245–329.

Matsumura, M. and Woody, C. D., 1982, Excitability changes of facial motoneurons of cats related to conditioned and unconditioned facial motor responses, in: *Conditioning: Representation of Involved Neural Functions* (C. D. Woody, ed.), Plenum Press, New York, pp. 451–457.

McCormick, D. A., Lavond, D. G., and Thompson, R. F., 1982, Concomitant classical conditioning of the rabbit nictitating membrane and eyelid responses: correlations and implications, *Physiol. Behav.* **28**:769–775.

McCormick, D. A. and Thompson, R. F., 1984, Cerebellum: Essential involvement in the classically conditioned eyelid response, *Science* **233**:296–299.

Moore, J. W. and Desmond, J. E., 1982, Latency of the nictitating membrane response to periocular electrostimulation in unanesthetized rabbits, *Physiol. Behav.* **28**:1041–1046.

Quinn, K. J., Disterhoft, J. F., and Weiss, C., 1982, Accessory abducens single unit activity during NM conditioning in the rabbit, *Neurosci. Abstr.* **8**:314.

Quinn, K. J., Kennedy, R. P., Weiss, C., and Disterhoft, J. F., 1984, Eyeball retraction latency in the conscious rabbit measured with a new photodiode technique, *J. Neurosci. Methods* **10**:29–39.

Spencer, R., Baker, R., and McCrea, R. A., 1980, Localization and morphology of cat retractor bulbi motoneurons, *J. Neurophysiol.* **43**:754–770.

Thompson, R. F., 1976, The search for the engram, *Am. Psychol.* **31**:209–227.

Thompson, R. F., 1980, The search for the engram, II, in: *Neural Mechanisms of Behavior* (D. McFadden, ed.), Springer-Verlag, New York, pp. 172–222.

Thompson, R. F., McCormick, D. A., Lavond, D. G., Clark, G. A., Kettner, R. E., and Mauk, M. D., 1983, The engram found? Initial localization of the memory trace for a basic form of associative learning, in: *Progress in Psychobiology and Physiological Psychology* (J. M. Sprague and A. N. Epstein, eds.), Academic Press, New York, pp. 167–196.

Weiss, C. and Disterhoft, J. F., 1985, Connections of the rabbit abducens nucleus, *Brain Res.* **326**:172–178.

12

Two Model Systems

JOHN W. MOORE

1. HERMISSENDA

Learning in *Hermissenda* largely conforms to expectations of what classical Pavlovian conditioning is supposed to look like, and the neural and biophysical substrates of learning have been well characterized in this system (e.g., Alkon, 1974; Crow and Alkon, 1978; Farley *et al.*, 1983). Features shared by conditioning in *Hermissenda* (or other invertebrate systems) and behavioral conditioning in vertebrates strengthens the assumption that mechanisms of learning in the former are applicable to the latter. What follows is a consideration of some of the characteristics of classical conditioning in *Hermissenda* that are often cited as relevant to the issue of whether this system can tell us much about neural mechanisms of classical conditioning in vertebrates.

Conditioned suppression of phototaxis (CSPT) reflects an association between light and rotation. Long-lasting Ca^{2+}-dependent depolarization of the Type B photoreceptor, increased membrane resistance, and accompanying alterations of Ia and Ib conductances all reflect this association, as their development parallels the acquisition of CSPT (Alkon, 1979; Alkon *et al.*, 1982; West *et al.*, 1982). That is, CSPT in the intact animal goes hand in hand with these biophysical effects, even when the latter are instilled by simulated light–rotation pairings.

CSPT develops progressively (e.g., Crow and Alkon, 1978, 1980). Its manifestations increase as a function of CS–US pairings; they do not increase and then decline (as in, e.g., sensitization or habituation). Nor is it the case that training simply enhances the rate of suppression of PT above that which would be expected by habituation. Early studies on learning and retention of CSPT by Alkon and Crow contained all the control groups a reasonable person would wish for, including random CS-alone presentations with no other treatment. A more recent study (Richards *et al.*, 1983) found no evidence of sensitization or habituation of PT. Nevertheless, our understanding of CSPT would be further enhanced if we knew more

JOHN W. MOORE ● Department of Psychology, University of Massachusetts, Amherst, Massachusetts 01003.

about the parameters that control sensitization and/or habituation of PT, assuming that one or both occur under some conditions.

Hermissenda investigators have been particularly sensitive to the problems of relying solely on an unpaired control procedure to counter interpretations of suppressed PT in terms of habituation (e.g., West *et al.*, 1982). Unpaired CS and US presentations can have consequences inconsistent with normal habituation: (1) sensitization (defined here as an enhanced original or alpha response to the CS—PT in this case—due merely to US occurrences, independent of pairing or context); (2) dishabituation (arrest or reversal of normal habituation due to unpredictable US occurrences within the context); (3) conditioned inhibition such that the light CS is associated with the absence of rotation, thereby giving an inappropriate baseline against which to assess CSPT as distinct from normal habituation of PT.

It now appears that CSPT undergoes extinction, provided the light CS is made sufficiently salient with respect to lighting under husbandry (Richards *et al.*, 1983). Earlier reports of failure to observe extinction raised strong doubts about the strength of the analogy between CSPT and vertebrate classical conditioning. However, spontaneous recovery has not been demonstrated, suggesting to Richards *et al.* (1983) that extinction of CSPT represents a reversal of original learning. Failure to observe spontaneous recovery across a range of conditions would lend further support to the unusual prospect of extinction-as-reversal; so, too, would evidence that reacquisition following extinction is as slow or slower than original learning.

It is interesting that the sort of reversal of associative strength suggested by the preliminary reports of extinction are precisely what would be predicted by the simplest linear learning models, including that of Rescorla and Wagner (1972). Spontaneous recovery and rapid reacquisition following extinction cannot be described by this class of models. Extinction has therefore been portrayed as involving processes (e.g., internal inhibition) related to the performance of a learned behavior, but not its associative undercarriage. Another suggested difference between CSPT and vertebrate learning has to do with the question of whether classical conditioning in the former is as sensitive to variation of CS–US interval as is generally the case with the latter. Grover and Farley (1983) report that a forward CS–US interval of 30 sec did not yield conditioning, whereas simultaneous light plus rotation for 30 sec per trial did. It would be premature to conclude that simultaneous pairings are actually more efficacious for learning than a possibly more judiciously chosen arrangement of CS and US in the forward paradigm. Nevertheless, it is interesting that some theorists have come to question the dogma that forward paradigms are optimal for associative learning. For example, Rescorla (1980) reports that simultaneous presentation of stimuli resulted in greater sensory preconditioning than did presentations in a forward-delay arrangement in flavor-aversion conditioning in rats. Wagner (1981) has presented a mathematical model that assumes that simultaneous pairing of a CS and US produces the strongest associative learning. I remain to be convinced that simultaneous conditioning is truly more congenial for the acquisition of CRs than is forward conditioning. My reluctance stems from deep-rooted convictions about the adaptive nature of CRs.

True CRs are anticipatory, and to be anticipatory implies an elapsed time between the signal and the anticipated event, the US. Moore and Stickney (1980,

1982, 1985) have followed some other real-time computational models in stressing this anticipatory nature of CRs (e.g., Sutton and Barto, 1981). In the case of the Moore–Stickney model the associative relationship between the CS and any other stimulus is characterized as a *predictive* relationship. One is drawn into this mind-set after countless observations of an eye blink or nictitating membrane extension emerging as a shadow of the UR cast in time toward the CS.

Izja Lederhendler, Serge Gart, and Daniel Alkon (personal communication, 1983) have recently discovered that it may be the same with CSPT in *Hermissenda*. They report that the animal's foot normally extends (increases in length) during a light step. By contrast, the normal unconditioned reaction to rotation is one of contraction of the foot. Pairing light with rotation leads to contraction of the foot in the presence of the light. This is the first clear indication that the CS elicits a shadow or "representation" of the US in this preparation. Most useful would be further details on the topography of the light-elicited foot contraction as it evolves over the course of acquisition training, extinction, etc.

1.1. Some Caveats

Farley *et al.* (1983) contend that changes in the Type B photoreceptor *cause* CSPT (Farley *et al.*, 1983). This article reports that the pairing of injected depolarizing current of the Type B receptor with a light step can substitute for normal light–rotation pairings to produce CSPT. Although this light-paired depolarization of the Type B photoreceptor (simulated rotation) is a *sufficient* condition ("cause") for learning, is it truly *necessary* as the paper goes on to suggest? The case for necessity is weak. One proof of necessity would be the observation of no learning under normally effective training protocols but with the Type B component somehow circumvented, e.g., by voltage clamping it so that it cannot undergo the depolarization that normally accompanies light–rotation pairing. "Lesioning" the Type B photoreceptor presents a similar approach to the problem, but both tacks have their difficulties. One wonders whether causality can even be proven, and single causes are notoriously the most difficult to pin down.

Hermissenda CSPT is highly regarded as a model system of learning because it is both associative and relatively long lasting. The distinction between associative and nonassociative phenomena can be misleading to investigators who are not abreast of recent developments in learning theory. Learning theorists nowadays recognize that all salient events occurring within a given context can be associated with each other and/or with contextual stimuli. Habituation, sensitization, and pseudoconditioning all have plausible interpretations within one associationistic theory or another. Differences between behavior that emerges from "associative" training and "nonassociative control" procedures may reflect different sorts of associations, often with conflicting implications, rather than a difference between association and nonassociation. It may also be incorrect to assume that long-term behavioral plasticity is always more important or interesting than short-term phenomena. Short-term (completely reversible and/or spontaneously decaying) behavioral changes may be more adaptive for a particular species in a particular niche than their long-term analogues. Long-term habituation, sensitization, and associative learning convey an aura of sophistication and cognitive agility, but under water hallmarks of intelligence may be radically different from this.

2. ANOTHER MODEL SYSTEM

The classically conditioned nictitating membrane (NM) response of the rabbit is a widely adopted model system for investigations of mammalian learning (Moore, 1979; Thompson, 1976; Woody, 1982). Historical and technical considerations too numerous to mention here have contributed to the current prominence of the rabbit NM and eye blink response as a system of investigating mammalian learning.

2.1. The Reflex Pathway

We employ electrical stimulation of the periocular region as the US in our research because it is easy to specify and control and because it can produce rapid CR acquisition. Electrical stimulation is applied via 9-mm wound clips crimped into the facial skin within 3 mm of the margin of the eye; one near the posterior (lateral) margin and the other in the anterior-inferior position. Facial fur is not removed. Current levels as low as 0.1 mA applied for a few msec can elicit NM responses in some rabbits. With current levels higher than this, e.g., 1 mA, the NM reflex attains its maximum extension of over 10 mm within 100 msec (Moore and Desmond, 1982).

The initiation of the response corresponds to the first detectable retraction of the eyeball, NM extension being a passive consequence of globe retraction (see, e.g., Berthier and Moore, 1980). By best current estimates, the minimum latency for initiation of eyeball retraction is slightly over 9 msec (Quinn et al., 1984). The time between stimulus onset and the firing of retractor bulbi motoneurons of the ipsilateral accessory abducens nucleus is approximately 4 msec, suggesting a disynaptic pathway mediated by rostral elements of the sensory trigeminal complex. The initial volley of sensory input reaches the semilunar ganglion in just over 1 msec and appears to be carried by A-alpha-beta fibers (Berthier and Moore, 1983).

The reflex pathway appears to be weakly crossed. High levels of stimulating current are required to elicit a detectable response form the contralateral eye. In addition, Desmond et al. (1983) observed only scatterings of labeled neurons in the contralateral sensory trigeminal complex following implantation of horseradish peroxidase (HRP) into the accessory abducens region. In marked contrast with this paucity of labeling within the contralateral sensory trigeminal complex, adjacent reticular formation contains many labeled neurons, particularly the supratrigeminal reticular formation (see Mizuno, 1970). The anatomical picture beginning to emerge suggests the presence of distinct zones adjacent to the rostral trigeminal system that project to both ipsilateral and contralateral accessory abducens nuclei. Physiological evidence suggests that these peritrigeminal regions receive sensory input from electrical stimulation of either eye (Desmond and Moore, 1983), probably via secondary sensory trigeminal neurons.

2.2. Premotor Components of the CR

Brain structures rostral to the red nuclei, including neocortex, are not essential for simple forward-delay conditioning (see Moore, 1979). This statement is a fair summary of the lesioning literature with the rabbit NM/eye blink preparation. It is, however, a bit misleading in that downstream influences from such forebrain systems as the septo-hippocampal complex and the basal ganglia can modulate the speed of acquisition of CRs (e.g., Kao and Powell, 1983; Prokasy et al., 1983; Moore and Solomon, 1984). However, the hippocampus may be essential for a variety of conditioning phenomena where information processing demands are greater than in the case of delay conditioning, e.g., trace conditioning (Solomon et al., 1983) and discrimination reversal (Berger and Orr, 1983).

The most significant development to emerge from studies of the neural substrates of classical conditioning of the rabbit NM response has been the discovery that discrete lesions of the cerebellum (e.g., Lincoln et al., 1982; Yeo et al., 1982) and pontine brain stem (Desmond and Moore, 1982; Lavond et al., 1981; Moore et al., 1982) can completely and irrevocably eliminate CRs without also affecting the UR. Desmond and Moore (1982) found that unilateral lesions of the dorsolateral pons in the parabrachial region and adjacent structures eliminated previously established CRs from the eye ipsilateral to the lesion or precluded their acquisition; URs and learning by the contralateral eye were unimpaired. Lesions for seven of the ten cases where the CR was eliminated clearly included portions of the superior cerebellar peduncle (brachium conjunctivum; henceforth BC), and BC lesions are now known to cause the elimination of CRs (McCormick et al., 1982). An additional 20 cases with pontine lesions showed no loss of CRs. All cases of CR-disrupting lesions in our original report involved supratrigeminal reticular formation to varying degrees, but so too did 9 of the 20 nondisrupted cases.

Implantation of HRP into the dorsolateral pons, including the supratrigeminal region, reveals projections from the contralateral supratrigeminal region, and HRP implanted into the accessory abducens region indicates bilateral projection from supratrigeminal regions (Desmond et al., 1983). Thus, the same population of neurons that project to the loci of motoneurons mediating eyeball retraction (accessory abducens area; see, e.g., Berthier and Moore, 1980, 1983) also projects to its contralateral homologue. It is not known whether single neurons within this population send axons to more than a single destination through axon collateralization.

The question of bilateral projection of US information is central for understanding why, once a CR has been well established for one eye, it is not unusual to observe a companion CR from the other eye (Desmond and Moore, 1983; Stickney and Donahoe, 1983) and why there is rapid transfer of CR acquisition when the US is switched from one eye to the other. Discrete brain lesions that eliminate or preclude CRs from one eye (but which leave the reflex pathway intact) need not eliminate CRs from the other eye nor preclude normal positive transfer of acquisition from one eye to the other (e.g., Desmond and Moore, 1982). These facts suggest that information carried by the US (or its association with CSs) is available to both sides of the brain and that each side has the necessary circuitry to produce CRs from either eye. Among the candidates for such bilateral representation of the US and CR generating capabilities are those reticular regions adjacent to (but separate from) the reflex pathway. Since supratrigeminal neurons receive bilateral input from the US (Desmond and Moore, 1983) and project bilaterally to the accessory abducens nuclei, they may be involved in mediating the transfer and eventual acquisition of contralateral CRs (see Desmond and Moore, 1982; Desmond *et al.*, 1983).

2.2.1. Red Nucleus

Lesions of the interpositus region of the cerebellum cause the elimination of CRs (Lincoln *et al.*, 1982; Yeo *et al.*, 1982). Interpositus neurons send axons to the red nuclei of the mesencephalon via BC, these fibers crossing en route, and lesions of magnocellular red nucleus disrupts contralateral conditioned responding (Haley *et al.*, 1983; Rosenfield and Moore, 1983). Desmond *et al.* (1983) showed that neurons of the red nucleus project caudally to the contralateral accessory abducens region (Desmond *et al.*, 1983). In a more recent study in our laboratory (Rosenfield *et al.*, 1985), HRP was implanted into magnocellular red nucleus in order to determine the course of the caudal-going projections (ultimately the rubrospinal tract) to the level of the accessory abducens nuclei. Only cases with heavy retrograde labeling of the contralateral interpositus region of the cerebellum were considered (see Figs. 1 and 2). Caudal-going rubral projection cross the midline in the ventral tegmental bundle just posterior to the third nerve and then assume a ventrolateral position beneath the fifth and seventh nerves. At the level of the

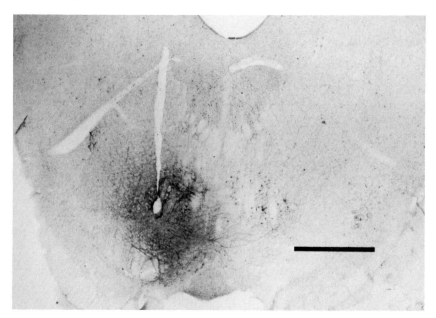

FIGURE 1. Photomicrograph showing HRP implantation site and diffusion in left magnocellular red nucleus (animal No. 30). Bar, 1mm. (For methodology, see Desmond *et al.*, 1983.)

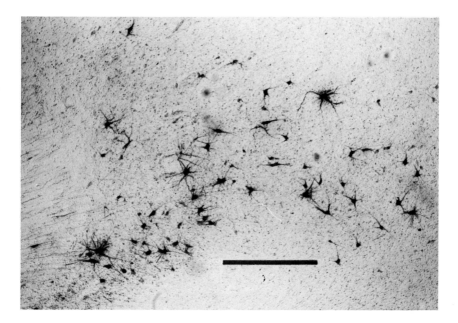

FIGURE 2. Photomicrograph showing retrograde HRP labeling of neurons of the right inter-positus region of the cerebellum (animal No. 30). This is a transverse section oriented at 45% such that dorsal is to the upper right and medial to the upper left. (calibration bar 0.5 mm.)

accessory abducens nuclei, fibers could be seen branching in a dorsomedial direction between the superior olive and the seventh nerve (see Fig. 3). We propose that some of the fibers terminate within the accessory abducens region and other motoneuron pools associated with eyeball retraction and/or defensive eye blink.

The anatomical evidence, therefore, indicates a doubly decussating circuit originating in the ipsilateral deep cerebellar region and running to the contralateral red nucleus via BC, crossing the midline once again as red nucleus neurons send axons caudally to the ipsilateral accessory abducens nucleus. Lesions anywhere in this circuit should cause a disruption of CRs from the ipsilateral eye, and this is precisely what several recent studies suggest. For example, Rosenfield *et al.* (1985) examined histological material from 70 animals with brain stem lesions, 28 of which caused CR disruption from one or both eyes. The phi correlation coefficient relating damage to a component of the circuit to CR disruption was 0.94 and highly statistically significant. By contrast, the value of phi relating damage of the supratrigeminal reticular formation to CR disruption, based on 54 animals from two relevant studies, was only 0.41 (also statistically significant). Clearly, the evidence from lesion studies implicates both anatomical entities in the CR, but the circuit involving BC and the rubrobulbar tract is the more strongly implicated at this juncture.

Haley *et al.* (1983), in their study reporting CR disruption following lesions of contralateral red nucleus, also noted disruption of URs. Rosenfield and Moore (1983) and C.H. Yeo (personal communication, 1983) have not observed deficits

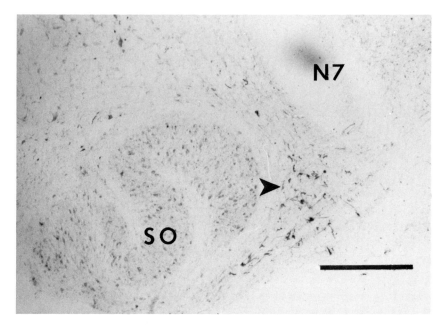

FIGURE 3. Photomicrograph of anterograde HRP labeling of fibers of the right rubrospinal tract as they appear to project toward the accessory abducens region (animal No. 26). Implantation of HRP was in the left magnocellular red nucleus, as in Fig. 1. Bar, .5mm.

in unconditioned responding following red nucleus lesions. The fact that Haley *et al.* (1983) used corneal air puff instead of electrical stimulation might account for this discrepancy between the two sets of studies: Red nucleus can involve the oculomotor nerve, altering the orbital position of the cornea and thereby mitigating the effect of the air puffs.

2.2.2. Cerebellar Cortex

Thompson has reported that, unlike nucleus interpositus, cerebellar cortex is not essential for the conditioned NM/eyelid response (e.g., McCormick and Thompson, 1983). In contrast, C.H. Yeo, M.J. Hardiman, M. Glickstein, and I. Steele Russell in London (personal communication, 1983) have found that a small portion of hemispheric lobus simplex of cerebellar cortex is necessary for this behavior. This area of cerebellar cortex receives all the sensory inputs that would be required for NM/eyelid conditioning and projects to the ipsilateral interpositus nucleus.

Cerebellar cortex contains ample machinery for associative learning and the performance of motor CRs (Marr, 1969; Albus, 1971), and Ito and his colleagues have begun to elaborate possible mechanisms that may underlie this type of learning, specifically the modulation of Purkinje cell excitability to parallel fiber input (e.g., Ito, 1982).

2.2.3. Red Nucleus and Supratrigeminal Region

Given a cerebellar-rubral circuit projecting to accessory abducens motoneurons, all components of which being essential for the generation of CRs, it is tempting to conclude that the supratrigeminal region is not importantly involved in NM conditioning and that its anatomical relationship to the accessory abducens nucleus serves some other function. The CR-disrupting lesions of the dorsolateral pons reported by Desmond and Moore (1982), in addition to being effective by involving BC, might have interrupted fibers passing through the lesioned zone from red nucleus to the accessory abducens region. The possibility that red nucleus fibers to the accessory abducens nuclei actually pass through the supratrigeminal zone is not supported by our HRP studies, as the rubrobulbar tract assumes a somewhat more ventrolateral position at the level of the fifth nerve. Lesions of the tract, however, do disrupt the CR without affecting the UR (Rosenfield *et al.*, 1985), as do lesions elsewhere in the circuit. The possible role of the supratrigeminal reticular formation in mediating transfer of conditioning from one eye to the other was discussed above. The contribution of this brain region to acquisition and expression of the CR and its relationship to the essential cerebellar-rubral circuit remains to be delineated.

2.3. Some Caveats

The foregoing discussion of rabbit NM/eye blink conditioning could not do justice to the important work that has been done in other laboratories. The combined efforts of the various groups suggest that a consensus concerning the anatomical substrates of simple forward conditioning is near at hand. However, physiological work designed to address questions of mechanisms has been sparse, and a great deal of work lies ahead.

ACKNOWLEDGMENT. This chapter is based on work supported by grants NSF BNS 8215816 and AFOSR 830215.

REFERENCES

Albus, J. S., 1971, A theory of cerebellar function, *Math. Biosci.* **10**:25–61.

Alkon, D. L., 1974, Associative training of *Hermissenda*, *J. Gen. Physiol.* **64**:70–84.

Alkon, D. L., 1979, Voltage-dependent calcium and potassium ion conductances: A contingency mechanism for an associative learning model, *Science* **205**:801–816.

Alkon, D. L., Lederhendler, I., and Shoukimas, J. J., 1982, Primary changes of membrane currents during retention of associative learning, *Science* **215**:693–695.

Berger, T. W. and Orr, W. B., 1983, Hippocampectomy selectively disrupts discrimination reversal conditioning of the rabbit nictitating membrane response, *Behav. Brain Res.* **8**:49–68.

Berthier, N. E. and Moore, J. W., 1980, Role of extraocular muscles in the rabbit (*Oryctolagus cuniculus*) nictitating membrane responses, *Physiol. Behav.* **24**:931–938.

Berthier, N. E. and Moore, J. W., 1983, The nictitating membrane response: An electophysiological study of the abducens nerve and nucleus and the accessory abducens nucleus in rabbit, *Brain Res.* **258**:201–210.

Crow, T. J. and Alkon, D. L., 1978, Retention of an associative behavioral change in *Hermissenda, Science* **201:**1239–1241.

Crow, T. J. and Alkon, D. L., 1980, Associative behavioral modification in *Hermissenda:* cellular correlates, *Science* **209:**412–414.

Desmond, J. E. and Moore, J. W., 1982, A brain stem region essential for the classically conditioned but not unconditioned nictitating membrane response, *Physiol. Behav.* **28:**1029–1033.

Desmond, J. E. and Moore, J. W., 1983, A supratrigeminal region implicated in the classically conditioned nictitating membrane response, *Brain Res. Bull.* **10:**765–773.

Desmond, J. E., Rosenfield, M. E., and Moore, J. W., 1983, An HRP study of the brainstem afferents to the accessory abducens region and dorsolateral pons in rabbit: Implications for the conditioned nictitating membrane response, *Brain Res. Bull.* **10:**747–763.

Farley, J., Richards, W. G., Ling, L. J., Liman, E., and Alkon, D. L., 1983, Membrane changes in a single photoreceptor cause associative learning in *Hermissenda, Science* **221:**1201–1202.

Grover, L. and Farley, J., 1983, Temporal order sensitivity of learning in *Hermissenda, Soc. Neurosci. Abstr.* **9:**915.

Haley, D. A., Lavond, D. G., and Thompson, R. F., 1983, Effects of contralateral red nucleus lesions on retention of the classically conditioned nictitating membrane response/eyelid response, *Soc. Neurosci. Abstr.* **9:**643.

Harvey, J. A., Marek, G. J., Johannsen, A. M., McMaster, S. E., Land, T., and Gormezano,I., 1983, Role of the accessory abducens nucleus in the nictitating membrane response of the rabbit, *Soc. Neurosci. Abstr.* **9:**330.

Ito, M., 1982, Synaptic plasticity underlying the cerebellar motor learning investigated in rabbit's flocculus, in: *Conditioning* (C. D. Woody, ed.), Plenum Press, New York, pp. 213–222.

Kao, K. T. and Powell, D. A., 1983, Substantia nigra lesions and Pavlovian conditioning of eyeblink and heart rate responses in the rabbit, *Soc. Neurosci. Abstr.* **9:**330.

Lavond, D. G., McCormick, D. A., Clark, G. A., Holmes, D. T., and Thompson, R. F., 1981, Effects of ipsilateral rostral pontine lesions on retention of the classically conditioned nictitating and eyelid responses, *Physiol. Psychol.* **9:**335–339.

Lincoln, J. S., McCormick, D. A., and Thompson, R. F., 1982, Ipsilateral cerebellar lesions prevent learning of the classically conditioned nictitating membrane/eyelid response, *Brain Res.* **242:**190–193.

Marr, D., 1969, A theory of cerebellar cortex, *J. Physiol.* **202:**437–470.

McCormick, D. A., Guyer, P. E., and Thompson, R. F., 1982, Superior cerebellar peduncle lesions selectively abolish the ipsilateral classically conditioned nictitating membrane/eyelid response of the rabbit, *Brain Res.* **244:**347–350.

McCormick, D. A. and Thompson, R. F., 1983, Cerebellum: Essential involvement in the classically conditioned eyelid response, *Science* **223:**296–299.

Mizuno, N., 1970, Projection fibers from the main sensory trigeminal nucleus and the supratrigeminal region, *J. Comp. Neurol.* **139:**457–472.

Moore, J. W., 1979, Brain processes and conditioning, in: *Mechanisms of Learning and Motivation: A Memorial Volume to Jerzy Konorski* (A. Dickinson and R. A. Boakes, eds.), Erlbaum, Hillsdale, New Jersey, pp. 111–142.

Moore, J. W. and Desmond, J. E., 1982, Latency of the nictitating membrane response to periocular electro-stimulation in unanesthetized rabbits, *Physiol. Behav.* **28:**1041–1046.

Moore, J. W., Desmond, J. E., and Berthier, N. E., 1982, The metencephalic basis of the conditioned nictitating membrane response, in: *Conditioning* (C. H. Woody, ed.), Plenum Press, New York, pp. 459–482.

Moore, J. W. and Solomon, P. R., 1984, Forebrain-brainstem interaction: Conditioning and the hippocampus, in: *The Neuropsychology of Memory* (N. Butters and L. R. Squire, eds.), Guilford, New York, pp. 462–472.

Moore, J. W. and Stickney, K. J., 1980, Formation of attentional-associative networks in real time: Role of the hippocampus and implications for conditioning, *Physiol. Psychol.* **8:**207–217.

Moore, J. W. and Stickney, K. J., 1982, Goal tracking in attentional-asociative networks: Spatial learning and the hippocampus, *Physiol. Psychol.* **10:**202–208.

Moore, J. W. and Stickney, K. J., 1985, Antiassociations: Conditioned inhibition in attentional-associative networks, in: *Information Processing in Animals: Conditioned Inhibition* (R. R. Miller and N. E. Spear, eds.), Erlbaum, Hillsdale, New Jersey, pp. 209–232.

Prokasy, W. F., Kesner, R. P., and Calder, L. D., 1983, Posttrial electrical stimulation of the dorsal hippocampus facilities acquisition of the nictitating membrane response, *Behav. Neurosci.* **97**:860–896.

Quinn, K. J., Kennedy, P., Weiss, C., and Disterhoft, J., 1984, Eyeball retraction latency in the conscious rabbit measured with a new technique, *J. Neurosci. Meth.* **10**:29–39.

Rescorla, R. A., 1980, Simultaneous and successive associations in sensory preconditioning, *J. Exp. Psychol: Anim. Behav. Processes* **6**:207–216.

Rescorla, R. A. and Wagner, A. R., 1972, A theory of Pavlovian conditioning: Variations in the effectiveness of reinforcement and nonreinforcement, in: *Classical Conditioning II: Current Theory and Research* (A. H. Black and W. F. Prokasy, eds.), Appleton-Century-Crofts, New York, pp. 64–99.

Richards, W., Farley, J., and Alkon, D. L., 1983, Extinction of associative learning in *Hermissenda*: Behavior and neural correlates, *Soc. Neurosci. Abstr.* **9**:916.

Rosenfield, M. E. and Moore, J. W., 1983, Red nucleus lesions disrupt the classically conditioned nictitating membrane response in rabbits, *Behav. Brain Res.* **10**:393–398.

Rosenfield, M. E., Dovydaitis, A., and Moore, J. W., 1985, Brachium conjunctivum and rubrobulbar tract: Brain stem projections of red nucleus essential for the conditioned nictitating membrane response, *Physiol. Behav.* **34**:751–759.

Solomon, P. R., Vander Schaaf, E. R., Nobre, A. C., Weisz, D. J., and Thompson, R. F., 1983, Hippocampus and trace conditioning of the rabbits' nictitating membrane response, *Soc. Neurosci. Abstr.* **9**:645.

Stickney, K. J. and Donahoe, J. W., 1983, Attenuation of blocking by a change in US locus, *Anim. Learn. Behav.* **11**:60–66.

Sutton, R. S. and Barto, A. G., 1981, Toward a modern theory of adaptive networks: Expectation and prediction, *Psychol. Rev.* **88**:135–170.

Thompson, R. F., 1976, The search for the engram, *Am. Psychol.* **31**:209–227.

Wagner, A. R., 1981, SOP: A model of automatic memory processing in animal behavior, in: *Information Processing in Animals: Memory Mechanisms* (N. E. Spear and R. R. Miller, eds.), Erlbaum, Hillsdale, New Jersey, pp. 5–47.

West, A., Barnes, E., and Alkon, D. L., 1982, Primary changes of voltage responses during retention of associative learning, *J. Neurophysiol.* **48**:1243–1255.

Woody, C. D., 1982, *Conditioning*, Plenum Press, New York.

Yeo, C. H., Hardiman, M. J., Glickstein, M., and Steele Russell, I., 1982, Lesions of cerebellar nuclei abolish the classically conditioned nictitating membrane response, *Soc. Neurosci. Abstr.* **8**:22.

13

How Can the Cerebellar Neuronal Network Mediate a Classically Conditioned Reflex?

MASAO ITO

In view of the remarkable possibility that the cerebellum is the site of the classically conditioned eyelid eye blink reflex, it would be interesting to speculate about how the currently known mechanisms of the cerebellar neuronal network account for this possibility.

Grossberg (1969) early suggested that the convergence of two distinct synaptic inputs to a Purkinje cell, one from parallel fibers (axons of granule cells) and the other from a climbing fiber (axon of inferior olive cell), represents an associative memory. If a climbing fiber conveys unconditioned stimulus signals, parallel fiber synapses simultaneously activated with conditioned stimulus signals will be facilitated so that thereafter the conditioned stimuli would be able to excite the Purkinje cell by themselves. The conjunctive stimulation of parallel fibers and a climbing fiber, however, has been found to induce only a long-term depression (LTD), but not any type of facilitation, in parallel fiber-Purkinje cell transmission (Ito *et al.*, 1982).

A question would follow: whether a cerebellar neuronal network with the LTD incorporated, but without any facilitation mechanism, can account for an associative memory that usually is ascribed to a sustained synaptic facilitation (Brindley, 1967). I wish to suggest one possibility below.

Let us assume that a signal flow pathway through cerebellar nuclei had been blocked by inhibitory action of Purkinje cells. These Purkinje cells would be activated by signals of the nuclear pathway, through mossy fibers and parallel fibers, and in turn would inhibit nuclear cells before the nuclear cells yield any significant outputs. When signals of a climbing fiber pathway induce the LTD in the parallel fiber-Purkinje cell synapses, the nuclear pathway would be released from Purkinje

MASAO ITO ● Department of Physiology, Faculty of Medicine, University of Tokyo, Bunkyo-ku, Tokyo 113, Japan.

cell inhibition. With the nuclear pathway responsible for conditioned response, and with the climbing fiber pathway conveying unconditioned stimulus signals, this cerebellar system would constitute a switching device that simulates an associative memory mechanism. However, it is important to note that in this model, the association is due to a release of a preexisting pathway from Purkinje cell inhibition; the acoustically conditioned eyelid eye blink response may be effected by release of an inherent startle response that had been suppressed by Purkinje cell inhibition.

The above possibility may not apply to all kinds of classically conditioned reflexes, a part of which may be positively formed with a facilitation process. Nevertheless, since the LTD is a remarkable phenomenon in the cerebellar cortex that accounts for cerebellar adaptation very well (Ito, 1984), its applicability to some cases of classically conditioned reflexes may deserve examination in a future investigation.

REFERENCES

Brindley, G. S., 1967, The classification of modifiable synapses and their use in models for conditioning, *Proc. R. Soc. London B* **168:**361–76.

Grossberg, S., 1969, On learning of spatiotemporal patterns by network with ordered sensory and motor components. I. Excitatory components of the cerebellum, *Studies Appl. Math.* **48:**105–132.

Ito, M., 1984, *The Cerebellum and Neural Control,* Raven Press, New York.

Ito, M., Sakurai, M., and Tongroach, P., 1982, Climbing fibre induced depression of both mossy fibre responsiveness and glutamate sensitivity of cerebellar Purkinje cells, *J. Physiol. (London)* **324:**113–134.

14

Mnemonic Interaction between and within Cerebral Hemispheres in Macaques

ROBERT W. DOTY, JEFFREY D. LEWINE, and JAMES L. RINGO

1. INTRODUCTION

Since its inception (Myers and Sperry, 1953) work on interhemispheric mnemonic transfer in animals has referred to the acquisition of a discrimination learned over many trials, first by one hemisphere and then by the other (see, e.g., Gazzaniga, 1970; Doty and Negrão, 1973; Hamilton, 1977; Butler, 1979). The experiments to be described herein utilize a significantly different procedure, in which macaques with transected optic chiasm are queried as to whether they can recognize with one eye and hemisphere visual images previously seen on but one occasion by the other eye and hemisphere. Using several thousand highly varied images, the capabilities of such interhemispheric comparison can be continually and repeatedly assessed, as can the level of such performance by each hemisphere individually. Thus, essentially for the first time, it will be possible to assay inter- and intrahemispheric processing in relation to memory for events, rather than, as heretofore, simply for rules.

2. METHOD

2.1. Animals

Five male *Macaca nemestrina* have been used in the experiments to date. RHD and HUD, studied for 6.5 years, were first used in experiments of Overman and Doty (1980, 1982). The optic chiasm was subsequently transected, after which they

ROBERT W. DOTY, JEFFREY D. LEWINE, and JAMES L. RINGO ● Center for Brain Research, University of Rochester, Rochester, New York 14642.

survived for 44 and 60 months, respectively. All of the corpus callosum (CC) was cut in RHD 15.5 months after the chiasm transection, leaving the anterior commissure (AC) intact, and he was then tested for 28 months more. The AC and rostral CC were cut in HUD 29 months after the chiasm transection, leaving only 4–5 mm of the splenium intact. Electrodes were implanted in the optic tract and splenium after 23 months more, and removed one month later when the remaining CC was also transected, making a fully "split-brain" animal. The right medioventral tip of the temporal lobe was removed 2.5 months later, and the left amygdala 2 months after that, following which he was studied for another 2.5 months. Histology on HUD is concordant with the surgical intent, but in RHD there were surviving fibers crossing in the optic chiasm.

DND was trained for 6 months preoperatively and tested for 18 months following transection of the optic chiasm, for 11 months of which all of the CC had been cut, leaving the AC as the only forebrain commissure. Histology confirmed the completeness of the transection of the CC and chiasm. TDY received 14 months of preoperative training and has been tested for 8 months subsequent to transection of the chiasm. All of the foregoing monkeys have been tested with the delayed match to sample (DMS) procedure (see below). Testing in the "List" mode has been used with RAO, who received 4 months of preoperative training before undergoing transection of the optic chiasm. After 25 months of testing in this condition, the posterior 9–10 mm of the CC was also transected, and there has now been a further 4 months of testing.

2.2. Surgery

Transphenoidal transection of the optic chiasm (Downer, 1959) has the advantage over a dorsal approach in leaving the CC untouched. The animal, anesthetized with secobarbital, is placed supine, and the nasopharynx entered through a "U"-shaped incision initiated at the posterior border of the hard palate. Hemorrhage can be profuse, and cautery may be essential. All the surgery is performed using $12 \times$ stereoscopic magnification with axial illumination. Bone is removed with an otological bur, the angle of attack being critical, otherwise the hypophysis, cavernous sinus, or interpeduncular fossa, rather than the chiasm, may be exposed. Bone underlying the chiasm is readily recognized by its contour and characteristic whiteness. About 2 mm of its central portion is removed, and when the dura mater is incised, roughly half the surface of the chiasm is immediately visible. An initial cut with an eye knife is extended easily with blunt dissection. However, the ventral posterior quadrant of the cut surface of the chiasm can never be fully visualized, and assurance that the transection is complete is gained only by continuing the dissection blindly in this sector until the cut surfaces "fall apart", i.e., separate entirely of their own accord, leaving a distinct gap between them. This has been the case for all of the animals described herein. The sphenoidal opening is occluded with an absorbable cellulose pledget emplaced with cyanoacrylate glue. This effectively eliminates significant loss of cerebrospinal fluid. The small palatal incision is closed with 5-0 silk, and the stitches are removed under halothane anesthesia 1 week later. The animal is kept on chloramphenicol for 5 days postoperatively.

Transection of the CC, or AC from the dorsal approach, closely follows the procedures developed in Sperry's laboratory (see, e.g., Gazzaniga, 1970), the only significant addition being use of a 40% urea solution intravenously, 2.5 ml/kg, to reduce brain volume and thus improve accessibility of midline structures.

2.3. Tests

The macaques were trained to accept daily capture and sufficient restraint to keep them positioned in front of the display panels. For monocular testing the animals with split chiasm wore a light-weight mask, equipped with rotary solenoid shutters (Doty, 1984). In the DMS task (see Overman and Doty, 1979, 1980, 1982) there were three panels, stacked vertically, each roughly 20° wide by 14° high, which could be transilluminated from their rear with high-quality photographic images under the control of three corresponding projectors. The central panel was first illuminated for a few seconds with a particular image, and the monkey rewarded with a few drops of juice for pressing it. It was then extinguished and a delay period, usually of 2–10 sec, ensued. Images then appeared on the upper and lower panels, one of which was identical to that just presented, and the monkey was rewarded with 1–2 or more ml of juice for pressing the panel on which that image appeared. Choice of the incorrect image could produce a puff of air directed at the top of the monkey's head, sounding of loud horn, and/or a 20–50 sec delay in presentation of the next "sample" (which would normally occur in 2–10 sec). A total of 50–100 trials was presented in each session. In most instances the images used were extremely varied, e.g., tools, chinaware, Christmas tree ornaments, electronic components, etc., photographed against a black background, or reproductions of magazine advertising and illustrations.

The same type of material was used for the "List" procedure (Gaffan, 1977). In this case there were two panels. Upon the upper panel a series of rear-projected images appeared at 10-sec intervals. The monkey was rewarded with a small quantity of juice for pressing this panel if this was the first time in that session that the image had appeared. At later, quasi-random positions in the sequence an image was re-presented, and on this occurrence the monkey was rewarded with 1–2 ml of juice if it pressed the blank bottom panel, and punished by air puff for pressing the top panel with the re-presented image. In most instances 280 images were presented in each session. Note that the "chance" level of recognition is here given by the monkey's "false positive" rate; i.e., how many times it misidentifies an image as having been presented previously when in fact it is the first presentation. This level was roughly 20% for RAO, a well-trained animal. Conceivably, it might be somewhat lower were the inventory of images sufficient that across sessions the same set of images was never used again. In actual practice at least 4–7 days elapsed before any given image was used in a subsequent session.

For both DMS and list procedures all parameters and performance were computer controlled and recorded.

3. RESULTS AND DISCUSSION

3.1. Interhemispheric Mnemonic Recognition of Visual Images

The major result is simply stated: using either the AC or the splenium of the CC, one eye and hemisphere can readily recognize images previously seen by the other, whereas if both forebrain commissures, or only the AC and splenium have been cut, this is no longer possible. With the DMS procedure the accuracy of this recognition, using colored images of objects, is 90% or better, but for the list procedure it is only about 70% even when the second presentation follows immediately upon the first (Lewine and Doty, 1983). It must be recalled, of course, that with a false positive rate of only 20%, a 70% level of correct identification of recurrences in the List still reflects a very high level of performance; however, the accuracy is almost 95% if each presentation is to the same eye. The reason for this discrepancy between the List and DMS procedures is not understood. It probably reflects the large difference inherent in the mnemonic task, although, if so, it is puzzling why this should not also hold for the intrahemispheric comparisons. Controls for the possibility that this poorer interhemispheric performance might be related to the split in the visual field (see Hamilton and Tieman, 1973) are still being pursued.

While Hamilton and his colleagues (Hamilton *et al.*, 1968; Hamilton and Brody, 1973; Tieman and Hamilton, 1973, 1974) had demonstrated that macaques with split chiasm were capable of making simultaneous interocular comparisons, they examined interhemispheric mnemonic comparison only for pure color, using a 3–sec delay between sample and match. For monkey RAO in the best direction of interhemispheric comparison (see below) performance was still above chance levels even with 46 intervening images and a delay of 12 min in the List procedure.

Perhaps most interesting is the facility of the AC alone for effecting such interhemispheric mnemonic comparisons, since there is presently considerable uncertainty regarding the human capacity to utilize this pathway in similar tasks (see, e.g., Zihl and von Cramon, 1980; McKeever *et al.*, 1981). There was, in fact, no distinguishable difference in the DMS performance of DND with only AC intact versus HUD with only the splenium present (Doty *et al.*, 1982; Doty, 1984), other than that the performance of DND was consistently better on the more difficult types of material.

When called upon for the first time to utilize a restricted component of the forebrain commissural system, only one of the animals showed any hesitation or confusion. This was RHD, 60 days after cutting of all of the CC, leaving only the AC (and some of the chiasm); his manifest uncertainty cleared within a few trials, so that he failed to respond to 13 of the 50 "matches" required but was correct on 97% of the remaining 37. However, when examined over a span of several weeks, it was apparent that all of the animals displayed some increment in the accuracy with which they came to make cross-commissural or callosal comparisons.

For animal HUD, an attempt was made to perturb interhemispheric comparisons by tetanizing the optic tract or splenium (the only remaining portion of his forebrain commissures) during the "match" phase of the DMS task (see Overman and Doty, 1979). No significant effect was obtained until it became obvious, either from forced movements or deterioration of performance for intrahemispheric comparisons, that the current was engaging structures other than those intended. For instance, concurrent stimulation at 1–2 mA, 100 Hz, with 1.0-msec pulses through three pairs of side-by-side "bipolar" electrodes in the 5 mm remaining of the splenium, timed to occur just as the images appeared for the "match" trial and continue until the choice was made, had no effect upon the 90% level of correct interhemispheric performance until intensities were reached at which intrahemispheric performance also became erratic.

3.2. Indications of Differences in the Performance of the Two Hemispheres

There are, at times, clear indications that one hemisphere is more proficient at one type of task than is the other. In so far as some asymmetry of performance might be expected simply because of the vagaries of the surgical procedures (e.g., loss of more optic tract fibers on one side consequent to transection of the chiasm, slight disruption of cortical vascular supply by midline surgery, and so on), such results are not always of interest. However, there are distinct instances in which such objections do not apply.

The role of "dominance", as evidenced by handedness, seems to offer no firm foundation or correlate for clarifying those signs of hemispheric specialization that are observed (see Hamilton and Vermeire, 1982). HUD, for instance, for a period of 2.5 years, including the six months following transection of the optic chiasm and while both CC and AC were intact, invariably used his left hand in all of a variety of lever- or panel-pressing situations in which he was trained. During the latter period, while his performance with intrahemispheric comparisons after 3- to 5-sec delays was roughly 90% correct for either hemisphere, all observers were agreed that he displayed much slower and more hesitant performance, with false starts, when working with the right eye open than when using the left, i.e., just the opposite of an a priori expectation for the left-handed performance. Also suggestive of some asymmetry between the hemispheres was the fact that for 500 trials each of viewing the "sample" with the right eye and choosing the "match" with the left, he made only 55 errors, whereas with the opposite direction of comparison (left eye, "sample," right eye, "match") he made 73 errors. Shortly thereafter he was observed for the first time to use the right hand to press the panels, and within a few days was using the right hand exclusively! Following this switch in hand use, all indications of asymmetry in left-to-right versus right-to-left comparisons disappeared.

Another monkey was noted for a while to switch hands depending upon the type of visual material presented, especially in relation to use of a particular eye. This occurred during six sessions with DND, when he still had both AC and CC fully intact and was receiving 20 trials per day with pure color on the DMS task. These color trials were intermixed randomly with 40 trials using images of complex colored objects. As had been his habit for months, every response to the latter material was made with the right hand, regardless of which eye was used for viewing. Several sessions after starting with the training on the task with pure color it was noted that DND had begun using his left hand on the color trials. Hand use was thus carefully noted from then on. The left hand use for color continued throughout six sessions, and thereafter the right hand was used constantly. For those six sessions, in which the right hand was always used for images, the left hand was used for color in 36 out of 80 choices with the left eye open and 37 of 38 with the right eye open. At this time the monkey clearly distinguished between images and pure color even though two of the images, a red rose and a red gladiolus flower, gave one a strong initial impression of color per se.

In all other cases examined, which hand was used, either voluntarily or forced by restraint, had no significant influence on accuracy or latency of response of either hemisphere or direction of comparison between hemispheres. Given full freedom, however, HUD, following transection of both AC and CC, routinely used the hand opposite to the viewing eye.

There were two other instances where a significant asymmetry was displayed depending upon the direction of interhemispheric comparison required. Since, again, in each case intrahemispheric comparisons were equally accurate, it seems unlikely that these examples of directionality in interhemispheric transfer can be attributed to inadvertent trauma. In both instances the most accurate comparison was made when the "sample" was observed with the right eye and the "match" made with the left. Each animal, RHD ($p < 0.005$, double-tailed) and DND ($p < 0.02$, double-tailed), was working with only the AC intact (i.e., CC cut, but RHD with some optic chiasm surviving), with plain color and human faces, respectively. While these individual examples are clearly real enough, there remains something like a 5% possibility that within all types of material presented such runs might occur by chance. Thus, claims of "specialization" in this regard must await duplication of the same phenomenon in more than one monkey.

Potentially the most important observation, unfortunately also awaiting confirmation in a second animal, is the difference observed between right and left hemispheres of RAO, using the List procedure. Accuracy of performance diminishes the longer the interval and the greater the number of intervening images prior to assaying recognition that a particular image is a re-presentation. The question can be asked as to whether these variables, time and intervening images, are dissociable. Thus RAO, with chiasm ~96% cut but CC and AC intact, was given an extensive series of tests, intermixing number of intervening items, elapsed time (varied independently of number of items), and viewing by the same or the other eye, in all totalling over 18,000 presentations. About 2400 trials each were accumulated for the situation where the left or right eye viewed the image initially and where the recognition then had to be accomplished with the same eye. The average delay between first and second presentations was roughly 3 min (range 8–718 sec), and the average number of intervening images was about 14 (range 0–46), about equally distributed between the two eyes. At the $p < 0.01$ level the decrease in performance using the left eye and hemisphere could be explained soley by considering the number of intervening images, whereas for the right eye and hemisphere a definite temporal factor was present; i.e., decrease in performance was to a significant degree dependent upon elapsed time as well as intervening trials. Obviously, if this seeming difference in "degree of temporal erosion" of the trace in the left versus right hemisphere should turn out to be a reproducible phenomenon, it might present some clue as to the basic difference in modus operandi for human right versus left hemisphere.

Further examples of hemispheric superiority were seen in HUD after fully transecting both AC and CC. Two of these were deliberately created by removal of the amygdala or medioventral temporal cortex. At first, on the right side, just the medial inferior tip of the temporal cortex was removed (by subpial suction). This reduced performance with that hemisphere on the DMS task from 90% to 72% correct at a 10-sec delay, without altering (actually slightly improving!?) performance with the left hemisphere. When all of the amygdala on the left was then removed (which, however, as histology revealed, was combined with degeneration of the left fornix undoubtedly consequent to midline surgery), performance by the left hemisphere was reduced nearly to chance levels for most of the remaining 75 days that the animal was studied. For the last three sessions, however, totaling 150 trials, HUD averaged 57% correct. Performance with the right hemisphere was unaffected. The importance of the amygdala and the fornix system (Gaffan, 1977; Mishkin, 1982; Zola-Morgan et al., 1982) thus seems confirmed in a situation affording some additional control over possibly extraneous motivational factors.

The other example of hemispheric superiority in HUD is more puzzling and again involves color. However, it is complicated by unknown factors associated either with the implantation and removal of electrodes in the left optic tract and splenium approached from the left side, by the completion of forebrain commissurotomy with transection of the splenium, and by the degeneration of the left fornix noted above. Prior to these surgical interventions (while the splenium was still intact but with left fornix probably gone), performance with colored images of complex objects at a 10-sec delay was roughly 96% correct with any combination of initially and subsequently viewing eyes. Interhemispheric transfer was entirely eliminated by this surgery, and performance with the left hemisphere became significantly less accurate than with the right, which had also suffered a significant diminution: 75% correct for the left, 90% for the right. It was reasoned that the electrodes in the optic tract might have produced some visual disturbance on the left, accounting for its pronounced deficiency. Wholly unexpected on this basis, however, was the difference in the opposite direction for performance on trials when featureless color had to be matched. This was always a difficult problem for HUD and thus no delay was used between disappearance of the "sample" and presentation of the pair of colors for the "match." The striking effect was that when pure color was viewed, the left hemisphere was correct 80% of the time, while the right, rather than the consistent 90% level with colored objects in preceding and subsequent sessions, was only 71% correct with the pure color ($p < 0.025$, double-tailed).

In the final situation with HUD, when the left hemisphere with amygdala and fornix missing could perform only near chance levels, and the right hemisphere with ventromedial temporal cortex gone performed overall at 70% correct, there was an interesting distribution of errors for this performance by the right hemisphere.

Rather than being randomly distributed in time, there was something of an oscillation between chance performance and excellent performance, as though the ability to make correct choices waxed and waned. Administration of the neotropic drug, Piracetam (Giurgea, 1981), in massize doses (120–500 mg/kg, IM, given 10–20 min, respectively, prior to the first trial) did not improve the accuracy nor, seemingly, alter the erratic nature of the behavior. In any event, such observations raise the question as to whether the "nonviewing" hemisphere may be periodically intruding some perturbation of the capabilities of the "viewing" hemisphere to which the performance is being attributed.

4. SUMMARY

Five macaques with optic chiasm transected have been observed for their ability to use the same versus the other eye and hemisphere for recognizing previously viewed images. Such interhemispheric mnemonic comparison was highly accurate and could be achieved equally well using only the anterior commissure or the splenium of the corpus callosum. After transection of both forebrain commissures, or of the splenium and anterior commissure, such interhemispheric recognition was no longer possible, although this in no way disturbed the animal's remembrance of the procedure when using either hemisphere. A number of instances are detailed in which one hemisphere or direction of interhemispheric comparison was superior to the other when working only with a particular type of material. So far, however, no systematic differences have been found, nor has handedness played any definitive role. One animal in which the amygdala and fornix were removed on one side, after cutting of both forebrain commissures, could perform only at levels slightly above chance with that hemisphere, while concurrently performing at a much higher level when using the other hemisphere.

ACKNOWLEDGMENT. The research reported herein has been accomplished with the support of Grant BNS-8208583 from the National Science Foundation.

REFERENCES

Butler, C. R., 1979, Interhemispheric transfer of visual information via the corpus callosum and anterior commissure in the monkey, in: *Structure and Function of the Cerebral Commissures* (I. Steele Russell, M. W. van Hof, and G. Berlucchi, eds.), Macmillan, London, pp. 342–357.

Doty, R. W., 1984, Some thoughts, and some experiments, on memory, in: *The Neuropsychology of Memory* (N. Butters and L. Squire, eds.), Guilford Press, New York, pp. 330–339.

Doty, R. W. and Negrão, N., 1973, Forebrain commissures and vision, in: *Handbook of Sensory Physiology, Volume VII/3B* (R. Jung, ed.), Springer-Verlag, Berlin, pp. 543–582.

Doty, R. W., Gallant, J. A., and Lewine, J. D., 1982, *Abstr. Soc. Neurosci.* **8**:628.

Downer, J. L. de C., 1959, Changes in visually guided behaviour following midsagittal division of optic chiasm and corpus callosum in monkey (*Macaca mulatta*), *Brain* **82**:251–259.

Gaffan, D., 1977, Monkeys' recognition memory for complex pictures and the effect of fornix transection, *Q. J. Exp. Psychol.* **29**:505–514.

Gazzaniga, M. S., 1970, *The Bisected Brain,* Appleton-Century-Crofts, New York, 172 pp.

Giurgea, C. E., 1981, *Fundamentals to a Pharmacology of the Mind,* Charles C Thomas, Springfield, Illinois, 446 pp.

Hamilton, C. R., 1977, Investigations of perceptual and mnemonic lateralization in monkeys, in: *Lateralization in the Nervous System* (S. Harnad, R. W. Doty, L. Goldstein, J. Jaynes, and G. Krauthamer, eds.), Academic Press, New York, pp. 45–62.

Hamilton, C. R. and Brody, B. A., 1973, Separation of visual functions within the corpus callosum of monkeys, *Brain Res.* **49:**185–189.

Hamilton, C. R. and Tieman, S. B., 1973, Interocular transfer of mirror image discriminations by chiasm-sectioned monkeys, *Brain Res.* **64:**241–255.

Hamilton, C. R. and Vermeire, B. A., 1982, Hemispheric differences in split-brain monkeys learning sequential comparisons, *Neuropsychologia* **20:**691–698.

Hamilton, C. R., Hillyard, S. A., and Sperry, R. W., 1968, Interhemispheric comparison of color in split-brain monkeys, *Exp. Neurol.* **21:**486–494.

Lewine, J. D. and Doty, R. W., 1983, Transcallosal mnemonic processing is inferior to intrahemispheric processing in *Macaca nemestrina, Abstr. Soc. Neurosci.* **9:**651.

McKeever, W. F., Sullivan, K. F., Ferguson, S. M., and Rayport, M., 1981, Typical cerebral hemisphere disconnection deficits following corpus callosum section despite sparing of the anterior commissure, *Neuropsychologia* **19:**745–755.

Mishkin, M., 1982, A memory system in the monkey, *Philos. Trans. Royal Soc. Lond.* **B298:**85–95.

Myers, R. E. and Sperry, R. W., 1953, Interocular transfer of a visual form discrimination in cats after section of the optic chiasm and corpus callosum, *Anat. Rec.* **115:**351–352.

Overman, W. H., Jr. and Doty, R. W., 1979, Disturbance of delayed match-to-sample in macaques by tetanization of anterior commissure versus limbic system or basal ganglia, *Exp. Brain Res.* **37:**511–524.

Overman, W. H., Jr. and Doty, R. W., 1980, Prolonged visual memory in macaques and man, *Neurosci.* **5:**1825–1831.

Overman, W. H., Jr. and Doty, R. W., 1982, Hemispheric specialization displayed by man but not macaques for analysis of faces, *Neuropsychologia* **20:**113–128.

Tieman, S. B. and Hamilton, C. R., 1973, Interocular transfer in split-brain monkeys following serial disconnection, *Brain Res.* **63:**368–373.

Tieman, S. B. and Hamilton, C. R., 1974, Interhemispheric communication between extraoccipital visual areas in the monkey, *Brain Res.* **67:**279–287.

Zihl, J. and von Cramon, D., 1980, Colour anomia restricted to the left visual hemifield after splenial disconnexion, *J. Neurol. Neurosurg. Psychiat.* **43:**719–724.

Zola-Morgan, S., Squire, L. R., and Mishkin, M., 1982, The neuroanatomy of amnesia: Amygdala-hippocampus versus temporal stem, *Science* **218:**1337–1339.

15

Passive Avoidance Training in the Chick

A Model for the Analysis of the Cell Biology of Memory Storage

STEVEN P. R. ROSE

1. INTRODUCTION

The young chick is a particularly appropriate model for the study of the cell biology of learning and memory. Work from our laboratory during the last 5 years has shown that, following a simple one-trial learning task in the day-old chick, region-specific synaptic events, measurable biochemically and morphologically, occur. These events are summarized herein, and evidence is discussed suggesting that they are not merely nonspecific concomitants of learning but are part of the biological language in which memory is coded in the central nervous system.

It is not enough merely to show that when an animal learns, biochemical and other changes occur in its brain, interesting though these may be. Nor is it enough to show that administration of exogenous drugs or analogues of neurotransmitters or neuromodulators affect acquisition or retention or recall processes, pharmacologically relevant and profitable as the many such observations have been. Such experiments reveal something of the processes that may be *necessary* for learning and memory to occur: they do not reveal the nature of the code that is the necessary, *sufficient* and *specific* (exclusive) correspondent in the cellular system of any particular memory for changed behavior in the organism. To use a biochemical analogy, they enable us to understand the role of ATP and the ribosomes in protein synthesis, but not that of the RNA message itself. These points have been discussed elsewhere (Rose 1981, 1982, 1984), where I have endeavored to specify the theoretical task

STEVEN P. R. ROSE ● Brain Research Group, The Open University, Milton Keynes MK7 6AA, United Kingdom.

and the criteria that must be met by experiments designed to approach it, in more precise detail. Here, I wish more fully to review our own experiments.

2. ORGANISM AND TASK

I was first attracted to working with the young chick in the late 1960s, when, in conjunction with the ethologist Pat Bateson and the neuroanatomist Gabriel Horn, I began a study of the biochemical sequelae of exposing the chick to imprinting stimuli. In a series of experiments we were able to show that, when imprinting occurred, there was enhanced RNA and protein synthesis in a particular brain region, later identified as the intermediate medial hyperstriatum ventrale (IMHV). This increased synthesis was not associated with concomitants of imprinting, such as motor activity or visual stimulation, and the extent of the biochemical changes were correlated with the "strength" of imprinting, measured as the bird's preference, when tested, for the stimulus on which it had been imprinted rather than a novel one. The analysis of the sequelae of imprinting has been continued in the last few years with great distinction by Bateson and Horn and the work has been reviewed elsewhere (Horn *et al.,* 1973; Rose, 1977; Horn, 1981).

Despite the considerable merits of imprinting as a model for learning, there are certain disadvantages to it from the point of view of the biochemist. The process of training by exposure to the stimulus is a relatively long one, and this makes it harder to distinguish the cellular events associated with putative memory storage processes from those that are the concomitants of the experience of training. Birds also show a degree of variability in their behavior during training and the strength of their later preference, which can be exploited experimentally but which also adds to the complexity of the analysis. Therefore, I sought an alternative task that could also make use of the great ontogenetic capacity for learning among very young birds but that might be acquired from brief exposure and be more reliable in terms of testable behavioral outcome.

The one-trial passive avoidance learning task, developed by Cherkin and Lee-Teng (Cherkin, 1969) and by Gibbs (Gibbs and Ng, 1977) seemed to offer such a prospect. This task exploits the tendency of young chicks to explore their environment by pecking at small bright objects in their field of view. Such pecking is clearly part of the ontogenetic learning about sources of food and drink, and unpleasant tasting objects, once explored by pecking, are avoided thereafter. In the experimental protocol, pairs of day-old birds are placed in small pens, and after a period of equilibration and three "pretraining" trials with a small (2.5 mm diameter) white bead are offered a bright chromed bead (4 mm diameter, attached to a thin rod as handle). More than 80% of birds will peck at least once at this bead within a 10-sec presentation period. If the bead has been coated with a bitter-tasting substance (we use methylanthranilate [MeA]) they show a characteristic "disgust" response, backing away, shaking their heads, swallowing vigorously, and wiping their beaks on the floor of the pen. More than 70% of the birds that have pecked at the MeA-coated bead will actively avoid a similar, but dry, bead when presented in a further 10-sec trial at times (in our experiments) from 15 min to 48 hr subsequently. By contrast, of birds that in the training trial have pecked at a water-coated bead, more than 90% will subsequently peck at a dry bead. We are thus able to directly compare cellular events occuring in two groups of birds, which we call MeA-trained (M) and water-control (W), for a number of biochemical and morphological measures, and at various times after training.

This training protocol, adapted from Gibbs (Gibbs and Ng, 1977) and described in full most recently in Lossner and Rose (1983), enables us to compare directly two groups of birds that are distinguished by specific different experiences and show a clear distinction in subsequent behavior; that is, M birds have learned to avoid the offered bead, where W birds continue to show their ontogenetically "natural" tendency to peck at it. However learning theorists may wish to categorize this experience—generally called passive avoidance learning (PAL)—its utility to the cell biologist interested in dissecting the sequelae of experience and their relationships to memory formation is apparent, and I do not wish to transgress into the terrain of animal psychology further than is strictly necessary here.

3. LOCALIZATION OF SITES OF CHANGE FOLLOWING PAL

In the initial studies on imprinting, we divded the brain by a rather gross dissection into regions including (1) optic lobes, (2) forebrain base, and (3) forebrain roof, later dividing the roof region between anterior and posterior portions (Bateson et al., 1975). Interesting biochemical effects were localized to the anterior forebrain roof and later shown autoradiographically to be concentrated to the IMHV (Horn et al., 1979). In our studies of PAL, we have followed a similar strategy. Initial studies found differences confined to the (anterior) forebrain roof in a number of biochemical markers; quinuclidinyl benzilate (QNB) binding to the presumed muscarinic cholinergic receptor (Rose et al., 1980) and [^{14}C]-leucine incorporation into the microtubular protein tubulin (Mileusnic et al., 1980). In later studies of [^{14}C]-fucose incorporation into glycoprotein (e.g., Rose and Harding, 1984) we have also found changes in forebrain base regions. To investigate the localization of metabolic change more precisely we have utilized the 2-deoxyglucose (2DG) autoradiographic technique described by Sokoloff et al. (1977). 2DG is a general metabolic marker for glucose utilization. Enhanced glucose utilization is likely to be a consequence of increased neuronal activity, whether because of increased firing rate or metabolic mobilization for biochemical and structural reshaping.

Chicks were pretrained, and just prior to training injected pericardially with 10 μCi [^{14}C]-2DG. They were trained on either W or M beads, tested 30 min later, the brains immediately frozen and coronal and parasaggital autoradiographic sections prepared (Kossut and Rose, 1984). Optical density measurements on 13 identified anatomical structures in brains from seven M and seven W birds were made using a computerized digital image analysis system. (In this, as in all our experiments, the morphological, autoradiographic, or biochemical measurements are made blind with respect to the treatment of the birds.) Optical densities in each autoradiogram section were normalized by comparison with reference structures chosen in each section, and the modal values for serial autoradiograms through each struc-

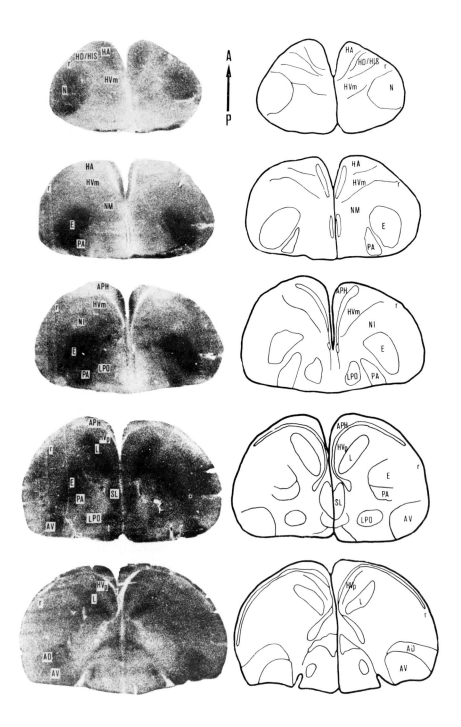

ture in each bird were compared (Fig. 1). The overall pattern of labeling was (not unexpectedly) similar in W and M birds, but quantitative analysis showed that 3 of the 13 regions examined, the palaeostriatum augmentatum (PA), hyperstriatum ventrale, posterior region (HVp), and lobus parolfactorius (LPO) showed increased metabolic activity, of 13% ($p < 0.001$), 10% ($p < 0.05$), and 11% ($p < 0.05$), respectively, in the M birds.

The hyperstriatum ventrale is located in the forebrain roof. It includes the region (IMHV) shown by Horn et al. (1979) to show increased uptake of uracil into RNA during exposure to the flashing light that forms the imprinting stimulus. Lesions in the HV are known to impair the performance of PAL and related tasks (Benowitz and Lee-Teng, 1973; Benowitz 1974), and lesions in the IMHV affect either capacity to imprint or recall for the imprinting stimulus, depending on where they are placed (Horn et al., 1983). The PA and LPO are located in the forebrain base. Both receive projections from the HV (Bradley and Horn, 1979; Benowitz, 1980), though the functional relationships of the LPO seem obscure.

This experiment locates regions of enhanced metabolic activity during training and its immediate sequelae in the M birds. It should be immediately apparent, though, that the changes could be consequent on aspects of the training experience—for instance, the taste of the MeA—as well as mobilization of these neuronal regions in the interests of memory storage. Also, the 2DG serves as a marker for short-term changes in metabolic activity. Can these be precursors to longer-term phenomena? In particular, most theories of memory storage processes are based on the assumption that they involve forms of synaptic remodeling. Based on the 2DG results, we have therefore explored the HV, PA, and LPO for evidence of longer-term changes in synaptic morphology as a consequence of training. In addition, in these experiments we were also able to take account of increasing evidence for the lateralization of memory trace formation in the chick (Rogers and Anson, 1979; Horn, 1981; Horn et al., 1983).

Chicks were trained on water or MeA, as in the 2DG experiments, but were held for 24 hr after training to allow time for any possible morphological restructuring to take place. At the end of this period, the birds were perfused, brain regions located stereotaxically, and blocks of the HV, LPO, and PA from left and right hemispheres taken separately for electron microscopy. Sections from eight M and eight W birds were randomly sampled and photographed or analyzed directly through a projection system. A variety of synaptic measurements were made using a Kontron

←───

FIGURE 1. Series of coronal sections from the brain of a single W bird. Each section is matched with a camera lucida drawing showing the extent of the regions taken for optical density measurement. 2DG autoradiograms were prepared, structures identified, and optical density measurements made as described in the text. Abbreviations for the several brain regions are as follows: AD, archistriatum dorsale; APH, area parahippocampalis; AV, archistriatum ventrale; E, ectostriatum; HA, hyperstriatum accessorium; HD/HIS, hyperstriatum dorsale/intercalatus; HVm, hyperstriatum ventrale (mediale); HVp, hyperstriatum ventrale (posteriore); L, area L_4; LPO, lobus parolfactorius; N, neostriatum laterale; NI, neostriatum intermediale; NM, neostriatum mediale; PA, palaeostriatum augmentatum; r, reference zone for optical density measurement; SL, nucleus septalis lateralis. Bar; 2mm. (From Kossut and Rose, 1984.)

Videoplan system, enabling us to measure stereologically the following synaptic parameters: length of postsynaptic thickening, number of synapses per unit volume of neuropil, volume density of the presynaptic bouton, and number of synaptic vesicles per unit volume of neuropil and presynaptic bouton. The details are described in Stewart *et al.* (1984b).

The salient morphological observations are as follows. First, in both groups of birds, W and M, there are hemispheric asymmetries in a number of synaptic measurements. For instance, in the MHV of the W birds, the length of the postsynaptic thickening was some 12% greater than in the same region in the left hemisphere ($p < 0.02$). Such differences were not wholly unexpected and are comparable to those reported by Horn *et al.* (1983; see also Rogers, 1982).

However, this asymmetry in the W birds was absent in the M birds: the postsynaptic thickenings in the right MHV were reduced in length to that in the left MHV. An analogous finding was made in the LPO (Stewart *et al.*, 1984a). There were also striking changes in the left hemisphere consequent on training. The number of synapses per unit volume of MHV neuropil increased by 23% compared with the right hemisphere, and most strikingly the number of vesicles per synapse in the left hemisphere MHV increased in the M birds by comparison with the right hemisphere by 61%; comparing left hemisphere vesicle number in M birds with those in the comparable region in the control bird, the increase was 72% (Fig. 2). All these changes are highly significant ($p < 0.02$ on ANOVA).

These changes refer to synaptic profiles of the MHV. By contrast, despite the

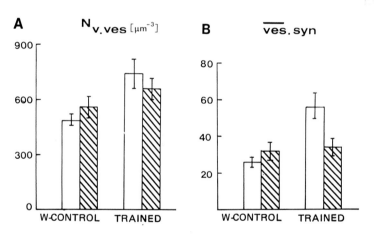

FIGURE 2. (a) Synaptic vesicle numerical density ($N_{V.ves}$) in the right and left MHV of W-control and MeA-trained chicks. Open bars, left hemisphere; cross-hatched bars, right hemisphere. Each bar is a mean value of measurements from eight birds and the vertical lines represent S.E.M.s. The effect of training on hemisphere is statistically significant. (b) The data in (a) have been transformed in order to permit the mean synaptic vesicle number per synapse ($\overline{ves}.syn$) to be expressed. The size of the difference between $\overline{ves}.syn$ in left and right hemispheres of trained chicks (61%) is such that an ANOVA now shows that differences between hemispheres are statistically significant, in addition to the effect of training on hemispheres. (From Stewart *et al.*, 1984b).

increased metabolic activity shown by the use of the 2DG marker, we were unable to find lasting structural changes in the PA (though this may be due to the fact that we sampled for electron microscopy only a small portion of a large and not necessarily homogenous structure). In the LPO comparable changes to those in the MHV were found (M. Stewart, unpublished results).

The implications of these observations seem striking. Following PAL, birds that have pecked at an MeA-coated bead show enhanced metabolic activity in three brain structures, HV, PA, and LPO; subsequently, in MHV and LPO, there are long-lasting changes in the length of synaptic apposition zone and, in addition, changes in the relative volume of the synapses and above all in the number of vesicles per synapse. It is obviously very tempting to see such changes as morphological evidence for a change in—presumably a strengthening of—synaptic connectivity in these regions consequent on the training. Before considering these implications further, however, it is necessary to say something more about the biochemistry of the processes involved.

4. BIOCHEMICAL SEQUELAE OF TRAINING.

4.1. The Question of Time Course

The changes in synaptic structures that were discussed in the preceding section may or may not require a net synthesis and lasting change in the concentrations of biochemical components: they could presumably result merely from the reorganization of existing membrane components and subunits. However, even if this were the case, a biochemical mobilization of enzyme systems associated with such reorganization would be required. The enhanced glucose metabolism indicated by the 2DG data also implies an activation of at least some biochemical processes. Our earlier imprinting studies had shown enhanced incorporation of precursors into RNA and protein, as well as changes in the enzymes of the cholinergic system (Rose, 1977). One might expect to find analogous changes in PAL, but the one-trial nature of the PAL task enables more pertinent questions about the time course of biochemical changes also to be asked. It is well known that the consolidation process involves more than one phase of short-term or labile memory (McGaugh, 1966; for a specific model, see Gibbs and Ng, 1977.) I have elsewhere pointed out that for a biochemical process to be regarded as a correspondent of memory formation, its time course must be compatible with that of the phenomenologically observed memory formation processes. In the chick, following PAL, there is a period of up to a minute or so during which the memory trace is electrically disruptible and of up to an hour or so during which it is disruptible by drugs such as ouabain. Long-term memory is blocked by inhibitors of protein synthesis such as cycloheximide (Gibbs and Ng, 1977), though this may not be directly a consequence of the drug's effect on protein synthesis but of damage resulting from the changed amino acid concentrations caused by the blocking of protein synthesis (Hambley and Rogers, 1979). At any event, it is appropriate to look for biochemical markers both of short and longer term sequelae of exposure to training on the PAL task.

4.2. Short-Term Changes

A variety of considerations led us to suspect that among the markers for short-term change would be alteration in aspects of neurotransmitter/receptor systems. Enhancement or inhibition of neurotransmitter function could in principle result from alteration in the level of transmitter (achieved by modifying synthetic or degradative enzyme activity), or its availability, perhaps achieved by altering the proportion bound in synaptic vesicles at the synapse, or its interaction with its receptor, achieved by altering either the amount or the binding capacity of receptor. The transmitter systems principally involved in neural connectivity in the HV, PA, and LPO are not, at present known. However, HV (especially MHV) and PA are rich in muscarinic cholinergic receptors, as indicated by autoradiographic mapping of the distribution of the binding ligands quinuclidinyl benzilate (QNB) and propyl benzylcholine mustard (PrBCM) (Coulter, 1982). Binding of the presumed nicotinic ligand α-bungarotoxin is one to two orders of magnitude lower. There is also a wide distribution of serotonin binding sites. The enzymes of acetylcholine synthesis and degradation are also especially enriched in the forebrain roof of the chick.

On this admittedly rather circumstantial basis, we examined the effect of PAL on the specific binding of the muscarinic ligand QNB, of the nicotinic ligand α-bungarotoxin, and of serotonin to chick brain regions at various times after training (Aleksidze *et al.*, 1981; Rose *et al.*, 1980). The results are summarized in Table I. Thirty minutes after training, there is a 22% increase in QNB binding activity in the forebrain roof of the M compared with the W birds. This increase is transient; it is not apparent 10 min after the onset of training and has disappeared by 3 hr after training. By contrast, the binding of α-bungarotoxin shows a comparable 17% *decrease* at 30 min in the M birds but is at control level again by 3 hr. Serotonin binding levels show an increase at 30 min that persists for the full 3 hr of the experiment. The reciprocal increase in QNB binding and decrease in α-bungarotoxin

TABLE I. Changes in Ligand Binding in Chick
Forebrain Roof Following Passive Avoidance
Training[a,b]

Time after training (min)	M/W × 100		
	QNB	αBT	5HT
10	110	—	—
30	122[c]	83[d]	114
180	101	98	115[d]

[a] From Rose *et al.* (1980); Aleksidze *et al.* (1981).
[b] Maximal specific binding of ligand to brain homogenates was measured for QNB (quinuclidinyl benzilate, for muscarinic cholinergic receptors), αBT (α-bungarotoxin, for nicotinic cholinergic receptors, and 5-HT (serotonin, for serotonergic receptors). Significant changes in ligand binding at various times after the training are indicated.
[c] $p < 0.001$.
[d] $p < 0.05$.

binding are thus compatible with their association with the short-term phase of memory storage, the serotonin binding increase with some more prolonged process.

4.3. Longer-Term Processes

We have, however, paid most attention to potential candidates for biochemical changes subserving long-term processes. Modification of synaptic membrane structure is likely, for instance, to involve changed production of both proteins and glycoproteins—generally regarded as serving as key recognition molecules at the synaptic membrane.

If a half-hour pulse of [^{14}C]-leucine is given by intraperitoneal injection to chicks at varying times after training, an increased incorporation occurs into TCA-precipitable proteins of the anterior forebrain roof of M compared with W birds. This increased incorporation persists for at least 24 hr after the training experience but drops back to control (W) levels by 48 hr. The increase of incorporation is into both soluble and insoluble proteins, but, with the half-hour pulse, the major effect is on soluble proteins. We have made some progress in identifying the proteins involved. For instance, one of the major constituents to show an increase in incorporation is the microtubular protein tubulin, whose concentration, determined by a colchicine binding assay, also shows a similar increase persisting for 24 hr, but at control levels by 48 hr (Mileusnic et al., 1981). Calmodulin, the calcium-binding protein, also shows increased turnover (P. Tillson and S. Rose, unpublished results), but actin does not (Tillson and Rose, 1981).

In order to investigate this increase in protein production further, we have recently developed an in vitro protein synthesizing system derived from chick brain slices, which can incorporate [^{14}C]-leucine into tissue protein at the rate of 2–3 nmoles/mg protein/hr over a period of at least 90 min (Schliebs et al., 1985). If slices are prepared from the chick brain an hour after training and the in vitro rate of protein synthesis measured, there is a 23% increase ($p < 0.01$) in synthetic rate in the forebrain roof of M compared with W birds (3.44 against 2.80 nmoles leu/mg protein/hr). This observation of enhanced in vitro incorporation (also predominantly into soluble protein), which matches the in vivo observation, is important because it rules out the possibility that increased incorporation observed in vivo is merely an artefactual consequence of changed blood flow, amino acid uptake, or other factors (see Rose and Haywood, 1976, for discussion). Also, one of the problems of in vivo studies has been that analysis of differentially radioactively labeled protein has been limited by the amount of radioactivity that can be got into the cells across the blood–brain barrier, even in the chick. With the availability of the in vitro system, this limitation has been transcended, and we are now in a much stronger position to analyse the protein products of the training experience. The persistence of the increase into an in vitro assay system must also imply a retained mobilization of protein synthetic machinery, presumably involving increased transcriptional rates and the activation of ribosomal systems, as a consequence of training. (In imprinting one of the earliest steps to occur after onset of stimulation is an enhanced nuclear RNA polymerase activity [Haywood et al., 1970].)

Our study of the involvement of glycoproteins has followed a parallel path to that of proteins. The chosen precursor is ^{3}H- or ^{14}C-labeled fucose, which is selectively incorporated into glycoproteins, but the analysis of its fate is harder in some respects than that of protein because incorporation is slow and fucose uptake across the blood–brain barrier certainly one limiting factor. With an experimental design that involved injecting the radiolabeled fucose at the time of training and analysing incorporation at various periods thereafter, we were able to show an enhanced incorporation into particulate glycoproteins of the anterior forebrain roof; this enhanced incorporation was concentrated to the synaptic membranes (Sukumar et al., 1980; Burgoyne and Rose, 1981). If the experimental design was changed so as to inject the [^{14}C]-fucose some time after training, effects were also found in the forebrain base (Rose and Harding, 1984). Proteins are fucosylated in the Golgi apparatus by pathways involving the enzymes fucosyl transferase and fucokinase. We were able to show that training increased the fucokinase activity in the forebrain base of M birds compared with W (Lossner and Rose, 1983). Further analysis of the synaptic membrane glycoproteins is underway. We need to know whether the increased production is confined to the glycoproteins of the junctional complex and if so, at which side of the cleft the glycoproteins lie. Our prospects will be enhanced if we can find an in vitro incorporation system that can generate labeled glycoprotein in amounts adequate for analysis and if we can go on from there to raise antibodies to specific membrane constituents.

What might be the relationship between these apparently diverse biochemical data and the morphological changes discussed in Section 3? Before I try to fit these observations together, I turn to one further, and perhaps crucial, aspect of our research strategy.

5. RELATIONSHIPS BETWEEN CELL BIOLOGICAL CHANGES AND MEMORY PROCESSES

The morphological and biochemical changes discussed in Sections 3 and 4 are all sequelae of exposure to the experience of pecking at a methylanthranilate—as opposed to a water-coated—bead on a training trial. There are many aspects to this experience, including of course the taste of the MeA, differential arousal, possibly fear, and so forth, which distinguish W from M birds; I have stated here and elsewhere (e.g., Rose, 1981, 1982) that to move from observation of sequelae of training to claims about relationships between these sequelae and memory storage processes requires rigorous controls.

One approach would be to attempt to decouple the experience of the taste of MeA from the association with pecking at the bead. For instance, if the bird's eyes are covered and MeA introduced into the beak, then the increase observed in QNB binding 30 min after training does not occur (Rose et al., 1980); but there are, of course, other obvious differences between the two types of experience. In the same series of experiments, we also observed that intracerebral injection of ouabain or cycloheximide drugs, which interfere with short- or long-term phases of memory formation, also prevent the training-induced increase in QNB binding. Such data too are suggestive, but scarcely conclusive.

Perhaps the most powerful attempt we have made to separate out the sequelae of the training experience from those of memory formation, however, takes advantage of the fact that brief subconvulsive transcranial electroshock administered within a minute after training renders the birds apparently amnestic when they are tested for recall (that is, avoidance of the bead) any time from half an hour to at least 24 hr subsequently. If the administration of the electroshock is delayed to 10 min after training, there is no such amnesia; birds avoid the bead on testing subsequently. If the electroshock is administered to birds trained on the water bead, there is no observable change in their pecking at the bead on test. We could thus carry out an experiment utilizing 6 groups of birds.

(a) Controls, unshocked which have pecked a water coated bead;
(b) Controls, immediate shocked;
(c) Controls, delayed shocked;
(d) Trained, unshocked which have pecked a MeA-coated bead;
(e) Trained, immediate shocked;
(f) Trained, delayed shocked.

Groups (d) and (f) avoid the bead on test; Group (e) pecks at the bead, as do control groups (a), (b) and (c). Groups (e) and (f) have had identical experiences; they have pecked MeA-coated beads and been shocked; the only difference is in the time of shock relative to test, and hence (e) behaves as if it is amnesic and (f) shows recall.

A biochemical change that is consequent upon some general aspect of training should appear in Groups (d), (e), and (f). If it is part of the memory storage process, it should be present in (d) and (f) compared with (a) and (c) but be absent in (e), which should be identical to (b).

We chose to use this experimental design with fucose incorporation in glycoproteins as our biochemical marker, since the elevated fucose incorporation persists beyond the immediate training period. To avoid the possibility that any immediate consequences of training and electroshock—such as blood flow changes—were responsible for any biochemical effect, the precursor was not administered until after all behavioral measures, including testing, had been carried out. Birds were trained, shocked or not, tested 30 min after training, and [^{14}C]-fucose injected intraperitoneally after a further 15 min. Birds were killed after a 3-hr incorporation period and fucose incorporation studied in several brain regions. The measure thus refers to cellular events taking place, not during training itself, but during a subsequent consolidation phase of memory formation.

The results of these experiments are summarized in Fig. 3. There were no differences of incorporation in W birds as a result of the shock. Unshocked M birds showed the expected increase in fucose incorporation in base and anterior roof. M birds rendered amnesic by immediate shock showed no increase in incorporation over W birds; delayed shocked, and therefore not amnesic, M birds showed a comparable increase in incorporation to the unshocked M birds.

The most parsimonious interpretation of this result must be that the experience of training, without the memory consolidation process occurring, is not sufficient to result in increased fucose incorporation in the base and anterior forebrain roof.

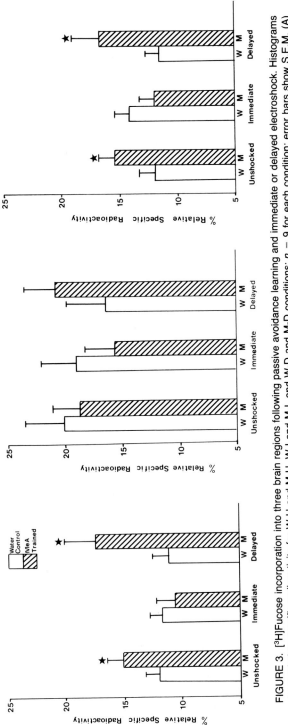

FIGURE 3. [³H]Fucose incorporation into three brain regions following passive avoidance learning and immediate or delayed electroshock. Histograms show relative specific radioactivity for W-U and M-U, W-I and M-I, and W-D and M-D conditions; n = 9 for each condition; error bars show S.E.M. (A) Forebrain base; (B) posterior roof; (C) anterior roof. Significant differences from corresponding water control (p < 0.05) shown by asterisks. Conditions: W-U, water control, unshocked; W-I, water control, immediate shocked; W-D, water control, 10 min delayed shocked; M-U, methylanthranilate trained, unshocked; M-I, methylanthranilate trained, immediate shocked; M-D, methylanthranilate trained, 10 min delayed shocked. (From Rose and Harding, 1984).

Hence this increase is likely to be part of the biochemical process involved in that consolidation; that is, it is a necessary and specific part of the consolidation process.

The fact that we have shown this reasonably convincingly for one biochemical process, that of fucose incorporation, does not allow us to conclude that all other biochemical or morphological sequelae of training we observe are equally specific. This is a problem we have met before in the context of the markers of imprinting (e.g., Rose 1977). Barring infinite time to repeat all possible controls with all possible markers, we can only offer the relative security produced by assembling a series of control experiments and hope that parsimony rules, O.K. If we are wrong, we will doubtless learn the hard way.

6. PUTTING IT ALL TOGETHER

The most surprising feature of our results is that they occur at all; that is, that the seemingly minor experience of pecking once at an MeA-coated as opposed to a water-coated bead and thereafter avoiding it, having (presumably) learned it to be distasteful, can result in a transient activation of cholinergic and other receptors, an increase in brain protein and glycoprotein synthesis that persists for 24 hr after the experience, and a lateralized change in synaptic volume and, above all, vesicle numbers in specific brain regions. The scale of these effects at first sight seems out of proportion to the experience. Yet we must remember that we are working with young birds for whom the testing and exploration of their environment is both a highly novel experience and one with a life-or-death survival value. Animals of this age have a lot to learn and must get it right to live.

Clearly several brain systems are involved in learning the association between bead and taste: visual and taste modalities and central connectivity systems must all take part. Just because the MHV, PA, and LPO show changed 2DG metabolism does not mean that these are the only regions relevant to the neurophysiology of the processes, nor indeed that there must be remodeling of connectivity within all of them to encode the experience. If for the moment, however, we accept the evidence of Section 5 at face value and conclude that the biochemical and morphological changes we have observed are connected with memory trace formation, what might they imply?

If we are at first surprised at the magnitude of the biochemical changes, the second puzzle is their apparent transience. The memory clearly persists, at least up to 48 hr and probably for a week or more after training, before it gets lost in the noise of other aspects of the young bird's experience. Yet the biochemical changes— even those in protein and glycoprotein synthesis—are transient. This must mean that they themselves are merely steps en route to other more lasting cellular changes. To remodel synapses, perhaps by reshaping or relocating them, would require only a transient metabolic change; once the remodeling had occurred, then the "normal" rate of metabolism would suffice to retain it. We do not yet know if the change in synaptic vesicle number implies some lasting change in the concentration of particular vesicle proteins or other constituents such as membrane lipids: we are urgently investigating the question.

However, it is possible to envisage a scenario that looks something like this: The arrival at a particular group of cells (in the left MHV and LPO?) of a coordinated set of novel input results in transient synaptic facilitation, involving increased receptor activity (triggered by opening new Ca^{2+} channels?). This enhanced activity signals to both pre- and postsynaptic cell nuclei, resulting in increased synthesis of new proteins, including those concerned with intracellular information flow (tubulin) and glycoprotein. The new glycoproteins are inserted into the synaptic membrane and possibly vesicular membranes, thereby lastingly altering synaptic efficacy. A particular pattern of strengthened synapses, diffusely distributed within and between brain regions, serves as the storage system for the information interpreted by the bird as: that object tastes bad; avoid it.

To go further raises questions of molecular biology (the signaling process that results in enhanced *de novo* protein and glycoprotine production); cell biology (the mechanism of directed flow of novel components to specific synapses); synaptology (the nature of the new channels involved in synaptic membrane modulation and of other vesicle systems involved in the response to training); neurophysiology (specification of the changed output of the cells whose connectivity has been modified); neuroanatomy (mapping of the MHV–LPO–PA pathways and exploring the lateralization phenomena); and behavior (how does a change in connectivity "correspond" to learning and memory processes? Are these mechanisms generalizable to other forms of learning?). It would be arrogant to claim that we can now solve all these questions. It would be immodest to deny that we intend to try.

NOTE ADDED IN PROOF

Since the preparation of this review we have been able to show: (a) that the 2-DG effects in MHV and LPO are confined to the left hemisphere (Csillag and Rose, 1985); (b) that increased glycoprotein incorporation can be observed *in vitro* (McGabe and Rose, 1985) and (c) that increases occur in synaptic vesicle numbers in left LPO as well as MHV (M. Stewart and S. P. R. Rose, manuscript in preparation).

ACKNOWLEDGMENTS. The experiments described here have been conducted with my colleagues in the Brain Research Group and valued visitors to our laboratories. I thank all those whose work is cited, both for experimental collaboration and many fruitful discussions. I also thank Pat Bateson for continued interactive discourse over the years. This work was carried out under grants from the MRC (1500BB/AMV/FR-15M) and NIH (1 RO1 NS19030-1), which are gratefully acknowledged.

REFERENCES

Aleksidze, N., Potempska, A., Murphy, S., and Rose, S. P. R., 1981, Passive avoidance in the young chick affects forebrain α-bungarotoxin and serotonin binding, *Abstr. 8th ISN,* p. 382.

Bateson, P. P. G., Horn, G., and Rose, S. P. R., 1975, Imprining: Correlation between behaviour and incorporation of ^{14}C-uracil in chick brain, *Brain Res.* **84**:202–220.

Benowitz, L., 1974, Conditions for the bilateral transfer of monocular learning in the chick, *Brain Res.* **65**:203–213.

Benowitz, L., 1980, Functional organization of the avian telencephalon, in: *Comparative Neurology of the Telencephalon* (S. Ebbeson, ed.), Plenum Press, New York.

Benowitz, L. and Lee-Teng, E. 1973, Contrasting effects of three forebrain ablations on discrimination learning and reversal in chickens *J. Comp. Physiol. Psychol.* **84**:391–397.

Bradley, P. and Horn, G. 1979, Efferent connections of hyperstriatum ventrale in the chick, *J. Anat.* **128**:414–415.

Burgoyne, R. D. and Rose, S. P. R. 1980, Subcellular localization of increased incorporation of ^{3}H-fucose following passive avoidance learning in chicks, *Neurosci. Lett.* **19**:343–348.

Cherkin, A., 1969, Kinetics of memory consolidation: role of amnestic treatment parameters, *Proc. Natl. Acad. Sci. USA* **63**:1094–1101.

Coulter, J. C., 1982, *Thesis:* Open University, Milton Keynes.

Gibbs, M. E. and Ng, K. T., 1977, Psychobiology of memory: Towards a model of memory formation, *Biobehav. Rev.* **1**:113–136.

Hambley, J. W. and Rogers, L. J., 1979, Retarded learning induced by amino acids in the neonatal chick, *Neuroscience* **4**:677–684.

Haywood, J., Rose, S. P. R., and Bateson, P. P. G., 1970, Effects of an imprinting procedure on RNA polymerase activity in the chick brain, *Nature* **228**:373–374.

Horn, G., 1981, Neural mechanisms of learning: an analysis of imprinting in the domestic chick, *Proc. R. Soc. Lond. B.* **213**:101–137.

Horn, G., Bateson, P. P. G., and Rose, S. P. R. 1973, Experience and plasticity in the nervous system, *Science* **181**:506–514.

Horn, G., McCabe, B. J., and Bateson, P. P. G., 1979, Imprinting: an autoradiographic analysis of changes in uracil incorporation into chick brain, *Brain Res.* **168**:361–379.

Horn, G., McCabe, B. J., and Cipolla-Neto, J., 1983, Imprinting in the domestic chick: The role of each side of the hyperstriatum ventrale in acquisition and retention, *Exp. Brain Res.* **53**:91–98.

Kossut, M. and Rose, S. P. R., 1984, Differential 2-deoxyglucose uptake into chick brain structures during passive avoidance training, *Neuroscience* **12**:971–977.

Lossner, B. and Rose, S. P. R. 1983, Passive avoidance training increases fucokinase activity in right forebrain base of day-old chicks, *J. Neurochem.* **41**:1357–1363.

McCabe, N. and Rose, S. P. R., 1985, Passive avoidance training increases fucose incorporation into glycoprotein in chick forebrain slices *in vitro, Neurochem Res.* (in press).

McGaugh, J., 1966, Time dependent processes in memory storage, *Science* **153**:1351–1358.

Mileusnic, R., Rose, S. P. R., and Tillson, P., 1980, Passive avoidance training results in changes in concentration of and incorporation into colchicine binding proteins in the chick forebrain, *J. Neurochem.* **34**:1007–1015.

Rogers, L. J., 1982, Light experience and asymmetry of brain function in chickens, *Nature* **297**:223–225.

Rogers, L. J. and Anson, J. N., 1979, Lateralization of function in the chick forebrain, *Pharmacol. Biochem. Behav.* **10**:679–686.

Rose, S. P. R., 1977, Early visual experience, learning and neurochemical plasticity in the rat and the chick, *Philos. Trans. R. Soc. Lond. (B)* **278**:307–318.

Rose, S. P. R., 1981, What should a biochemistry of learning and memory be about?, *Neuroscience* **6**:811–821.

Rose, S. P. R., 1982, From causations to translations: A dialectical solution to a reductionist enigma, in: *Towards a Liberatory Biology* (S. P. R. Rose, ed.), Allison & Busby, London, pp. 10–25.

Rose, S. P. R., 1984, Strategies in studying the cell biology of learning and memory, in: *The Neuropsychology of Memory* (L. R. Squire and N. Butters, eds.), Guilford Press, New York, pp. 547–559.

Rose, S. P. R. and Csillag, A., 1985, Passive avoidance training results in lasting changes in deoxy-glucose metabolism in left hemisphere regions of chick brain, *Behav. Neural Biol.* (in press).

Rose, S. P. R. and Harding, S., 1984, Training increases ^{3}H-fucose incorporation in chick brain only if followed by memory storage, *Neuroscience* **12**:663–667.

Rose, S. P. R. and Haywood, J., 1976, Experience, learning and brain metabolism in: *Biochemical Correlates of Brain Structure and Function* (A.N. Davison, ed.), Academic Press, London, pp. 249–292.

Rose S. P. R., Gibbs, M. E., and Hambley, J. W., 1980, Transient increase in forebrain muscarinic cholinergic receptors following passive avoidance learning in the young chick, *Neuroscience* **5**:169–172.

Schliebs, R., Rose, S. P. R., and Stewart, M. G., 1985, Effect of passive avoidance training on *in vitro* protein synthesis in forebrain slices of day old chicks, *J. Neurochem.* **44**:1014–1028.

Sokoloff, L., Reivich, M., Kennedy, C., Des Rosiers, M. H., Patlak, C. S., Pettigrew, K. D., Sakurada, O., and Shinohara, M., 1977, the ^{14}C-deoxyglucose method for the measurement of local cerebral glucose utilisation: Theory, procedure and normal values in the conscious and anaethetized albino rat, *J. Neurochem* **28**:897–916.

Stewart, M. G., Rose, S. P. R., and King, T. S., 1984a, A stereological investigation of synapses in chick palaeostriatum augmentatum and lobus parolfactorius following training on a passive avoidance task, *Acta Stereologica* **21**(Suppl. I):227–230.

Stewart, M. G., Rose, S. P. R., King, T. S., Gabbott, P. L. A., and Bourne, R., 1984b, Hemispheric asymmetry of synapses in chick medial hyperstriatum ventrale following passive avoidance training: a stereological investigation, *Devel. Brain Res.* **12**:261–269.

Sukumar, R., Rose, S. P. R., and Burgoyne, R. D., 1980, Increased incorporation of ^{3}H-fucose into chick brain glycoproteins following training on a passive avoidance task, *J. Neurochem.* **34**:1000–1006.

Tillson, P. and Rose, S. P. R., 1981, Passive avoidance training results in region specific changes in incorporation of ^{14}C-leucine into chick forebrain total protein but not into actin, *Abstr. 8th I.S.N.*, p. 399.

Membrane Physiology

Role of Calcium Ions in Learning

K. KRNJEVIĆ

1. INTRODUCTION

The title of this chapter may well seem inappropriate. No one will dispute the basic premise: taking part in so many membrane and internal cellular processes (Rasmussen, 1981; Rasmussen and Barrett, 1984), Ca^{2+} can hardly fail to be involved in learning. On the other hand, the title seems to imply a *particular* role, both essential and well defined. To claim that such a role has been identified would be patently untrue. Nevertheless, it may be useful to review briefly the facilitatory processes—not dependent on structural changes, such as sprouting of new connections—that have been recognized in the CNS and to discuss ways in which Ca^{2+} may be of importance. Special reference will be made to the hippocampus, where direct measurements of Ca^{2+} levels have recently revealed some remarkable changes during "burst" activity.

2. MECHANISMS OF FACILITATION

There are many ways in which neural activity can be potentiated and almost as many ways in which Ca^{2+} may be involved. Of the many ongoing studies of learning, three have been outstanding in the range of investigations attempted, from the behavioral to the cellular and molecular level: those on *Hermissenda* by Alkon and his colleagues (Alkon, 1982), on *Aplysia* by Kandel and colleagues (Kandel *et al.*, 1983), and the studies on long-term potentiation (LTP) in the mammalian hippocampus by Lynch and colleagues (Lynch and Baudry, 1984). In each case, a crucial role of activity-linked Ca^{2+} influx has been postulated, but at different sites and in a different manner: in *Hermissenda,* increased photoreceptor responses in conditioned learning are believed to be caused by intracellular accumulation of Ca^{2+}, which depresses a fast-adapting K^+ current that normally reduces the intensity

K. KRNJEVIĆ • Departments of Anaesthesia Research and Physiology, McGill University, Montréal, Quebec H3G 1Y6, Canada.

of responses; in *Aplysia*, Ca^{2+} influx may selectively enhance serotonin-mediated heterosynaptic facilitation, which operates by reducing a cyclic AMP-sensitive K^+ current; while, in the hippocampus, long-term potentiation is thought to depend on increased postsynaptic responses to the neurotransmitter glutamate, initiated by Ca^{2+} influx, the activation of a Ca^{2+}-sensitive peptidase, and a resulting increase in the number of available membrane receptors for glutamate.

In view of the widely varied suggested mechanisms, it is of interest to consider more generally mechanisms of facilitation that could be the basis of learning. They are summarized in tabular form in Table I.

2.1. Presynaptic Mechanisms

It has long been accepted that posttetanic potentiation (PTP) has a presynaptic mechanism, which is caused by a temporary increase in transmitter release (Eccles, 1964). Since transmitter release is triggered by Ca^{2+}, PTP can be ascribed to a rise in internal Ca^{2+} concentration $[Ca]_i$ which may reflect an increase in Ca^{2+} influx (Stinnakre and Tauc, 1973), persistence of a raised $[Ca]_i$ because of slower Ca^{2+} sequestration or outward transport, or more effective coupling between Ca^{2+} and transmitter release. There is reason to believe that the influx of Na^+ may be a significant factor in enhancing $[Ca]_i$ (e.g., Erulkar and Rahamimoff, 1978; Atwood *et al.*, 1983). One cannot exclude the possibility that Ca^{2+} influx, by a direct activation of relevant enzymes, also promotes the synthesis of transmitter and so contributes to enhanced release.

Of course, most investigators consider PTP as only a possible model of learning, probably essentially different from LTP not only by its transience but probably also in its mechanisms—though it is by no means a foregone conclusion that LTP

TABLE I. Summary of Mechanisms of Facilitation in CNS Which Could Explain Long-term Potentiation

I. *Presynaptic*
 1. Enhanced release of excitatory transmitter (as in PTP): owing to greater Ca^{2+} influx, mobilization of internal Ca^{2+} by Na^+ influx, change in pH, etc., or increased synthesis.
 2. Diminished release of inhibitory transmitter: owing to depletion of transmitter, smaller Ca^{2+} influx, selective inhibition of inhibitory neurons.

II. *Postsynaptic*
 1. Change in transmitter effectiveness (increase at excitatory synapses, decrease at inhibitory synapses): owing to changes in receptor synthesis and turnover, sensitization or desensitization of receptors, synergistic or antagonist effect of other agents (? peptides or ions) released by tetanic stimulation, or increased or reduced rate of transmitter removal (by uptake or enzymes).
 2. Enhanced electrical excitability, owing to suppression of outward currents:
      (a) G_K lower (M,C or A currents); mediated by ACh, 5HT, NA, peptides, $[CA]_i$, etc.
      (b) G_{Cl} lower (IPSPs); mediated by ACh or peptides.
 3. Increased electrical interactions: ephaptic or via electrical junctions.

III. *Intracellular*
    Is facilitation made permanent by activation of intracellular messengers, such as Ca^{2+} or cyclic nucleotides and corresponding protein kinases?

is predominantly or exclusively a postsynaptic phenomenon (Skrede and Malthe-Sørenssen, 1981; Dolphin, 1983).

2.1.1. Heterosynaptic Facilitation or Depression

An interaction between two nerve inputs at a presynaptic site—is obviously important, because it provides for very selective sensitization of one sensory input by another. The interaction may be positive or negative. A particularly well-known and much studied example is the serotonergic presynaptic facilitation originally observed by Shimahara and Tauc (1975) and later extensively investigated in a learning context (Kandel *et al.*, 1983). As already mentioned above, Ca^{2+} influx is a crucial factor for the selective conditioning of a given input.

Negative heterosynaptic interactions are of course well known as presynaptic inhibition. Although less prominent in recent discussions of learning, there is no reason why specific and long-term modulation of presynaptic inhibition could not be an important mechanism of disfacilitation or disinhibition. Several agents have significant presynaptic effects, notably acetylcholine (ACh), which appears to depress GABA release at inhibitory synapses in the hippocampus (Krnjević *et al.*, 1981; Ben Ari *et al.*, 1981), and GABA itself, when it acts presynaptically. The latter is of particular interest because it generates primary afferent depolarization by activating Cl⁻ channels via "GABA$_A$" receptors but also, and perhaps more importantly, by interfering with Ca^{2+} influx in nerve terminals (Dunlap and Fischbach, 1978) via "GABA$_B$" receptors (Bowery *et al.*, 1984).

2.2. Postsynaptic Mechanisms

2.2.1. Increased Sensitivity to the Excitatory Transmitter

Such a mechanism has been proposed as mainly responsible for hippocampal LTP (Lynch & Baudry, 1984). As already emphasized, a key role has been postulated for postsynaptic Ca^{2+} influx as the trigger for the chain of intracellular events that results in a higher density of membrane glutamate receptors.

2.2.2. Increased Electrical Excitability by Reduction of Outward Curents

Excitability reflects the ease with which self-regenerative inward currents (of Na^+ or Ca^{2+}) can be developed. It is normally kept at a relatively low level by the generation of opposing outward currents. These may be generated intrinsically or extrinsically to the cell in question.

2.2.2a. Intrinsic Currents. These are K^+-mediated, and they may be mainly voltage-dependent (like the fast adapting A current or the slow adapting M current) or mainly Ca^{2+}-dependent (C current). A block of such intrinsic outward currents facilitates cell firing. An example has already been mentioned, the depression of A current in *Hermissenda* photoreceptors that accompany conditioned learning (Alkon, 1982). In the vertebrate CNS, a block of K^+ outward currents is now a well-established facilitatory mechanism (Krnjević et al., 1971; Benardo and Prince, 1982; Halliwell and Adams, 1982), possibly involved in long-term conditioning (Woody et al., 1978). There is reason to believe that ACh depresses both M and C currents (Benardo and Prince, 1982; Cole and Nicoll, 1984), though it is not clear whether the depression of the C current is caused mainly by a direct effect on the relevant K^+ channels or by a block of the initial Ca^{2+} influx.

Facilitation by a block of K^+ outward currents is not a unique characteristic of cholinergic inputs: a variety of other modulator substances act in a very similar fashion, including peptides such as substance P (Krnjević, 1977; Nowak and Macdonald, 1982; Murase and Randić, 1984), gonadotrophin-releasing hormone and angiotensin (Adams and Brown, 1980), 5HT (Vandermaelen and Aghajanian, 1982), and noradrenaline (Madison and Nicoll, 1982).

2.2.2b. Extrinsic Currents. Outward currents of Cl^- are generated exclusively by synaptic inhibition, mediated most widely by GABA-releasing interneurons. Because of the ubiquitous distribution of inhibitory synapses, characterized by a high level of both tonic and phasic activity, this is a powerful mechanism of control, but one which is particularly susceptible to modulation in several ways. $GABA_A$ receptors are closely connected with benzodiazepine receptors, through which their efficacy can be markedly raised or lowered (Haefely et al., 1983). Endogenous agonists have not yet been identified, but if such agents were released by certain nerve fibers, they could provide the basis for selective facilitations.

Outward currents of Cl^- can also be diminished indirectly by agents such as ACh or angiotensin that depress GABA release (Haas et al., 1980; Krnjević et al., 1981; Ben Ari et al., 1981; Haas, 1982) or opioid peptides that inhibit inhibitory neurons (Zieglgänsberger et al., 1979; Dunwiddie et al., 1980).

2.2.3. Increased Electrical Interactions

Though perhaps less likely, a significant role of "passive" electrical interaction in learning cannot be excluded. At least two types of phenomena come under this category: coupling through specialized, high or low resistance junctions (Bennett, 1977; Dudek et al., 1983) and ephaptic (electrical field) interactions, which may be either excitatory or inhibitory (Korn and Faber, 1980; Taylor and Dudek, 1982, 1984; Taylor et al., 1984). The effectiveness of both types can be modulated by transmitter action (Bennett, 1977; Dalkara et al., 1983) and coupling through gap junctions by variations in $[Ca]_i$ (Rose and Loewenstein, 1976) or pH (Turin and Warner, 1977). In addition, local changes in tissue hydration, extracellular ionic mobility, or the electrical properties of the investing glial network, which tend to make nerve cells electrically closer, could greatly enhance electrical coupling.

3. CHANGES IN $[Ca]_o$ AND $[Ca]_i$ RESULTING FROM Ca^{2+} INFLUX

The introduction of aequorin and other Ca^{2+}-sensitive dyes made possible for the first time systematic measurements of $[Ca]_i$, inevitably in relatively large invertebrate neurons (Baker, 1972; Blinks et al., 1982). The recording of changes in [Ca] in vertebrate tissue had to await the development of Ca^{2+}-sensitive microelectrodes. At first only extracellular measurements were possible (Nicholson, 1980). In regions such as the cerebellar cortex, fluctuations in [Ca]$_o$ were small (except during a grossly abnormal state like spreading depression), indicating only modest Ca^{2+} fluxes, likely to be of minor significance.

The results of the first intracellular recordings in the mammalian CNS were in keeping with these expectations: only small increases in [Ca]$_i$ typically by 10–20% over the baseline level, could be evoked in spinal motoneurons by maximal tetanic activation, antidromic or orthodromic (Krnjević et al., 1983; Morris et al 1985). Judging by these observations, intracellular sequestration is a very efficient process, which effectively minimizes changes in [Ca]$_i$, except perhaps in the region immediately subjacent to the cell membrane. Though we do not know precisely how large a change of [Ca]$_i$ is needed to induce long-lasting effects in cellular function, it is unlikely that fluctuations in the order of 10^{-7} M could be of major consequence. This would support the idea that motoneurons are not of primary importance for the initiation (as opposed to the implementation) of long-term changes in neural activity required for learning.

On the other hand, preliminary data from spinal interneurons indicate much greater activity-related increases in [Ca]$_i$ (Morris et al., 1985). Even more striking, however, are the changes in [Ca]$_i$ observed in the hippocampus. As illustrated by the upper trace of Fig. 1, extracellular recordings first revealed surprisingly large falls in [Ca]$_o$ in the stratum pyramidale (by 50–70%) during burst-type firing induced by quite low frequencies of stimulation (Krnjević et al., 1980, 1982,a,b; Benninger et al., 1980). This suggested that hippocampal cells (especially cell bodies) can generate Ca^{2+} currents that are far more intense than in motoneurons, which could be expected to produce correspondingly much greater increases in [Ca]$_i$. This was subsequently confirmed by intracellular recording (Morris et al., 1983): though technically even more challenging and therefore obtained under poorer conditions (unstable resting potentials, etc.), the observations demonstrated remarkably large increases in [Ca]$_i$ evoked by brief periods of low-frequency repetitive stimulation (about 10 Hz). Like the associated burst-firing, such increases could be evoked either during the tetanic stimulation, or as a delayed phenomenon, typically 30–60 sec after the end of the tetanus (as in the lower trace of Fig. l). Reaching a peak at 10^{-5}–10^{-4} M, these increases in [Ca]$_i$ were 100- to 1000-fold greater than those evoked by maximal tetanic stimulation in motoneurons.

4. SIGNIFICANCE OF LARGE ACTIVITY-EVOKED CHANGES IN [Ca]$_i$

There is no reason to suspect that Ca^{2+} sequestration is vastly less efficient in hippocampal cells than in spinal motoneurons. It is more likely that hippocampal cells can generate particularly large Ca^{2+} fluxes (as suggested also by the correspondingly large fall in [Ca]$_o$) whenever they are activated so as to fire in a "bursting" mode. This type of activity is observed without electrical stimulation even in freely behaving animals (Ranck, 1973; Buzsaki et al., 1983). One can therefore postulate

HIPPOCAMPUS

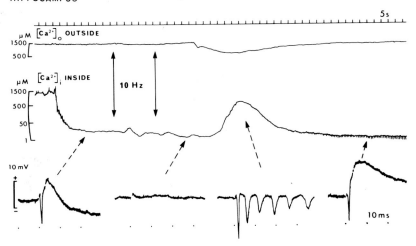

FIGURE 1. Delayed changes in extracellular and intracellular free Ca^{2+} concentration $[Ca^{2+}]_i$ in hippocampal CA2-3 region following repetitive stimulation of the fimbria. Upper $[Ca^{2+}]_o$ trace: *extracellular* recording with Ca^{2+}-sensitive micro-electrode. Lower $[Ca^{2+}]_i$ trace: *intracellular* recording with same electrode: note large fall in $[Ca]_i$ when electode penetrated cell. Oscilloscope traces (at bottom) were recorded at times indicated by broken arrows. Initially the fimbrial stimulation evoked an antidromic spike and a partly reversed IPSP. During the 10-Hz tetanus (between arrows), there were only small fluctuations in $[Ca^{2+}]_i$ (reference barrel contained 3 M KCl), but there followed a period of posttetanic depression, characterized by an absence of responses (including IPSPs) to the same fimbrial stimulation. About 30 sec after the end of the tetanus, paroxysmal responses suddenly appeared, in the form of bursts of population spikes. They were accompanied by a huge increase in $[Ca]_i$ (to a peak of about 700 µM) that lasted about 1 min. The return of $[Ca]_i$ to the baseline level (close to 1 µM) was followed by gradual return of the IPSP (now fully reversed).

The upper $[Ca]_o$ trace shows a comparably delayed large fall in extracellular $[Ca]$ evoked in a second run by a similar tetanic stimulation shortly after the end of intracellular recording. Data were obtained *in situ,* from a rat under urethane anaesthesia.

that it has a certain functional connotation, which is reflected in increases in $[Ca]_i$ sufficient to initiate whatever chain of intracellular events is necessary to imprint a memory trace. A well-established route (Cheung, 1982; Nestler and Greengard, 1983; Rasmussen and Barrett, 1984) is much discussed elsewhere in this volume: the activation of calmodulin and related protein kinases and the consequent phosphorylation of functionally or structurally significant proteins (enzymes, ionic channels, membrane receptors, etc.). It may be objected that the observed increases in $[Ca]_i$ are far greater than the threshold for activating calmodulin ($<10^{-6}$ M). Indeed, this suggests that some less sensitive Ca^{2+}-activated mechanism is involved. The observations are therefore in keeping with Lynch and Baudry's (1984) evidence that LTP is generated by the activation of a membrane-bound protease capable of "uncovering" occluded glutamate receptors. This protease (calpain) is activated by $[Ca]_i$ of 10 µM or more, in the range of $[Ca]_i$ evoked by repetitive stimulation.

A final point of interest is that the slow but rapidly reversible fall in extracellular [Ca] (Krnjević *et al.*, 1980, 1982a,b) may be of more than transient significance: the extracellular matrix is rich in ependyminlike protein that is highly, and irreversibly, responsive to a reduction in [Ca] (Shashoua, 1982; see Chapter 3 in present volume). This could also provide the elements of a permanent memory trace, by altering in a functionally meaningful way the physicochemical environment at strategic sites near synapses or membrane channels.

ACKNOWLEDGMENTS. The author's research is financially supported by the Medical Research Council of Canada.

REFERENCES

Adams, P. R. and Brown, D. A., 1980, Luteinizing hormone-releasing factor and muscarinic agonists act on the same voltage-sensitive K$^+$ current in bullfrog sympathetic neurones, *Br. J. Pharmacol.* **68:**353–355.

Alkon, D. A., 1982, A biophysical basis for molluscan associative learning, in: *Conditioning* (C. D. Woody, ed.) Plenum Press, New York, pp. 147–170.

Atwood, H. L., Charlton, M. P., and Thompson, C. S., 1983, Neuromuscular transmission in crustaceans is enhanced by a sodium ionophore, monensin, and by prolonged stimulation, *J. Physiol. (London)* **335:**179–195.

Baker, P. F., 1972, Transport and metabolism of calcium ions in nerve, *Progr. Biophys. Mol. Biol.* **24:**177–223.

Benardo, L. S. and Prince, D. A., 1982, Cholinergic pharmacology of mammalian hippocampal pyramidal cells, *Neuroscience* **7:**1703–1712.

Ben-Ari, Y., Krnjević, K., Reinhardt, W., and Ropert, N., 1981, Intracellular observations on the disinhibitory action of acetylcholine in the hippocampus, *Neuroscience* **6:**2475–2484.

Bennett, M. V. L., 1977, Electrical transmission: A functional analysis and comparison to chemical transmission, in: *Handbook of Physiology, Section 1: The Nervous System,* Vol. 1, Part 1 (J. M. Brookhart, V. B. Mountcastle, E. R. Kandel, and S. R. Geiger, eds.), American Physiological Society, Bethesda, Maryland, pp. 357–416.

Benninger, C., Kadis, J., and Prince, D. A., 1980, Extracellular calcium and potassium changes in hippocampal slices, *Brain Res.***187:**165–182.

Blinks, J. R., Wier, W. G., Hess, P., and Prendergast, F. G. 1982, Measurement of Ca^{2+} concentrations in living cells, *Progr. Biophys, Mol. Biol.* **40:**1–114.

Bowery, N. G., Price, G. W., Hudson, A. L., Hill, D. R., Wilkin, G. P., and Turnbull, M. J., 1984, GABA receptor multiplicity. Visualization of different receptor types in the mammalian CNS, *Neuropharmacology* **23:**219–231.

Buzsaki, G., Leung, L.-W. S., and Vanderwolf, C. H., 1983, Cellular bases of hippocampal EEG in the behaving rat, *Brain Res. Rev.* **6:**139–171.

Cheung, W. Y., 1982, Role of calmodulin in brain function, *Progr. Brain Res.* **56:**237–253.

Cole, A. E., and Nicoll, R. A., 1984, Characterization of a slow cholinergic post-synaptic potential recorded in vitro from rat hippocampal pyramidal cells, *J. Physiol. (London)* **352:**173–188.

Dalkara, T., Ropert, N., Yim, C. Y., and Krnjević, K., 1983, Mechanisms of facilitation of antidromic population spikes by iontophoretic applications of acetylcholine into hippocampal CA3 region *in situ, Soc. Neurosci. Abst.* **9:**968.

Dolphin, A. C., 1983, The excitatory amino-acid antagonist γ-D-glutamyl-glycine masks rather than prevents long term potentiation of the perforant path, *Neuroscience* **10:**377–383.

Dudek, F. E., Andrew, R. D., MacVicar, B. A., Snow, R. W., and Taylor, C. P., 1983, Recent evidence for and possible significance of gap junctions and electrotonic synapses in the mammalian brain, in: *Basic Mechanisms of Neuronal Hyperexcitability* (H. H. Jasper and N. M. van Gelder, eds.), Alan R. Liss, New York, pp. 31–73.

Dunlap, K. and Fischbach, G. D., 1978, Neurotransmitters decrease the calcium component of sensory nerve action potentials, *Nature* **276**:837–839.

Dunwiddie, T., Mueller, A., Palmer, M., Stewart, J., and Hoffer, B., 1980, Electrophysiological interactions of enkephalins with neuronal circuitry in the rat hippocampus. I. Effects on pyramidal cell activity, *Brain Res.* **184**:311–330.

Eccles, J. C., 1964, *The Physiology of Synapses,* Springer Verlag, Berlin, 316pp.

Erulkar, S. D. and Rahamimoff, R., 1978, The role of calcium ions in tetanic and post-tetanic increase of miniature end-plate potential frequency, *J. Physiol. (London)* **278**; 501–511.

Haas, H. L., 1982, Cholinergic disinhibition in hippocampal slices of the rat, *Brain Res.* **233**:200–204.

Haas, H. L., Felix, D., Celio, M. R., and Inagami, T., 1980, Angiotensin II in the hippocampus. A histochemical and electrophysiological study, *Experientia* **36**:1394–1395.

Haefely, W., Polc, P., Pieri, L., Schaffner, R., and Laurent, J.-P., 1983, Neuropharmacology of benzodiazepines: Synaptic mechanisms and neural basis of action, in: *The Benzodiazepines: From Molecular Biology to Clinical Practice* (E. Costa, ed.), Raven Press, New York, pp. 21–66.

Halliwell, J. V. and Adams, P. R., 1982, Voltage clamp analysis of muscarinic excitation in hippocampal neurons, *Brain Res.* **250**:71–92.

Kandel, E. R., Abrams, T., Bernier, L., Carew, T. J., Hawkins, R. D., and Schwartz, J. H., 1983, Classical conditioning and sensitization share aspects of the same molecular cascade in *Aplysia, Cold Spring Harbor Symp. Quant. Biol.* **48**:821–830.

Korn, H. and Faber, D. S., 1980, Electrical field effect interactions in the vertebrate brain, *Trends Neurosci.* **3**:6–9.

Krnjević, K., 1977, Effects of substance P on central neurons in cats, in: *Substance P* (U. S. von Euler, and B. Pernow, eds.), Raven Press, New York, pp. 217–230.

Krnjević, K., Morris, M. E., and Reiffenstein, R. J., 1980, Changes in extracellular Ca^{2+} and K^+ activity accompanying hippocampal discharges, *Can J. Physiol. Pharmacol.* **58**:579–583.

Krnjević, K., Reiffenstein, R. J., and Ropert, N., 1981, Disinhibitory action of acetylcholine in the rat's hippocampus: Extracellular observations, *Neuroscience* **12**:2465–2474.

Krnjević, K., Morris, M. E., and Reiffenstein, R. J., 1982a, Stimulation-evoked changes in extracellular K^+ and Ca^{2+} in pyramidal layers of the rat's hippocampus, *Can. J. Physiol. Pharmacol.* **60**:1643–1657.

Krnjević, K., Morris, M. E. Reiffenstein, R. J., and Ropert, N., 1982b, Depth distribution and mechanism of changes in extracellular K^+ and Ca^{2+} concentrations in the hippocampus, *Can J. Physiol. Pharmacol.* **60**:1658–1671.

Krnjević, K., Morris, M. E., and MacDonald, J. F., 1983, Free Ca^{2+} inside cat motoneurons at rest and during activity, *Can. J. Physiol. Pharmacol.* **61**:Axiii–Axiv.

Krnjević, K., Pumain, R., and Renaud, L., 1971, The mechanism of excitation by acetylcholine in the cerebral cortex, *J. Physiol. (London)* **215**:247–268.

Lynch, G. and Baudry, M., 1984, The biochemistry of memory: A new and specific hypothesis, *Science* **224**:1057–1063.

Madison, D. V. and Nicoll, R. A., 1982, Noradrenaline blocks accommodation of pyramidal cell discharge in the hippocampus, *Nature* **299**:636–638.

Morris, M. E., Krnjević, K., and MacDonald, J. F., 1985, Changes in intracellular free Ca ion concentration evoked by electrical activity in cat spinal neurons in situ, *Neuroscience* **14**:563–580.

Morris, M. E., Krnjević, K., and Ropert, N., 1983, Changes in free Ca^{2+} recorded inside hippocampal pyramidal neurons in response to fimbrial stimulation. *Soc. Neurosci. Abst.* **9**:395.

Murase, K. and Randić, M., 1984, Actions of substance P on rat spinal dorsal horn neurones, *J. Physiol. (London)* **346**:203–217.

Nestler, E. J. and Greengard, P., 1983, Protein phosphorylation in the brain, *Nature* **305**:583–588.

Nicholson, C., 1980, Modulation of extracellular calcium and its functional implications, *Fed. Proc.* **39**:1519–1523.

Nowak, L. M., and MacDonald, R. L., 1982, Substance P: Ionic basis for depolarizing responses of mouse spinal cord neurons in cell culture, *J. Neurosci.* **2**:1119–1128.

Ranck, J. B., 1973, Studies on single neurons in dorsal hippocampal formation and septum in unrestrained rats. Part I. Behavioural correlates and firing repertoires, *Exp. Neurol.* **41**:461–531.

Rasmussen, H., 1981, *Calcium and cAMP as Synarchic Messengers,* John Wiley & Sons, New York, 370 pp.

Rasmussen, H. and Barrett, P. Q., 1984, Calcium messenger system: An integrated view, *Physiol. Rev.* **64:**938–984.

Rose, B. and Loewenstein, W. R., 1976, Permeability of a cell junction and the local cytoplasmic free ionized calcium concentration: A study with aequorin, *J. Membrane Biol.* **28:**87–119.

Shashoua, V. E., 1982, The role of specific brain proteins in long-term memory formation, in: *Changing Concepts of the Nervous System* (A. R. Morrison and P. L. Strick, eds.), Academic Press, New York, pp. 681–716.

Shimahara, T. and Tauc, L., 1975, Heterosynaptic facilitation in the giant cell of *Aplysia, J. Physiol. (London)* **247:**321–341.

Skrede, K. K. and Malthe-Sørenssen, D., 1981, Increased resting and evoked release of transmitter following repetitive electrical tetanization in hippocampus: A biochemical correlate to long-lasting synaptic potentiation, *Brain Res.* **208:**436–441.

Stinnakre, J. and Tauc, L., 1973, Calcium influx in active *Aplysia* neurones detected by injected aequorin, *Nature New Biol.* **242:**113–115.

Taylor, C. P. and Dudek, F. E., 1982, Synchronous neural after discharges in rat hippocampal slices without active chemical synapses, *Science* **218:**810–812.

Taylor, C. P. and Dudek, F. E., 1984, Excitation of hippocampal pyramidal cells by an electrical field effect, *J. Neurophysiol.* **52:**126–142.

Taylor, C. P., Krnjević, K., and Ropert, N., 1984, Facilitation of hippocampal CA3 pyramidal cell firing by electrical fields generated antidromically, *Neuroscience* **11:**101–109.

Turin, L. and Warner, A., 1977, Carbon dioxide reversibly abolishes ionic communication between cells of early amphibian embryo, *Nature* **270:**56–57.

Vandermaelen, C. P. and Aghajanian, G. K., 1982, Serotonin-induced depolarization of rat facial motoneurones *in vivo:* comparison with amino acid transmitters, *Brain Res.* **239:**139–152.

Woody, C. D., Swartz, B. E., and Gruen, E., 1978, Effects of acetylcholine and cyclic GMP on input resistance of cortical neurons in awake cats, *Brain Res.* **158:**373–395.

Zieglgänsberger, W., French, E. D., Siggins, G. R., and Bloom, F. E., 1979, Opioid peptides may excite hippocampal pyramidal neurons by inhibiting adjacent inhibitory interneurons, *Science* **205:**415–417.

17

Calcium-Dependent Regulation of Calcium Channel Inactivation

R. ECKERT and J. E. CHAD

1. INTRODUCTION

Ionized calcium acts as an intracellular "messenger" or regulatory agent controlling a variety of cell functions, including exocytosis, motility, enzyme activity, membrane conductance, and others (reviewed by Katz, 1969; Meech, 1978; Llinás, 1980; Llinás *et al.*, 1981; Reuter, 1983). Calcium, upon entering the cell, also contributes to further membrane depolarization, which supports a positive feedback loop counteracting repolarization. Without any conteracting processes this would produce uncontrolled entry of Ca^{2+}, a situation incompatible with the regulatory function of the calcium ion. An important phenomenon preventing uncontrolled entry of Ca^{2+}, which has been demonstrated in a number of diverse tissues including nerve cells, is a Ca^{2+}-dependent inactivation of the voltage-activated calcium-channel. This form of inactivation appears to be widespread in excitable tissues, and may play an important role in basic neural function.

Observations on dialyzed snail neurons first led to the suggestion that the accumulation of Ca^{2+} during flow of the calcium current might act back on the calcium channels to limit the current (Kostyuk and Krishtal, 1977). Observations on Ca^{2+}-dependent locomotory responses of cilia to membrane depolarization in both intact and EGTA-injected paramecia produced similar speculation (Eckert, 1977; Brehm and Eckert, 1978a; Brehm *et al.*, 1978). The possibility that the Ca^{2+} conductance becomes inactivated in response to accumulation of calcium ions during current flow was first examined under voltage clamp in *Paramecium* (Brehm and Eckert, 1978b; 1979) and *Aplysia* neurons (Tillotson, 1979; Tillotson and Eckert, 1979; Eckert and Tillotson, 1979). In both preparations, the initial evidence indicated that inactivation was dependent on a specific intracellular action of Ca^{2+} accumulating in the cell during current flow (Eckert and Brehm, 1979; Brehm *et*

R. ECKERT and J. E. CHAD ● Department of Biology and Ahmanson Laboratory of Neurobiology, University of California, Los Angeles, Los Angeles, California 90024.

al., 1980; Tillotson, 1980; Eckert, 1981; Eckert *et al.*, 1981, 1983). Similar findings
were subsequently obtained in other tissues, including snail neurons (Standen, 1981;
Doroshenko *et al.*, 1982), insect muscle (Ashcroft and Stanfield, 1980, 1981,
1982b), frog atrium, calf Purkinje fibers, rat ventricular muscle (Giles *et al.*, 1980;
Fischmeister *et al.*, 1981; Fischmeister and Horackova, 1982a,b; Hume and Giles,
1983; Marban and Tsien 1981, 1982a,b; Tsien and Marban, 1982), squid presynaptic
terminal (Augustine *et al.*, 1981) and rod inner segment (Corey *et al.*, 1982), and
sympathetic ganglion cells (Adams, 1981). Here we review some recent studies of
calcium-dependent inactivation of calcium current.

2. EVIDENCE FOR Ca^{2+} DEPENDENCE

Several diagnostic criteria can be listed for distinguishing purely Ca^{2+}-depen-
dent from purely voltage-dependent inactivation. Thus, if the inactivation depends
on a specific action of intracellular Ca^{2+} rather than on a direct effect of membrane
potential on the channel mechanism, it should exhibit the following characteristics:

1. The degree and rate of development of inactivation will increase with
   increasing Ca^{2+} entry and accumulation irrespective of membrane potential.
2. The inactivation will depend on the species of ion carrying current through
   the membrane, Ca^{2+} being more effective than Sr^{2+} or Ba^{2+}.
3. Inactivation will be diminished, and its rate of removal will be accelerated
   by any means that decreases Ca_i or hastens its decline.
4. The rate of development of inactivation will be independent of membrane
   potential except as the latter influences the availability of Ca^{2+} to the Ca^{2+}-
   binding site that mediates inactivation.
5. Inactivation will develop in the absence of membrane depolarization in
   response to elevation of Ca_i by injection of Ca^{2+} or other means.

2.1. Relation to Membrane Voltage

An effect that depends on the entry of Ca^{2+} during depolarization rather than
on the depolarization itself should increase and then diminish along the voltage axis
according to the voltage dependence of Ca^{2+} entry (Katz and Miledi, 1966, 1967;
Baker *et al.*, 1971; Meech and Standen, 1975; Eckert and Lux, 1976). In *Paramecium* (Brehm and Eckert, 1978b; Brehm *et al.*, 1980), molluscan neurons (Tillotson, 1979; Eckert and Tillotson, 1981; Plant and Standen, 1981b), insect muscle
(Ashcroft and Stanfield, 1980, 1981, 1982b), and in several cardiac tissues (Fischmeister *et al.*, 1981; Tsien and Marban, 1982), the degree of inactivation has a
bell-shaped relation to prepulse potential, being maximal at intermediate potentials
that produce maximal Ca^{2+} entry and tailing off toward zero as the prepulse approaches E_{Ca}, at which Ca^{2+} entry is blocked in spite of strong depolarization
(Fig. 1).

Characteristic of voltage-dependent inactivation is a dependence of the rate of
removal of inactivation on membrane potential (Hodgkin and Huxley, 1952). In

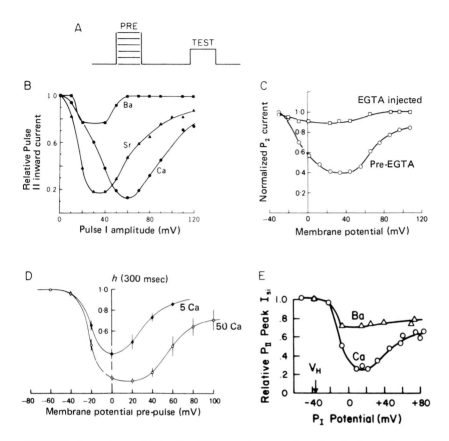

FIGURE 1. Dependence of test pulse Ca²⁺ current on prepulse voltage in diverse tissues. (A) Voltage clamp protocol. Prepulse voltage was varied while test pulse voltage was held constant. In each plot the ordinate gives the ratio of the test pulse current intensity without prepulse to the intensity with prepulse. (B) *Paramecium.* Relations in Ba²⁺-, Sr²⁺-, and Ca²⁺-containing solutions (Brehm and Eckert, 1978b). (C) *Aplysia* neuron: before and after injection of EGTA (Eckert and Tillotson, 1981). (D) Stick insect muscle: in 5 mM and 50 mM Ca²⁺ solutions (Ashcroft and Stanfield, 1981). (E) Cardiac cell: in Ca²⁺- and Ba²⁺-containing solutions (Tsien and Marban, 1982).

Paramecium (Brehm and Eckert, 1978b) and *Aplysia* neurons (Eckert and Tillotson, 1981), however, neither hyperpolarization nor depolarization to about E_{Ca} between the prepulse and the test pulse produced any change in the test pulse current. The effect of membrane depolarization on inactivation of Ca²⁺ current in *Aplysia* neurons is to diminish the inactivation and its rate of development.

2.2. Relation to Ca²⁺ Entry and Accumulation

If inactivation depends on Ca²⁺ entry and accumulation rather than on membrane voltage, it should be possible to achieve varying degrees of inactivation by changing the Ca^{2+} current, I_{Ca}, through means independent of membrane voltage. This was done by varying the extracellular calcium concentration, Ca_o, and hence I_{Ca} without changing the clamp potential (Brehm et al., 1980; Eckert and Tillotson, 1981; Plant and Standen, 1981a; Ashcroft and Stanfield, 1982b), and the rate of inactivation was found to increase with increased current strength. In a related approach Ca_o was kept constant, while the Ca^{2+} current in *Helix* or *Aplysia* neurons was reduced by means of a Ca^{2+}-blocking agent such as Cd^{2+} (Plant and Standen, 1981b; Eckert et al., 1982; Chad et al., 1983). Reduction in Ca^{2+} current strength caused a decrease in rate of relaxation of the current. The rates of inactivation exhibited by currents obtained under differing conditions of voltage or partial current block all correlated closely with current strength irrespective of membrane voltage.

2.3. Inactivation is Suppressed by Injected EGTA

The injection of EGTA partially suppresses the inactivation of the Ca^{2+} current in *Paramecium* (Brehm and Eckert, 1978b; Brehm et al., 1980) and molluscan neurons (Eckert and Tillotson, 1979, 1981; Plant et al., 1983a,b). The suppression of inactivation is manifested both as diminished reduction in amplitude of test pulse Ca^{2+} current following a prepulse (Fig. 1C) and as a decrease in the rate of relaxation of the Ca^{2+} current during a depolarizing step (Fig. 2A). Since injection of EGTA causes the rate of relaxation to decrease while the size of the current increases, the relaxation of calcium current cannot be simply attributed to depletion of Ca^{2+} from the extracellular space in these tissues, although extracellular depletion does affect the current in some cells (Fox and Krasne, 1982). Injection of EGTA also substantially increases the rate of removal of inactivation remaining from a prepulse as tested by application of test pulses following increasing intervals (Brehm et al., 1980; Eckert and Ewald, 1983b; Plant et al., 1983a,b; Deitmer and Eckert, 1984).

2.4. Injection of Ca^{2+} Produces Inactivation

Microinjection of calcium ions into intact cells by pressure or ionophoresis causes a reduction of Ca^{2+} current in *Helix* (Standen, 1981; Plant et al., 1983a,b) and *Aplysia* neurons (Eckert and Ewald, 1983b). This effect could be reversed by subsequent injection of EGTA.

2.5. Specificity of Ca^{2+} Relative to Sr^{2+}, Ba^{2+}, and H^+

The three divalent cations all carry current through Ca^{2+} channels (Hagiwara, 1975), but in some cells their respective currents differ significantly in the rate at which they undergo inactivation. In *Paramecium* (Brehm and Eckert, 1978b), *Aplysia* neurons (Tillotson, 1979; Eckert and Tillotson, 1981), insect muscle (Ashcroft and Stanfield, 1981, 1982a,b) and cardiac muscle (Mentrard et al., 1984) Sr^{2+} and Ba^{2+} are less effective than Ca^{2+} in producing inactivation. Ba^{2+} current undergoes a much smaller inactivation than Ca^{2+} current, and inactivation of Sr^{2+} current is intermediate (Fig. 1B,E). Since the Ba^{2+} current was both larger and slower to relax than Ca^{2+} currents under similar conditions, it must produce significantly greater intracellular ion (free plus bound) accumulation under similar depolarizations

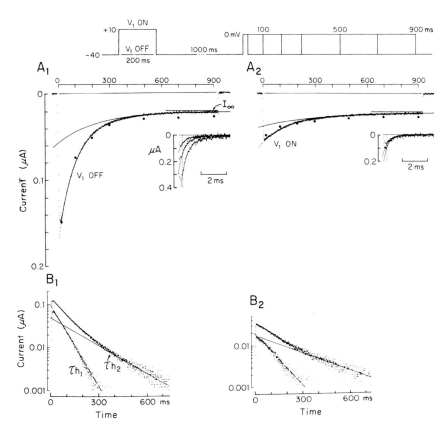

FIGURE 2. Inactivation of Ca²⁺ current in *Aplysia* neuron. (A₁) Voltage clamp step to 0 mV ($V_h = -40$) for 900 msec elicited a current that relaxed toward a steady-state asymptote, I_∞. The dashed lines are the computer-generated least-squares fits of a biexponential ($\tau_1 + \tau_2 + I_\infty$). In this example, τ_1 and τ_2 were 90 msec and 250 msec, respectively. (Inset) Tail currents recorded following pulses of 20, 100, and 500 msec duration, measured at 400 μsec (dashed vertical line) from computer-generated fits. Tail current amplitudes (×0.5) are indicated as solid circles for comparison with current trajectory. (B₁) Semilog plot of the current shown in (A₁). After subtraction of I_∞, log I_{Ca} was plotted against time and τ_2 determined from slope of the plot between 350 and 900 msec. This was peeled off to determine τ_1. These values were checked by fitting the calculated biexponential curve to the current trajectory in (A₁). (A₂, B₂) The same as (A₂) and (B₁), except that the test pulse, V_2, was preceded by a 200 msec conditioning pulse, V_1, as shown in the protocol above. Inset shows tail currents taken at 20 and 500 msec. (Chad *et al.*, 1984.)

than the Ca²⁺ current. Barium appears to be buffered less effectively in the cytoplasm than Ca²⁺, for measurements of cytoplasmic Ca²⁺ and Ba²⁺ with arsenazo III indicate that Ba²⁺ produces stronger and more slowly decaying signals following its entry (Ahmed and Connor, 1979; Connor and Ahmed, 1984). Since Ca²⁺ entry more effectively inactivates the channels than Ba²⁺ entry does, Ca²⁺ appears to exert a more specific action. That is to say, it exhibits a higher potency for producing inactivation than Ba²⁺.

Intracellular pH, pH$_i$, has been found to drop in response to Ca²⁺ entry in molluscan cells (Meech and Thomas, 1977, 1980; Ahmed and Connor, 1980). Lowering of pH_i elicits a reduction in calcium current in *Paramecium* (Umbach, 1982) and perhaps in neurons of *Pleurobranchaea* (Gillette, 1983). Thus, Ca^{2+} influx might affect Ca^{2+} conductance through a drop in pH_i. This is unlikely, however, for the injection of EGTA on the one hand enhances the drop in pH_i that accompanies Ca^{2+} entry in molluscan neurons (Ahmed and Connor, 1980) and, on the other hand, counteracts Ca^{2+}-dependent inactivation. Furthermore, experimental reduction of pH_i does not cause Ca^{2+} inactivation in *Helix* neurons (Plant *et al.*, 1983a).

2.6. Sensitivity of the Ca^{2+} Channel to Ca_i

Injections of calcium-EGTA buffer into intact cells appear to provide the most reliable figures for the Ca_i sensitivity of the Ca^{2+} current (Standen, 1981; Plant *et al.*, 1983a,b). Thus, injections of Ca^{2+} or Calcium-EGTA buffers that elevate Ca_i from a steady-state level of 10^{-7} M to 10^{-6} M to somewhat less than 10^{-5} M were reported to produce substantial reductions ($\approx 40\%$) in strontium or calcium currents in *Helix*, even though the attending reduction in driving force could account for less than 1% of the measured drop in current. The intracellular action of injected Ca^{2+} on the Ca^{2+} current therefore must have been due to a reduction in Ca^{2+} conductance. Metabolic poisons that interfere with mitochondrial function increased rather than decreased the effect of Ca^{2+} injection (Plant *et al.*, 1983a). This argues against a nonspecific effect of reduced cytosolic pH resulting from H^+/Ca^{2+} exchange during mitochondrial uptake of Ca^{2+}.

3. KINETICS OF Ca^{2+}-DEPENDENT INACTIVATION

Depolarizations of only a few millivolts from holding potentials of up to -55 mV can produce small, steady Ca^{2+} currents in molluscan neurons. These small currents exhibit little or no inactivation over periods of at least seconds (Eckert and Lux, 1975, 1976). This suggests that a Ca^{2+} current may flow continuously at resting potentials more positive than about -55 mV and that the small, steady influx of Ca^{2+} may be modulated by slow changes in resting potential. Larger step depolarizations in molluscan neurons elicit transient Ca^{2+} currents that decay with a time course containing one or two phases (Adams and Gage, 1979; Plant and Standen, 1981b; Eckert and Tillotson, 1981; Chad *et al.*, 1984). The inactivation that terminates the transient phase(s) of the current is incomplete, however, and the transient current is followed by a small, steady current, I_∞ (Fig. 2), which appears to be equivalent to the persistent current recorded during very small depolarizations (Eckert and Lux, 1975, 1976).

3.1. Two Phases of Inactivation

The presence of a fast (τ_1) and a slow (τ_2) phase in snail neurons led to the suggestion that inactivation of the Ca^{2+} current may occur as two separate processes

(Magura, 1977), raising the possibility of more than one population of Ca^{2+} channels (Kostyuk, 1980). Evidence reviewed below obtained in *Aplysia* neurons indicates, however, that the fast and slow components of inactivation need not represent separate populations or processes.

The rapid phase of inactivation is most pronounced in currents of large amplitude. The relative contribution of the fast component of inactivation is diminished by any maneuver reducing the peak amplitude of the Ca^{2+} current, while the slower phase is less sensitive to peak amplitude. Thus, presentation of a prepulse, lowering of the holding potential, or other means of raising Ca_i and hence increasing inactivation prior to the test pulse, will decrease the peak current and thus selectively depress the fast phase of inactivation (Fig. 2A₂). Likewise, under conditions of sufficiently weak activation or of sufficient block of I_{Ca}, the inactivation proceeds with only the slow phase. Maneuvers such as increased activation, elevated Ca_o, and diminished background inactivation, which increase the peak current, also increase the prominence of the fast phase of inactivation (Figs. 2 and 3). The two phases of inactivation are both slowed by injection of EGTA. This, in addition to other evidence (Eckert and Ewald, 1982b; Chad *et al.*, 1984), indicates that both phases of inactivation in *Aplysia* neurons arise from a Ca^{2+}-dependent process.

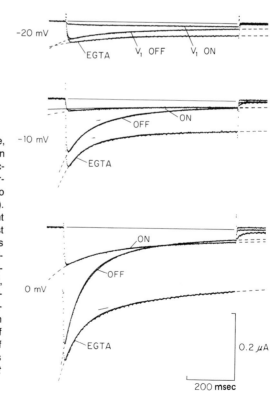

FIGURE 3. Effects of voltage, prepulse, and EGTA injection on kinetics of Ca^{2+}-dependent inactivation in *Aplysia* neuron. Currents during 700-msec steps to -20, -10, and 0 mV ($V_h = -40$). Each set shows three current traces. The one with the smallest peak amplitude labelled V_1 "on" was obtained 1000 msec following presentation of a 200-msec conditioning pulse, V_1 to $+10$ mV. The next, labeled V_1 "off," is the control current, obtained without presentation of V_1. The largest current in each set was obtained with V_1 off following inotophoretic injection of EGTA. Least squares computer fits are shown as in Fig. 1A. (Chad *et al.*, 1984.)

3.2. The Noninactivating Fraction of Current

Injection of EGTA causes a substantial increase in the intensity of the steady-state current, I_∞ (Fig. 3), which suggests that the level of I_∞ is normally limited, via negative feedback, by the accumulation of free Ca^{2+}. The amplitude of I_∞ may normally depend on an interplay between voltage-dependent activation and inactivation dependent on Ca^{2+} accumulation. The Ca_i near the inner surface of the membrane should approach a steady state in which the rate of Ca^{2+} entry equals the rate of Ca^{2+} removal from the region of the membrane. In that somewhat idealized state, Ca^{2+}-dependent inactivation should neither increase nor decrease with time, thus permitting the flow of steady, noninactivating Ca^{2+} current.

3.3. Current Dependence of Inactivation Kinetics

To examine the current dependence of Ca^{2+} inactivation in the voltage-clamped *Aplysia* neuron, the peak current intensity during depolarizing steps was altered by two distinct methods: a change in test pulse voltage and a partial competitive blockade of the Ca^{2+} current with cadmium ions (Chad *et al.*, 1984).

First, a family of currents with a broad range of amplitudes was generated by voltages ranging from -26 to 0 mV (Fig. 4A). More positive potentials were avoided to minimize contamination by outward currents. As the amplitude of the depolarization and hence the current increased, the early peak current followed by the rapid phase of inactivation, initially absent at small depolarizations, appeared and grew disproportionately large relative to the later current. Subsequently, 0.5 mM Cd^{2+} was added to the bath, producing a gradual block of I_{Ca} (Fig. 4B) during repeated potential steps to 0 mV. As the currents became progressively smaller, the rate of inactivation slowed, and the fast phase of inactivation was lost. Matching of currents of similar amplitude produced by altered voltage in the absence of Cd^{2+} with the currents produced by progressive Cd^{2+} block at a fixed voltage indicates that inactivation kinetics were closely correlated with the peak current intensity, irrespective of membrane voltage (Fig. 4C). Similar dependency of inactivation kinetics on current strength was seen when the test current amplitude was altered by presentation of a prepulse (Figs. 1 and 2) or alterations in Ca_o (Ashcroft and Stanfield, 1980; Eckert and Tillotson, 1981).

4. INACTIVATION MODELED AS A Ca^{2+}-MEDIATED PROCESS

A model of Ca^{2+} current inactivation has been proposed (Eckert *et al.*, 1982, 1983; Chad *et al.*, 1983, 1984) that in most respects is similar to one developed independently (Standen and Stanfield, 1982; Plant *et al.*, 1983a). The basic assumptions for the model are:

1. Activation has at least three states and can be approximated with a Hodgkin-Huxley voltage-dependent m^2 process (Kostyuk *et al.*, 1975; Byerly and Hagiwara, 1982). This formalism may not be fully appropriate, but it allows

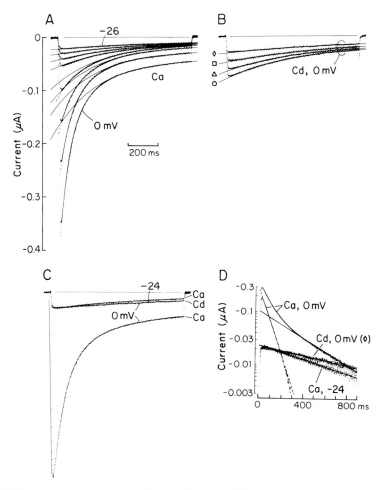

FIGURE 4. Current dependence of inactivation during 900-msec steps to various potentials (V_h = − 40 mV). Bath contained 5 mM 4-amino-pyridine plus 200 mM TEA. (A) Currents elicited in control artificial sea water (ASW) by pulses to − 26, − 24, − 22, − 20, − 15, − 10, − 5, and 0 mV. Computer fits as in Fig. 1A, except that τ_2 alone is shown by the smooth solid traces. (B) Currents obtained at 0 mV during developing block by 0.5 mM Cd²⁺. The four smaller currents, indicated here and in subsequent figures by the symbols, ○, △, □, and ◇, were recorded at intervals of 20 sec as cadmium block developed. (C) Superposition of three traces selected from (A) and (B). The two smaller traces, one at − 24 mV in cadmium-free ASW, the other at 0 mV after partial cadmium block of Ca²⁺ current, were selected and matched for similar current peak. The larger current was recorded at 0 mV before addition of cadmium. (D) Semilog display of currents in (C). The time constants τ_1 and τ_2 in Ca at 0 mV were 65 and 300 msec, respectively. τ_2's in Ca at − 24 mV and in Cd at 0 mV were 650 and 900 msec, respectively. (Chad et al., 1984.)

considerable simplification and does not greatly affect the result for inactivation.

2. Free Ca^{2+} within the cell regulates the inactivation of Ca^{2+} channels so as to produce inactivation with $1 : 1$ stoichiometry.

3. Relative to time scale of the observed macroscopic kinetics, inactivation effectively proceeds instantaneously. Thus, the general case is a six-state scheme in which Ca^{2+} causes the transition of any state to an inactivated state. If the processes of activation and inactivation are assumed to be parallel and independent, simplifications can be made that minimize the number of rate constants.

$$
\begin{array}{ccccccc}
 & & k_1 & & & k_2 & \\
C_1 & \rightleftharpoons & & C_2 & \rightleftharpoons & & O \\
 & & & & & & \\
k_{-3} \;\updownarrow & k_3 \;\begin{array}{c}k_2\\k_1\end{array}\; k_{-3} & & k_3 \;\begin{array}{c}k_{-2}\\k_2\end{array}\; k_{-3} & & & \updownarrow \;k_3 \\
 & & & & & & \\
C_1^* & \rightleftharpoons & & C_2^* & \rightleftharpoons & & C^* \\
 & & k_{-1} & & & k_{-2} &
\end{array}
$$

In this scheme horizontal transitions are voltage dependent, while vertical transitions are Ca^{2+} dependent. The asterisks denote the inactivated states.

4.1. Voltage-Dependent Activation

In the absence of inactivation, the current at time t is given by the expression

$$
I_{Ca} = I_{max} \, [m_\infty - (m_\infty - m_O) \, e^{-t/\tau_m}]^2 \tag{1}
$$

in which I_{max} represents the calcium current that would flow with maximal activation of the channel population and m_O and m_∞ represent probabilities at the holding potential and after infinite time at the test potential, respectively. The time constant τ_m is inversely proportional to the rate of change of probabilities between the two values (Hodgkin and Huxley, 1952).

I_{max} was assumed to be constant at any given potential during current flow and, in the voltage range used ($< +10$ mV), would be predicted to decrease nearly linearly with depolarization. In the absence of accurate determinations of I_{max}, a fixed value of I_{max} was used, and m_∞ was varied to represent changes in the product $I_{max} \cdot m_\infty^2$ at different membrane potentials. The value of m_∞ was arbitrarily set to unity for the largest current modeled.

4.2. Relationship of Ca_i to I_{Ca}

The fraction of entering Ca^{2+} remaining free to inactivate Ca^{2+} channels depends primarily on cytoplasmic buffering of free Ca^{2+}. A simple buffering system can be represented as

$$
Ca^{2+} + B^{2-} \underset{y}{\overset{x}{\rightleftharpoons}} BCa_i
$$

The free Ca^{2+} concentration at time t is given as $[Ca_i]_t$, while the total Ca^{2+} free plus bound, at time t is denoted $[Ca_i]_{tot}$. The total concentration of buffer, invariant with time, is given as $[B]_{tot}$, whereas the time-varying free buffer concentration is termed $[B]_t$. The ratio of rate constants, $y : x$, gives the dissociation constant K_A. Assuming rapid equilibration of the system, the probability of a single entering calcium ion being bound by buffer at time t, $P_B(t)$, is given by

$$P_B(t) = \frac{[Ca_i]_{tot} - [Ca_i]_t}{[Ca_i]_{tot}} \tag{2}$$

and it can be shown that

$$P_B(t) = \frac{[B]_t}{[B]_t + K_A} \tag{3}$$

Thus, if the buffer is far from saturation and influx of Ca^{2+} is small, the probability of buffering will be nearly constant. A fixed value for probability of buffering was used by Standen and Stanfield (1982) and Plant et al. (1983a), although with large currents and long pulses the value of $[B]_t$, and hence P_B, should decrease. Hence, the value $[B]_t$ is calculated and related to physiological buffers in the present model. Thus, if a simple single buffer compartment is assumed,

$$[B]_t = \frac{K_A \cdot [B]_{tot}}{[Ca_i]_t + K_A} \tag{4}$$

the change in probability of buffering can be estimated from values of buffer concentration and affinity and the concentration of free calcium ions. Buffering values used in modeling were within the physiological range established for a Ca^{2+}-binding protein which has been identified in neurons of Aplysia ($[B]_{tot} \approx 4 \times 10^{-4}$ M, $K_A \approx 2.0 \times 10^{-6}$ M, initial $[Ca_i^{2+}] \approx 0.1 \times 10^{-6} M$) (Breddermann and Wasserman, 1974; Baimbridge et al., 1982; Christakos et al., 1983). The intracellular movement of calcium is restricted by buffering (Rose and Loewenstein, 1975; Connor et al., 1981; Connor and Ahmed, 1984). It therefore appears that physiological rates of Ca^{2+} entry through Ca^{2+} channels produce immediate increases in Ca_i limited to a region believed to be restricted to within about 1 μm of the cytoplasm face of the membrane as estimated from modeling studies (Smith and Zucker, 1980; Connor and Nikolakopoulou, 1982; Zucker and Stockbridge, 1983). As a first approximation the effective volume, v, is taken to consist of a uniform 1-μm-thick shell* immediately under the membrane of a 100-μm-radius spherical neuron, from which there is a slow diffusional loss to the cell interior. Loss of Ca^{2+} from this arbitrary volume is modeled as a simple first-order diffusion process represented by the single rate constant D. Thus, if the free calcium ion activity,

---

* It is more likely that the volume v consists of the sum of numerous hemispherical "domains" of elevated Ca^{2+} centered on active Ca^{2+} channels (Chad and Eckert, 1984).

Ca_i, is denoted S, starting from an initial value of S_O, the relationship to calcium current is represented as

$$S = S_O + \int_0^t \left[(1 - P_B) \cdot I_{Ca} \cdot \frac{1}{-2Fv} - D \cdot S \right] dt. \tag{5}$$

4.3. Relationship of Inactivation to Ca_i

The inactivation of the open channel by calcium can be represented as

$$\underset{\text{open}}{O} + Ca \underset{b}{\overset{a}{\rightleftharpoons}} \underset{\text{inactivated}}{C^*}$$

The system is assumed to be in equilibrium, the total number of voltage-activated channels is given as $[O]_{tot}$, and the number of voltage-activated, noninactivated (open) channels is given as $[O]_t$. The ratio of rate constants, $a : b$, is represented as the rate constant K, also termed the potency parameter. Therefore at equilibrium

$$K \cdot [O]_t \cdot [Ca_i] = [C^*] \tag{6}$$

and

$$[O]_{tot} = [O]_t + [C^*] \tag{7}$$

Thus, by substitution and rearrangement

$$[O]_{tot}/[O]_t = 1 + K[Ca_i] \tag{8}$$

and hence the probability P_n, of the channel being open (i.e., activated but not inactivated) is given by

$$P_n = \frac{1}{1 + K \cdot Ca_i} \tag{9}$$

4.4. Mathematical Model of the Calcium Current

Equations representing voltage-dependent activation (Eq. 1), the relationship of Ca_i ($= S$ in the model) to the calcium current (Eq. 5), and the dependence of inactivation on Ca_i (Eq. 9) are combined to produce an expression for the progress of the calcium current through time during a step depolarization,

$$I_{Ca} = I_{max}[m_\infty - (m_\infty - m_0) \cdot e^{-t/\tau_m}]^2 \cdot P_n \tag{10}$$

This model is not exclusive; the final expression also describes the Ca^{2+} current predicted for a four-state linear scheme in which only the open state becomes inactivated (Chad et al., 1983, 1984), providing inactivation is rapid compared to the voltage-dependent steps. In addition, the action of Ca^{2+} in mediating the inactivation may contain intermediary steps, but if Ca$_i$ is rate limiting, the additional steps will have little effect on the modeled currents.

5. COMPUTER SIMULATION OF CURRENTS

The model described above appears plausible because it readily reproduces the basic kinetics of the Ca^{2+} current of *Aplysia* neurons. The parameters used in each case were based on computer fits to currents recorded from neurons during voltage steps to 0 mV (I_{max}, 420 nA; m_∞, 1.0; τ_m, 4.3 msec; K, 1 $\times$ 10^6 M^{-1}; B_{tot}, 4 $\times$ 10^{-4} M; S_O, 0.1 μM) except where otherwise stated. The calcium influx was assumed to diffuse into and rapidly equilibrate with the buffer within the effective volume. Subsequent loss of Ca^{2+} from this volume was not included in order to show that Ca^{2+}-mediated inactivation alone can produce the basic kinetics observed.

5.1. The Biphasic Time Course

As in the recorded current, the time course of the modeled current decays in two phases that can be approximated by the sum of two exponentials (τ_1 and τ_2). The basic relation underlying these kinetics is shown in Fig. 5A, in which the probability of a channel being not inactivated, P_n, is plotted against Ca$_i$ (Eq. 10; the value of K used was 10^6 M^{-1}, which corresponded to values obtained with model fits to recorded currents). This relationship describes a rectangular hyperbola with two limbs (*a* and *b*) connected by a marked transition. The slope (dP_n/dS) decreases with increased levels of Ca$_i$. The "resting" inactivation predicted for a background Ca$_i$ of 0.1 μM is shown by the arrow.

Plots of the inverted modeled current are shown in Figs. 5B and 5C. Curve (i) represents current expected from m^2 activation alone (Eq. 1) while curve (ii) includes the effect of modeled Ca^{2+}-mediated inactivation (Eq. 10). The two phases of inactivation (*a'*, *b'* in Fig. 5B) are related to the two limbs (*a,b*) in plot (A). The rapid ($\tau_1 \approx a'$) phase of inactivation occurs when the slope dP_n/dCa_i is large (limb *a*), whereas the slower phase ($\tau_2 \approx b'$) occurs when the slope is smaller (limb *b*).

The presence of one or two phases of inactivation depends primarily on the growth of Ca$_i$ during current flow, namely, whether one or both of the limbs *a* and *b* in Fig. 5A are traversed. Two phases of inactivation are thus implicit in the hyperbolic relation between the proportion of channels remaining not inactivated and the buildup of free Ca^{2+} during current flow (Eq. 9). As Ca$_i$ increases along

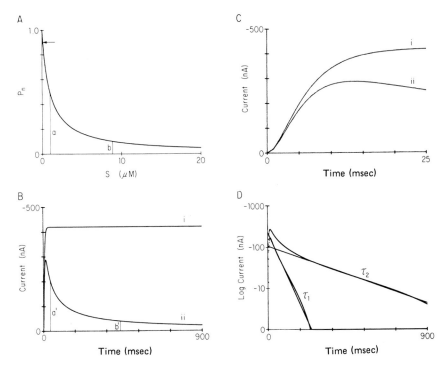

FIGURE 5. Computer simulations of the model of Ca^{2+}-dependent inactivation. (A) Probability of a channel being not inactiviated, P_n, plotted against internal free Ca^{2+} activity, Ca_i (Eq. 9), showing marked transition in slope with increased Ca^{2+}. The arrow indicates P_n at physiological background level of Ca_i. (B) Graph of inverted simulated Ca^{2+} current for voltage step to 0 mV: i, without inactivation (Eq. 2); ii, including Ca^{2+}-mediated inactivation (Eq. 10). a, a' and b, b' indicate equal degrees of inactivation (P_n) and equal levels of Ca_i. (C) Same as (B), but with time scale expanded to show effect of inactivation developing during activation. (D) Semilog plot of current in (B) after subtraction of I_∞ of 18 nA. Two quasi-exponential phases are present. (From Chad et al., 1984).

the steep limb of the relation (Fig. 5A), there is at first a strong effect on channel closing by each increment in Ca_i. This is followed by a transition to the shallow limb of the relationship, along which the effect of further increasing Ca_i is much weaker.

The τ_1 and τ_2 phases in the recorded currents appear to be fit by the sum of two exponentials (Fig. 2B), which might be taken as evidence for the presence of two separate first-order processes. However, the simulated currents show a small discrepancy in the fit to a biexponential (Fig. 5D). Such a discrepancy between the recorded current and their fitted biexponentials would be hidden in the recording noise. We suggest, then, that the fast and slow phases of inactivation seen in the recorded currents neither represent pure exponentials nor separate processes.

5.2. The Steady-State Persistent Current

If activation remains constant during a prolonged depolarization (Fig. 5B), a steady current, I_∞, should persist due to the failure of Ca^{2+}-dependent inactivation to go to completion. This can be understood from simple feedback considerations if we assume that Ca^{2+} diffuses away from the membrane to the interior of the cell. The fraction of channels remaining open in the steady state should depend on the steady-state Ca$_i$, as expressed in Eq. 9 and Fig. 5A. Thus, as diffusional loss ($D \cdot S$) approaches influx ($1/2F \cdot I_{Ca}$), S will cease to increase (Eq. 5), and hence I_{Ca} will cease to decrease (Eqs. 9 and 10).

5.3. Inactivation by Prepulse

The effect of prior Ca^{2+} entry and hence elevation of S_O on the modeled current is a reduction in peak amplitude and a preferential loss of the τ_1 phase of inactivation; at large values of S_O, inactivation proceeds with a single slow ($=\tau_2$) component (Fig. 6A; compare Fig. 2A$_2$). This preferential loss of the rapid phase results from the relation of P_n to Ca$_i$, for a prepulse increasing Ca$_i$ beyond the $a \rightarrow b$ transition in Fig. 5A will lead to a time course of inactivation dominated by limb b alone.

5.4. Varied Membrane Potential

Increased depolarization is simulated by an increase in the value of m_∞ and in the rate of change between probabilities ($1/\tau_m$), as in the model for sodium current activation (Hodgkin and Huxley, 1952). The values here were determined from fits of modeled currents to recorded currents. As the value for m_∞ increased, the peak current amplitude increased and the rapid phase of inactivation became increasingly prominent (Fig. 6B; compare with Fig. 3). The slow phase is less affected. Again, the prominence of the rapid phase relative to the slow phase of inactivation depends on the extent of Ca$_i$ buildup (Eq. 9).

5.5. Partial Current Block

The Cd^{2+} blockade of Ca^{2+} channels at a fixed membrane potential was simulated based on competition of Cd^{2+} and Ca^{2+} for a binding site at the Ca^{2+} channel, according to the relationship established by Hagiwara and Takahashi (1967). The binding affinity of Cd^{2+} ($K_D = 10^{-5}$ M) was determined from fits of the modeled currents to recorded currents. The effect of increased channel blockade on inactivation kinetics for a fixed voltage step in the modeled current is a preferential depression of the peak current (due to blocking of open channels) and a loss of the rapid phase of inactivation, leaving only a slowed τ_2 phase at reduced currents (compare Fig. 6C with Fig. 4B,C). This effect is similar to that produced by reducing current strength by other means such as elevated Ca$_i$ (Fig. 6A) or lower stimulus voltage (Fig. 6B).

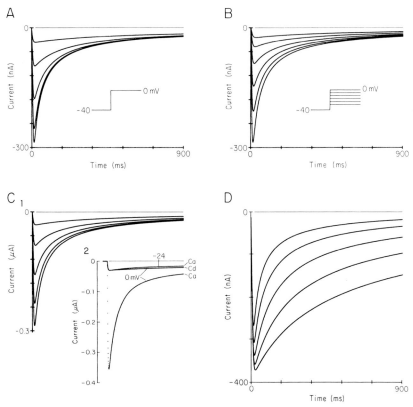

FIGURE 6. Effects on computer-generated Ca^{2+} currents of changing experimental parameters. (A) Effect of initial Ca_i (S_O) on simulated current in response to a step to 0 mV. The ascending family of curves correspond to S_O values of 0.1, 0.3, 1.0, 3.0, and 10 μM. (B) Changes in activation with increasing depolarization (-25 mV, $m\infty$ 0.26, τ_m 6.1 msec; -20 mV, $m\infty$ 0.37, τ_m 5.6 msec; -15 mV, $m\infty$ 0.52, τ_m 5.2 msec; -10 mV, $m\infty$ 0.68, τ_m 5.0 msec; -5 mV, $m\infty$ 0.84, τ_m 4.8 msec; 0 mV, $m\infty$ 1.0, τ_m 4.3 msec). (C) Simulation of competitive blockade. (C_1) Blocker concentrations of 0, 0.012, 0.04, 0.12, and 0.4 mM (affinity 1.0×10^{-5} M). (C_2) Effect of blockade (0.5 mM) compared to the effect of reduced voltage. The fitted values of K were 0.245 and 0.7 ($\times 10^6$ M^{-1}) for 0 and -24 mV, respectively. Pulse duration was 900 msec in each. (D) Effect of increased intracellular Ca^{2+} buffering. The descending family of curves correspond to values of B_{tot} of 0.4, 0.8, 1.6, 3.2, and 6.4 mM. Values for S_O were 0.1, 0.05, 0.025, 0.0125, and 0.00625 μM. (From Chad et al., 1984.)

5.6. Increased Ca^{2+} Buffering

Increasing the buffering capacity ($[B]_{tot}$) in the model produced a progressive slowing of the fast and slow phases of inactivation, a reduction in the extent of the fast phase, and a marked increase in I_∞ (Fig. 6D; compare with Fig. 3). An important effect of increased Ca^{2+} buffering is to retard, during a depolarization, the progression along the plot describing P_n (Fig. 5A). Another effect is to lower background Ca_i and hence the steady-state inactivation of the resting cell.

6. PHYSIOLOGICAL SIGNIFICANCE

Since the Ca^{2+}-dependent inactivation of Ca^{2+} channels occurs in a variety of tissues, it is likely to have physiological importance. Several proposed functions of such inactivation are discussed below.

6.1. Feedback Control of Ca^{2+} Entry

Ca^{2+}-dependent inactivation appears to be part of a negative feedback loop that limits the elevation of Ca$_i$, slowing Ca^{2+} entry by lowering membrane permeability to Ca^{2+}. Thus, as Ca$_i$ increases, there is a reduction in the percentage of Ca^{2+} channels available for carrying Ca^{2+} into the cell under any given membrane potential. Control of Ca^{2+} entry also arises from another feedback loop, namely, through the activation of $g_{K(Ca)}$ (Meech, 1978). Since E_K is generally more negative than potentials that activate I_{Ca}, this feedback loop fosters *de*activation of the Ca^{2+} conductance. In this regard it is interesting to note the different voltage sensitivities of the two feedback loops. The activation of $g_{K(Ca)}$ is greatest at high positive potentials whereas Ca^{2+}-dependent Ca^{2+} inactivation is greatest at negative potentials.

6.2. Modulation of Ca$_i$

The low-gain negative feedback that characterizes the Ca^{2+}-dependent inactivation allows continual, weak Ca^{2+} entry as a persistent current even with small depolarizations. It has been suggested (Eckert and Lux, 1976) that the slowly modulated persistent Ca^{2+} current exhibits two features of possible significance for regulatory functions of a continuous nature, namely, its persistence during prolonged depolarization and its activation at relatively high (up to -55 mV in snail neurons) membrane potentials. Thus, small but continuous modulation of Ca^{2+} influx and Ca$_i$ near the membrane is possible by small changes in membrane potential near rest.

6.3. Modulation of Membrane Potential

Regulation of Ca$_i$ near the membrane by removal mechanisms such as diffusion, buffering, and active pumping, can influence the membrane potential through modulation of Ca^{2+}-sensitive K$^+$ channels (Meech, 1978; Gorman *et al.*, 1981). Since small Ca^{2+} currents flowing with the membrane potential at or near rest resist full inactivation (Eckert and Lux, 1975, 1976), a small steady entry of Ca^{2+} may activate a small but significant Ca^{2+}-dependent K$^+$ conductance contributing to the resting potential. Dependence of resting conductance on Ca^{2+} entry and $g_{K(Ca)}$ was recently reported in *Aplysia* neurons (Johnson and Thompson, 1983).

Ca^{2+}-dependent modulation of the Ca^{2+} current in principle can also directly affect the membrane potential. Thus, the membrane potential following a period of depolarization and strong Ca^{2+} entry may undergo changes that depend in part on the removal of Ca^{2+} inactivation and hence return of the Ca^{2+} current as Ca$_i$

drops near the membrane following repolarization. Such a mechanism has been recently implicated in the origin of the pacemaker potential in burst-generating *Aplysia* neurons (Adams and Levitan, 1981; Kramer and Zucker, 1983).

7. CONCLUSIONS

Several criteria have proven useful in recognizing Ca^{2+}-dependent inactivation in certain tissues. (1) Inactivation of the Ca^{2+} current is current dependent, increasing with increasing current strength. (2) Inactivation depends on the species of ion carrying current through the membrane, Ca^{2+} being more effective than Sr^{2+} or Ba^{2+}. (3) Inactivation is diminished, and its rate of removal is accelerated by any means that decreases Ca_i or hastens its decline. (4) The inactivation and its kinetics are independent of membrane voltage, although certain secondary effects of potential are manifested. (5) Inactivation develops in the absence of membrane depolarization in response to elevation of Ca_i by various means such as injection of Ca^{2+}. In light of criterion (3), it is difficult to identify or characterize Ca^{2+}-dependent inactivation in preparations where powerful Ca^{2+}-chelating agents have been introduced intracellularly, as in cell dialysis or whole-cell patch-clamp studies.

Ca^{2+}-dependent inactivation has been modeled using the premise that the Ca^{2+} channel passes to the inactivated state by a process dependent upon an action of Ca^{2+} that exhibits a $1:1$ stoichiometry with channel inactivation. The model incorporates the buffering properties of known cytoplasic Ca^{2+}-binding proteins and assumes the buffer to be saturable. When an expression for the probability of channel activation was multiplied by a factor proportional to the probability of a channel being not inactivated by Ca^{2+} binding, modeled currents were generated that exhibit the temporal features characteristic of the recorded Ca^{2+} currents, including current-dependent kinetics, fast and slow phases of inactivation, and late steady-state current. In addition, the simulated currents behave like the real currents in response to changing "experimental" parameters.

An important conclusion derived from the modeling study is that the fast and slow phases of inactivation generally seen during sustained depolarization can occur as a consequence of a single Ca^{2+}-dependent mechanism of inactivation; thus, neither the existence of two populations of channels nor two distinct processes of inactivation are indicated or required.

Another general concept, derived from experiments and modeling studies, is that the efficiency and capacity of the cytoplasmic Ca^{2+} buffer will determine the current dependence of Ca^{2+}-dependent inactivation. Thus, identical Ca^{2+} channels should exhibit different inactivation kinetics depending on the effectiveness of the buffer in retarding the rise in Ca_i. This may explain some observed differences in the rates of inactivation of Ca^{2+} currents in different cells.

ACKNOWLEDGMENTS. We are grateful to Drs. G. J. Augustine and J. A. Connor for helpful discussion and comments and to Ms. D. Kuper for skillful preparation of the typescript. The work from our laboratory reviewed herein was supported by

USPHS NS 8364, NSF BNS 80-12346, and BNS 82-03843, the Muscular Dystrophy Foundation, and the Epilepsy Foundation of America.

REFERENCES

Adams, D. J. and Gage, P. W., 1979, Characteristics of sodium and calcium conductance changes produced by membrane depolarization in an *Aplysia* neurone, *J. Physiol. (London)* **289**:143–161.

Adams, P. R., 1981, The calcium current of a vertebrate neurone, *Adv. Physiol. Sci.* **4**:564–578.

Adams, W. B. and Levitan, I. B., 1981, Ionic dependence and charge carriers of the currents underlying bursting in *Aplysia* neuron R15, *Soc. Neurosci. Abstr.* **5**:239.

Ahmed, Z. and Connor, J. A., 1979, Measurement of calcium influx under voltage clamp in molluscan neurones using the metallochromic dye arsenazo III, *J. Physiol. (London)* **286**:61–82.

Ahmed, Z. and Connor, J. A., 1980, Intracellular pH changes induced by calcium influx during electrical activity in molluscan neurons, *J. Gen. Physiol.* **75**:403–426.

Alvarez-Leefmans, F. J., Rink, T. J., and Tsien, R. Y., 1981, Free calcium ions in neurones of *Helix aspersa* measured with ion-selective micro-electrodes, *J. Physiol. (London)* **315**:531–548.

Ashcroft, F. M. and Stanfield, P. R., 1980, Inactivation of calcium currents in skeletal muscle fibres of an insect depends on calcium entry, *J. Physiol. (London)* **308**:36P.

Ashcroft, F. M. and Stanfield, P. R., 1981, Calcium dependence of the inactivation of calcium currents in skeletal muscle fibers of an insect, *Science* **213**:224–226.

Ashcroft, F. M. and Stanfield, P. R., 1982a, Calcium and potassium currents in muscle fibres of an insect (*Carausius morosus*), *J. Physiol. (London)* **323**:93–115.

Ashcroft, F. M. and Stanfield, P. R., 1982b, Calcium inactivation in skeletal muscle fibres of the stick insect *Carausius morosus, J. Physiol. (London)* **330**:349–372.

Augustine, G., Eckert, R., and Zucker, R., 1981, Presynaptic calcium channel inactivation at the squid giant synapse, *Soc. Neurosci. Abstr.* **7**:442.

Baimbridge, K. G., Miller, J. J., and Parkes, C. O., 1982, Calcium-binding protein distribution in the rat brain, *Brain Res.* **239**:519–525.

Baker, P., 1976, The regulation of intracellular calcium, in: *Calcium in Biological Systems,* Cambridge University Press, Cambridge.

Baker, P., Hodgkin, A. L., and Ridgeway, E. B., 1971, Depolarization and calcium entry in squid giant axons, *J. Physiol. (London)* **218**:709–755.

Bredderman, P. J. and Wasserman, R. H., 1974, Chemical composition, affinity for calcium, and some related properties of the vitamin D dependent calcium-binding protein, *Biochemistry* **13**:1687–1694.

Brehm, P. and Eckert, R., 1978a, An electrophysiological study of the regulation of ciliary beating frequency in *Paramecium, J. Physiol. (London)* **283**:557–568.

Brehm, P. and Eckert, R., 1978b, Calcium entry leads to inactivation of calcium channel in *Paramecium, Science* **202**:1203–1206.

Brehm, P. and Eckert, R., 1979, Elevation of intracellular free Ca^{2+} is required for inactivation of Ca conductance in *Paramecium, Soc. Neurosci. Abstr.* **5**:290.

Brehm, P., Dunlap, K., and Eckert, R., 1978, Ca-dependent repolarization in *Paramecium, J. Physiol. (London)* **274**:639–654.

Brehm, P., Eckert, R., and Tillotson, D., 1980, Calcium-mediated inactivation of calcium current in *Paramecium, J. Physiol. (London)* **306**:193–203.

Byerly, L. and Hagiwara, S., 1982, Calcium currents in internally perfused nerve cell bodies of *Limnea stagnalis, J. Physiol. (London)* **322**:503–528.

Chad, J. E. and Eckert, R., 1984, Calcium 'domains' associated with individual channels may account for anomalous voltage relations of Ca-dependent responses, *Biophys. J.* **45**:993–999.

Chad, J., Eckert, R., and Ewald, D., 1983, Kinetics of calcium current inactivation simulated with an heuristic model, *Biophys. J. 41:*61a.

Chad, J., Eckert, R., and Ewald, D., 1984, Kinetics of Ca-dependent inactivation of calcium current in neurones of *Aplysia* californica, *J. Physiol. (London)* **347**:279–300.

Christakos, S., Van Eldik, L. J., Bruns, M. E., Mehru, A., and Feldman, S., 1983, Calmodulin and mammalian vitamin D dependent calcium binding proteins: A comparison, *Fed. Proc.* **42**:961.

Connor, J. A. and Ahmed, Z., 1984, Diffusion of ions and indicator dyes in neural cytoplasm, *Cell. Molec. Neurobiol.* **4**:53–56.

Connor, J. A. and Nikolakopoulou, G., 1982, Calcium diffusion and buffering in nerve cytoplasm, *Lec. Math. Life Sci.* **15**:79–101.

Connor, J. A., Ahmed, Z., and Ebert, G., 1981, Diffusion of Ca^{2+}, Ba^{2+}, H^+ and arsenazo III in neural cytoplasm, *Soc. Neurosci. Abstr.* **7**:15.

Corey, D. P., Dubinsky, J., and Schwartz, E. A., 1982, The calcium current of rod-photoreceptor inner segments recorded with a whole-cell patch clamp, *Soc. Neurosci. Abst.* **8**:944.

Deitmer, J. W. and Eckert, R., 1984, Relaxation of two calcium-dependent membrane processes following Ca^{2+} influx in neurones of *Aplysia californica*, in preparation.

Doroshenko, P. A., Kostyuk, P. G., and Martynyuk, A. I. 1982, Inactivation of calcium currents in the somatic membrane of molluscan neurones, *Neirofiziologiya (Kiev)* **14**:532–538.

Eckert, R., 1977, Genes, channels and membrane currents in *Paramecium, Nature* **268**:104–105.

Eckert, R., 1981, Calcium-mediated inactivation of voltage-gated Ca channels, in: *The Mechanism of Gated Calcium Transport Across Biological Membranes* (S. T. Ohnishi and M. Endo, eds.), Academic Press, New York, pp. 63–70.

Eckert, R. and Brehm, P., 1979, Ionic mechanisms of excitation in *Paramecium, Ann. Rev. Biophys. Bioeng.* **8**:353–383.

Eckert, R. and Ewald, D., 1982, Fast and slow components of calcium inactivation in *Aplysia* neurons both exhibit current dependence, *Soc. Neurosci. Abstr.* **8**:943.

Eckert, R. and Ewald, D., 1983, Inactivation of calcium conductance characterized by tail current measurements in neurones of *Aplysia californica, J. Physiol. (London)* **345**:549–565.

Eckert, R. and Lux, H. D., 1975, A non-inactivating inward current recorded during small depolarizing voltage steps in snail pacemaker neurons, *Brain Res.* **83**:486–489.

Eckert, R. and Lux, H. D., 1976, A voltage-sensitive persistent calcium conductance in neuronal somata of *Helix, J. Physiol. (London)* **254**:129–151.

Eckert, R. and Tillotson, D., 1979, Intracellular EGTA interferes with inactivation of the Ca current in *Aplysia* neurons, *Soc. Neurosci. Abstr.* **5**:291.

Eckert, R. and Tillotson, D., 1981, Calcium-mediated inactivation of the calcium conductance in caesium-loaded giant neurones of *Aplysia californica, J. Physiol. (London)* **314**:265–280.

Eckert, R., Tillotson, D., and Brehm, P., 1981, Calcium mediated control of Ca and K currents, *Fed. Proc.* **40**:2226–2232.

Eckert, R., Ewald, D., and Chad, J., 1982, A single Ca-mediated process can account for both rapid and slow phases of inactivation exhibited by a single calcium conductance, *Biol. Bull.* **163**:398.

Eckert, R., Ewald, D., and Chad, J., 1983, Calcium-mediated inactivation of calcium current in neurons of *Aplysia californica,* in: *The Physiology of Excitable Cells* (A. D. Grinnell and W. Moody, eds.), Alan Liss, New York, pp. 25–38.

Fischmeister, R. and Horackova, M., 1982a, Slow inward Ca current in frog heart: Voltage-dependent or Ca-mediated inactivation? *Biophys. J.* **37**:323.

Fischmeister, R. and Horackova, M., 1982b, Slow inward Ca current in frog heart: theoretical evidence against a voltage-dependent inactivation, *Can. J. Physiol. Pharmacol.* **60**:1185–1192.

Fischmeister, R., Mentrard, D., and Vassort, G., 1981, Slow inward current inactivation in frog heart atrium, *J. Physiol. (London)* **320**:27–28P.

Fox, A. P. and Krasne, S., 1982, Relaxation due to depletion in an egg cell calcium current, *Biophys. J.* **37**:20a.

Giles, W., Hume, J., and Noble, S., 1980, The ionic mechanism underlying the interval-duration relationship in bullfrog atrium, *J. Physiol. (London)* **300**:62P.

Gillette, R., 1983, Intracellular alkalinization potentiates slow inward current and prolonged bursting in a molluscan neuron, *J. Neurophysiol.* **49**:509–515.

Gorman, A. L. F., Thomas, M. V., and Hermann, A., 1981, Intracellular calcium and the control of neuronal pacemaker activity, *Fed. Proc.* **40**:2233–2239.

Hagiwara, S., 1975, Ca-dependent action potential, in: *Membranes,* Vol. 3 (G. Eisenman, ed.), Marcell Dekker, New York, pp. 359–381.

Hagiwara, S. and Takahashi, K., 1967, Surface density of calcium ions and calcium spikes in the barnacle muscle fiber membrane, *J. Gen. Physiol.* **50:**583–601.

Hodgkin, A. L. and Huxley, A. F., 1952, The dual effect of membrane potential on sodium conductance of the giant axon of *Loligo, J. Physiol. (London)* **116:**497–506.

Hume, J. R. and Giles, W., 1983, Ionic currents in single isolated bullfrog atrial cells, *J. Gen. Physiol.* **81:**153–194.

Johnson, J. W. and Thompson, S. H., 1983, Calcium dependence of resting neuronal conductance, *Soc. Neurosci. Abstr.* **9:**1187.

Katz, B., 1969, *The Release of Neural Transmitter Substances,* Charles Thomas, Springfield.

Katz, B. and Miledi, R., 1966, Input-output relation of a single synapse, *Nature* **212:**1242–1245.

Katz, B. and Miledi, R., 1967, A study of synaptic transmission in the absence of nerve impulses, *J. Physiol. (London)* **192:**407–436.

Kostyuk, P. G. 1980, Calcium ionic channels in electrically excitable membranes, *Neuroscience* **5:**945–959.

Kostyuk, P. G. and Krishtal, O. A., 1977, Effects of calcium and calcium-chelating agents on the inward and outward current in the membrane of mollusc neurones, *J. Physiol. (London)* **270:** 569–580.

Kostyuk, P. G., Krishtal, O. A., and Pidoplichko, V. I., 1975, Effect of internal fluoride and phosphate on membrane currents during intracellular dialysis of nerve cells, *Nature (London)* **257:**691–693.

Kramer, R. H. and Zucker, R. S., 1983, Inactivation of persistent inward current mediates post-burst hyperpolarization in *Aplysia* bursting pacemaker neurons, *Soc. Neurosci. Abstr.* **9:**510.

Llinás, R., 1980, A model of presynaptic Ca^{++} current and its role in transmitter release, in: *Molluscan Nerve Cells: From Biophysics to Behavior* (J. Koester and J. H. Byrne, eds.), Cold Spring Harbor Laboratory, Cold Spring Harbor.

Llinás, R., Steinberg, I. Z., and Walton, K., 1981, Relationship between presynaptic calcium current and postsynaptic potential in squid giant synapse, *Biophys. J.* **33:**323–352.

Magura, I. S., 1977, Long-lasting inward current in snail neurons in barium solutions in voltage-clamp conditions, *J. Memb. Biol.* **35:**239–256.

Marban, E. and Tsien, R. W., 1981, Is the slow inward current of heart muscle inactivated by calcium? *Biophys. J.* **33:**143a.

Marban, E. and Tsien, R. W., 1982a, Enhancement of calcium current during digitalis inotropy in mammalian heart: Positive feed-back regulation by intracellular calcium? *J. Physiol. (London)* **329:**589–614.

Marban, E. and Tsien, R. W., 1982b, Effects of nystatin-mediated intracellular ion substitution on membrane currents in calf purkinje fibres, *J. Physiol. (London)* **329:**569–587.

Meech, R. W., 1978, Calcium-dependent potassium activation in nervous tissues, *Ann. Rev. Biophys. Bioeng.* **7:**1–18.

Meech, R. and Standen, N., 1975, Potassium activation in *Helix* neurones under voltage clamp: A component mediated by calcium influx. *J. Physiol. (London)* **249:**211–239.

Meech, R. W. and Thomas, R. C., 1977, The effect of calcium injection on the intracellular sodium and pH of snail neurones, *J. Physiol. (London)* **265:**867–879.

Meech, R. W. and Thomas, R. C., 1980, The effect of measured calcium chloride injections on the membrane potential and internal pH of snail neurones, *J. Physiol. (London)* **298:**111–129.

Mentrard, D., Vassort, G., and Fischmeister, R., 1984, Calcium-mediated inactivation of the calcium conductance in caesium-loaded frog heart cells, *J. Gen. Physiol.* **83:**105–131.

Plant, T. D. and Standen, N. B., 1981a, Calcium current inactivation in *Helix aspersa* neurones studied using potassium current blockers, *J. Physiol. (London)* **316:**4P.

Plant, T. D. and Standen, N. B., 1981b, Calcium current inactivation in identified neurones of *Helix aspersa, J. Physiol. (London)* **321:**273–285.

Plant, T. D., Standen, N. B., and Ward, T. A., 1983a, The effects of injection of calcium ions and calcium chelators on calcium channel inactivation in *Helix* neurones, *J. Physiol. (London)* **334:**189–212.

Plant, T. D., Standen, N. B., and Ward, T. A., 1983b, Calcium injection and calcium channel inactivation, in: *The Physiology of Excitable Cells* (A. D. Grinnell and W. Moody, eds.), Alan R. Liss, New York, pp. 39–49.

Reuter, H.,, 1983, Calcium channel modulation by neurotransmitters, enzymes and drugs, *Nature* **301:**569–574.

Rose, B. and Lowenstein, W. R., 1975, Calcium ion distribution in cytoplasm visualized by aequorin: Diffusion in cytosol restricted by energized sequestering, *Science* **190:**1204–1206.

Smith, S. J. and Zucker, R. S., 1980, Aequorin response facilitation and intracellular calcium accumulation in molluscan neurones, *J. Physiol. (London)* **300:**167–196.

Standen, N. B., 1981, Ca channel inactivation by intracellular Ca injection into *Helix* neurones, *Nature* **293:**158–159.

Standen, N. B. and Stanfield, P. R., 1982, A binding-site model for calcium channel inactivation that depends on calcium entry, *Proc. R. Soc. Lond. B* **217:**101–110.

Tillotson, D., 1979, Inactivation of Ca conductance dependent on entry of Ca ions in molluscan neurons, *Proc. Natl. Acad. Sci. U.S.A.* **77:**1497–1500.

Tillotson, D., 1980, Ca^{++}-dependent inactivation of Ca^{++} channels, in: *Molluscan Nerve Cells* (J. Koester and J. H. Byrne, eds.), Cold Spring Harbor Laboratory, Cold Spring Harbor.

Tillotson, D. and Eckert, R., 1979, Ca inactivation in *Aplysia* neurons is quantitatively related to prior Ca entry, *Soc. Neurosci. Abstr.* **5:**296.

Tsien, R. W. and Marban, E., 1982, Digitalis and slow inward current in heart muscle: Evidence for regulatory effects of intracellular calcium on calcium channels, in: *Advances in Pharmacology and Therapeutics* II, Vol. 3 (H. Yoshida, Y. Hagihara, and S. Ebashi, eds.), Pergamon Press, Oxford, pp. 217–225.

Umbach, J., 1982, Changes in intracellular pH affect calcium currents in *Paramecium caudatum, Proc. R. Soc. Lond. B.* **216:**209–224.

Zucker, R. S. and Stockbridge, N., 1983, Presynaptic calcium diffusion and the time courses of transmitter release and synaptic facilitation at the squid giant synapse, *J. Neurosci.* **3:**1263–1269.

18

Calcium Action Potential Induction in a "Nonexcitable" Motor Neuron Cell Body
A Study with Arsenazo III

T. SHIMAHARA, G. CZTERNASTY, J. STINNAKRE, and J. BRUNER

1. INTRODUCTION

It is now well documented that the membrane of many neurons and of heart cells present two types of voltage gated channels that carry Na^+ or Ca^{2+}. In most cases, activation of Na^+ channels is faster than that of Ca^{2+} channels so that the Ca^{2+} current is delayed relatively to the Na^+ current (Hagiwara and Byerly, 1981). Recently it has been observed that in response to a depolarization, mammalian thalamic neurons *in vitro* show Na^+ spikes when the membrane potential is more positive than -60 mV, and Ca^{2+} action potential when it was more negative than -65 mV (Llinás and Jahnsen, 1982; Jahnsen and Llinás, 1984a,b). Such a change in the ionic selectivity of a membrane has also been reported in the "non spiking" somata of crayfish motor giant neuron (MoG). In this preparation, no regenerative spike is observed when the cell is depolarized from the resting potential. However, if the cell is hyperpolarized to about -90 mV, a brief depolarizing pulse triggers a fast (Na^+ dependent) action potential. Conversely, when the membrane potential is depolarized to about -50 mV, or more, the same pulse induces a slow Ca^{2+} action potential (SAP) (Czternasty and Bruner, 1981).

In this preparation, as in many others, it has been suggested that hyperpolarization removes the Na^+ inactivation that otherwise prevents the development of Na^+ action potential (Czternasty et al., 1982a,b). The mechanism involved in the

T. SHIMAHARA, G. CZTERNASTY, J. STINNAKRE, and J. BRUNER ● Laboratoire de Neurobiologie Cellulaire, C.N.R.S., 91190-Gif sur Yvette, France.   *Present address* for G. C. and J.B. Laboratoire de Neurobiologie Cellulaire, Université de Picardie, 80039-Amiens, France.

initiation of the Ca^{2+} spike is likely to be different. One hypothesis might be that the predepolarization inactivates K^+ channels, allowing the development of a Ca^{2+} action potential; indeed, in the presence of a K^+ channel blocker, a Ca^{2+} spike may also be triggered at the resting potential (Czternasty and Bruner, 1981). Alternatively, the predepolarization might facilitate the subsequent increase in Ca^{2+} conductance due to the triggering pulse, leading to a long-lasting and overshooting Ca^{2+} spike. To answer these questions, we have measured directly the intracellular free Ca^{2+} concentration using the Ca^{2+} sensitive dye Arsenazo III (AzIII; see Thomas, 1982). Preliminary reports of this work have been presented in abstract form (Shimahara *et al.,* 1983a,b).

2. MATERIALS AND METHODS

Experiments were performed on somata of the MoG from the third and fourth abdominal ganglion of *Procambarus clarkii* as described elsewhere (Czternasty *et al.,* 1984), except that the AzIII absorbance was measured differentially at the 650–572 nm pair, which minimizes the Mg^{2+} interference. Considering the morphological study of Mittenthall and Wine (1978), the area analyzed for light transmission was set smaller than the soma diameter to exclude the initial part of the axon from the measured field, using a field diaphragm. Electrophoretic dye injection was stopped when the intracellular concentration of the dye reached 0.2–0.25 mM. Concentration was calculated from the absorbance change at 572 nm, using an extinction coefficient of 29,800 ℓ mole^{-1} cm^{-1} (Smith and Zucker, 1980). A third electrode filled with 3 M KCl was used to voltage-clamp the neurones.

3. RESULTS

Application of a constant depolarizing current to the somatic membrane of the MoG produced a jump of the membrane potential, which then slowly drifted to a more depolarized level as shown in Fig. 1A. A slow increase of the $[Ca^{2+}]_i$ also became apparent after about 30 sec. Two test pulses applied at -40 and -34 mV, respectively, were ineffective in producing a regenerative response but gave a small, then a slightly larger Ca^{2+} entry. A third pulse applied soon after the second one triggered a slow action potential, which was accompanied by a large intracellular Ca^{2+} transient, as observed by Czternasty *et al.* (1984). When the long depolarization was maintained, a single slow action potential occurred without a test pulse. As said earlier, the cause for the occurrence of the slow action potential may be this slow facilitating Ca^{2+} entry during the predepolarization or an increase in the membrane resistance that occurs during the same period (Fig. 1B).

To study the changes induced by the predepolarization, the AzIII absorbance was measured under voltage clamp (Fig. 2). Pulsing the membrane potential to 0 mV (Fig. 2A2) produced a transient increase of the intracellular Ca^{2+} concentration, which appeared with a latency of about 50 msec and rose continuously until the cessation of the pulse. Recovery of the AzIII signal was slow (not shown). Only

FIGURE 1. Simultaneous recording of
membrane potential (upper traces) and of
AzIII absorbance (lower traces) during depolarization of the MoG soma membrane. In
(A), a steady depolarizing current of about
10 nA was applied to the MoG membrane
(resting potential: -65 mV), then three short
depolarizing pulses were given. The arrows
show the change in [Ca^{2+}]$_i$ that they produced. Only the last pulse triggered the SAP
accompanied by a large AzIII transient (arrow 3). In (B) (another preparation, resting
potential: -61 mV), short hyperpolarizing
pulses were given regularly (1/sec) to measure the membrane resistance. The depolarizing current produced a quick drop in input membrane resistance followed by a partial
recovery. In this preparation, the [Ca^{2+}]$_i$ rose
without significant latency; note that fluctuations in the Ca^{2+} signal are correlated with
the repetitive pulses. In this and next figures, an upward deflexion of the AzIII trace corresponds
to an increase in absorbance.

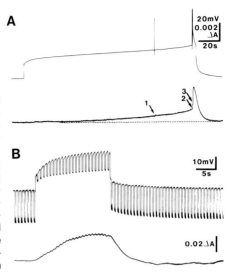

outward current was recorded during the pulse, and it reached its maximum within
5 msec after the onset of the pulse and decreased to a lower level with a half-time
of about 40 msec. Presumably, this decrease was due to an inactivation of the K$^+$
conductance and to an external accumulation of K$^+$ (see Aldrich et al., 1979). If
a predepolarizing pulse was given (Fig. 2A1), the same test pulse gave a 50% larger
Ca^{2+} transient that started without a significant latency and rose more steeply. After
the end of the pulse, the slope of the calcium signal decreased but remained positive.
Again, no net inward current was recorded during the pulse but the peak amplitude
of the outward current was greatly reduced. The current decreased during the pulse
to the same fraction and with the same time course as in Fig. 2A2. Conversely,
the tail current, which was inward, increased in spite of the fact that the membrane
potential was repolarized to -30 mV instead of -70 mV. This behavior may be
related to either a large drift of the equilibrium potential for K$^+$ or to a sustained
Ca^{2+} entry, as suggested by the AzIII trace.

 Ionophoretic injection of tetraethylammonium (TEA) ions into the cell dramatically altered the recordings in a reproducible way (Fig. 2B): (1) the AzIII
responses rose without an appreciable latency even in the absence of a prepulse;
(2) the slope of the AzIII signal decreased progressively during the test pulse; (3)
the prepulse did not increase the amplitude of the Ca^{2+} signal. Instead, a 10%
decrease was observed. In addition, the current was inward during the pulse and
was not appreciably modified by the predepolarization. However, it decreased
almost to zero at the end of the pulse. Returning to the holding potential gave a
tail current that was the same in the two records.

 Figure 3 shows the effects of the test potential on the amplitude of the AzIII
peak change of light absorbance (ΔA). A transient increase in ΔA, and presumably

A1   **B1**

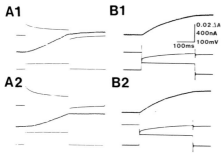

A2   **B2**

FIGURE 2. AzIII response in two different voltage-clamped MoGs (A, B). From the holding potential, a 300-msec depolarizing pulse to 0 mV was applied with (A1, B1) or without a 8-sec predepolarization (A2, B2). (A) Control responses, from top to bottom traces are membrane current, absorbance change, membrane voltage; holding potential, −70 mV; prepulse potential, −30 mV. (B) Responses after intracellular injection of TEA: holding potential, −60 mV; prepulse potential, −40 mV. Note that the positions of the current and of the absorbance traces are reversed.

in intracellular Ca^{2+} concentration, was detected during a 300-msec pulse above −44 mV. This signal increased as the voltage was made more positive and peaked around +10 mV (Fig. 3A). Beyond this value, a slight reduction was observed, but the signal could not be suppressed even if the pulse potential was brought up to +150 mV (not shown), which is likely close to the Ca^{2+} equilibrium potential. When a predepolarization was present (Fig. 3A, solid squares), the Ca^{2+} signal was larger at any one membrane potential between −40 and +40 mV. In this case also a "suppression potential" could not be reached. In a TEA-injected MoG, the effect of a prepulse was no longer seen. The AzIII response decreased to nearly 0 around +130/+140 mV (Fig. 3B).

4. DISCUSSION

It is now well accepted that AzIII accurately monitors the intracellular free Ca^{2+} concentration (see Thomas, 1982). The results presented in Fig. 2A and Fig. 3A suggest that a predepolarization of the MoG soma membrane potentiates the Ca^{2+} entry induced by a test depolarizing pulse. Indeed, facilitation of Ca^{2+} entry by a depolarization has been reported in several preparations (Eckert and Ewald, 1983; Fenwick *et al.*, 1982). However the results obtained here in the presence of intracellular TEA do not disclose any facilitation of Ca^{2+} entry when a prepulse is given: neither the AzIII transient nor the inward current was increased when the prepulse was present; instead a small decrease of the peak AzIII response was observed.

How could TEA have abolished the facilitation of the Ca^{2+} influx induced by the predepolarization? A simple explanation may be that in the absence of TEA, isopotentiality of the membrane was not achieved because of the large K^+ conductance: the reduction of the potassium current by the predepolarization (Figs. 1 and 2) allowed a better control of the membrane potential, which could now be closer to the command potential (i.e., more positive), giving an artifactual increase

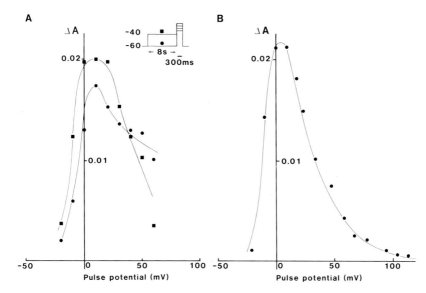

FIGURE 3. Relationship between the membrane potential imposed during the test pulse (abscissae) and the peak light absorbance change (ordinates). The inset shows the parameters of the pulse protocol. Two different preparations: the cell in B was injected with TEA.

in Ca^{2+} entry. On the contrary, in the presence of TEA, the prepulse could no longer reduce the K$^+$ current and therefore had no action.

This interpretation is supported by the observation that TEA, and probably the prepulse as well (see filled squares in Fig. 3A), allow to observe a Ca^{2+} "suppression potential." Figure 3 shows that in the absence of either TEA or prepulse, the Ca^{2+} signal remained almost unchanged above $+40$ mV; this means that when we pulsed the membrane to high positive voltages, the potential sensed by the Ca^{2+} channels did not exceed $+40/+50$ mV, although the space clamp was apparently correct. Indeed, using a third microelectrode inserted in the soma, we checked membrane isopotentiality during a clamp pulse: for any imposed potential, the difference between the two voltage-recording electrodes, which were inserted on opposite sides of the soma, never exceeded 1 mV.

The same events probably occur in current-clamp conditions so that the appearance of the SAP in the MoG somatic membrane results from the reduction of the K$^+$ outward current and not from a voltage of a time-dependent Ca^{2+} facilitation. Presumably, when the K$^+$ conductance is sufficiently reduced, the triggering pulse is able to switch the membrane to a predominantly Ca^{2+} conducting state.

Our results imply also that it is not possible to achieve a satisfactory control of the potential sensed by the membrane channels in this preparation unless the K$^+$ current has been substantially reduced (see Stevens, 1980, for further discussion). This situation may result from the following: (1) the largely infolded somatic membrane of this neuron, as revealed by electron microscopy (J. Cuadras, personal communication), which prevents an effective control of the membrane potential over the whole soma membrane; (2) that the initial part of the axon also escapes from voltage control while substantially contributing to the Ca^{2+} influx. We favor the first hypothesis because the diameter of the initial part of the axon in this preparation is quite small (Mittenthall and Wine, 1978). Furthermore, this part of the cell was certainly left out of the measuring beam. Thus, when interpreting experiments performed on highly convoluted cell membranes it should be taken into account that the test for space clamp by a third microelectrode may not give a reliable indication of the isopotentiality.

5. SUMMARY

In the giant motor neuron of the crayfish, a calcium-dependent slow action potential can be obtained when the cell has been previously submitted to a pre-depolarization. In voltage clamp, a predepolarization "facilitated" the calcium entry measured by AzIII and decreased the outward current due to a test depolarization. After TEA injection into the cell, the "facilitation" of calcium entry was abolished. The relationship between the recorded membrane potential and the AzIII signal studied in different conditions suggest that the "facilitation" of Ca^{2+} entry results from better control of the membrane potential when the K^+ conductance is reduced. It is concluded that (1) the initiation of the SAP is correlated to the reduction of the K^+ conductance and not to a facilitation of a Ca^{2+} conductance *per se*. (2) In normal conditions, the soma membrane infoldings likely escape from voltage control.

ACKNOWLEDGMENTS. We are indebted to Dr. R. T. Kado for critical reading of the first draft of this article. This work was supported in part by grants from Institut National de la Santé et de la Recherche Médicale (INSERM, grants 836004 and 836017).

REFERENCES

Aldrich, R. W., Getting, P. A., and Thompson, S. H., 1979, Inactivation of delayed current in molluscan neurones somata, *J. Physiol. (London)* **291:**507–530.
Czternasty, G. and Bruner, J., 1981, Two types of action potential recorded in giant motoneuron somata of crayfish, *Neurosci. Lett. Suppl.* **7:**379.
Czternasty, G., Kado, R. T., and Bruner, J., 1982a, Voltage-clamp studies of the sodium and calcium inward currents in the giant motoneuron of crayfish, *Neurosci. Lett. Suppl.* **10:**127.
Czternasty, G., Kado, R. T., and Bruner, J., 1982b, Slow action potential in the giant motoneuron of crayfish: conditions for triggering, ionic mechanism and localization, *Soc. Neurosci. Abstr.* **8:**126.
Czternasty, G., Thieffry, M., and Parker, I., 1984, Calcium transient in a crustacean motoneuron soma: Detection with arsenazo III, *Experiencia* **40:**106–108.
Eckert, R. and Ewald, D., 1983, Inactivation of calcium conductance characterized by tail current measurements in neurones of *Aplysia californica, J. Physiol. (London)* **345:**549–565.

Fenwick, E. M., Marty, A., and Neher, E., 1982, Sodium and calcium channels in bovine chromaffin cells, *J. Physiol. (London)* **331**:599–635.

Hagiwara, S. and Byerly, L., 1981, Calcium channels, *Ann. Rev. Neurosci.* **4**:69–125.

Jahnsen, H. and Llinás, R., 1984a, Electrophysiological properties of guinea-pig thalamic neurones: An *in vitro* study, *J. Physiol. (London)* **349**:205–226.

Jahnsen H. and Llinás R., 1984b, Ionic basis for the electroresponsiveness and oscillatory properties of guinea-pig thalamic neurones *in vitro*, *J. Physiol. (London)* **349**:227–247.

Llinás, R. and Jahnsen, H., 1982, Electrophysiology of mammalian thalamic neurons *in vitro*, *Nature (London)* **297**:406–408.

Mittenthall, J. E. and Wine, J. J., 1978, Segmental homology and variation in flexor motoneurones of the crayfish abdomen, *J. Comp. Neurol.* **177**:311–334.

Shimahara, T., Czternasty, G., Stinnakre, J., and Bruner, J., 1983a, Ca spike initiation in the somata of crayfish giant motor neuron: Study with arsenazo III, *Soc. Neurosci. Abstr.* **9**:499.

Shimahara, T., Czternasty, G., Stinnakre, J., and Bruner, J., 1983b, Intracellular calcium spike in the giant motor neurone of crayfish measured by the metallochromic indicator dye arsenazo III, *Neurosci. Lett. Suppl.* **10**:197.

Smith, S. J. and Zucker, R. S., 1980, Aequorin response facilitation and intracellular calcium accumulation in Molluscan neurones, *J. Physiol. (London)* **300**:167–196.

Stevens, C. F., 1980, Ionic channels in neuromembranes; methods for studying their properties, in: *Molluscan nerve cells: From Biophysics to Behavior* (J. Koestler and J. H. Byrne, eds.), Cold Spring Harbor Laboratory, Cold Spring Harbor, New York.

Thomas, M.V., 1982, *Techniques in Calcium Research,* Academic Press, London.

19

Persistent Changes in Excitability and Input Resistance of Cortical Neurons in the Rat

LYNN J. BINDMAN and C. A. PRINCE

1. INTRODUCTION

Changes in the excitability of cortical neurons persisting undiminished for hours can be elicited in anesthetized animals by a number of experimental procedures that alter the firing rate of the cells for a few minutes (e.g., Burns, 1957; Bindman, et al., 1964b; see Chap. 17 in Bindman and Lippold, 1981, for review). Evidence that the long-lasting increases in firing were not dependent on continuous neuronal activity in reverberating circuits was obtained by Gartside (1968a), who showed that the increased excitability in the rat survived the temporary abolition of neuronal firing produced by either whole body cooling or spreading depression.

Although most of the experiments were performed in anesthetized animals, prolonged increases in firing have been obtained in unanesthetized, unrestrained rats following the brief application of extracellular polarizing current or local iontophoretic application of glutamate (McCabe, 1972, 1973). However, it is possible that changes in posture of the animals affected the firing rate of the cells in the sensorimotor cortex whose activity was being monitored.

One study of possible mechanisms involved in the production of persisting increases in excitability of cortical neurons used memory disrupting drugs, which include inhibition of protein synthesis and depression of central levels of amines among their actions (see Day et al., 1977). Neomycin or cycloheximide, when allowed to diffuse directly into the rat cerebral cortex beforehand, prevented the establishment of a long-term increase in firing. The drugs did not themselves alter cortical firing at the doses used, nor did they interfere with the increase of firing elicited during subsequent passage of polarizing current, a stimulus that reliably

LYNN J. BINDMAN and C. A. PRINCE ● Department of Physiology, University College London, London WC1E 6BT, England.

evoked a prolonged increase of firing in the absence of the drug (Gartside, 1968b, 1971, 1975). Similarly, Bindman and Moore (1980) found that the probability of producing long-lasting increases in cortical firing following noxious somatosensory stimuli was greatly reduced by cycloheximide applied to the pial surface 30 min prior to tail stimulation. The cycloheximide affected neither the spontaneous firing nor the responses of the neurons to the somatic stimulation.

The site of the persisting changes in the experiments mentioned above could have been presynaptic, postsynaptic, or both. The involvement of a postsynaptic mechanism was demonstrated by experiments in the cat, using repetitive, antidromic stimulation of pyramidal tract neurons as conditioning stimuli and blocking synaptic transmission throughout the cortex with a locally applied $MgCl_2$ solution. The response to test shocks delivered to the pial surface showed that an increase in excitability of the population of pyramidal tract neurons could be produced by the antidromic stimulation (at 100 Hz for 0.5 sec every sec, over several min) which persisted, undiminished, for hours (Bindman et al., 1976a; 1979).

Prolonged decreases in excitability were also observed following stimulation of the pyramidal tract, but only in experiments where synaptic transmission was not blocked by additional $MgCl_2$. The prolonged decreases were induced most readily by stimulation of the contralateral tract (Bindman et al., 1976b, 1979, 1982).

It was considered unlikely that local changes of blood flow, cortical impedance, or ionic environment could account for the persisting changes in excitability following antidromic stimulation; when consecutive responses to a repeated cortical test shock were recorded from each pyramidal tract, prolonged increases were found only in the ipsilateral pyramidal tract, which was the one subjected to the conditioning stimulation. Other control experiments excluded the axons as the site of the persisting changes (Bindman et al., 1979).

We considered that further investigation of the underlying mechanisms would best be pursued by using intracellular recording and stimulating techniques. Woody and his colleagues demonstrated that the input resistance and the excitability to direct current stimulation of neurons in motor cortex of cats were raised in the population of neurons involved in the production of a particular conditioned movement (Woody and Engel, 1972; Woody and Black-Cleworth, 1973). In view of their results, we decided to follow the time course of changes in excitability and input resistance of cortical neurons after procedures that we expected to elicit long-lasting effects.

Initially we chose to mimic the antidromically evoked discharge of cells by stimulation with intracellular current application. Although Woody et al. (1978) reported that increased activity induced in 15 cells by intracellular current alone did not give rise to a prolonged increase in input resistance, the stimulation they used (10 Hz, 10-msec pulses) probably drove the cells at much lower rates than the stimulation used in the experiments with antidromic firing. Preliminary experiments showed that it was feasible to maintain stable intracellular recordings in cortical cells in the anesthetized rat for periods of time sufficient to examine the after-effects of high frequency firing (Bindman and Prince, 1983). We show here that stimulation of single cells can give rise to alterations in their excitability and input resistance, which persist for minutes or tens of minutes after the end of stimulation.

2. METHODS

2.1. Preparation

Specific pathogen-free (SPF grade IV) male albino rats, and cats were anesthetized with urethane (1.8 g/kg). The skull overlying the sensorimotor cortex was exposed and the bone thinned with a drill so that a piece of <1 mm dia. could be lifted and removed. A slit of about 0.3 mm was made in the dura mater to allow microelectrode insertion; keeping the slit small was an important factor in minimizing arterial and respiratory pulsations. Fine dental needles were inserted under the skin of the contralateral forepaw for electrical stimulation of the afferent nerves (0.05-msec pulse, at voltage just above threshold for muscle twitch).

2.2. Recording

Glass microelectrodes containing a single fiber were filled with 3 M KCl or 4 M KAc; for stable recordings of >10 min we found that electrode resistances had to be in excess of 40 MΩ (KCl) or 65 MΩ (KAc). The mean tip potential of the KCl electrodes was 9.38 ± 1.2 mV (1 S.E.) for a mean electrode resistance of 51.9 ± 2 MΩ, $n = 16$. Ag/AgCl wires were used to connect the microelectrode, and the indifferent (earthed) electrode on the preparation, to the headstage of a Neurolog 102 pre-amplifier; current was injected via a bridge circuit into the microelectrode.

Microelectrodes were advanced using a Clarke microdrive with a 2μm stepping motor. Impalement of cells, lying at depths between 240 and 1900 μm below the pial surface was usually achieved with a brief + 10 to + 30 nA current pulse (Fig. 1, top left).

A four-channel Racal tape recorder was used to store (1) the recorded voltage, (2) applied current, (3) pulses indicating stimuli to contralateral forepaw, and (4) trigger pulses, for later off-line analysis.

2.3. Measurements

Voltages and currents were measured from a storage oscilloscope display (Tektronix 5111) or from photographed records. Voltage and current were also displayed continuously on a pen recorder. The rate of firing of the unit was counted electronically and also displayed on the pen recorder.

Changes in apparent input resistance of a neuron were estimated in three ways:

1. The voltage changes in response to repeated current pulses (<1 nA) were measured 20 to 40 msec after onset (time constant of cells about 5 to 10 msec) and

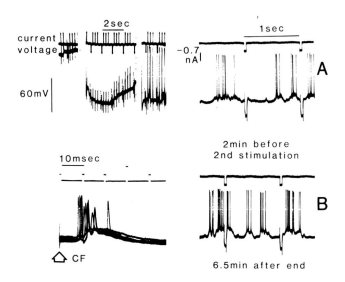

FIGURE 1. Recordings from neuron 1290 μm below pial surface in sensorimotor cortex of rat anesthetized with urethane. Upper traces, current injected into microelectrode; lower traces, voltage recorded from the same electrode. Current and voltage calibrations refer to all four pairs of records; time calibration is shown separately for penetration (top left), short latency response evoked by contralateral forepaw shock at arrow (bottom left), and spontaneous firing (right, top, and bottom) recorded 2 min before (A) and 6.5 min after (B) the second period of stimulation.

the resistance, R_i, was calculated. Samples were only taken if the current pulse fell in a period between bursts of firing, when the membrane potential was stable, i.e., in the absence of obvious synaptic potentials (see Results, Section 3.1). In some experiments, additional anesthetic was administered in order to prolong the interburst intervals. The amplitude of the voltage response to the current pulse was corrected for residual bridge imbalance by subtracting the fast component, (see also Purves, 1981, p. 86). The current pulse was chosen to fall within a linear range of the cell's voltage response to applied current. The mean and S.E. of samples of measurements were calculated, and tests of significance were applied to the measurements obtained before and after high-frequency stimulation by intracellular current.

2. Changes in input resistance were also estimated by measuring the slope when the resting potential was altered by ramp currents, before and after stimulation. Appropriate corrections were made for electrode resistance at the various current levels. The best fit slopes were calculated and 95% confidence limits examined.

3. Changes in amplitude of the action potential during applied depolarizing current were measured, and the slope calculated before and after stimulation (Frank and Fuortes, 1956). The estimates of input resistance obtained by this method were lower than with (1) or (2) but served to confirm the direction of change of apparent cell resistance produced by stimulation.

3. RESULTS

3.1. Background Cortical Activity

The location of neurons within the sensorimotor cortex, identified on anatomical grounds, could be confirmed by a short-latency evoked response to contralateral paw stimulation; it can be seen in Fig. 1 (bottom left) that the cell was driven at about 8-msec latency following shocks to the contralateral forepaw.

Under urethane anesthesia, many neurons in the cerebral cortex fire spontaneously, in bursts separated by silent intervals (Fig. 1A,B). The pattern of firing and the associated potential changes that we recorded intracellularly were very similar, although opposite in polarity, from recordings made extracellularly with NaCl-filled micropipettes (e.g., Bindman *et al.*, 1964a).

The depolarization from the resting potential required to reach the firing threshold of the neurons varied considerably among cells and was between a few millivolts and about 30 millivolts. It was about 14 mV more depolarized than the resting potential in the cell of Fig. 1.

3.1.1. Stability of Firing

It has already been established with extracellular recording techniques in the rat anesthetized with urethane that the mean firing rate of groups of spontaneously active cells is steady over several hours in the absence of extraneous stimuli (Bindman *et al.*, 1964a; Gartside and Lippold, 1967). The cortical neuronal excitability to applied current in the cat anesthetized with urethane was also stable over several hours (Bindman *et al.*, 1979).

Immediately following penetration of cortical neurons, in the absence of clear signs of injury, we found that the firing rate declined and the resting potential became more polarized over the course of several minutes. Some cells continued to fire spontaneously; others only fired when depolarizing current pulses (10 or 20 msec) were applied. Only recordings from cells that remained in a stable state for tens of minutes were used to examine the after-effects of intracellular stimulation.

3.2. After-Effects of High-Frequency Intracellular Stimulation

We report here preliminary results obtained from a sample of ten neurons in which stable recordings were maintained in excess of 30 min. The recordings were obtained from one cat and eight rats. The mean resting potential of the sample was 76.1 mV $\pm$ 2.9 (1 S.E.): mean spike amplitude (threshold to peak) was 72.6 mV $\pm$ 2.9; and the mean input resistance was 20.7 MΩ $\pm$ 3.5.

Prolonged changes in excitability, ranging from a few minutes to tens of minutes after the end of stimulation, were obtained in all the cells as a result of driving them at high rates, i.e., in excess of 20 Hz for a few minutes (usually >40 Hz for 0.5 sec each sec). By excitability we mean one or more of the following: the spontaneous firing rate of the cell, its rate of firing in response to fixed depo-

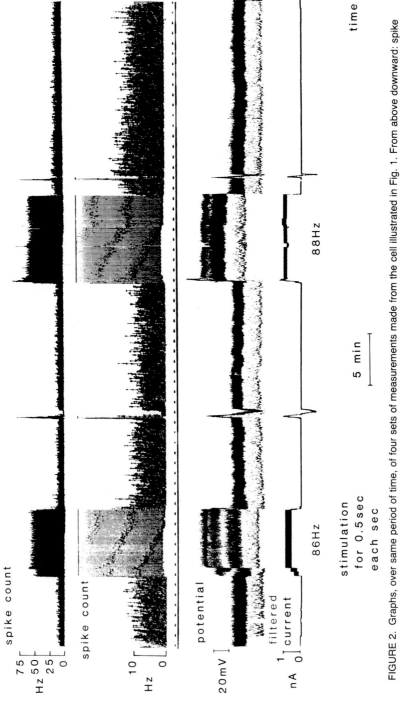

FIGURE 2. Graphs, over same period of time, of four sets of measurements made from the cell illustrated in Fig. 1. From above downward: spike count at low gain; spike count at higher gain; time trace giving 1 min marks; d.c. voltage; current injected across bridge circuit into cell via microelectrode, filtered (RC 0.47 sec). During each stimulation period, a steady depolarizing current was applied with superimposed depolarizing current pulses (10 msec, 86 Hz, first stimulation; or 5 msec, 88Hz, second stimulation; for 0.5 sec in each second). Ramp currents were also applied at 13 min before and 2 min after the second stimulation.

larizing current pulses, and/or the number of action potentials evoked by constant shocks delivered to a contralateral paw. The effects of more than one period of stimulation were observed in some cells, so that in our sample of ten long-term, stable recordings a total of 13 long-lasting changes were produced by 16 periods of stimulation. Eight increases in excitability were observed in seven cells, and five decreases of excitability in four cells; in two of the cells it was possible to induce either a prolonged increase or a decrease by using different stimulation regimes.

3.2.1. Prolonged Increases in Excitability

The eight increases in excitability persisted from 3 min to more than 40 min after the end of stimulation. A mean value was estimated for each increase over its total duration. The mean increase in excitability for the sample of eight increases was 42% of control.

An example is shown in Figs. 1–6. Figure 2 shows the time courses of the following: (from above downwards) the measured spike count at low and high gain; the potential, showing fluctuations between the resting potential (base of dark line) and the peak of slow depolarizing waves; and the filtered, applied intracellular current. In order to drive the cell at a high rate in the stimulation periods a steady depolarizing current and superimposed depolarizing pulses were used. The mean rate of firing of the unit during the first stimulation period was about 58 Hz; only a transient increase (<1 min) was observed after the end of stimulation. Consequently, we used a greater steady depolarizing current in the second stimulation period and drove the unit at a higher mean rate (of about 63 Hz) for a longer time. The firing rate then remained above the control level for about 18 min after the end of the stimulation period.

We cannot tell whether it was the more intense and prolonged firing in the second stimulation period that was important in producing the long-lasting change, or the repetition itself.

In our sample of eight prolonged increases, there was only one that returned to the control level. The others persisted until the stability of recording was lost. Five examples were longer than 10 min, the longest in excess of 40 min.

3.2.2. Increases in Input Resistance

In each of the eight examples of prolonged increases in firing, there was an increase in the input resistance of the cell (mean increase 13%). The degree of association between increased excitability and increased resistance was very highly significant (Bindman and Prince, 1984).

An example of such changes is shown in Figs. 3 and 4. Measurement of the voltage changes in response to repeated 0.7 nA hyperpolarizing current pulses of 40-msec duration (using only pulses arriving during the absence of obvious synaptic potentials) showed that a very highly significant increase in input resistance occurred after the second stimulation period. Figure 3 shows examples of the voltage changes produced by the current pulses.

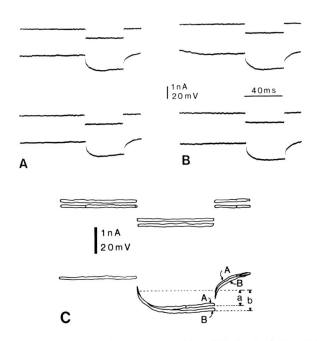

FIGURE 3. Examples of the voltage changes produced by -0.7-nA pulses, 40 msec in duration, used to measure R_i as for the graph in Fig. 4; each record shows current above and voltage below. (A) Two examples obtained prior to second period of stimulation; (B) two obtained after second period of stimulation. The measurements of R_i were obtained at 40 msec after onset of pulse, using a storage oscilloscope at constant intensity. The samples were chosen having eliminated responses occurring during obvious synaptic potentials. (C) Tracings of the lower record in (A) superimposed on the lower record of (B) using a photographic enlarger and arranging the records so that the prepulse voltage levels were identical. The shoulder on the record between the fast component (due to electrode resistance) could be distinguished from the slow component (due to cell resistance), which had a time constant of about 5 msec. Thus the distance betwen the horizontal dotted lines indicates the measured amplitude, a, of the voltage trace from A and of b from the trace in B.

Figure 4 (lowest trace) shows the time course of change in calculated resistance, R_i, throughout the recording. (Note that the pulses on the voltage record of this graph do not give a good indication of cell resistance because the variable electrode component cannot be seen.) Pooling the data from 60 measurements made prior to the second stimulation, a mean of 16.0 MΩ $\pm$ 0.17 S.E. was calculated. By comparison, for the 60 measurements after the second stimulation (i.e., from 1 to 18 min after the end of stimulation) the mean was 18.4 MΩ $\pm$ 0.21 S.E.; using an unpaired t test, the difference was significant at $p < 0.001$ level.

The slopes of the resting potential change produced by ramp currents (-0.9 to $+1.0$ nA) were compared 13 min before and 2 min after the second stimulation period (Figs. 5 and 6 respectively). The calculated best fit for the slopes obtained before the second stimulation period was 13.1 MΩ for hyperpolarizing current and

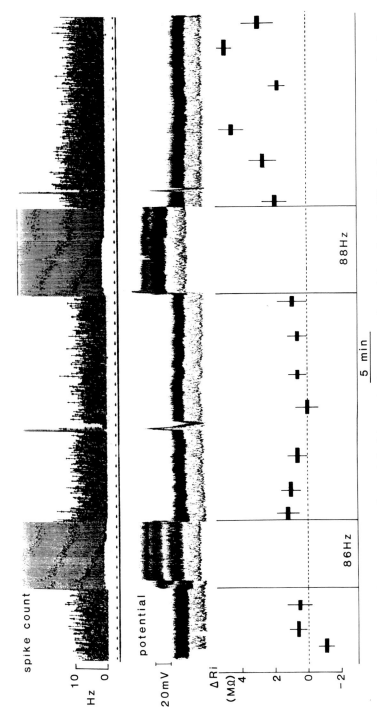

FIGURE 4. Graphs, each over the same time period, of three sets of measurements made from the cell of Fig. 1. From above downward: spike count at high gain, voltage; both as in Fig. 2; changes in resistance, R_i, each horizontal bar giving the mean of 10 measurements and the duration over which the sample was taken. Verical lines above and below each horizontal bar give ±1 S.E. For details of R_i measurements, see legend of Fig. 3. The dotted horizontal line is the mean of the resistance measurements in the period before the first stimulation.

16.4 MΩ for depolarizing current, with $r^2 = 0.99$ in each case. The slope resistances increased after the second stimulation: with hyperpolarizing current, by about 2 MΩ, to 14.8 MΩ, a value in agreement with the change observed around this period of time using the negative current pulses. In the depolarizing range there was a greater increase in slope resistance, of about 7 MΩ to 23.8 MΩ. r^2 was 0.985 in each case. There was no overlap of the 95% confidence limits of the slopes of Fig. 5 with the 95% confidence limits of the slopes of Fig. 6 when current levels were greater than $+0.3$ nA for depolarizing current and -0.6 nA for hyperpolarizing current.

The amplitudes of the spontaneous action potentials during the application of the depolarizing currents were also measured (Frank and Fuortes, 1956) and the slopes compared before and after the second stimulation period. An increase in input resistance was confirmed by these measurements.

3.2.3. Changes in Resting Potential Associated with Increased Excitability

The observed increases in input resistance can be assumed to be due to a change in membrane conductance of the cells. We hoped that our recordings of the resting potentials would provide a clue to the ionic conductance concerned; for example, a decreased gK would be expected to be accompanied by a depolarization of the membrane. However, no consistent change in resting potential was found. Accompanying the eight prolonged increases in excitability, there were four cases

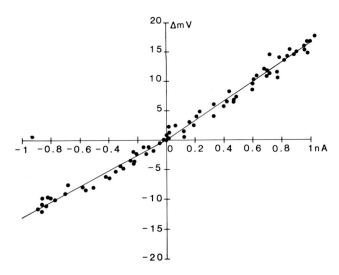

FIGURE 5. Current–voltage plot of measurements taken during application of ramp depolarizing current 13 min prior to the second stimulation period. The resting potential change was calculated from the measured voltage change by correcting for the voltage drop across the uncompensated electrode resistance, at the various current levels. The slopes are calculated and the values and coefficients of determination are given in the text.

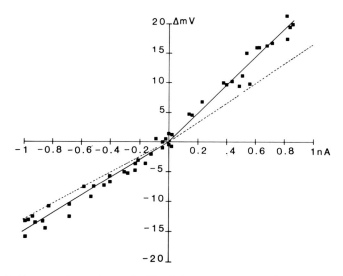

FIGURE 6. Current–voltage plot, as for Fig. 5, for ramp current applied 2 min after end of second stimulation period. Calculated values in text. The slopes of Fig. 5 are shown by the dotted lines.

of depolarization (1–7 mV), two cases with no change in potential, and two cases in which the resting potential showed a hyperpolarization.

In the cell illustrated in Fig. 2, there was a small but significant hyperpolarization. Comparing 12 min prior to the second stimulation with 12 min after it and sampling the resting potential three times a minute, the mean change was a hyperpolarization of 1.6 mV ($p < 0.001$). The hyperpolarization was maintained at the same level over the following 6 min. It can be seen from the slope resistance of this cell, shown in Fig. 5, that this hyperpolarization was within a linear portion of the cell's current/voltage relation, and therefore the potential change is not likely to be responsible for the increase in input resistance.

It is unlikely that this sustained hyperpolarization is brought about by an electrogenic pump. In many of the cells, immediately after a period of stimulation during which the cell fired at a high rate, there was a brief period of inhibition of firing, with a hyperpolarization of the resting potential. The firing rate and the potential recovered in a roughly exponential fashion over the next minute or two. It is possible that these brief posttetanic hyperpolarizations were due to electrogenic pump activity. No such change was observed in the cell illustrated here.

We do not know for certain why the resting potential did not show consistent changes associated with the 8 increases in excitability and input resistance. However we suspect the hyperpolarization in the experiment of Figure 2 is a consequence of a fall in the electrode resistance, possibly causing an increased flow of KCl into the cell from the electrode. Not surprisingly, the increases in excitability were greater in cells where a depolarization occurred together with the increase in input resistance.

3.2.4. Prolonged Decreases in Excitability

Five decreases lasting from 3 min to >10 min were found, with a mean decrease of excitability in the sample of 40%. Some decreases returned to the control level; others persisted until the recording was lost or another experimental procedure carried out.

3.2.5. Decreased Input Resistance

A decrease in input resistance was found to be associated with each example of decreased excitability. However, in one cell, the decrease in input resistance returned to the control level while the decrease in firing rate persisted, suggesting that an effect may have been produced at a cell remote from the one in which the recording was being made.

3.2.6. Changes in Resting Potential Associated with Decreased Excitability

A decreased excitability was always accompanied by membrane hyperpolarization (mean in the sample of five prolonged decreases $=3$ mV).

4. DISCUSSION

We have found that prolonged increases in the excitability of single neurons in the sensorimotor cortex of the anesthetized rat are associated with long-lasting increases in input resistance, and decreases in excitability of the neurons are accompanied by decreases in input resistance. The distribution of the changes in excitability against changes in resistance showed a very highly significant association (Bindman and Prince, 1984).

Prolonged increases in excitability accompanied by prolonged increases in input resistance have been reported previously, following the iontophoretic application of acetylcholine extracellularly, or of cGMP intracellularly to cortical neurons in awake cats (Woody *et al.,* 1978). Woody and Black-Cleworth (1973) have also reported a change in the excitability and input resistance of cells in the particular population of neurons in the motor cortex of the cat that are involved in producing a classically conditioned movement of facial muscles. Excitability and resistance of neurons before and after the conditioning procedure were sampled. In our experiments we have been able to follow continuously the excitability and resistance changes in single neurons, following high-frequency firing induced by intracellularly applied currents.

From the preliminary experiments reported in this chapter, we have no evidence to suggest whether the production and/or the maintenance of changes in input resistance and excitability require an alteration in synaptic transmission, or are independent of synaptic activity. If altered synaptic input is responsible for the prolonged changes, then the increases in excitability and resistance could be produced by disinhibition. Alternatively, they could be produced by release of excitatory transmitter: possible candidates that have been shown to increase excitability and apparent input resistance are ACh in neocortex (Krnjevic et al., 1971; Woody et al., 1978) and amino acids in hippocampus (Dingledene, 1983). The prolonged decreases in excitability and resistance could be produced by an increase in recurrent inhibitory synaptic inputs, possibly involving GABA (Krnjevic and Schwartz, 1967).

However, increases of resistance and excitability of cellular origin have also been described (e.g., Alkon, 1982). A postsynaptic mechanism has been implicated in experiments in which synaptic transmission was blocked, where long-lasting increases in excitability were produced in cortical neurons of the cat (Bindman et al., 1979). We have yet to carry out the experiments with stable intracellular recording and stimulation, in the presence of sufficient additional extracellular Mg^{2+} ions to block all synaptic inputs to the cells.

Since we found an increase in neuronal input resistance, it is not likely that the increased excitability produced by the high firing rates of the neurons was caused by an accumulation of K^+ extracellularly. A fall in input resistance was found when extracellular $[K^+]$ was raised in hippocampal slices (Halliwell and Adams, 1982; Dingledine, 1983) and in cortical neurons in tissue culture (Dichter, 1983).

We do not know why an induced increase in firing rate produces opposite after-effects on different occasions. We have observed both directions of change in the same cell following different rates and durations of stimulation. In the previous observations on pyramidal tract cells both directions of change of excitability were observed following stimulation of the pyramidal tract: prolonged decreases were found when synaptic inputs alone were activated, while prolonged increases were produced following antidromic activation when synaptic transmission was blocked. The pyramidal tract stimulation could give rise to either increases or decreases of excitability when antidromic plus synaptic inputs were activated (Bindman et al., 1982). It was inferred that prolonged increases were cellular in origin while the prolonged decreases were due to persistent activity in inhibitory synaptic inputs onto the cells. A similar explanation might be applicable to our results. Alternatively, different networks could be activated by the different rates and durations of stimulation.

5. SUMMARY

We have used intracellular recording and stimulating techniques, in rats or cats anesthetized with urethane, to examine the effects of electrical stimulation of single neurons in the sensorimotor cortex. When the firing rate of a cell was increased by depolarizing current to rates in excess of 35 Hz for a few minutes, prolonged changes of excitability were found in the stimulated cell; the after-effects were from a few minutes to tens of minutes in duration. In some cells, more than one period of stimulation was required to produce a prolonged change in excitability. In a sample of ten neurons in which stable recordings were maintained for more than 30 min, 16 stimulation periods gave rise to eight prolonged (>3 min) increases, and five prolonged decreases in excitability.

In each of the examples of prolonged increases in excitability, there was an associated increase in the input resistance of the cell. Decreased excitability was associated with a decreased input resistance.

The change in input resistance may reflect a cellular mechanism underlying the prolonged changes in excitability. Alternatively, synaptic mechanisms may be involved, for example, disinhibition in the case of prolonged increases in excitability and recurrent inhibition for prolonged decreases in excitability.

ACKNOWLEDGMENTS. C.A. Prince is an MRC scholar. We thank M. Duchen for helpful comments on the manuscript. Work supported by MRC project grant to LJB.

REFERENCES

Alkon, D. L., 1982, A biophysical basis for molluscan associative learning, in: *Conditioning* (C. D. Woody, ed.), Plenum Press, New York, pp. 147–170.

Bindman, L. and Lippold, O., 1981, *The Neurophysiology of the Cerebral Cortex*, Ed. Arnold, London; Texas University Press, Austin.

Bindman, L. J. and Moore, R. B., 1980, The effect of cycloheximide on the production of prolonged increases in firing rate of cortical neurones by somatic stimulation in the anaesthetized rat, *J. Physiol. (London)* **305**:34–35P.

Bindman, L. J. and Prince, C. A., 1983, Intracellular recording from neurones in the cerebral cortex of the anaesthetized rat, *J. Physiol. (London)* **341**:7–8P.

Bindman, L. J. and Prince, C. A., 1984, Intracellular current stimulation produces changes in excitability and input resistance of cortical neurones in the anaesthesized rat, *J. Physiol. (London)* **357**:35P.

Bindman, L.J., Lippold, O. C. J., and Redfearn, J. W. T., 1964a, Relation between the size and form of potentials evoked by sensory stimulation and the background electrical activity in the cerebral cortex of the rat, *J. Physiol. (London)* **171**:1–25.

Bindman, L.J. Lippold, O. C. J., and Redfearn, J. W. T., 1964b, The action of brief polarizing currents on the cerebral cortex of the rat, (1) during current flow and (2) in the production of long-lasting after-effects, *J. Physiol. (London)* **172**:369–382.

Bindman, L. J., Lippold, O. C. J., and Milne, A.R., 1976a, Long-lasting changes of postsynaptic origin in the excitability of pyramidal tract neurones, *J. Physiol. (London)* **258**:71–72P.

Bindman, L. J., Lippold, O. C. J., and Milne, A. R., 1976b, Prolonged decreases in excitability of pyramidal tract neurones, *J. Physiol. (London)* **263**:141–142P.

Bindman, L. J. Lippold, O. C. J., Milne, A. R., 1979, Prolonged changes in excitability of pyramidal tract neurones in the cat, *J. Physiol. (London)* **286**:457–477.

Bindman, L. J., Lippold, O. C. J., and Milne, A.R., 1982, A postsynaptic mechanism underlying long-lasting changes in the excitability of pyramidal tract neurones in the anaesthetized rat, in: *Conditioning* (C. D. Woody, ed.), Plenum Press, New York, pp. 171–178.

Burns, B. D., 1957, Electrophysiologic basis of normal and psychotic function, in: *Psychotropic Drugs* (S. Garattini and V. Ghetti, eds.), Elsevier, Amsterdam.

Day, T. A., Overstreet, D. H. and Schiller, G. D., 1977, Centrally administered cycloheximide in rats: Behavioural concomitants and modulation of amnesic effects by biogenic amines, *Pharmacol. Biochem. Behav.* **6**:557–565.

Dichter, M. A., 1983, Cerebral cortex tissue culture, in: *Current Methods in Cellular Neurobiology.* IV. (J. L. Barker and J. F. McKelvy, eds.) John Wiley and Sons, New York, pp. 81–106.

Dingledine, R., 1983, N-Methyl aspartate activates voltage-dependent calcium conductance in rat hippocampal pyramidal cells, *J. Physiol.* **343**:385–405.

Frank, K. and Fuortes, M. G. F., 1956, Stimulation of spinal motoneurones with intracellular electrodes, *J. Physiol. (London)* **134**:451–470.

Gartside, I. B., 1968a, Mechanisms of sustained increases of firing rate of neurones in the rat cerebral cortex after polarization: Reverberating circuits or modification of synaptic conductance? *Nature* **220**:382–383.

Gartside, I. B., 1968b, Mechanisms of sustained increases of firing rate of neurones in the rat cerebral cortex after polarization: Role of protein synthesis, *Nature,* **220**:383–384.

Gartside, I. B., 1971, Is the inhibition by cycloheximide of induced long-term changes in cortical activity due to inhibition of protein synthesis? *Nature* **232**:47–48.

Gartside, I. B., 1975, Long-term increases in cortical neuronal activity and protein synthesis, *J. Physiol. (London)* **246**:94P.

Gartside, I. B. and Lippold, O. C. J., 1967, The production of persistent changes in the level of neuronal activity by brief cooling of the cerebral cortex of the rat, *J. Physiol. (London)* **189**:475–487.

Halliwell, J. V. and Adams, P. R., 1982, Voltage-clamp analysis of muscarinic excitation in hippocampal neurons, *Brain Res.* **250**:71–92.

Krnjevic, K. and Schwartz, S., 1967, The action of γ-aminobutyric acid on cortical neurones. *Exp. Brain Res.* **3**:320–336.

Krnjevic, K., Pumain, R., and Renaud, L., 1971, The mechanism of excitation by acetylcholine in the cerebral cortex, *J. Physiol. (London)* **215**:247–268.

McCabe, B. J., 1972, Iontophoresis and persisting changes in neuronal firing rate in the cerebral cortex of the unrestrained rat, *J. Physiol. (London)* **224**:6–7P.

McCabe, B. J., 1973, Production of prolonged changes in cortical neuronal activity by iontophoresis of L-glutamate in anaesthetized and unanaesthetized rats, Ph.D. Thesis, University of London.

Purves, R. D., 1981, *Microelectrode Methods for Intracellular Recording and Iontophoresis,* Academic Press, London.

Woody, C. D. and Black-Cleworth, P., 1973, Differences in excitability of cortical neurons as a function of motor projection in conditioned cats, *J. Neurophysiol.* **36**:1104–1116.

Woody, C. D. and Engel, J. Jr., 1972, Changes in unit activity and thresholds to electrical microstimulation at coronal pericruciate cortex of cat with classical conditioning of different facial movements, *J. Neurophysiol.* **35**:230–241.

Woody, C. D., Swartz, B. E., and Gruen, E., 1978, Effects of acetylcholine and cyclic GMP on input resistance of cortical neurons in awake cats, *Brain Res.* **158**:373–395.

20

A Critique of Modeling Population Responses for Mammalian Central Neurons

WAYNE E. CRILL

We must still be extremely cautious in accepting the conclusions reached by modeling the responses of neurons in the central mammalian nervous system. Although we know a great deal about the properties of mammalian central neurons, very little quantitative information is available. For example, although the passive membrane properties of motoneurons have been analyzed in great detail (Rall, 1977), there are now new experiments suggesting that the estimates of membrane resistivity made a decade ago (Barrett and Crill, 1974) may be too low. Experimental results from Robert Burke's laboratory are best explained by nonuniform passive properties over the soma and dendritic tree (Fleshman et al., 1982; Rall, 1982). The point is that we do not even have reliable quantitative values for these relatively simple linear properties of central neurons.

One of the most exciting areas of recent research with regard to the behavior of mammalian central neurons is the investigation of active membrane properties. It is clear that the spike-generating mechanism is similar in all mammalian central neurons examined so far. The all-or-nothing response is caused by the regenerative relationship between the voltage-dependent increase in sodium conductance and membrane potential (Hodgkin and Huxley, 1952). Action potential repolarization occurs because the depolarization also activates potassium conductance mechanisms and because the increase in sodium conductance also shows voltage-dependent inactivation (Hodgkin and Huxley, 1952). These conductance systems have been measured quantitatively in cat spinal motoneurons (Barrett and Crill, 1980). The quantitative detail even in this preparation is potentially erroneous because of the problems of space-clamping a neuron with complex geometry. For the Hodgkin-Huxley-like reconstruction (Hodgkin and Huxley, 1952) to give a response similar

WAYNE E. CRILL • Department of Physiology and Biophysics, University of Washington, Seattle, Washington 98195.

to that measured experimentally the detailed impulse response of the neuron had to be measured (Barrett *et al.*, 1980). The response properties of the model are extremely sensitive to the experimentally measured characteristics of the involved active and passive ionic conductance systems (Schwindt, unpublished results).

Modeling central neuron responses is further complicated by presence of conductance systems in the subthreshold voltage range in addition to those responsible for spike generation. In motoneurons and other central neurons examined, outward potassium currents with relatively slow kinetic properties have been measured when the neuron is depolarized only a few millivolts above resting potential (Barrett *et al.*, 1980; Schwindt and Crill, 1981, 1982). Motoneurons also have a noninactivating inward current activated in the subthreshold voltage range. This current is probably carried primarily by calcium ions (Schwindt and Crill, 1980). Simulating synaptic currents with the tonic application of intracellular current to spinal motoneurons reveals a progressive increase in firing level caused by accommodation of the initial segment region (Schwindt and Crill, 1982). This increase in spike threshold allows summation of synaptic currents over a relatively large range of membrane potential and also insures the tonic activation of the conductance systems that are activated in the subthreshold region. Because the persistent inward current causes the slope conductance to decrease in the subthreshold region, the effectiveness of synaptic input changes at different membrane potentials.

The response properties, that is, the transduction of synaptic current into spike trains for transmission down the axon will depend upon the magnitude and dynamic properties of the subthreshold currents. For example, spinal motoneurons characteristically fire at relatively slow rates. This is caused by the activation and dominance of the slow potassium conductance system activated in the subthreshold region (Schwindt and Crill, 1982). Betz cells of the cat neocortex fire with a frequency–current relationship that has a slope 10–20 times greater than motoneurons. This markedly different response property compared to spinal motoneurons is caused by the presence of a relatively much larger persistent inward current activated in the subthreshold region. In Betz cells the subthreshold inward current is tetrodotoxin sensitive and therefore carried by sodium ions (Stafstrom *et al.*, 1982). The persistent subthreshold current in Betz cells is activated within 2–4 msec and can amplify the cells response even to single excitatory postsynaptic potentials near threshold. Electroresponses have also been measured in guinea pig neocortex (Connors *et al.*, 1982) and Purkinje cells (Llinas and Sugamori, 1980) that probably reflect similar conductance mechanisms. R.K.S. Wong has, (unpublished) shown voltage clamp records from isolated hippocampal pyramidal neurons demonstrating that they also have a subthreshold persistent sodium conductance system.

An additional complication in understanding neuronal responses is the recent description of neurotransmitter effects upon voltage-dependent conductance systems. Adams and his colleagues have shown that muscarinic agonists block a voltage dependent potassium conductance, I_M, (Brown, 1983; Brown and Adams, 1980; Halliwell and Adams, 1982). This will markedly alter the response properties of the neuron to excitatory synaptic input (Brown, 1983). It has been shown that activation of receptors for excitatory amino acids activates a highly voltage-dependent current carried by sodium and calcium ions (Dingledine, 1983; Flatman *et al.*, 1983; MacDonald *et al.*, 1982).

Our understanding of the quantitative aspects of synaptic transmission in the mammalian central nervous system is also far from complete. The effectiveness of synaptic inputs depends upon the type, number, and location of synaptic inputs. Moreover the response to many inputs is not stationary because of temporal factors controlling the release of transmitter and the summation of transmitter effects (Curtis and Eccles, 1960).

It is this lack of quantitative detail about both the membrane and synaptic properties that makes the interpretation of model responses for either single cells or groups of neurons in the mammalian central nervous system so difficult. Traub and Wong (1983) recognize these major limitations. The Traub–Wong model does show that, given the rigid constraints of their system, a decrease in inhibition can produce behavior similar to that observed experimentally. Whether or not the behavior in the experimental preparation can be explained by similar mechanisms remains to be determined. It is an exciting time in neurobiology. The properties of circuits and neuronal elements are much more complex than we had imagined. Nevertheless, techniques are rapidly being developed that will allow us to answer many questions about the cellular properties of neurons.

ACKNOWLEDGMENT. Supported by NIH Grant NS 16792.

REFERENCES

Barrett, E. F., Barrett, J. N., and Crill W. E., 1980, Voltage-sensitive outward currents in cat motoneurones, *J. Physiol. (London)* **304**:251–276.

Barrett, J. N. and Crill, W. E., 1974, Specific membrane properties of cat motoneurons, *J. Physiol. (London)* **239**:301–324.

Barrett, J. N. and Crill, W. E., 1980, Voltage clamp of cat motoneurone somata: properties of a fast inward current, *J. Physiol. (London)* **304**:231–249.

Brown, D. A., 1983, Slow cholinergic excitation—a mechanism for increasing neuronal excitability, *Trends Neurosci* **6**:302–306.

Brown, D. A. and Adams, P. R., 1980, Muscarinic suppression of a novel voltage-sensitive K^+ current in a vertebrate neurone, *Nature (London)* **283**:673–676.

Brown, D. A. and Griffith, W. H., 1983, Persistent slow inward calcium current in voltage-clamped hippocampal neurones of guinea-pig, *J. Physiol. (London)* **337**:303–320.

Conners, B. W., Gutnick, M. J., and Prince, D. A., 1982, Electrophysiological properties of neocortical neurons in vitro, *J. Neurophysiol.* **4**:81302–1320.

Crill, W. E. and Schwindt, P. C., 1983, Active currents in mammalian central neurons, *Trends Neurosci.* **6**:236–240.

Curtis, D. R. and Eccles, J. C., 1960, Synaptic action during and after repetitive stimulation, *J. Physiol. (London)* **150**:374–398.

Dingledine, R., 1983, N-methyl aspartate activates voltage-dependent calcium conductance in rat hippocampal pyramidal cells, *J. Physiol. (London)* **343**:385–405.

Flatman, J., Schwindt, P. C., Crill, W. E., and Stafstrom, C. E., 1983, Multiple actions of N-methyl-D-aspartate on cat neocortical neurons in vitro, *Brain Res.* **266**:169–173.

Fleshman, J. W., Burke, R. E., Glenn, L. L., Lev Tov, A., and Miller J. P., 1982, Cell size and specific membrane resistivity of type-identified cat motoneurons: morphological, physiological and modeling studies, *Abstr. Soc. Neurosci.* **8**:414.

Halliwell, J. V. and Adams, P. R., 1982, Voltage-clamp analysis of muscarinic excitation in hippocampal neurons, *Brain Res.* **250**:71–92.

Hodgkin, A. L. and Huxley, A. F., 1952, Currents carried by sodium and potassium ions through the membrane of giant axon of Loligo, *J. Physiol. (London)* **116**:449–472.

Johnston, D., Hablitz, J. J., and Wilson, W. A., 1980, Voltage clamp discloses slow inward current in hippocampal burst-firing neurons, *Nature (London)* **286**:391–393.

Llinas, R. and Sugamori, M., 1980, Electrophysiologic properties of in vitro purkinje cell somata in mammalian cerebellar slices, *J. Physiol. (London)* **305**:171–195.

MacDonald, J. F., Porietis, A. V., and Wojtowicz, J. M., 1982, Aspartic acid induces a region of negative slope conductance in the current-voltage relationship of cultured spinal cord neurons, *Brain Res.* **237**:248–253.

Rall, W., 1977, Core conductor theory and cable properties of neurons, in: *Handbook of Physiology,* Volume 1 (E. Kandel, ed.), American Physiological Society, Bethesda, pp. 39–98.

Rall, W., 1982, Theoretical models which increase Rm with dendritic distance help fit lower value of Cm, *Abstr. Soc. Neurosci.* **8**:414.

Schwindt, P. C. and Crill, W. E., 1980, Properties of a persistent inward current normal and TEA-injected motoneurons, *J. Neurophysiol.* **43**:1700–1724.

Schwindt, P. C. and Crill, W. E., 1981, Differential effects of TEA and cations on the outward ionic currents of cat motoneurons, *J. Neurophysiol.* **46**:1–16.

Schwindt, P. C. and Crill, W. E., 1982, Factors influencing motoneuron rhythmic firing: results from a voltage clamp study, *J. Neurophysiol.* **48**:875–890.

Stafstrom, C. E., Schwindt, P. C., and Crill, W. E., 1982, Negative slope conductance due to a persistent subthreshold sodium current in cat neocortical neurons in vitro, *Brain Res.* **236**:221–226.

Traub, R. D. and Wong, R. K. S., 1983, Synchronized burst discharge in disinhibited hippocampus slice. II. Model of cellular behavior, *J. Neurophysiol.* **49**:459–471.

21

Hippocampal Pyramidal Cells: Ionic Conductance and Synaptic Interactions

R. K. S. WONG, R. E. NUMANN, R. MILES, and R. D. TRAUB

1. INTRODUCTION

The burst firing pattern of the hippocampal pyramidal cells was first described by Kandel and Spencer in their intracellular studies using the *in vivo* cat preparation (Kandel and Spencer, 1961). Subsequently, the ionic basis for action potential generation in the hippocampal pyramidal cells has been extensively studied in the hippocampal slice. Data derived from the *in vitro* preparation also demonstrated that the bursting pattern provided a basis for the generation of synchronized population oscillation in the hippocampus. In this chapter we describe the membrane conductance system of the pyramidal cells that allows burst generation. In addition, we summarize the way synaptic interaction can occur between these bursting cells to bring about population synchrony.

2. FIRING PATTERN OF THE HIPPOCAMPAL PYRAMIDAL CELLS

Bursts recorded from the pyramidal cells consist of a train of 2–6 action potentials riding on a depolarizing envelope (Wong and Prince, 1978). The event usually lasts about 30 msec. Often intracellular records show spontaneous rhythmic

R. K. S. WONG, R. E. NUMANN, and R. MILES ● Department of Physiology and Biophysics, University of Texas Medical Branch, Galveston, Texas 77550.   R. D. TRAUB ● IBM T. J. Watson Research Center, Yorktown Heights, New York 10598, and Neurological Institute, New York, New York 10032.

bursting occurring at frequencies of 0.2–5 Hz. The interburst interval is determined by the development and decay of postburst membrane hyperpolarizations.

The voltage-dependent inward currents sustaining action potential in these cells can be differentiated into two types: a tetrodotoxin (TTX)-sensitive component that is carried by Na^+ and a calcium component that is insensitive to TTX but is suppressed by Co^{2+} or Mn^{2+} (Schwarzkrion and Slawsky, 1977; Wong and Prince, 1978). Experiments in the slice preparation also show that one component of the outward currents elicited during a burst is activated by increases in intracellular calcium and is mediated by K^+ (Hotson and Prince, 1980; Alger and Nicoll, 1980). This calcium-activated K^+ conductance decays slowly and appears to be the primary component underlying the postburst hyperpolarization. These data from the slice suggest the following scheme for burst generation: membrane depolarizations above threshold elicit the upstroke of the action potential primarily caused by an influx of Na^+; this depolarization activates the calcium conductance, which deactivates slowly to sustain a secondary depolarization following the action potential (the depolarizing after potential; DAP). The amplitude of the DAP reaches threshold in these bursting cells and in such a way a sequence of action potentials is generated. The concentration of intracellular calcium gradually elevates during burst firing and in turn produces an accumulative activation of K^+ conductance. The amplitude of the K^+ conductance finally becomes sufficient to terminate the burst and sustain a slowly decaying afterhyperpolarization.

Intradendritic recordings from the hippocampal pyramidal cells show that the dendrites of these cells can function as independent sites of burst generation (Wong *et al.*, 1979). The distribution of active membrane sites in the soma-dendritic complex is particularly interesting for pyramidal cells in the CA1 region. Here intrasomatic recordings often reveal solitary spiking activity. Intracellular recordings

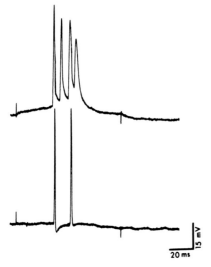

FIGURE 1. Differential firing patterns recorded intracellularly from the dendrite (top trace) and soma (lower trace) of hippocampal CA1 pyramidal cell. The recorded elements were electronically coupled, raising the possibility that they are obtained from the same neuron. Depolarizing current was injected into the dendritic recording site.

15 mV

20 ms

from the distal dendrites however show that the predominant pattern of activity is burst firing. Figure 1 shows intracellular records obtained form the soma and dendritic sites in the CA1 region. Membrane hyperpolarization of one of the sites produced an electrotonically induced hyperpolarization of the other raising the possibility that the recordings were obtained from the dendrite and soma of a single neuron. It was observed that depolarization of the dendrites produced burst firing and such activity induced solitary action potentials recorded in the soma. Depolarization of the soma on the other hand elicited repetitive firing of solitary action potentials and did not trigger bursts in the dendrites. These results suggest that the communication between the dendrites and soma is facilitated by the bursting capacity of the dendrites. This fact takes on special significance when one considers that powerful excitatory input impinges onto the pyramidal cells in the distal portion of the apical dendrites. If dendritic bursts are triggered by these inputs, a significant amplification of the afferent signals will occur in the postsynaptic cell. Burst firing can be envisaged as a device for securing the transmission of signals from cell to cell within a synaptically connected network.

3. IONIC CONDUCTANCE OF THE HIPPOCAMPAL CELLS

The ionic conductance of the pyramidal cell has been further examined by a voltage-clamp approach using the slice preparation. These studies confirmed the presence of an inward Ca^{2+} current (Johnston et al., 1980; Brown and Griffith, 1983b) and the Ca^{2+}-mediated K^+ currents in the pyramidal cells (Brown and Griffith, 1983a), and they provided additional information on the kinetic and pharmacological characteristics of these currents. We have now developed an acutely isolated cell preparation for studies on the ionic conductances of hippocampal neurons (see Numann and Wong, 1984, for details). Slices of the hippocampus are treated with a proteolytic enzyme (papain) followed by mechanical dispersion. Single neurons prepared in this way can be studied immediately by electrophysiological approaches. We have applied voltage-clamp analysis by means of a single, low-resistance, suction electrode. The results reveal the presence of at least three kinetically or pharmacologically distinct inward currents and three outward currents.

Upon a 10- to 20-mV depolarization from a holding potential of -50 to -70 mV, a fast activating and inactivating inward current of large amplitude (up to 2 nA) is elicited. The time course of the current lasts for about 10 msec. When TTX is added to the perfusing solution, this current is blocked indicating that Na^+ is the charge carrier.

To further examine the properties of the inward currents, Cs^+-containing electrodes were used in order to suppress outward currents activated by depolarization. Figure 2 shows the inward current activated by a depolarizing step of 35 mV from a holding potential of -35 mV. The fast Na^+ current described above is inactivated at this voltage, and the remaining inward current is distinct in having a very slow inactivation time course. Addition of TTX under this condition show that part of the inward current is suppressed leaving a component that is insensitive

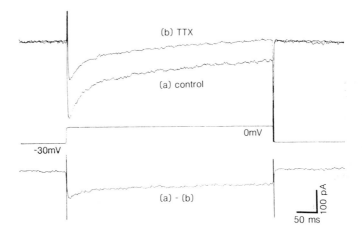

FIGURE 2. (a) shows the slowly inactivating current recorded from an isolated pyramidal cell bathed in normal solution and the shifted response after addition of TTX. Holding potential was at -35 mV. The cell was depolarized to 0 mV. (b) shows the difference in current amplitude recorded in the normal and TTX conditions and represents the amplitude and time course of inward current carried by Na$^+$ through TTX-sensitive channels.

to the toxin. This TTX-insensitive component is probably carried by Ca^{2+} since it can be blocked by Co^{2+} or Mn^{2+}.

The outward currents consist of the following (Fig. 3): (1) A transient outward current is activated upon depolarization from holding potentials of -40 to -100 mV. The current activates within 10 msec and inactivates more slowly, with a half-decay time of about 25 msec. (2) A later outward current is evoked by prolonged depolarization and is generally sustained during pulses of 500 msec or more. The rate of activation of the late component increases with increasing depolarization. This tends to obscure the transient outward current for large depolarizations. This later outward current is sensitive to Mn^{2+} and is probably activated by intracellular Ca^{2+}. (3) In the presence of Mn^{++} the cells generate outward currents upon depolarization from holding potentials of -30 mV or above. The transient outward current is inactivated at these holding potentials. The rate of activation of this remaining outward current increases with large depolarization steps. In addition, this current shows a decline when the depolarization is sustained for more than 500 msec. The rate of inactivation also increases with increased depolarizations. A transient outward current has also been described in studies using the slice preparation (Gustafsson *et al.*, 1982). Two time constants of inactivation has been described. Our data show that the inactivating outward currents can be separated into two types with distinctly different kinetic properties. A detailed description of these outward currents seems to be important since there are now evidence suggesting that the kinetic properties of the outward currents can be modified by a variety of neurotransmitters (Halliwell and Adams, 1982; Cole and Nicoll, 1983; Madison and Nicoll, 1982).

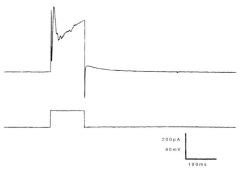

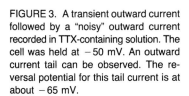

FIGURE 3. A transient outward current followed by a "noisy" outward current recorded in TTX-containing solution. The cell was held at −50 mV. An outward current tail can be observed. The reversal potential for this tail current is at about −65 mV.

200 pA
80 mV
100 ms

4. INTEGRATIVE FUNCTION OF BURST FIRING IN THE HIPPOCAMPUS

It is clear that the intrinsic membrane properties of the hippocampal pyramidal cells can sustain burst firing. The excitability of the cells to synaptic input is further enhanced by the presence of multiple bursting sites on the soma-dendritic membrane. Our studies show that these properties of the neurons provide the basic step in the generation of synchronized discharge in the hippocampus (Wong and Prince, 1979; Traub and Wong, 1982). Such a synchronized discharge represents a simple kind of epileptiform event.

The synchronization process is elicited when GABA antagonists are added to the hippocampus. The discharge is dependent on chemical synaptic transmission and is blocked in the presence of gamma-d-glutamyl-glycine (Miles *et al.*, 1984), a presumed antagonist for glutaminergic excitatory synapses. Our studies also show that recurrent excitatory synapses between pyramidal cells in the CA2-3 region are importantly involved in the synchronization process (Miles and Wong, 1983). Figure 4 shows that burst firing generated in a CA3 neuron can trigger a burst in the postsynaptic cell via a monosynaptic connection. Such connections between the pyramidal cells may allow activity in a single neuron to initiate and reset the rhythm of synchronized discharge of thousands of cells in the population (Miles and Wong, 1983).

The population discharge can occur spontaneously or it can be triggered by activities in any one of the afferent inputs to the population. For the evoked event the latency of onset is usually prolonged (30–100 msec) and shows considerable variability. Population discharges have refractory periods typically in excess of 2 sec. Thus, when a stimulus is applied at frequencies in excess of 0.5 Hz, the population discharge can be observed to occur with alternate stimuli in an all-or-none fashion (Schwartzkroin and Prince, 1980; Wong and Traub, 1983). Our original hypothesis on synchronization has provided explanations for most of these observations. These initial studies of synchronization involved the simulation of a network of 100 bursting neurons (Traub and Wong, 1982, 1983). Two basic pre-

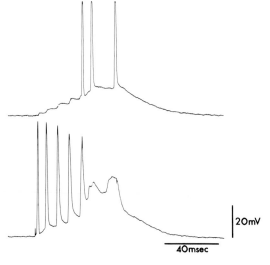

FIGURE 4. Recurrent excitatory connection between pyramidal cells. Each action potential in the presynaptic cell triggered an EPSP in the follower cell eventually leading to a burst of action potentials. Synaptic transmission is obligatory.

dictions of the model are: (1) that a burst elicited in one cell will be obligatorily transmitted to the postsyaptic cell to elicit bursting; (2) that each pyramidal cell is connected, on the average, to more than one postsynaptic cell. With these properties the simulated network provided a detailed description of the synchronization process (Fig. 5). Activity in any one cell in the network will elicit bursting in a few (more than one) postsynaptic neurons. These postsynaptic cells in turn will excite a few more neurons and in this way an increasing number of neurons will be activated eventually resulting in a synchronized discharge. The long-onset latency of the event recorded by extracellular electrodes is probably due to the fact that in the initial phase of generation only a few cells are active in the population and that the signal is below noise level. An electrical signal can only be recorded later in the event when the majority of neurons become active.

Experiments using the slice preparation also suggest an important role of synaptic inhibition in regulating synchronized discharge generation (Wong and Prince, 1979; Wong *et al.,* 1979). Inhibition in the hippocampus is activated via disynaptic connections through a feedforward or feedback arrangement (Andersen *et al.,* 1963; Alger and Nicoll, 1982; Miles and Wong, 1984). Consequently, excitatory afferent volleys directly eliciting an excitation of the pyramidal cells will also activate a disynaptic IPSP. This pattern of evoked response allows suprathreshold afferent input to activate a single action potential but not the endogenous burst due to the occurrence of the concomitant IPSP. Convulsant agents with a common property of suppressing IPSPs allow the elicitation of postsynaptic bursts and thereby release the synchronization process.

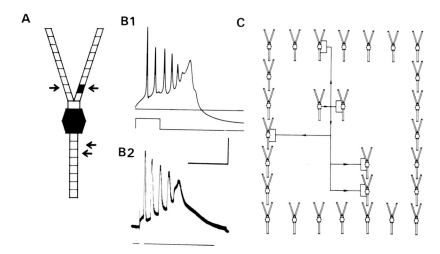

FIGURE 5. Features of the model for synchronization. (A) Electronic structure of a single neuron divided into compartments of 0.1 space constant. Shaded components contain active ionic conductances. Arrow indicate location of synaptic inputs. (B) Intracellular activity elicited by a short duration depolarizing current pulse in a model neuron (upper record) and in a pyramidal cell (lower record). (C) Connectivity of the model network. Each cell excites 50% of the other neurons in the network. (From Traub and Wong, 1982.)

5. SUMMARY

It is clear that the intrinsic membrane properties of the hippocampal pyramidal cells can sustain burst firing activities. Experimental data and computer simulation studies suggest that these properties of the neuron together with the recurrent excitatory connections allow the generation of population synchronized discharge. Our initial model for synchronization suggest a few neurons or even a single neuron can trigger a stereotypically patterned population discharge, and this is now supported by experimental evidence. The primary purpose of the simulation approach is to provide insight to the synchronization mechanism in the hippocampal slice, and the results are largely independent of many of the details of the conductance mechanism and synaptic properties of the network. In this way the assumptions and predictions of the simulation study have provided a guide to the planning of additional experiments. We have also found that the experimental results have already verified some of the basic assumptions and predictions of the simulation studies.

ACKNOWLEDGMENT. This work is supported in part by DHHS grant NS13778. Computer simulation work is done at the IBM T. J. Watson Research Center.

REFERENCES

Alger, B. E. and Nicoll, R. A., 1980, Epileptiform burst afterhyperpolarization: calcium-dependent potassium potential in hippocampal pyramidal cells studied in vitro, *Science* **210**:1122–1124.

Alger, B. E. and Nicoll, R. A., 1982, Feed-forward dendritic inhibition in rat hippocampal pyramidal cells studied *in vitro*, *J. Physiol. (London)* **328**:105–123.

Andersen, P., Eccles, J. D., and Loyning, Y., 1963, Recurrent inhibition in the hippocampus with identification of the inhibitory cell and its synapses, *Nature* **198**:540–542.

Brown, D. A. and Griffith, W. H., 1983a, Calcium activated outward current in voltage-clamped hippocampal neurones of the guinea-pig, *J. Physiol. (London)* **337**:287–301.

Brown, D. A. and Griffith, W. H., 1983b, Persistent slow inward calcium current in voltage-clamped hippocampal neurones of the guinea-pig, *J. Physiol. (London)* **337**:303–320.

Cole, A. E. and Nicoll, R. A., 1983, Acetylcholine mediates a slow synaptic potential in hippocampal pyramidal cells, *Science* **221**:1299–1301.

Gustafsson, B., Galvan, M., Grafe, P., and Wigstrom, H., 1982, A transient outward current in a mammalian central neurone blocked by 4-aminopyridine, *Nature* **299**:252–254.

Halliwell, J. V. and Adams, P. R., 1982, Voltage-clamp analysis of muscarinic excitation in hippocampal neurons, *Brain Res.* **250**:71–92.

Hotson, J. R. and Prince, D. A., 1980, A calcium activated hyperpolarization follows repetitive firing in hippocampal neurons, *J. Neurophysiol.* **43**:409–419.

Johnston, D., Hablitz, J. J., and Wilson, W. A., 1980, Voltage-clamp discloses slow inward current in hippocampal burst firing neurons, *Nature* **286**:391–393.

Kandel, E. R. and Spencer, W. A., 1961, Electrophysiology of hippocampal neurons. II. Afterpotentials and repetitive firing, *J. Neurophysiol.* **24**:243–259.

Madison, D. V. and Nicoll, R. A., 1982, Noradrenaline blocks accommodation of pyramidal cell discharge in the hippocampus, *Nature* **299**:636–638.

Miles, R. and Wong, R. K. S., 1983, Single neurones can influence synchronized population discharge in the CA3 region of the guinea pig hippocampus, *Nature* **306**:371–373.

Miles, R. and Wong, R. K. S., 1984, Unitary inhibitory synaptic potentials in the guinea pig hippocampus *in vitro*, *J. Physiol. (London)* **356**:97–113.

Numann, R. E. and Wong, R. K. S., 1984, Voltage-clamp study on GABA response desensitization in single pyramidal cells dissociated from the hippocampus of adult guinea-pigs, *Neurosci. Lett.* **47**:289–294.

Schwartzkroin, P. A. and Prince, D. A., 1980, Changes in excitatory and inhibitory potentials leading to epileptogenic activity, *Brain Res.* **183**:61–76.

Schwartzkroin, P. A. and Slawsky, M., 1977, Probable calcium spikes in hippocampal neurons, *Brain Res.* **135**:157–161.

Traub, R. D. and Wong, R. K. S., 1982, Cellular mechanism of neuronal synchronization in epilepsy, *Science* **216**:745–747.

Traub, R. D. and Wong, R. K. S., 1983, Synchronized burst discharge in disinhibited hippocampal slice. II. Model of cellular mechanism, *J. Neurophysiol.* **49**:442–458.

Wong, R. K. S. and Prince, D. A., 1978, Participation of calcium spikes during intrinsic burst firing in hippocampal neurons, *Brain Res.* **159**:385–390.

Wong, R. K. S. and Prince, D. A., 1979, Dendritic mechanism underlying penicillin-induced epileptiform activity, *Science* **204**:1228–1231.

Wong, R. K. S. and Traub, R. D., 1983, Synchronized burst discharge in the disinhibited hippocampal slice. I. Initiation in the CA2-CA3 region, *J. Neurophysiol.* **48**:938–951.

Wong, R. K. S., Prince, D. A., and Basbaum, A. I., 1979, Intradendritic recordings from hippocampal neurons, *Proc. Natl. Acad. Sci. U.S.A.* **76**:986–990.

22

Mechanisms Underlying Long-Term Potentiation

PHILIP A. SCHWARTZKROIN and JEFFREY S. TAUBE

The phenomenon of long-term potentiation (LTP) has become one of the most popularly studied candidates for a neural mechanism involved in learning and memory. LTP is an enduring change in the synaptic efficacy of a stimulus based upon history of activity at the synapse and seems to be relatively specific to the afferent synapses initially involved in the input. Because of its specificity, because of its long-term nature, and because it can be produced with "physiological" stimulus parameters, many laboratories have focused attention on the mechanisms underlying LTP. Although originally reported in experiments on intact animal hippocampus (Bliss and Gardner-Medwin, 1973; Bliss and Lømo, 1973), it was soon discovered that the LTP phenomenon could be replicated using the *in vitro* hippocampal slice preparation (Schwartzkroin and Wester, 1975). This *in vitro* model has enabled investigators to study basic mechanisms that would have been difficult or impossible to approach using *in vivo* preparations of mammalian brain.

The phenomenon of LTP itself is very hardy, especially in hippocampus. However, it has been surprisingly difficult to elucidate the cellular changes concomitant with, and/or responsible for, the changes in field responses often measured. At the field potential level, the major reported observations are: (1) an increase in population spike amplitude, decrease in population spike latency (to peak), and occasional development of additional population spikes (as recorded at the cell body level); and (2) an increase in amplitude of the population EPSP and an increase in rate of rise of the population EPSP (as recorded at the level of the dendrites).

One of the mysteries of LTP has been the observation that the population EPSP potentiates relatively little compared to the population spike. This discrepancy has been seen both *in vivo* (Bliss and Lømo, 1973) and *in vitro* (Schwartzkroin and

PHILIP A. SCHWARTZKROIN ● Department of Neurological Surgery, University of Washington, Seattle, Washington 98195.   JEFFREY S. TAUBE ● Departments of Physiology and Biophysics, University of Washington, Seattle, Washington 98195.

Wester, 1975; Andersen *et al.*, 1980; see also Swanson *et al.*, 1982) and has led investigators to question whether changes at the synapse could "explain" changes in cellular propensity to produce action potentials following a LTP conditioning train. Most workers, however, believe that the LTP phenomenon is due to an increase in synaptic efficacy and have focused their research on elucidating underlying synaptic mechanisms (either pre- or post-synaptic). Numerous studies now support a synaptic localization. The evoked potentiated responses appear to be confined to the orthodromic pathway receiving the conditioning train (i.e., LTP is homosynaptic) (Andersen *et al.*, 1977; McNaughton and Barnes, 1977; Alger *et al.*, 1978). Further, intracellular studies indicate that intrinsic cellular properties, such as membrane resting potential, input resistance, and action potential threshold are not altered following a LTP conditioning tetanus (Andersen *et al.*, 1980).

    The finding that the population spike is increased more substantially that the population EPSP may not, at first, be disconcerting, since only a small percentage increase in the EPSP may be needed to bring a large population of cells to discharge threshold. This EPSP–spike relationship can be seen clearly in the steep "input–output" curve that relates input magnitude to response amplitude (Fig. 1). Over a large region of the curve, only a small increase in EPSP amplitude can cause a large increase in population spike (Fig. 1B). However, Wilson (1981; Wilson *et al.*, 1981) has found that changes in the population EPSP cannot account for the magnitude of the observed changes in population spike. If mechanisms responsible

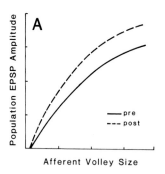

Afferent Volley Size

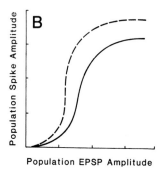

Population EPSP Amplitude

FIGURE 1. Theoretical input–output curves relating (A) stimulus input magnitude to population EPSP amplitude and (B) population EPSP amplitude to population spike amplitude. Solid lines in (A) and (B) show "control" relationships, whereas the dashed lines illustrate the shift in curves following LTP-inducing tetanization. If an increase in EPSP amplitude sufficiently explained LTP, then a leftward shift of curves should be seen only in (A). Experimental data show, however, a shift also in the (B) curve, thus suggesting an alteration in EPSP/spike coupling.

for producing population spike potentiation were confined solely to increases in synaptic amplitude, then one would expect tetanization to produce a leftward shift in the curve relating input to EPSP amplitude (Fig. 1A), but not in the curve relating EPSP amplitude to population spike amplitude (Fig. 1B). However, studies have shown that, following LTP-inducing tetanization, both relationships are shifted, thus indicating that the increase in population spike amplitude cannot be attributed entirely to the increase in population EPSP. Andersen et al. (1980) labeled the form of potentiation seen in Fig. 1A as V–E potentiation (volley–EPSP) as opposed to the E–S potentiation (EPSP–Spike) seen in Fig. 1B. Data from the early studies of LTP by Bliss and Lømo (1973) are consistent with this dissociation; they reported occasional population spike potentiation in the absence of population EPSP potentiation.

What are the intracellular data that support the hypothesis that LTP is a reflection of increased synaptic efficacy? Do intracellular recordings show the expected increase in EPSP amplitude? There have been surprisingly few intracellular studies of the LTP phenomenon. Andersen et al. (1980) reported increased EPSP amplitude in some CA1 neurons in hippocampal slices evidencing LTP at the field potential level. However, the EPSP changes were rather small and inconsistent. In reexamining their figures, it also seems that there is some contamination from field potentials in their intracellular records; it is possible that ephaptic influences could be contributing to apparent changes in intracellular EPSPs (Turner et al., 1984). Recording from CA3 pyramidal cells in hippocampal slices, Misgeld et al. (1979) and Yamamoto and Chujo (1978) reported similar inconsistencies. In these latter studies, alterations in IPSPs as well as in EPSPs were encountered. Therefore, it was unclear whether tetanization produced a potentiation of excitatory potentials or whether the conditioning stimulus produced a decrease in the underlying IPSP, thus resulting in an *apparent* increase in EPSP amplitude. Assaf (personal communication), studying LTP in the dentate granule cells, has been unsuccessful in discovering any changes in intracellular EPSP following LTP, even though the population spike shows consistent and significant enhancement.

A number of recent studies have to some extent clarified, but largely added to, this confusion. Wigström and Gustafsson (1983) used picrotoxin (10 μM) to block IPSPs seen in intracellular studies and found that this treatment did not abolish EPSP potentiation (as reflected in the population EPSP), thus showing that alterations in GABA-mediated IPSPs could not account for the apparent EPSP changes. This manipulation was also used by Brown and colleagues (Barrionuevo et al., 1983) to show that both synaptic current (seen under voltage clamp conditions) and synaptic voltage were increased in both CA1 and CA3 neurons during LTP conditions; the current increase was far greater, however, than the change in EPSP amplitude. Yamamoto and Sawada (1981) have similarly seen potentiation of the population spike when using bicuculline (1 μM). However, these authors did not demonstrate that the IPSP was actually blocked by this drug concentration; Alger and Nicoll (1982) have reported that bicuculline concentrations much in excess of 1 μM are necessary to block hippocampal IPSPs. Lynch and colleagues (1983) have reported tetanus-induced changes in intracellularly recorded EPSP amplitude in CA1 neurons, but only when dendritic field EPSPs were also potentiated. Their study, therefore, does not exclude the possibility that LTP, as defined as an increase in the population spike, may occur even when no potentiation occurs in the dendritic population EPSP.

Researchers have differed on whether postsynaptic cell firing is necessary to produce LTP. Using extracellular techniques in CA1, Scharfman and Sarvey (1983) blocked cell discharge during the tetanization period by three different methods (TTX application, long-duration GABA ejections, and administration of pentobarbital) and found there was no subsequent development of LTP. In contrast, Wigström *et al.* (1982) recorded intracellularly in CA1 neurons and blocked cell discharge by hyperpolarizing the postsynaptic cell during tetanization; this procedure did *not* block development of LTP. Similarly, McNaughton (McNaughton *et al.*, 1978) and Douglas (Douglas *et al.*, 1982) were unable to prevent dentate LTP when granule cell discharge was blocked by stimulating the inhibitory commissural/associational pathway. These latter two studies suggested that postsynaptic discharge was not coupled to the development of LTP.

Another area of confusion in the LTP literature is the degree to which calcium is required, and the site at which it acts, to insure development of LTP. Several experiments have shown its presence is crucial (Dunwiddie *et al.*, 1978; Dunwiddie and Lynch, 1979; Wigström *et al.*, 1979; Turner *et al.*, 1982), but data indicate that calcium's involvement in LTP may go beyond its role in synaptic transmission/transmitter release. Dunwiddie and Lynch (1979) suggested a possible postsynaptic calcium action in LTP, and Lynch *et al.* (1983) have recently claimed that calcium chelation, by intracellular EGTA injections into the *post*synaptic cell, blocks LTP in the treated neuron. Calcium specificity for such mechanisms must be questioned in light of experiments by Wigström and Swann (1980), where strontium was substituted for calcium in the extracellular medium and found to support LTP. Strontium is known to substitute for calcium in synaptic transmission, but these experiments indicate that either (1) strontium can also substitute for calcium in LTP postsynaptic mechanisms or (2) calcium is not required postsynaptically for the generation of LTP. Also of interest is these authors' observation that the strontium produced an E–S potentiation that was more pronounced than that observed in normal medium.

In contrast to the prevailing notion that there is a calcium-mediated postsynaptic component of LTP, Sastry and colleagues (Chirwa *et al.*, 1983) demonstrated that extracellular concentration of calcium did not change following a 100-Hz conditioning train that led to the development of LTP. However, if the frequency of the conditioning train was low (20 Hz), extracellular calcium concentration was reduced, and the evoked response was depressed rather than enhanced. Recording intracellularly with ion-sensitive microelectrodes, these investigators found parallel results—that low frequency stimulation elevated intracellular calcium levels while the high frequency trains had no effect on calcium levels. Sastry and colleagues interpret their findings as suggesting that postsynaptic neuronal accumulation of calcium leads to depression, not potentiation. They have further supported their argument against a postsynaptic calcium action in LTP in studies in which verapamil, a calcium channel blocker (claimed by the authors to be selective for postsynaptic channels), did not prevent development of LTP (Sastry *et al.*, 1984). Furthermore, verapamil was capable of unmasking the potentiation initially blocked by the *N*-methyl-aspartate antagonist D.L 2-amino-5-phosphonovalerate (APV). They suggested that APV enhanced a postsynaptic calcium influx that led to a postsynaptic depression; application of verapamil inhibited this calcium influx, blocked the postsynaptic depression, and consequently unmasked the potentiation. Several authors have presented evidence that LTP is due to a presynaptic mechanism, entailing terminal hyperpolarization (Sastry, 1982) and increase of transmitter release (Skrede and Malthe-Sorenssen, 1981).

The variety of observations and discrepancies with regard to LTP intracellular reflections led us to a reexamination of LTP. Using the *in vitro* hippocampal slice preparation and intracellular techniques, we attempted to assess increases in EPSP amplitude following tetanizing stimulation by recording PSPs intradendritically. Recordings were obtained from the CA1 region of hippocampus; with one electrode we monitored field potential (either in the dendritic region to record field EPSPs or at the cell body level to record population spikes), and with another electrode we simultaneously recorded intradendritically. A tetanizing train of stimuli was delivered through bipolar electrodes to the *en passant* fibers coursing through stratum radiatum, contacting the apical dendrites of the CA1 pyramidal cells. Stimulus parameters were: 100 Hz stimulation for 1 sec or 20 Hz stimulation for 5 sec; 50-μsec pulses; stimulus intensity of the pulse adjusted so that it was subthreshold for spike generation in the intracellularly recorded neuron (at this intensity, a minimal population spike was usually visible in the field electrode recording).

Our results, rather than clarifying the issue of potentiation of the intracellular EPSP, have added to the confusion. In many cases, there was no evidence that the dendritically recorded EPSP increased in amplitude or rise time (Fig. 2). This lack of intracellular EPSP potentiation could not be attributed to the fact that the recording electrode was electrotonically remote from the synapses, for the recordings were made intradendritically (at least 100 μm from the soma level). The EPSP changes were not simply masked by IPSPs, for similar "negative" results were obtained when the GABA blocker picrotoxin (50 μM) was added to the bathing medium to block IPSPs. In all cases that we evaluated, there was a clear potentiation of the population spike recorded at the cell body level. Potentiation of the field EPSP was not so clear. When field EPSP potentiation occurred, there was usually some minimal potentiation of the intracellular EPSP. However, it was clear that a potentiated EPSP—extracellular or intracellular—was not necessary to produce a potentiated population spike. EPSPs initially subthreshold for spike initiation often triggered action potentials following tetanization, even though EPSP amplitude and rise time were unchanged. This result supports the hypothesis that a separate E–S potentiation underlies at least part of the LTP phenomenon. These results do not, of course, indicate the EPSP—field or intracellular—may not sometimes be potentiated by the tetanizing stimulation. These results do question the interpretation, however, that PSP changes are a necessary prerequisite of LTP (i.e., that the PSP change represents the basic mechanism underlying the LTP phenomenon).

Our results are in agreement with those of Haas and Rose (1982) who showed that the role of inhibition in the generation of LTP was minor, and that noninhibitory mechanisms must be responsible. In our studies, the IPSP recorded intracellularly

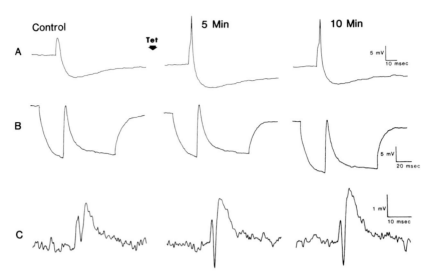

FIGURE 2. Absence of potentiation in the intradendritic EPSP during population spike potentiation. (A) Intracellular recordings were from a CA1 pyramidal cell responding to stimulation in
stratum radiatum. The left-hand traces show the control response; middle and right-hand traces
show responses 5 and 10 min after tetanization. No increase in EPSP was noted although the
stimulus effectively triggered action potentials after the tetanus. (B) Same as (A), except responses are embedded in a 0.5-nA hyperpolarizing current pulse. (C) Extracellular field responses recorded in stratum pyramidale. Tetanization was at 20 Hz for 5 sec. All traces are
averages of five responses.

in the EPSP/IPSP evoked response was either unchanged or enhanced following
tetanization. This occurred simultaneously with a large enhancement of the population spike in the pyramidale field recording (Fig. 3). Our experiments cannot
identify the cause of the IPSP potentiation since we could not distinguish between
(1) actual enhancement of the IPSP due to alterations in interneuron function and
(2) increased recurrent inhibition resulting from a prior increased discharge of
pyramidal cells. Recordings from interneurons showed no decrease in their evoked
response following a conditioning train, further showing that LTP was not generated
as a result of decreased inhibition.

Such results regarding changes in EPSP are problematic in evaluating the
hypothesis presented by Baudry, Lynch and colleagues (Baudry and Lynch, 1980,
1983) for LTP generation. These investigators have proposed that LTP reflects a
calcium-dependent uncovering of glutamate receptors in the postsynaptic membrane.
If such a hypothesis were to be correct, one would expect an increase in EPSP
amplitude during LTP, for the liberation of the glutamatelike transmitter in the CA1
system would have opportunity to bind to more receptors and thus produce a larger
PSP. One would also predict an increase in the postsynaptic cell sensitivity to
exogenously applied glutamate. That the latter condition is not met was first demonstrated by Lynch himself several years ago (Lynch *et al.*, 1976), using field
potential techniques. In fact, just the opposite was observed—a depression in the

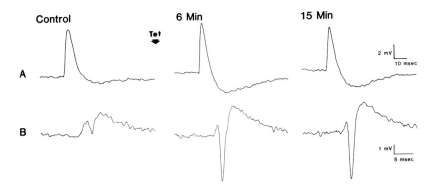

FIGURE 3. Potentiation of IPSPs by LTP-inducing tetanization. (A) Intradendritic recordings from a CA1 pyramidal cell showing the EPSP–IPSP response to stimulation in stratum radiatum. The left-hand trace shows the control response; middle and right-hand traces show responses 6 and 15 min after tetanization. The IPSP grew in amplitude following the tetanus and became more effective in curtailing the depolarizing PSP (the EPSP duration is shorter after the tetanus). (B) Extracellular field responses recorded in pyramidale. Tetanization was at 20 Hz for 5 sec. All traces are averages of five responses.

glutamate response following tetanization. We have also reexamined this possibility, using intrasomatic recording and micropressure ejection of glutamate in the apical dendrites of the CA1 pyramidal neurons. Sodium glutamate (1.0 mM) was ejected from micropipettes (resistances of about 30 MΩ, 30 psi applied to the pipette) in 5- to 50-msec pulses. This manner of glutamate ejection produced consistent responses when pulses were delivered with an interpulse interval of 5 sec. In most cells, a depolarizing glutamate response could be easily established with ejection times of 20 msec or less; larger ejections would invariably lead to repetitive action potential discharge. Our studies have shown that cell sensitivity to glutamate applications is not altered by LTP-inducing tetanization. There is virtually no change in the cells' response to glutamate under these conditions. These data do not, of course, exclude the possibility that there is some change in receptor configuration during the LTP process, but our results do not support the hypothesis that an increase in number of glutamate receptors underlies LTP (Baudry *et al.,* 1980).

What mechanisms other than facilitation of synaptic transmission might be involved in LTP? What can account for the EPSP/spike coupling (E–S) potentiation? Two possibilities that have been tested experimentally are a decrease in inhibition and/or a change in intrinsic membrane properties. As indicated above, however, neither of these explanations have proven satisfactory. No consistent decrease in inhibition has been observed following LTP-inducing tetanization; studies of cellular properties (such as input resistance, threshold, and resting membrane potential) have shown no significant changes in somatically measured parameters. Our intra-dendritic experiments have also shown no consistent changes in cellular characteristics. Another factor recently suggested as relevant to field potential potentiation is ephaptic recruitment among hippocampal neurons. Discharge of a pyramidal cell population could lead, through ephaptic interaction, to synchronous firing of cells only marginally excited by the stimulated input. Although such recruitment might account for some component of population spike potentiation during LTP, it does not explain the initial enhancement of the stimulated input, nor does it account for the E–S potentiation. Why isn't the population EPSP also enhanced by ephaptic mechanisms? Why should there be a more potent ephaptic effect following tetanization than before? LTP-induced ephaptic effects might be produced via a localized change in the extracellular resistance that would lead to an increase in extracellular voltage, and thus larger transmembrane potentials. However, Heinemann has found no significant changes in extracellular volume (and, by extrapolation, in extracellular resistance) following a conditioning stimulus train (personal communication; see also Dietzel *et al.*, 1982). Finally, another possibility, still unexplored, is that E–S potentiation is produced by some alteration in the distribution of sinks/sources on these hippocampal neurons. For example, changes in the density and/or location of dendritic calcium and sodium channels (Wong *et al.*, 1979; Benardo *et al.*, 1982) could lead to altered sites and thresholds for spike initiation.

The confusing state of present work on LTP is not confined to those laboratories attempting to elucidate cellular mechanisms underlying the phenomenon. The interest in LTP has been heightened by its possible link to learning/memory mechanisms, and several laboratories have pursued this link. The results of a recent NRP Workshop on LTP and its implications for memory (Swanson *et al.*, 1982) were equivocal. At the time of the Workshop, there were few convincing data to connect LTP to learning. Recently, however, Berger presented the results of a study that showed that an LTP-inducing tetanizing stimulus improved performance in a classical eye-blink conditioning paradigm (Berger, 1983). This improvement was seen only in those animals in which LTP could be clearly demonstrated; animals that received a similar stimulus train, but showed no hippocampal LTP, did not exhibit facilitated learning. The investigator suggested that establishment of LTP "preconditioned" a set of synapses that were subsequently used in the classical conditioning study. While these results appear to be rather exciting, it is difficult to know how to interpret them, given an apparently opposing finding by Barnes and McNaughton (1983). These latter investigators showed that LTP stimulation led to poorer learning/memory performance in animals dealing with a spatial task. They suggested that LTP "saturated" the synaptic circuits needed for the spatial task, so that animals found it more difficult to establish the correct circuitry. Both of these behavioral studies are open to considerable interpretative freedom and thus establish no compelling connection between LTP and learning.

A fundamental issue that now needs clarification is whether any LTP-like phenomenon actually occurs in awake, functioning animals. Although LTP can be produced in awake animals using experimentally manipulated inputs (Bliss and Gardner-Medwin, 1973; Douglas and Goddard, 1975), it has not been shown that LTP occurs "naturally." The stimulus parameters used to elicit LTP are arguably within physiological limits. However, the stimulating conditions are such that several hundred fibers are simultaneously activated. Does such synchrony occur in the awake, functioning animal? Can LTP occur at the level of an individual neuron under normal behavioral conditions?

Long-term potentiation remains a fascinating physiological phenomenon in search of both underlying mechanisms and significance. The LTP process represents one of the most dramatic examples of physiological plasticity in the mammalian CNS. However, as should be expected of a complex nervous system, the relation of LTP to complex behaviors is not straightforward. Further, the mechanisms underlying the phenomenon may be variable and numerous. Synaptic changes undoubtedly can occur during LTP-inducing stimulation, but it appears that other changes (at sites other than the pre- or postsynaptic membrane) must also contribute to LTP development.

ACKNOWLEDGMENTS. The work from this laboratory was supported by NINCDS-NIH grants NS 00413, NS 15317, and NS 17111 (PAS) and training grant GM 07108 (JST).

REFERENCES

Alger, B. E. and Nicoll, R. A., 1982, Pharmacological evidence for two kinds of GABA receptor on rat hippocampal pyramidal cells studied in vitro, *J. Physiol. (London)* **328**:125–141.

Alger, B. E., Megela, A. L., and Teyler, T. J., 1978, Transient heterosynaptic depression in the hippocampal slice, *Brain Res. Bull.* **3**:181–184.

Andersen, P., Sundberg, S. H., Sveen, O., and Wigström, H., 1977, Specific long-lasting potentiation of synaptic transmission in hippocampal slices, *Nature* **266**:736–737.

Andersen, P., Sundberg, S. H., Sveen, O., Swann, J. W., and Wigström, H., 1980, Possible mechanisms for long-lasting potentiation of synaptic transmission in hippocampal slices from guinea pig, *J. Physiol. (London)* **302**:463–482.

Barnes, C. A. and McNaughton, B. L., 1983, Where is the cognitive map? *Neurosci. Abstr.* **9**:649.

Barrionuevo, G., Kelso, S., and Brown, T. H., 1983, Voltage-clamp analysis of long-term synaptic potentiation, *Neurosci. Abstr.* **9**:103.

Baudry, M. and Lynch, G., 1980, Hypothesis regarding the cellular mechanisms responsible for long-term synaptic potentiation in the hippocampus, *Exp. Neurol.* **68**:202–204.

Baudry, M. and Lynch, G., 1983, A specific hypothesis concerning the biochemical substrates of memory, *Neurosci. Abstr.* **9**:480.

Baudry, M., Oliver, M., Creager, R., Wieraszko, A., and Lynch, G., 1980, Increase in glutamate receptors following repetitive electrical stimulation in hippocampal slices, *Life Sci.* **27**:325–330.

Benardo, L. S., Masukawa, L. M., and Prince, D. A., 1982, Electrophysiology of isolated hippocampal pyramidal dendrites, *J. Neurosci.* **2**:1614–1622.

Berger, T., 1983, "Long-term potentiation of hippocampal synaptic transmission accelerates behavioral learning," poster presented at a *Symposium on Neural Mechanisms of Conditioning*, Marine Biological Laboratory, Woods Hole, Mass.

Bliss, T. V. P. and Gardner-Medwin, A. R., 1973, Long-lasting potentiation of synaptic transmission in the dentate area of the unanaesthetized rabbit following stimulation of the perforant path, *J. Physiol. (London)* **232**:357–374.

Bliss, T. V. P. and Lømo, T., 1973, Long-lasting potentiation of synaptic transmission in the dentate area of the anaesthetized rabbit following stimulation of the perforant path, *J. Physiol. (London)* **232**:331–356.

Chirwa, S. S., Goh, J. W., Maretic, H., and Sastry, B. R., 1983, Evidence for a presynaptic role in long-term potentiation in the rat hippocampus, *J. Physiol. (London)* **339**:41P–42P.

Dietzel, I., Heinemann, U., Hofmeier, G., and Lux, H. D., 1982, Changes in the extracellular volume in the cerebral cortex of cats in relation to stimulus induced epileptiform afterdischarges, in:

Physiology and Pharmacology of Epileptogenic Phenomena (M. R. Klee, H. D. Lux, and E. J. Speckmann, eds.), Raven Press, New York, pp. 5–12.

Douglas, R. M. and Goddard, G. V., 1975, Long-term potentiation of the perforant path granule cell synapse in the rat hippocampus, *Brain Res.* **86:**205–215.

Douglas, R. M., Goddard, G. V., and Riives, M., 1982, Inhibitory modulation of long-term potentiation: Evidence for a postsynaptic locus of control, *Brain Res.* **240:**259–272.

Dunwiddie, T. V. and Lynch, G., 1979, The relationship between extracellular calcium concentrations and the induction of hippocampal long-term potentiation, *Brain Res.* **169:**103–110.

Dunwiddie, T. V., Madison, D., and Lynch, G., 1978, Synaptic transmission is required for initiation of long-term potentiation, *Brain Res.* **150:**413–417.

Haas, H. L. and Rose, G., 1982, Long-term potentiation of excitatory synaptic transmission in the rat hippocampus: The role of inhibitory processes, *J. Physiol. (London)* **329:**541–552.

Lynch, G., Gribkoff, V. K., and Deadwyler, S. A., 1976, Long-term potentiation is accompanied by a reduction in dendritic responsiveness to glutamic acid, *Nature* **276:**151–153.

Lynch, G., Larson, J., Kelso, S., Barrionuevo, G., and Schottler, F., 1983, Intracellular injections of EGTA block induction of hippocampal long-term potentiation, *Nature* **305:**719–721.

McNaughton, B. L. and Barnes, C. A., 1977, Physiological identification and analysis of dentate granule cell response to stimulation of the medial and lateral perforant pathways in the rat, *J. Comp. Neurol.* **175:**439–454.

McNaughton, B. L., Douglas, R. M., and Goddard, G. V., 1978, Synaptic enhancement in fascia dentata: Cooperativity among coactive afferents, *Brain Res.* **157:**277–293.

Misgeld, U., Sarvey, J. M., and Klee, M. R., 1979, Heterosynaptic postactivation potentiation in hippocampal CA3 neurons: Long-term changes of the postsynaptic potentials, *Exp. Brain Res.* **37:**217–229.

Sastry, B. R., 1982, Presynaptic change associated with long-term potentiation in hippocampus, *Life Sci.* **30:**2003–2008.

Sastry, B. R., Goh, J. W., and Pandanoboina, M. M., 1984, Verapamil counteracts the masking of long-lasting potentiation of hippocampal population spike produced by 2-amino-5-phosphonoval-erate, *Life Sci.* **34:**323–329.

Scharfman, H. E. and Sarvey, J. M., 1983, Inhibition of postsynaptic firing in the hippocampus during repetitive stimulation blocks long-term potentiation, *Neurosci. Abstr.* **9:**677.

Schwartzkroin, P. A., and Wester, K., 1975, Long-lasting facilitation of a synaptic potential following tetanization in the in vitro hippocampal slice, *Brain Res.* **89:**107–119.

Skrede, K. K. and Malthe-Sørenssen, D., 1981, Increased resting and evoked release of transmitter following repetitive electrical tetanization in hippocampus: A biochemical correlate to long-lasting synaptic potentiation, *Brain Res.* **208:**436–441.

Swanson, L. W., Teyler, T. J., and Thompson, R. F., 1982, Hippocampal long-term potentiation: Mechanisms and implications for memory, *Neurosci. Res. Prog. Bull.* **20:**613–769.

Turner, R. W., Baimbridge, K. G., and Miller, J. J., 1982, Calcium induced long-term potentiation in the hippocampus, *Neuroscience* **7:**1411–1416.

Turner, R. W., Richardson, T. L., and Miller, J. J., 1984, Ephaptic interactions contribute to paired pulse and frequency potentiation of hippocampal field potentials, *Exp. Brain Res.* **54:**567–570.

Wigström, H. and Gustafsson, B., 1983, Facilitated induction of hippocampal long-lasting potentiation during blockade of inhibition, *Nature* **301:**603–604.

Wigström, H. and Swann, J. W., 1980, Strontium supports synaptic transmission and long-lasting potentiation in the hippocampus, *Brain Res.* **194:**181–191.

Wigström, H., Swann, J. W., and Andersen, P., 1979, Calcium dependency of synaptic long-term potentiation in the hippocampal slice, *Acta Physiol. Scand.* **105:**126–128.

Wigström, H., McNaughton, B. L., and Barnes, C. A., 1982, Long-term synaptic enhancement in hippocampus is not regulated by postsynaptic membrane potential, *Brain Res.* **233:**195–199.

Wilson, R. C., 1981, Changes in translation of synaptic excitation to dentate granule cell discharge accompanying long-term potentiation. I. Differences between normal and reinnervated dentate gyrus, *J. Neurophysiol.* **46:**324–338.

Wilson, R. C., Levy, W. B., and Steward, O., 1981, Changes in translation of synaptic excitation to dentate granule cell discharge accompanying long-term potentiation. II. An evaluation of mecha-

nisms utilizing dentate gyrus dually innervated by surviving ipsilateral and sprouted cross tem-
porodentate inputs, *J. Neurophysiol.* **46:**339–355.

Wong, R. K. S., Prince, D. A., and Basbaum, A. I., 1979, Intradendritic recordings from hippocampal
neurons, *Proc. Natl. Acad. Sci. USA* **76:**986–990.

Yamamoto, C. and Chujo, T., 1978, Long-term potentiation in thin hippocampal sections studied by
intracellular and extracellular recordings, *Exp. Neurol.* **58:**242–250.

Yamamoto, C. and Sawada, S., 1981, Important factors in induction of long-term potentiation in thin
hippocampal sections, *Exp. Neurol.* **74:**122–130.

23

Modifiability of Single Identified Neurons in Crustaceans

H. L. ATWOOD

1. INVERTEBRATE NEURONS

The ability to use identified neurons of inverbrates as model systems for study of plastic or adaptive changes, even those associated with conditioning, confers a great advantage to the experimentalist. Selection of the recorded neurons is eliminated as an experimental variable, and defined circuits can be studied.

Although much recent work on invertebrates has been directed at events taking place in the peripheral nervous system (e.g., eye of *Hermissenda*), the membrane changes of peripherally located cells, which may possibly be involved in behavior that can be conditioned (Alkon, 1980), are similar in their general nature to membrane changes reported in central neurons of *Aplysia* (Kandel and Schwartz, 1982). Modifications of K^+ and Ca^{2+} channels have been reported, with important functional implications. Thus, it may not be unreasonable to postulate that some cellular processes important in conditioning are represented in peripheral neurons of invertebrates. Development of much larger numbers of neurons in central nervous systems of vertebrates may be accompanied by generally greater specialization of the peripheral nervous system and by relatively less representation of central-type cellular mechanisms.

An example to illustrate this contention is evident through comparison of synaptic performance of motor neurons of crustaceans (Atwood, 1976, 1982) and of higher vertebrates (Hubbard, 1970). Plastic phenomena such as short-term facilitation and long-term potentiation can be demonstrated at vertebrate neuromuscular junctions (Magleby and Zengel, 1975, 1976), but usually only by artificially depressing transmitter output to a low level. These synapses are specialized to release large numbers of transmitter quanta with each impulse and under normal conditions show depression with maintained stimulation. In contrast, neuromuscular junctions of crustaceans normally release small numbers of transmitter quanta with

H.L. ATWOOD ● Department of Physiology, Faculty of Medicine, University of Toronto, Toronto, Ontario, Canada M5S 1A8.

each impulse. Many synapses show facilitation and, in some cases, long-term potentiation with repeated stimulation. These facilitative changes can be demonstrated in the intact animal and probably are important in its normal functioning (Jacobs and Atwood, 1981). Further examples of peripheral modulation of crustacean motor synapses are found in the occurrence of presynaptic inhibition (Dudel and Kuffler, 1961) and in the responses to neurohormones and peptides (Cooke and Sullivan, 1982). Central-type "philosophy" seems to exist peripherally and to play a role in normal function of crustacean motor neurons.

2. NEURONAL MODIFICATION

Much of the work on central neurons, both invertebrate and vertebrate, involves recording from or manipulating an entire cell (including cell body with nucleus and associated organelles, dendrites, axons). Thus, it is possible that both nuclear-mediated and non-nuclear-mediated effects could be involved in changes associated

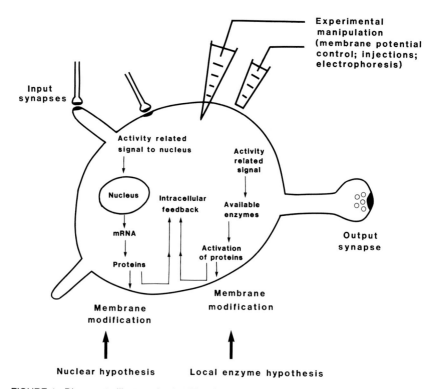

FIGURE 1. Diagram to illustrate in simplified form two general routes for production of membrane-related changes in a central neuron. Experimental manipulation, or activity set up by conditioning, may affect one or both of these. In addition to membrane-related changes, intracellular changes may be produced that result in short-term or long-term alterations in cellular performance (e.g., transmitter synthesis or mobilization).

with conditioning (Fig. 1). We can distinguish these two possibilities as "nuclear" and "local enzyme" hypotheses. At one time or another, both have been investigated for invertebrate neurons (e.g., Strumwasser, 1967; Kandel and Schwartz, 1982). Currently, variants of the "local enzyme" hypothesis are very fashionable among experimentalists, as a result of important recent discoveries relating to calmodulin-controlled (cf. Alkon, Chapter 1, this volume) and cyclic AMP controlled (cf. Byrne *et al.*, this volume) enzyme systems. These findings provide mechanisms for adapting membrane properties to changes in neuronal activity.

The range of responsiveness of the neuron is determined ultimately by the genome. Given that individual neurons have been endowed with certain components by operation of the genome during the course of development, there may be considerable built-in ability for the neuron to respond adaptively to electrical, hormonal, or synaptic activity, including activity associated with conditioning situations.

However, if the experimentalist wishes to distinguish changes associated with altered nuclear activity from those involving local enzyme responses, criteria must be sought to allow these possibilities to be defined or eliminated.

In some cases, the kinetics of the adaptive change may be sufficiently rapid to rule out the nuclear pathway. In other cases, a more effective criterion would be separation of the nuclear part of the neuron from the rest to determine whether a particular adaptive response can be retained when the nucleus is not present.

3. CRUSTACEAN MOTOR NEURONS

Crayfish motor neurons lend themselves well to the latter approach and could be very useful for investigation of adaptive mechanisms mediated either by the neuron as a whole or by parts of the neuron. The long axon, with its extensive peripheral branches richly endowed with central-type synapses, provides a means of isolating the synaptic output region from the cell body (Fig. 2). Thus, the

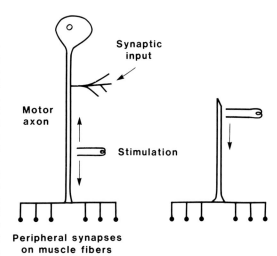

FIGURE 2. Diagram of a crustacean motor neuron (crayfish opener motor neuron). An extensive peripheral output region is separated from the cell body by a long axon. Stimuli applied to the intact axon cause impulses to propagate both centripetally and centrifugally. Blocking the axon in one spot can eliminate one set of impulses. Cutting the axon, for example, permits investigation of the effects of impulse activity on the output region of the neuron, with no involvement of the cell body. The separated peripheral region is known to remain physiologically potent for months.

Synaptic input

Motor axon

Stimulation

Peripheral synapses on muscle fibers

crustacean motor neuron provides an excellent model for investigation of the adaptive responses of a single neuron to effects of activity, with or without the cell body.

In addition, it is technically possible to follow changes in the synaptic performance and impulse activity of an identified neuron in the intact animal over long periods of time. A convenient way to do this is to record the myogram of muscles, such as the opener or closer of the claw, which receive only one or two excitatory motor axons. Each myogram potential represents one impulse in the innervating motor axon. Changes in relative amplitude of the myogram with repetitive activity indicate facilitation or depression (Jacobs and Atwood, 1981).

Once a conditioned change in the motor axons's impulse activity or synaptic performance has been followed in an identified neuron of an experimental animal, an acute preparation can be made to define the changes at the level of individual synapses.

4. LONG-TERM FACILITATION

Homosynaptic long-lasting potentiation of transmission has been studied in the isolated crustacean neuromuscular preparation. Prolonged stimulation of a tonic crustacean motor axon (the excitatory axon of the opener muscle in crayfish) at low frequencies leads to a phenomenon originally termed *long-term facilitation* (LTF). This phenomenon, first described at crustacen neuromuscular synapses (Sherman and Atwood, 1971), is seen as a gradually developing enhancement of transmission that appears after many impulses and decays, with cessation of stimulation, in two phases, an initial rapid one and much slower one; the latter may persist for hours (Atwood *et al.*, 1975). A similar phenomenon (but without the long-lasting aftereffect) has been described at magnesium-poisoned vertebrate neuromuscular junctions (Magleby and Zengel, 1975, 1976).

Several lines of evidence indicate that the slow development of long-term facilitation is dependent upon accumulation of sodium ions in the presynaptic terminal. For example, application of ouabain (to block extrusion of Na^+) speeds up development of LTF and retards its decay, even in the absence of external calcium (Swenarchuk and Atwood, 1975). Also, treatment of nerve terminals with Monensin, an ionophore with a high selectivity for sodium, produces an effect very similar to LTF, even in the absence of external calcium (Atwood *et al.*, 1982). Currently, it is thought that elevated intraterminal Na^+ releases calcium from intracellular bound pools, thus enhancing secretion of transmitter. Similar evidence in other secreting systems supports this hypothesis (Lowe *et al.*, 1976). It seems widely accepted at present that both intracellular Ca^{2+} and intracellular Na^+ can influence transmitter release (Rahaminoff *et al.*, 1980).

Recently, it has been possible to record from nerve terminals close to the sites of output synapses (Wojtowicz and Atwood, 1983a). During stimulation leading to LTF, the action potential becomes smaller and slower, while the steady-state membrane potential becomes hyperpolarized following stimulation. These changes are consistent with build-up of Na^+ in the nerve terminal during stimulation. Reduction of E_{Na} leads to changes in the action potential, while sodium loading activates an electrogenic sodium pump, leading to hyperpolarization. Injection of Na^+ into the terminal produces changes in the action potential, steady-state membrane potential, and synaptic transmission that are very similar to those seen during maintained stimulation (Wojtowicz and Atwood, 1983b).

It is important to note that the changes in action potential and steady-state membrane potential are reversed after a relatively brief time, while the changes in synaptic transmission persist, sometimes for many hours (Fig. 3). All evidence at present suggests that ionic changes are rapidly reversed but leave a persistent aftereffect. Thus, a local enzyme mechanism in the terminal triggered by ionic changes, could be involved in long-lasting synaptic modification (Fig. 4).

Enhanced transmission following maintained stimulation of a "tonic" motor axon could result either from enhanced probability of release at existing synapses or from recruitment of existing but previously inactive synapses on the same terminal. Enhanced probability of release could result from increased synthesis and availability of transmitter (Birks, 1977) or from modification of membrane conductance channels (Ca^{2+} and/or K^+) at or near the synapse. Recruitment of new synapses could be achieved by insertion or unmasking of functionally necessary molecules in the presynaptic membrane. In this connection, a recent study by Chiang (1983) strongly indicates that presynaptic dense bodies (release zones) increase among synapses of lobster terminals during imposition of sodium loading (which leads to long-term facilitation).

An observation that suggests recruitment of new synaptic release sites as a possibility is that the ultrastructural features of individual release sites on a given

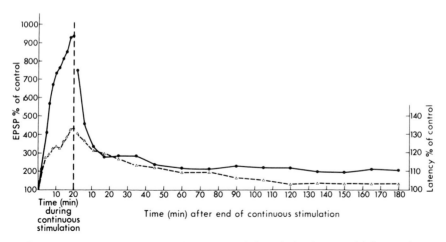

FIGURE 3. Time course of long-term facilitation and of terminal action potential changes (crayfish opener muscle). Growth of the synaptic potential during maintained stimulation at 15 Hz (15°C) is shown, together with decay in amplitude of a test response following stimulation. In addition, changes in conduction velocity of the action potential are shown: This measure of nerve terminal performance recovers more rapidly than does synaptic transmission. (From Atwood et al., 1975.)

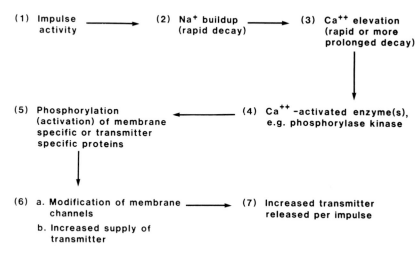

FIGURE 4. Possible scheme for long-term facilitation in an isolated neuromuscular preparation. Only the initial part of the mechanism is well established experimentally.

terminal show varying degrees of maturation (Jahromi and Atwood, 1974). It is possible that a large "pool" of relatively inactive release sites is available for recruitment, either during short-term facilitation or, on a more permanent basis, during long-term facilitation (Atwood and Marin, 1983). Morphological changes in synapses, e.g., active zone addition or subtraction or appearance of new membrane particles (Tokunaga *et al.*, 1979), can apparently occur rapidly. Also, it is quite possible that a single quantum of transmitter saturates the postsynaptic receptors of a single synaptic contact in the crayfish neuromuscular junction (Atwood, 1982); thus, a larger postsynaptic potential may be generated by recruiting release at additional contact points rather than by releasing more quanta at a single site. The model proposed (Korn *et al.*, 1981) for boutons in the central nervous system (0 or 1 quantum released per impulse per bouton) is likely to apply also to individual synaptic contacts on crayfish neuromuscular terminals.

Measurement of quantal statistics will provide data that may support or negate this model. From binomial statistics, it is possible to estimate the probability of release of an individual quantal unit (p) and also the "number of responding units" (n). The latter factor has recently been shown to correspond to the number of synaptic boutons in central neurons (Korn *et al.*, 1981), and a similar relationship was postulated some time ago for crustacean neuromuscular synapses (Zucker, 1973).

5. LONG-LASTING ADAPTIVE MODIFICATION OF SYNAPSES RELATED TO NEURONAL ACTIVITY

The observations on long-term facilitation in isolated neuromuscular preparations suggested that if stimulation of a neuron results in persistent after-effects, then when the performance of a single neuron is monitored in the intact animal, changes in synaptic performance may be produced by altering the amount of nerve impulse activity experienced by that neuron.

A "phasic" motor neuron innervating the crayfish claw (the "fast" motor axon, which normally is silent most of the time) was stimulated for a short period each day, by means of chronically implanted electrodes (Lnenicka and Atwood, 1983). The synaptic performance was monitored through electrodes implanted in the muscle, and the phasic neuron was recruited at a low threshold by stimulation through electrodes implanted in the motor nerve. The performance of the stimulated neuron was followed on a day-to-day basis. Extra stimulation was given to the neuron on one side of the animal, while that on the other side served as a nonstimulated control. Definitive intracellular measurements of synaptic potentials were obtained from many acute preparations after a conditioning effect had been established.

Under normal conditions, synaptic transmission of this neuron depresses rapidly (Wiersma, 1961; Atwood, 1973). When we tested depression of synaptic transmission at 5 Hz, we found that the experimental neuron developed resistance to depression within a few days, while the control neuron remained quite depressible (Fig. 5). This alteration of synaptic performance occurred more readily in intermediate to small animals. The transmission pattern of the stimulated neuron came to resemble that of younger animals (Lnenicka and Atwood, 1983). Preliminary results indicate that immobilization of the limb to reduce impulse activity leads to changes in the opposite direction to those seen with extra activity. Thus, the overall synaptic performance appears linked to impulse traffic in an adaptive fashion. Synapses can be permanently altered to meet functional demands.

Further preliminary work has indicated that the conditioning effect can be produced more readily in regenerated limbs (in which the terminals are younger than the soma of the same neuron).

The work to date has clearly shown that initial transmitter output and rate of depression of transmission in an identified motor neuron can be modified in an adaptive fashion by neuronal activity, with a time course of 1–3 days. Once the effect has been established, it persists for at least two weeks without further extra-impulse activity. The effect is different from LTF, since initial transmitter output is lower in the "conditioned" synapses than in control synapses of the contralateral axon in the same animal (Fig. 5).

The slower time course of this adaptive effect, in comparison to LTF, suggests that the neuronal cell body may be involved in mediating the response. Further

FIGURE 5. Synaptic potentials of the fast closer axon (intermediate sized crayfish) recorded at the beginning and at the end of 30 min continuous stimulation at 5 Hz. Control claw shows initially large potentials which depress with stimulation. Conditioned claw shows initially smaller potentials which do not depress. Calibration: 20 msec, 4 mV. (From Lnenicka and Atwood, 1983.)

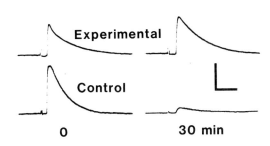

work, in which either the cell body or the terminal arborization is stimulated independently, must now be completed. Preliminary results from immobilization experiments favour the "nuclear" hypothesis. During immobilization over a period of many days, impulse activity in the phasic axon is reduced, but it is normally at a low level, so the reduction only amounts to a few impulses every hour. However, a sizeable increase in synaptic depression occurs. *A priori,* it seems unlikely that this effect could be due to the rather small observed decrease in number of impulses reaching the terminals. It is more likely that overall electrical activity in the central part of the neuron is reduced, due to curtailment of sensory feedback. Thus, subthreshold electrical events in the central part of the neuron may play an important role in determining its adaptive responses.

The picture that emerges from the studies of adaptive modification of the phasic neuron is that the neuron can, under direction from the cell body, adapt its synaptic performance to meet new conditions of activity. Neurons with more recently formed synapses can do this more readily; thus, the age of synaptic terminals may limit ability to undergo adaptive modification.

6. CONCLUSION

Comparison of the two types of synaptic modification in crustacean neurons shows that both intermediate modification (LTF) and more permanent modification (long-term adaptation to altered levels of impulse activity) may be brought into play. Local enzyme mechanisms seem to be involved during LTF. The cell body may be involved in longer-lasting adaptations, but the mechanisms are presently unknown.

The long-term adaptation of a phasic motor neuron to increased impulse activity appears to force synaptic performance into a more tonic mode. This change makes the neuron perform in a manner more closely resembling younger stages of the same neuron.

The significance of these synaptic modifications in the life of the animal have yet to be worked out. LTF may play a role in adaptation to environmental conditions (Jacobs and Atwood, 1981). Long-term adaptation to altered neuronal activity may play a role in adjusting neuronal performance within genetically allowed limits to meet situations arising during the lifetime of the individual.

ACKNOWLEDGMENTS. Dr. G. Lnenicka and Dr. Martin Wojtowicz have contributed greatly to recent experimental work on the problems outlined above. MRC (Canada) and NSERC (Canada) supported the research.

REFERENCES

Alkon, D. S., 1980, Cellular analysis of a gastropod (*Hermissenda crassicornis*) model of associative learning, *Biol. Bull.* **159**:505–560.

Atwood, H. L., 1973, Crustacean motor units, in: *Control of Posture and Locomotion* (R. B. Stein, K. B. Pearson, R. S. Smith, J. B. Redford, eds.), Plenum Press, New York, pp. 87–104.

Atwood, H. L., 1976, Organization and synaptic physiology of crustacean neuromuscular systems, *Progr. Neurobiol.* **7**:291–391.

Atwood, H. L., 1982, Synapses and neurotransmitters, in: *Neurobiology, Structure and Function, Biology of Crustacea,* Vol. 3 (H. L. Atwood and D. C. Sandeman, eds.), Academic Press, New York, pp. 105–150.

Atwood, H. L. and Marin, L., 1983, Ultrastructure of synapses with different transmitter-releasing characteristics on motor axon terminals of a crab, *Hyas areneus, Cell Tiss. Res.* **231**:103–115.

Atwood, H. L., Swenarchuk, L. E., and Gruenwald, C. R., 1975, Long-term synaptic facilitation during sodium accumulation in nerve terminals, *Brain Res.* **100**:198–204.

Atwood, H. L., Charlton, M. P., and Thompson, C. S., 1982, Neuromuscular transmission in crustaceans is enhanced by a sodium ionophore, monensin, and by prolonged stimulation, *J. Physiol. (London)* **335**:179–197.

Birks, R. I., 1977, A long-lasting potentiation of transmitter release related to an increase in transmitter stores in a sympathetic ganglion, *J. Physiol. (London)* **271**:847–862.

Chiang, R. G., 1983, Changes in nerve terminal physiology and ultrastructure at neuromuscular junctions of the lobster, *Homarus americanus,* caused by long-term facilitation or short-term denervation. Ph.D. Thesis, University of Toronto.

Cooke, I. M. and Sullivan, R. E., 1982, Hormones and neurosecretion, in: *Neurobiology: Structure and Function, Biology of Crustacea,* Vol. 3 (H. L. Atwood and D. C. Sandeman, eds.), Academic Press, New York, pp. 205–290.

Dudel, J. and Kuffler, S. W., 1961, Presynaptic inhibition at the crayfish neuromuscular junction, *J. Physiol. (London)* **155**:543–562.

Hubbard, J. I., 1970, Mechanism of transmitter release, *Prog. Biophys. Mol. Biol.* **21**:33–124.

Jacobs, J. R. and Atwood, H. L., 1981, Effects of thermal history on long-term neuromuscular facilitation in intact crayfish and isolated claw preparations, *J. Comp. Physiol.* **143**:53–60.

Jahromi, S. S. and Atwood, H. L., 1974, Three-dimensional ultrastructure of the crayfish neuromuscular apparatus, *J. Cell Biol.* **63**:599–613.

Kandel, E. R. and Schwartz, J. H., 1982, Molecular biology of learning: Modulation of transmitter release, *Science* **218**:433–443.

Korn, H., Triller, A., Mallet, A., and Faber, D. J., 1981, Fluctuating responses at a central synapse: n of binomial fit predicts number of stained presynaptic boutons, *Science* **213**:898–901.

Lnenicka, G. and Atwood, H. L., 1983, Age-dependent conversion of presynaptic properties at the crayfish neuromuscular junction through altered motoneuron activity, *Soc. Neurosci. Abstr.* **9**:53.

Lowe, D. A., Richardson, B. P., Taylor, P., and Donatsch, P., 1976, Increasing intracellular sodium triggers calcium release from bound stores, *Nature (London)* **260**:337–338.

Magleby, K. C. and Zengel, J. E., 1975, A quantiative description of tetanic and post-tetanic potentiation of transmitter release at the frog neuromuscular junction, *J. Physiol. (Lond.)* **245**:183–208.

Magleby, K C. and Zengel, Z. E., 1976, Long term changes in augmentation, potentiation, and depression of transmitter relase as a function of repeated synaptic activity at the frog neuromuscular junction, *J. Physiol (London)* **257**:471–494.

Rahaminoff, R., Lev-Tov, A., and Meiri, H., 1980, Primary and secondary regulation of quantal transmitter release: Calcium and sodium, *J. Exp. Biol.* **89**:5–18.

Sherman, R. G. and Atwood, H. L., 1971, Synaptic facilitation: Long-term neuromuscular facilitation in crustaceans, *Science* **171**:1248–1250.

Strumwasser, F., 1967, Types of information stored in single neurons, in: *Invertebrate Nervous Systems* (C. A. G. Wiersma, ed.), University of Chicago Press, Chicago, pp. 241–319.

Swenarchuk, L. E., 1975, Long-term facilitation at crayfish neuromuscular synapses, Ph.D. Thesis, University of Toronto.

Swenarchuk, L. E. and Atwood, H. L., 1975, Long-term facilitation with minimal calcium entry, *Brain Res.* **100**:205–208.

Tokunaga, A., Sandri, C., and Akert, K., 1979, Increase of large intramembranous particles in the presynaptic active zone after administration of 4-aminopyridine, *Brain Res.* **174**:207–219.

Wiersma, C. A. G., 1961, The neuromuscular system, in: *The Physiology of Crustacea,* Vol. 2 (T. H. Waterman, ed.), Academic Press, New York, pp. 191–240.

Wojtowicz, J. M. and Atwood, H. L., 1983a, Maintained depolarization of synaptic terminals facilitates nerve-evoked transmitter release at a crayfish neuromuscular junction, *J. Neurobiol.* **14:**385–390.

Wojtowicz, J. M. and Atwood, H. L., 1983b, Presynaptic mechanism of long-term potentiation at the crayfish neuromuscular junction involves sodium ions, *Soc. Neurosci. Abstr.* **9:**169.

Zucker, R. S., 1973, Changes in the statistics of transmitter release during facilitation, *J. Physiol. (London)* **229:**787–810.

24

Acetylcholinesterase and Synaptic Efficacy

P. FOSSIER, G. BAUX, and L. TAUC

1. INTRODUCTION

AChE has long been implicated in the control of neurotransmission at cholinergic synapses, where it assumes the important function of hydrolyzing ACh released from nerve terminals. Since cholinergic neuronal systems are considered to be involved in many essential brain activities, including behavioral changes such as agressivity, reward and punishment, or learned approach and avoidance behavior (for review, see Hingtgen and Aprison, 1976), the precise definition of the role of AChE in synaptic transmission is of particular interest.

The physiological function of AChE was mostly disclosed by studies using application of drugs that inhibited the AChE enzymatic activity in a reversible or irreversible manner. Prominent effects of AChE, inhibitors (AChEIs) are observed at the skeletal neuromuscular junction, where the amplitude and the duration of the end-plate potential (EPP) and of the miniature EPP are increased (e.g., Katz and Miledi, 1973). This effect was considered to be a consequence of an increase of ACh concentration in the synaptic cleft resulting from the blocking of AChE activity (Laskowski and Dettbarn, 1979; Morrison, 1977; Skliarov, 1980). Katz and Miledi (1973) hypothesized that a single ACh molecule can successively bind to several postsynaptic receptors ("rebinding") and thus account for the increase in duration of the postsynaptic response.

At vertebrate ganglionic cholinergic synapses (Eccles, 1944), however, the postsynaptic response is not modified when AChE is blocked, indicating that, at these synapses, AChE does not play a major role in the inactivation of released ACh. It appears that the main reason for this difference lies in the different geometry of the end plate compared to that of a neuroneuronal synapse: ACh can accumulate within the cleft of the neuromuscular junction whereas at a neuroneuronal synapse,

P. FOSSIER, G. BAUX, and L. TAUC ● Laboratoire de Neurobiologie Cellulaire, Centre National de La Recherche Scientifique, F-91190 Gif sur Yvette, France

it diffuses rapidly into the intercellular space. Only repetitive preganglionic stimulation in the presence of AChE showed that AChE limits intraganglionic diffusion of ACh (Bennett and McLachlan, 1972).

We have found, however, that a central inhibitory cholinergic synapse of *Aplysia,* AChEIs clearly increased the unitary postsynaptic response. The response to ionophoretic application of ACh was also facilitated. This could not be explained by the inhibition of the ACh hydrolyzing function of the enzyme, as the response to ionophoretic injection of carbachol was also potentiated by the AChEIs, and carbachol is well known as not being hydrolyzed by AChE. Experimental analysis presented in this chapter indicates that the facilitation of the postsynaptic response and of the responses to ACh and to carbachol by AChEIs may result from a change in a molecular inhibitory action of AChE on the acetylcholine receptor (AChR) rather than from a direct action of AChEIs on the AChR.

2. MATERIAL AND METHODS

Experiments were performed on isolated and desheathed ganglia of *Aplysia californica* (Pacific Bio Marine Company, California). We used two identified cholinergic interneurons that induce inhibitory Cl⁻ dependent postsynaptic responses (H-type response) (Tauc and Gerschenfeld, 1962) in several identified postsynaptic cells in the buccal ganglion (Gardner, 1971; Gardner and Kandel, 1977) and R_{15}, which is situated in the abdominal ganglion and which has cholinergic receptors opening cationic channels (D-type response) (Tauc and Gerschenfeld, 1962).

Current recordings of postsynaptic responses evoked by a presynaptic spike or ionophoretic application of the agonist were performed using a classical voltage clamp. Because in these central cells it is not possible to record individual postsynaptic currents resulting from the release of quanta from a given interneuron, quantal aspects of the transmission in the buccal ganglion were obtained by an indirect method as previously described (Simonneau *et al.,* 1980a; Simonneau *et al.,* 1980b). Briefly, both pre- and postsynaptic neurons were simultaneously voltage-clamped to holding potentials of -50 mV and -80 mV, respectively. When the voltage-dependent Na⁺ conductance was blocked by tetrodotoxin (TTX), a depolarization of the presynaptic neurone gave rise to a prolonged release of the transmitter from the terminal located a few hundreds of micrometers from the soma. The response recorded in the postsynaptic cell showed fluctuations or noise resulting from the summation of discrete events, representing miniature postsynaptic currents (MPSCs). Using a computer, it was then possible to apply to this response statistical analysis and calculate from Campbell's theorem and the power density spectra (Katz and Miledi, 1972) the amplitude of a single miniature postsynaptic response and the time constant of its decay. Similarly, the Cl⁻ channel parameters were calculated using a fast Fourier transform from the response to prolonged ionophoretic applications of ACh or carbachol onto the somatic receptors (Simmoneau *et al.,* 1980b; Gardner and Stevens, 1980).

As in most *Aplysia* central neurons (Tauc and Geschenfeld, 1962), AChRs of the buccal postsynaptic cells are not confined to the synapse but are also distributed on the soma, which is devoid of synaptic contacts. ACh and carbachol were alternately applied at the same membrane spot using a constant current source and a double-barreled electrode or two single electrodes filled with the agonists at 1 M concentration. Braking current was applied to the electrodes not in use. Before application of the drugs, the position of the ionophoretic electrodes was adjusted to obtain the maximal response for a given injecting current, and extreme care was taken to ascertain that, in the absence of additional experimental manipulations, repeated injections gave uniform responses.

In all experiments, the Cl^- reversal potential of the postsynaptic cells was monitored frequently, as was the temperature. Current amplitudes were routinely transformed into conductances. The preparation was continuously perfused with normal saline or saline to which drugs were added.

AChEs inhibitors used were: phospholine at a concentration of 5×10^{-4} M; parathion at 3×10^{-4} M; MPT (O-ethyl 5-2-diisopropyl-amino-ethyl methylphosphonothioate) at 2×10^{-4} M; prostigmine at 5×10^{-6} M. Contrathion (pralidoxime sulfomethylate) at 10^{-3} M was used as a reactivator of AChE. Tetrodotoxin (10^{-4} M) was obtained from Sigma. Triton X100 was used in the range 0.0005%–0.00025% and sodium deoxycholate in the range 10^{-7} M–10^{-9} M. Normal saline composition was: NaCl, 460 mM; KCl, 10 mM; $CaCl_2$, 11 mM; $MgCl_2$, 25 mM; $MgSO_4$, 28 mM; Tris-HCl, 10 mM, pH 7.8. The action of each AChE inhibitor was studied on at least ten preparations (28 for phospholine) for both ACh and carbachol.

3. RESULTS

When AChEIs were applied to the buccal ganglion preparation, the postsynaptic current (PSC) response to evoked spike was potentiated. With organophosphate inhibitors that are known to have a reversible curarelike action when present in the bath (Fossier *et al.*, 1983a), it was first necessary to wash the preparation for about 10 min to remove the depressing effect of the drug on the AChR and to observe the potentiation of the response (Fig. 1). Also in this case it was possible by applying to the preparation an oxime, contrathion (10^{-3} M), and then washing it with artificial sea water, to restore the test amplitude of the response (Fig. 1). The carbamate prostigmine at the concentration used (5×10^{-6} M) only showed a facilitatory effect (Fig. 1). The postsynaptic response could also be facilitated by the oxime contrathion (5×10^{-5} M), which upon application first increased the PSC (Fig. 2B) and then exerted a curarelike depressive action (Fossier *et al.*, 1983a).

Using the above described method, quantal analysis of the postsynaptic responses submitted to AChEIs showed that the increase of the postsynaptic response was not due to an increase in the number of quanta liberated but to an increase in the size of individual miniature postsynaptic currents (MPSCs) (Fossier *et al.*, 1983a).

Current responses to ionophoretically applied ACh on the somatic H receptors were depressed by organophosphate inhibitors. Upon washing the preparation, the amplitude of the response increased as much as 300% of the test response. This

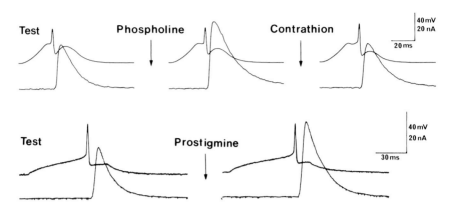

FIGURE 1. Effects of AChEIs on the H-type synapse. Upper traces, direct spikes in the pre-synaptic neurones; lower traces, evoked presynaptic currents recorded in a postsynaptic cell voltage clamped at -80 mV. The postsynaptic response was potentiated in the presence of prostigmine (5×10^{-6} M) or by phospholine (10^{-3} M) followed by washing. The oxime, contra-thion (10^{-3} M), restored the test amplitude of the postsynaptic response after phospholine treatment.

response returned to control level when the preparation was perfused with the reactivator contrathion for 10 min followed by prolonged washing (Fig. 3). To obtain the reactivation it was necessary, however, to avoid "aging" of the AChE–organophosphorus complex and apply rapidly the oxime without waiting sufficient time to completely wash out the "curarelike" effect of AChEIs. This explains the relatively small potentiation of the response in Fig. 3. The current responses to ACh ionophoretic application were also potentiated in the presence of prostigmine (Fig. 4) and contrathion (Fig. 2A).

The observed potentiations could be due to the inhibition of the ACh-hydro-

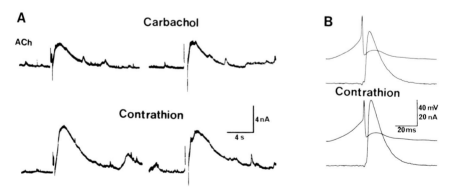

FIGURE 2. The oxime contrathion could act as an AChEI on H-type cells. Contrathion at 5×10^{-5} M and 10^{-4} M, respectively, increased the size of the postsynaptic response (B) as well as the amplitude of the response to ionophoretic application of ACh or carbachol (A).

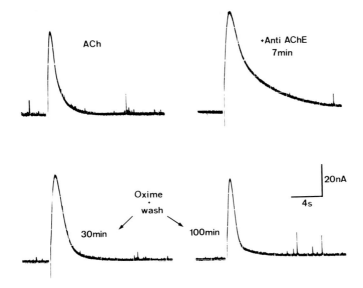

FIGURE 3. Ionophoretic injection of ACh on the somata of a postsynaptic cell (H cell) voltage clamped at -80 mV in the buccal ganglion: increase of the response by ecothiopate iodide $(2.10^{-4}$ M) and reactivation by treatment with contrathion $(10^{-3}$ M) during 10 min and wash.

lyzing function of AChE, thus leading to an increase in available ACh. However, when carbachol was applied and the preparation submitted to the same treatments, the current responses were also potentiated (Figs. 2,4) (Fossier *et al.*, 1983b). The potentiation of the carbachol response cannot be due to an increase of available agonist because carbachol is not hydrolyzed by AChE. Also, because there is no synapse on the soma, an indirect effect of AChE resulting in ACh leakage or activation of some presynaptic endings is unlikely. Carbachol was applied to the soma, which was freely exposed to the perfusing fluid, so that the distribution of

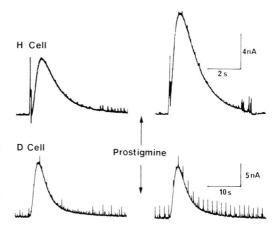

FIGURE 4. The AChEI prostigmine $(5 \times 10^{-6}$ M) potentiated the response to ionophoretic application of carbachol on H-type cell of the buccal ganglion (upper line), whereas it had no effect on carbachol response in a D-type cell of the abdominal ganglion (lower line).

concentrations of the drug over the injected region at different moments was probably identical whether AChE was active or inhibited. Furthermore, none of the observed changes could be attributed to a modification of the Cl⁻ reversal potential, as this was monitored throughout all experiments.

Thus, the potentiation of the responses could be attributed to a change in the properties of the ACh receptor, resulting in either a change in Cl⁻ channel characteristics or in an increased number of activated AChRs. When the mean currents induced by ACh and carbachol were identical, the single channel Cl⁻ conductance for channels opened by carbachol was greater than for those opened by ACh (Baux and Tauc, 1983). With a mean response of 20 nS, the channel conductance calculated was 3.4 ± 0.8 pS for ACh and 5.2. ± 1.1 pS for carbachol. The power density spectrum of the current noise produced by application of carbachol was shifted towards higher frequencies with respect to the ACh spectrum (Fig. 5). Whatever the reason for these differences in calculated conductances and open times for ACh and carbachol, we found that the channel parameters were not changed significantly by organophosphorus compounds or prostigmine. Channel conductance was 3.5 ± 0.7 pS for ACh and 4.7 ± 1.0 pS for carbachol in eight experiments after AChE inhibition using phospholine.

Thus, as the channel characteristics were unmodified when AChE was inactivated, it seems likely that the potentiated response to carbachol following AChE inhibition was due to "recruitment" of an increased number of AChRs. This might be due to a change in receptor affinity so that more channels opened for a given dose of agonist.

The potentiating effects of AChE inhibitors were not observed in the R_{15}

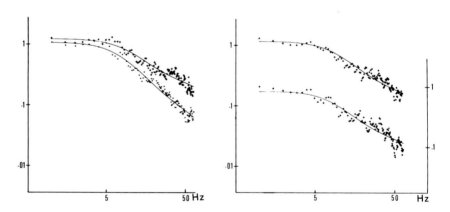

FIGURE 5. AChR channel properties. (Left curves) spectral density calculated from a fast Fourier transform of Cl⁻ channel noise: ionophoretic application on the same membrane spot of ACh (lower trace) and of carbachol (upper trace). Double Lorentzians (solid lines) were fitted to the data points. The open time of the slow component was 21 msec for ACh and 17 msec for carbachol (temperature 20°C). (Right curves) spectral density of carbachol Cl⁻ channel noise before (upper trace) and after application of phospholine (2×10^{-4} M) and prolonged wash (lower trace). The two power spectra are superimposable, indicating that the channel parameters were not changed by the organophosphate AChEI.

neuron, which contains D-type ACh receptor-opening cationic, mostly sodium-selective channels (Gerschenfeld *et al.*, 1967; Stinnakre, 1970; Tauc and Gerschenfeld, 1962). In this cell, the evoked postsynaptic response, as well as the response to the ionophoretic application of carbachol, was not modified by any of the AChE inhibitors used (Fig. 4). This absence of action not only indicated differences in functional receptor properties between R_{15} and the postsynaptic buccal ganglionic neurons but also could be considered as a good control: it shows that AChE inhibitors did not act nonspecifically on the neuronal membrane and that the potentiation was not due to an experimental artifact such as local movements of the ionophoretic micropipettes.

Because all kinds of AChEIs produce a similar facilitation of the agonist responses in spite of quite different molecular constitution, it seems unlikely that AChEIs act directly on the AChR. Our results are rather in agreement with a hypothesis that would postulate the existence of a molecular relationship between AChE and the neighboring AChR, in which AChE exerts an action on some property of the AChR that modulates its readiness to be activated by ACh. Such an action would differ whether AChE was in active or inactive state, active AChE exerting an inhibitory effect.

To test this hypothesis we attempted to change this assumed molecular interaction between AChE and AChR by perturbing the lipidic surroundings in which both macromolecules are embedded. The experiments using the detergents Triton X-100 and sodium deoxycholate confirmed the proposed hypothesis.

Detergents at concentrations greater than 0.0005% for Triton X-100 and 10^{-7} M sodium deoxycholate depressed current responses to ionophoretically applied ACh or carbachol for both D- or H-type receptors. This depression most probably was due to a direct action of the detergents on AChRs and was previously observed on neuromuscular junction (Anwyl and Narahashi, 1980). On the contrary, lower concentrations of the detergents produced a clear increase of the responses, but this increase was seen only for H-type receptors (Figs. 6 and 7). Triton X-100 at low concentration also facilitated the evoked postsynaptic current at the H-type synapse but was without effect at D-type synapses.

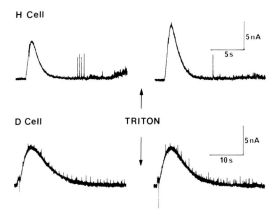

FIGURE 6. The bath applied detergent Triton X-100 (0.0005%) increased the size of the response to ionophoretic application of carbachol in a H-type cell (upper recordings), whereas it did not change the carbachol response in a D-type cell (lower recordings).

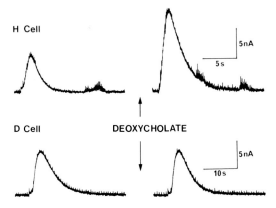

FIGURE 7. The detergent sodium deoxycholate (10^{-9} M) acted differently on H-type or D-type cells. It potentiated the response to ionophoretic application of carbachol onto H-type cell (upper line), but no change was observed when a D-type cell was used (lower line).

Moreover, no cumulative effect of AChEIs and detergents was observed: when the maximal potentiating effect of one compound has been obtained, the other compound did not additionally increase the response, whatever the order of application. This result indicates that both AChE and detergents probably act on the same mechanism. This latter could be the membrane fluidity if AChEIs acted also as detergents. However, with 30-min washing, the facilitatory effect of detergents was reversible, whereas that of organophosphate inhibition was not, unless AChE reactivators were used (Fossier *et al.*, 1983b).

4. DISCUSSION

To interpret our experimental results the following points have to be underlined:
In H-type cells:

1. AChEIs potentiated PSC and MPSC; the quantal content of PSC remained unchanged.
2. AChEIs also potentiated responses not only to ACh but also to carbachol ionophoretic application on the AChR. Yet carbachol is not hydrolyzed by AChE.
3. The potentiations were independent of the nature of AChEI used: liposoluble and non-lipo-soluble organophosphate compounds, carbamates, oximes.
4. When organophosphate AChEIs were used the reactivation of AChE by the oximes brought the response to control size. Such a reactivation is known as a very specific reaction (Wilson and Ginsburg, 1955).
5. The potentiation of the responses was due to an increased number of activated AChRs.

6. Detergents mimic the action of AChEIs.
7. The maximal potentiations of the responses by detergents and by AChEIs were not cumulative.

In D-type cells:
No potentiation was observed with either AChEIs or detergents.

The depression of synaptic or agonist responses with high concentrations of AChEIs or detergents in both H- and D-type cells resulted most probably from a direct action of these compounds on the AChR, as the specific potentiation of the H-type AChRs was only obtained with very low concentrations. It should also be noted that the facilitation of the responses induced by organophosphate inhibitors was measured following washout of the inhibitor and was irreversible, whereas washing did remove the facilitation produced by detergents. The irreversibility of organophosphates action indicates that most probably these AChEIs did not incorporate in the lipidic membrane and did not act directly on the membrane fluidity in a way similar to detergents. Also, it would be difficult to explain how the membrane fluidity would be directly modified by AChEIs such as pholine or prostigmine, which are not lipo-soluble.

Considering the combined results obtained with AChEIs (Fossier *et al.*, 1983b) and with the detergents on H- and D-type cells it seems unlikely that the facilitation of the responses to agonists is due to a direct action of these compounds on the AChR. As an alternative, we propose that the probability of the AChR entering into its active state can be modulated by its molecular environment. This may be represented by some protein-to-protein interaction, in which the conformational aspect of the AChE molecule in its active or inactive state might exert an inhibitory action on the AChR.

The hypothesis assumes that AChE is present in the postsynaptic membrane and that AChE and AChR are arranged in a specific spatial relationship. It is known that AChE is present in *Aplysia* ganglia, that it is the most potent esterase (Dettbarn and Rosenberg, 1962), and that it is present in the somatic membrane of both H and D cells, together with AChR (Fig. 8).

The role of the lipidic environment surrounding the AChE and AChR molecules is certainly of importance and interactions between the AChR and "boundary lipids" have been described (Neubig *et al.*, 1979; Klymkowski *et al.*, 1980; Gonzalez-Ros *et al.*, 1982). It is not impossible that such protein–lipid interactions may also exist between AChE and surrounding lipids.

Two models can be proposed: both conform to our experimental results. In the first model, a conformational change in the AChE molecule induced by an AChEI could induce a local increase in the membrane fluidity which affects the properties of the neighbouring AChR (Fig. 9). Detergents would similarly affect the membrane fluidity and thus mimic the effect of AChEIs. It may be of some importance to mention that the fluidity of *Aplysia* neuronal membranes is normally very low due to a large content of cholesterol (Lamar-Stephens and Shinitzky, 1977; Shinitzky and Inbar, 1976).

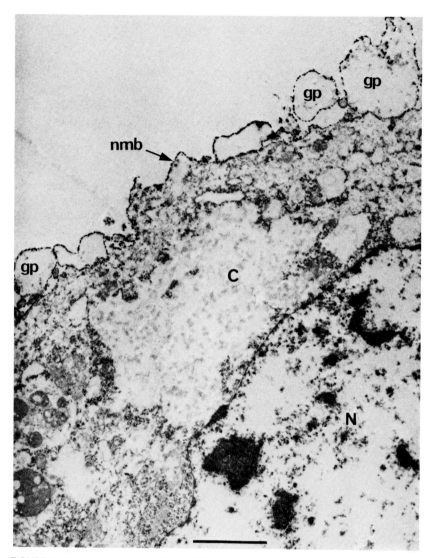

FIGURE 8. Electron micrograph of a small H cell of the buccal ganglion of Aplysia. The preparation was histochemically treated to reveal AChE according to Koelle's method. The labeling
of the membrane of the neuron and of glial membranes is clearly visible on the top of the
micrograph. gp, glial process; nmb, neuronal membrane; N, neuron nucleus; C, neuron cytoplasm. Bar, 2 μm.

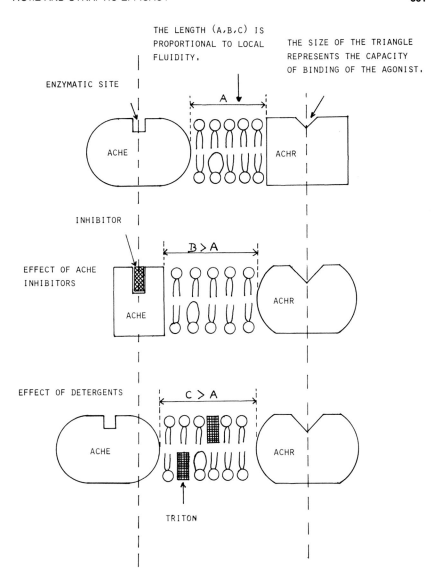

FIGURE 9. Scheme of a possible model explaining the facilitation of AChR in which a hypo-
thetical conformational change of inhibited AChE molecule affects the distance between the
enzyme and AChR, thus modifying molecular forces between the two molecules. The distance
would similarly be increased by inclusion of detergents in the surrounding lipidic membrane. In
an alternative model, the faculty of AChR to be activated by ACh or ACh agonist is dependent
on local membrane fluidity; this latter may be locally influenced by the activity of the AChE
molecule.

The schematic action would be as follows:

$$AChE \rightarrow membrane\ fluidity \rightarrow AChR$$

The absence of action of AChEIs and of detergents on D-type receptors might then be explained by a small dependence on membrane fluidity of the probability of AChR entering into its active state.

In the second model, the lipidic environment would have a relatively passive role: a change in fluidity could increase the distances or change some molecular forces between neighboring AChE and AChR molecules and thus remove the inhibitory action that AChE might normally exert on the AChR. The conformational change of AChE induced by the action of an AChEI would similarly remove the inhibitory effect. The interaction is then more direct: $AChE \rightarrow AChR$. The absence of effect of AChEIs or detergents on D-type receptors may be then due, in addition to the specific properties of D-type receptors, to a difference in AChE distribution or to a difference in positioning of AChE with respect to the AChR.

Whichever of these two models is applicable, our results suggest an experimental model of molecular interaction between neighboring membrane proteins that depends on their states of activity and on their immediate lipidic environment. This kind of behavior is probably a very common property of macromolecular components of the cytoplasmic membrane. However, it is rarely observed, as the experimental demonstration of such interaction is conditional on the presence of a measurable parameter. This is the case here for the proposed relationship between the AChE and AChR molecules of H-type cells.

Our experiments were made at neuroneuronal synapses and on somatic membranes where AChE is membrane-bound (Giller and Schwartz, 1971). This situation is different from that for the neuromuscular junction, where the ultrastructural organization is distinct and more complex. It would then be expected that only some types of central or ganglionic synapses would show properties similar to *Aplysia* H-type junctions. Yet whatever are the limitations and whatever is the basis of modifications which we have described in the present study, our results point to a new possible mechanism that can control the efficacy of a cholinergic synapse. Given the fact that AChE activity changes during maturation (Kullberg *et al.,* 1980; Black, 1978; Burt, 1968) and in learning situations, the existence of such a modulating factor may be of central importance.

ACKNOWLEDGMENTS. We are grateful to Dr. K. Takeda for helpful comments. This work was supported by Grants DRET No. 83/1124 and ATP No. 950501 to L.T.

REFERENCES

Anwyl, K. and Narahashi, T., 1980, Comparison of desensitization and time-dependent block of the acetylcholine responses by chloropromazine, cytochalasin B, Triton X-100 and other agents, *Br. J. Pharmacol.* **69**(1):99.

Baux, G. and Tauc, L., 1983, Carbachol can be released at a cholinergic ganglionic synapse as a false transmitter, *Proc. Natl. Acad. Sci. USA* **80**:5126–5128.

Bennett, M. R. and McLachlan, E. M., 1972, An electrophysiological analysis of the storage of acetylcholine in preganglionic nerve terminals, *J. Physiol. (London)* **221**:657–668.

Black, I. B., 1978, Regulation of autonomic development, *Annu. Rev. Neurosci.* **1**:183–214.

Burt, A. M., 1968, Acetylcholinesterase and choline acetyltransferase activity in the developing chick spinal cord, *J. Exp. Zool.* **169**:107–112.

Dettbarn, W. D. and Rosenberg, P., 1962, Acetylcholinesterase in *Aplysia. Biochim. Biophys. Acta* **65**:362–363.

Eccles, J. C., 1944, The nature of synaptic transmission in a sympathetic ganglion, *J. Physiol. (London)* **103**:27–54.

Fossier, P., Baux, G., and Tauc, L., 1983a, Direct and indirect effects of an organophophorus acetylcholinesterase inhibitor and of an oxime on a neuro-neuronal synapse, *Pflügers Arch.* **396**:15–22.

Fossier, P., Baux, G., and Tauc, L., 1983b, Possible role of acetylcholinesterase in regulation of postsynaptic receptor efficacy at a central inhibitory synapse of *Aplysia, Nature* **301**:710–712.

Gardner, D., 1971, Bilateral symmetry and interneuronal organization in the buccal ganglia of *Aplysia, Science* **173**:550–553.

Gardner, D. and Kandel, E. R., 1977, Physiological and kinetic properties of cholinergic receptors activated by multiaction interneurons in buccal ganglia in Aplysia, *J. Neurophysiol.* **40**:333–348.

Gardner, D. and Stevens, C. F., 1980, Rate-limiting step of inhibitory post-synaptic current decay in *Aplysia* buccal ganglia. *J. Physiol. (London)* **304**:145–164.

Gerschenfeld, H. M., Ascher, P., and Tauc, L., 1967, Two different excitatory transmitters acting on a single molluscan neurone, *Nature* **213**:358–359.

Giller, E. Jr. and Schwartz, J. H., 1971, Acetylcholinesterase in identified neurons of abdominal ganglion of *Aplysia californica, J. Neurophysiol.* **34**:108–115.

Gonzalez-Ros, J. M., Llanillo, M., Paraschos, A., and Martinez-Carrion, M., 1982, Lipid environment of acetylcholine receptor from *Torpedo californica. Biochemistry* **21**:3467–3474.

Hingten, J. N. and Aprison, M. H., 1976, Behavioral and environmental aspects of the cholinergic system, in: *Biology of Cholinergic Function* (A. M. Goldberg and I. Hanin, eds.), Raven Press, New York, pp. 515–566.

Katz, B. and Miledi, R., 1972, The statistical nature of the acetylcholine potential and its molecular components, *J. Physiol. (London)* **224**:665–699.

Katz, B. and Miledi, R., 1973, The binding of acetylcholine to receptors and its removal from the synaptic cleft, *J. Physiol. (London)* **231**:549–574.

Klymkowski, M. W., Heuser, J. E., and Stroud, R. M., 1980, Protease effects on the structure of acetylcholine receptor membranes from *Torpedo californica, J. Cell Biol.* **85**:823–838.

Kullberg, R. W., Mikelberg, F. S., and Cohen, M. W., 1980, Contribution of cholinesterase to developmental decrease in the time course of synaptic potentials at an amphibian neuromuscular junction, *Develop. Biol.* **75**:255–267.

Lamar Stephens, C. and Shinitzky, M., 1977, Modulation of electrical activity in *Aplysia* neurones by cholesterol, *Nature* **270**:267–268.

Lakowski, M. B. and Dettbarn, W. D., 1979, An electrophysiological analysis of the effects of paraoxon at the neuromuscular junction. *J. Pharmacol. Exp. Ther.* **210**:269–274.

Morrison, J. D., 1977, The generation of nerve and muscle repetitive activity in the rat phrenic nerve-diaphragm preparation following inhibition of cholinesterase by ecothiopate, *Br. J. Pharmacol.* **60**:45–53.

Neubig, R. R., Krodel, E. K., Boyd, N. D., and Cohen, J. B., 1979, Acetylcholine and local anesthetic binding to Torpedo nicotinic postsynaptic membranes after removal of non receptor peptides, *Proc. Natl. Acad. Sci. USA* **76**:690–694.

Shinitzky, M. and Inbar, M., 1976, Microviscosity parameters and protein mobility in biological membranes, *Biochim. Biophys. Acta* **433**:133–149.

Simonneau, M., Tauc, L., and Baux, G., 1980a, Quantal release of acetylcholine examined by current fluctuation analysis at an identified neuro-neuronal synapse of *Aplysia, Proc. Natl. Acad. Sci. USA* **77**:1661–1665.

Simonneau, M., Baux, G., and Tauc, L., 1980b, Quantal analysis of transmitter release at an identified synapse, in: *Ontogenesis and Functional Mechanisms of Peripheral Synapses*, INSERM Symposium, Volume 13 (J. Taxi, ed.), Elsevier/North-Holland Biomedical Press, Amsterdam, pp. 179–189.

Skliarov, A. I., 1980, The effect of anticholinesterase drugs on postjunctional potentials of skeletal muscle, *Gen. Pharmacol.* **11**:89–95.

Stinnakre, J., 1970, Action de l'hémicholinium sur une synapse centrale d'Aplysie, *J. Physiol. (Paris)* **62**(Suppl. 3):452–453.

Tauc, L. and Gerschenfeld, H. M., 1961, Cholinergic transmission mechanisms for both excitation and inhibition in molluscan central synapses, *Nature* **192**:366–367.

Tauc, L. and Gerschenfeld, H. M., 1962, A cholinergic mechanism of inhibitory synaptic transmission in a molluscan nervous system, *J. Neurophysiol.* **25**:236–262.

Wilson, I. B. and Ginsburg, S., 1955, A powerful reactivator of alkylphosphate inhibited acetylcholinesterase, *Biochim. Biophys. Acta* **18**:168–170.

25

Segregation of Synaptic Function on Excitable Cells

D. O. CARPENTER, J. M. H. FFRENCH-MULLEN, N. HORI, C. N. SINBACK, and W. SHAIN

1. INTRODUCTION

The neuron has long been considered the fundamental "unit" of the brain, functioning as a go–no-go switch. In many ways this assumption is not inaccurate, particularly with regard to the axon and the process of spike generation and transmission. This assumption is also not incompatible with the individual neuron's role as an integrator of synaptic activity, where the go–no-go signal is determined by the admixture of synaptic excitation and inhibition.

This view of the neuron, however, ignores the possibility that the synaptic inputs may not be distributed equally over the soma and dendrites—that inputs may in fact be specifically localized. If this is true, the neuron itself may be correspondingly complex, with various regions having specialized functions. There may then be levels of integration of information between such regions of the synaptic area that are totally unseen by a probing microelectrode, which can detect only the net potential at one point in the cell.

Perhaps the clearest example of a cell with an extreme specialization is the B-type retinal horizontal cell (Nelson *et al.*, 1975). This cell has an extensive axonal elaboration, which receives input only from rods, while the cell body receives input only from cones. The two dendritic systems appear to be electrically isolated from each other. Thus the only purpose of the connection is nutritive, and the two parts function independently.

While most neurons probably do not have as extreme segregation of function

D. O. CARPENTER, J. M. H. FFRENCH-MULLEN, N. HORI, C. N. SINBACK, and W. SHAIN ● Center for Laboratories and Research, New York State Department of Health, Albany, New York 12201. *Present address* for N. H.: Department of Pharmacology, Kyushu University School of Dentistry, Fukuoka, Japan. *Present address* for C.N.S.: Laboratory of Cell Biology, National Cancer Institute, National Institutes of Health, Bethesda, Maryland 20205.

and as clear an anatomic basis for the segregation, localization of synaptic function can be indicated in other anatomic and physiologic ways. In some large neurons, such as cerebellar Purkinje cells or pyramidal cells of cortex, all neurons are similarly oriented, and known synaptic inputs go to specific regions of the cell. For example, in Purkinje cells the climbing fibers innervate the soma and proximal dendrites, while the parallel fibers innervate the more distal dendrites. The fibers of the lateral olfactory tract (LOT) terminate only in the region of the most distal dendrites of the pyramidal neurons of prepyriform cortex (Shepherd, 1979).

The experiments we report here are concerned with specific localization of transmitter receptors on portions of excitable cells. Segregation of receptors is another indication of localized functions, particularly when a single transmitter elicits responses of opposing polarity on different parts of the same cell.

2. METHODS

Two preparations were used for these studies. The cell culture experiments were performed on human oviduct smooth muscle cells from a continuous cell line, prepared and studied as described by Sinback and Shain (1979, 1980). In the other studies slices of rat prepyriform cortex were prepared and studied as described by Hori *et al.* (1982) and ffrench-Mullen *et al.* (1983).

3. RESULTS

3.1. Transmitter Receptors on Smooth Muscle Cells

Figure 1 shows the variety of responses obtained from a continuous line of cultured human smooth muscle cells when histamine, acetylcholine (ACh), or noradrenaline was applied by ionophoresis. Each transmitter elicited three types of responses: depolarizing, hyperpolarizing, and biphasic. Thus, even on a single muscle cell, which is not integrative in the way neurons are, one transmitter can elicit both excitation and inhibition.

Figure 2 shows a careful analysis of the distribution of responses of another muscle cell to histamine. This cell is flat and its large surface area allows one to record from the central area near the nucleus while applying histamine by ionophoresis successfully at a number of sites. Application to one side of the cell gave depolarizing responses; application to the other side gave hyperpolarizing responses. The responses at the boundaries of these sites were biphasic—either depolarizing, hyperpolarizing, or hyperpolarizing-depolarizing, depending upon location.

Although the physiologic significance of this receptor distribution is not clear, the responses of this smooth muscle cell demonstrate that (1) there can be receptor localization on a cell; (2) a single cell may have localized receptors for a single transmitter, which elicit different ionic responses; and (3) when receptors for two different ionic responses exist on a single cell one may see only one or the other, depending upon the position of the ionophoretic electrode.

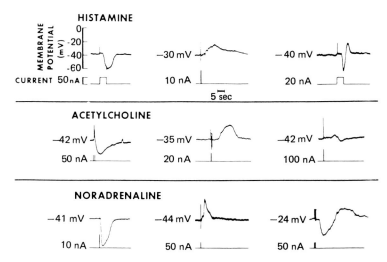

FIGURE 1. Responses of human smooth muscle cells in culture to ionophoretic application of histamine, ACh, or noradrenaline. In each record the upper trace is the intracellular recording, and the lower trace indicates the time of the ionophoretic application. Values for resting membrane potential and ionophoretic current are indicated to the left of each trace. Each record is from a different cell, and for all three transmitters depolarizing, hyperpolarizing, and biphasic responses could be recorded. (From Sinback and Shain, 1980; reproduced with permission of the Wistar Press.)

3.2. Asymmetric Distribution of Receptors on Mammalian Neurons

Figure 3 shows responses of an identified pyramidal neuron recorded from a slice of rat prepyriform cortex. Because this slice was cut parallel to the brain surface and was about 450 μm thick, we could apply transmitters to various portions of the cell with considerable confidence as to where the ionophoretic electrode was positioned.

Pyramidal neurons are all oriented with the cell bodies at a depth of 300–400 μm from the pial surface. They have an extensive apical dendritic tree, which ascends toward the pial surface and often runs laterally for a considerable distance. The fibers of the LOT terminate on these distal apical dendrites (Shepherd, 1979). Since the pyramidal neurons are the only cell type receiving monosynaptic excitation from the LOT, this excitation is a physiologic method for identification of a pyramidal neuron. These neurons also have distinct basal dendrites, which project from the cell body to deeper layers for a distance of at least 50 μm.

This particular neuron was tested for responses to glutamate, aspartate, N-methyl-D-aspartate (NMDA), homocysteate, and ACh, with the ionophoretic electrode placed first at 50 μm from the cut surface (approximately 400 μm from the pial surface) and then 300 μm from the cut surface (approximately 150 μm from the pial surface). The first location corresponded to a site in the region of the basal dendrites and/or the cell body; the second was in the area of the apical dendrites. At both locations the responses to the amino acids were characterized by short-

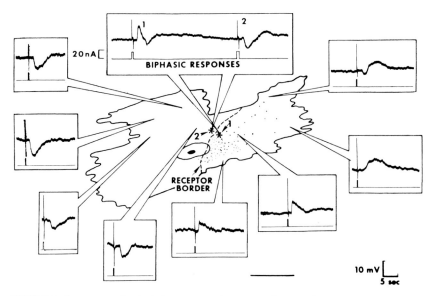

FIGURE 2. Responses of a single human smooth muscle cell to ionophoresed histamine applied at various sites. This cell was recorded from a site near the nucleus, and the ionophoretic electrode was positioned at various sites over the cell, which is greater than 50 μm wide. The ionophoretic current and the distance from the cell to the ionophoretic electrode were constant at sites 1 and 2, with only the location changed. The depolarizing responses at the right were obtained with a lower ionophoretic current. (From Sinback and Shain, 1980; reproduced with permission of the Wistar Press.)

latency and high-frequency discharges. In the basal, but not the apical, dendrites ACh elicited an excitatory response that was considerably longer in both latency and duration than the response to the amino acids. When the LOT was stimulated with two pulses, short-latency excitation was seen.

While responses to the amino acids were readily obtained in all neurons recorded, the ACh response was more variable. Therefore, we used the amino acid responses to search for effects of ACh that might be subthreshold for excitation alone. Figure 4 illustrates the results obtained in a neuron that showed no excitation by ACh. An application of aspartate was used to test the cell's excitability. In the basal dendrites the aspartate ionophoretic current was adjusted so that only two spikes were produced. After application of ACh the aspartate response was markedly facilitated for over 40 sec, indicating an augmenting action of ACh. When the ionophoretic electrode was placed in the apical dendrites, there was no trace of ACh-induced facilitation.

A systematic study of the distribution of ACh receptors on basal and apical dendrites was performed by extracellular recordings from 19 neurons. ACh and either aspartate or glutamate were applied at both sites alone and in combination to test for direct excitation by ACh and potentiation of the amino acid response by ACh. Appropriate placement of the ionophoretic electrode in proximity to the dendritic trees was monitored by the response to aspartate or glutamate. Although

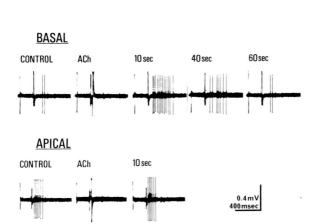

BASAL DENDRITE

| Glu (50 nC) | Asp (50 nC) | NM (50 nC) | HC (10 nC) |

ACh (100 nC)   500 μV 2 sec

LOT   400 μV 20 msec

FIGURE 3. Pattern of responses to amino acids and ACh on basal and apical dendrites of one neuron from rat prepyriform cortex. From the cut surface the ionophoretic electrode was placed 50 μm deep for the basal and 300 μm deep for the apical recordings. Although the relative sensitivities of the amino acid responses are not the same at the two sites, there are brisk responses at both places. ACh produces a delayed but prolonged excitation of the basal dendrites but is without effect on apical dendrites. Glu, glutamate; Asp, Aspartate; NM, NMDA; and HC, homocysteic acid. (From ffrench-Mullen *et al.*, 1983.)

APICAL DENDRITE

| Glu (250 nC) | Asp (10 nC) | NM (3 nC) | HC (8 nC) |

ACh (500 nC)   500 μV 2 sec

LOT   1 mV 20 msec

BASAL

CONTROL   ACh   10 sec   40 sec   60 sec

APICAL

CONTROL   ACh   10 sec

0.4 mV 400 msec

FIGURE 4. Effects of ACh on aspartate responses in basal and apical dendrites of the neuron shown in Fig. 5A. The control responses are to 200 and 75 nA aspartate, applied to basal and apical dendrites, respectively, in 200-msec pulses every 10 sec. ACh was applied at 40 nA for 200 msec, and the aspartate response followed at 10-sec intervals. (From ffrench-Mullen *et al.*, 1983.)

not all neurons were maintained for the full study, there were no exceptions to the patterns of responses obtained. When the ionophoretic electrode was in the region of the basal dendrites direct excitation by ACh was seen in only two of 17 cells, but the remaining 15 showed clear potentiation of the aspartate or glutamate response. None of eight neurons showed either excitation or potentiation by ACh when the ionophoretic electrode was in the apical dendrites.

In order to confirm that receptors are located on basal dendrites and/or cell bodies, but not on apical dendrites, we injected horseradish peroxidase (HRP) intracellularly in as many as possible of the 17 neurons in the systematic study above and in some other neurons that were excited monosynaptically by LOT stimulation. After processing we recovered all or part of more than 20 pyramidal neurons. Figure 5 shows micrographs of two neurons, which confirm the neuronal structure expected from the descriptions of Shepherd (1979). The cell in Fig. 5A, which is the neuron shown in Fig. 4, has a cell body near the cut surface and has clear apical and basal dendrites. The full extent of the apical dendrites of this cell is not seen, since the distal parts were not included in this histological section. The neuron in Fig. 5B has its cell body at a more superficial level (about 100 μm from the cut surface) and although the plane of section has cut some of the basal dendrites, the apical dendrites are intact. All the neurons recovered were of the forms illustrated by these two cells, although most cell bodies were located deeper from the pial surface than in Fig. 5B. These neurons correspond to the deep pyramidal cells described by Shepherd (1979) in that all recovered cells had clear basal and apical dendrites.

In order to characterize the ACh response pharmacologically we selected neurons that showed excitation by ACh or facilitation of an amino acid response by ACh and bath-perfused them with either curare (a nicotinic ACh antagonist) or atropine (a muscarinic ACh antagonist). Figure 6 shows such an experiment in the unusual circumstance where a single electrode placement recorded activity from two different neurons, which had different spike amplitudes. The small neuron was more responsive to glutamate, NMDA, and ACh, although in the records shown the response to glutamate is hidden by that of the larger unit. Perfusion of curare had no significant effect on any of the responses, but atropine totally blocked the ACh responses of both units without significant alteration of the glutamate and NMDA responses.

The next question was whether the ACh effects were direct or indirect: that is, were they due to ACh receptors on pyramidal neurons or to ACh-induced synaptic activity? We studied this by perfusing a slice with a low-Ca^{2+}, high-Mg^{2+} solution, which resulted in a blockade of transmitter release, as confirmed by the ability of LOT stimulation to excite the pyramidal cells. Figure 7 shows the results from a preparation in which we studied ACh potentiation of a glutamate response. Although the low-Ca^{2+}, high-Mg^{2+} medium reduced the excitability somewhat, ACh still potentiated the glutamate response. This observation indicates that the ACh effect is direct and that the receptors are indeed on the basal dendrites and possibly on the cell body of the pyramidal cells.

In order to determine the mechanism whereby ACh exerts these effects, we performed intracellular recordings, applied transmitters by ionophoresis, and mon-

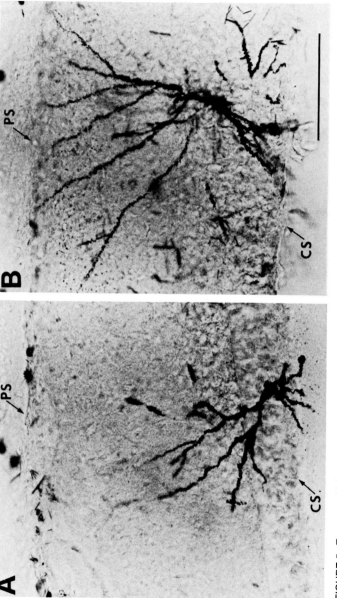

FIGURE 5. Two pyramidal neurons of prepyriform cortex labeled with intracellularly injected HRP. PS, pial surface; CS, cut surface. Because the calibration does not consider the approximately 30% shrinkage of the tissue during fixation, the cell body in (B) is actually greater than 100 μm from the cut surface and nearly 300 μm from the pial surface. (From ffrench-Mullen et al., 1983.)

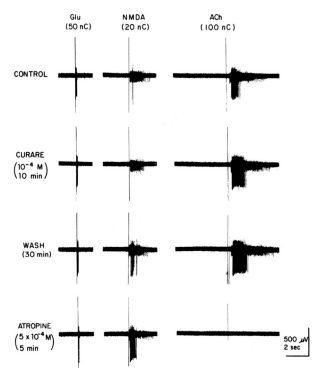

FIGURE 6. Effects of nicotinic and muscarinic antagonists on responses to glutamate (Glu), NMDA, and ACh in two prepyriform neurons, with the ionophoretic electrode in the basal dendritic region. The two neurons are distinguished by spike amplitudes, apparent only with the NMDA and ACh responses. Only the muscarinic antagonist atropine blocked the ACh response, but neither curare or atropine altered the responses to glutamate or NMDA.

itored membrane potential and resistance. Figure 8 shows on experiment where ACh caused a clear facilitation of the glutamate response. However, as seen in this figure, it was usually difficult to record very dramatic effects of ACh on membrane potential and resistance at the resting potential of the cell (usually -65 to -70 mV).

Figure 9 shows plots of the voltage and resistance changes to ACh ionophoresis at resting potential and with a steady DC depolarizing current. The magnitude of the depolarizing response to ACh was greater at depolarized potentials. This finding is consistent with the observations of Brown and Adams (1980), who described a voltage-dependent ACh response in bullfrog sympathetic ganglion that was due to an increase in membrane resistance similar to that observed in this cell (Fig. 9B). Brown and Adams named the channel responsible the "M" channel, since it was altered by muscarine. They demonstrated that this K^+ channel is normally activated by depolarization to potentials more depolarized than -60 mV, that it is distinct from other known K^+ channels, and that the effect of ACh is to prevent the channel from opening in the depolarized voltage range. A principal effect of ACh is consequently an augmentation of the response to any depolarizing stimulus and an

A) CONTROL

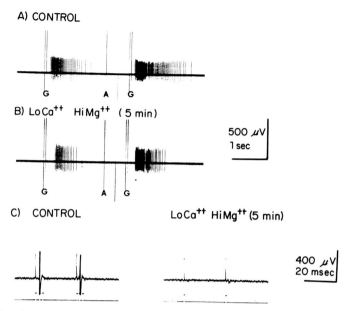

B) LoCa⁺⁺ HiMg⁺⁺ (5 min)

500 μV
1 sec

C) CONTROL   LoCa⁺⁺ HiMg⁺⁺ (5 min)

400 μV
20 msec

FIGURE 7. Effects of perfusion of a low-Ca^{2+}, high-Mg^{2+} medium on ACh (A) potentiation of a glutamate (G) response. Glutamate was applied at 50 nC and ACh at 200 nC to the cut surface. The durations of the ionophoretic application are shown by the long shock artifacts. While ACh did not produce a response directly, it caused an increase in both frequency and duration of the glutamate response (A) in the control medium (2.4 mM Ca^{2+}, 1.3 mM Mg^{2+}), and this was not significantly altered in the low-Ca^{2+} (1.0 mM), high Mg^{2+} (6.3 mM) solution (B). In contrast, the monosynaptic excitation produced by stimulation of the LOT was blocked by this perfusion (C). (From ffrench-Mullen *et al.*, 1983.)

Glu   ACh   Glu

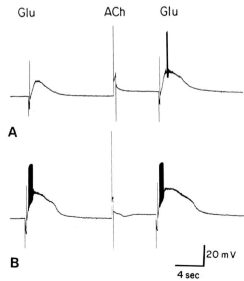

FIGURE 8. Potentiation by ACh of a response to glutamate (Glu). In (A) glutamate was applied at 100 nC and ACh at 400 nC. In (B) glutamate was applied at 200 nC. Ionophoresis was at the cut surface. Membrane potential was −65 mV. These ACh applications did not induce discharge. These records were obtained by playing back taped data at a slower than recorded speed onto a Gould pen recorder. There is some distortion of the spikes, giving a smaller than actual spike amplitude. (From ffrench-Mullen *et al.*, 1983.)

A

B

20 mV
4 sec

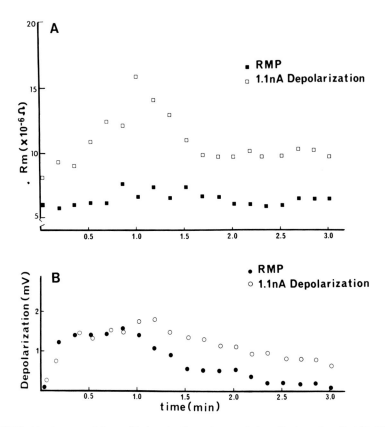

FIGURE 9. Membrane resistance (Rm) and voltage changes induced by ionophoretic ACh. The neuron had a resting potential of -68 mV. (A) Resistance changes as a function of time after a 5-sec pulse of ACh (200 nA), applied first at resting membrane potential (■, RMP), then in the presence of a constant depolarizing current of 1.1 nA (□). The resistance was measured from the voltage shift produced by a 1-nA depolarizing pulse, 30 msec in duration. (B) Voltage shift produced by the same applications as a function of time. (From ffrench-Mullen *et al.*, 1983.)

increased tendency to repetitive discharge. Figure 10 shows the current–voltage curve of the cell illustrated in Fig. 9 with and without ACh at an ionophoretic dose sufficient to potentiate the response to aspartate. The effect of ACh was to alter the resistance only at the most depolarized levels, where resistance was increased considerably.

Figure 11 shows the effects of ACh ionophoresis on a subthreshold response to aspartate and a depolarizing current pulse. After an ionophoretic pulse of ACh, both were equally facilitated. This is consistent with the conclusion that ACh acts to turn off a voltage-sensitive conductance such that no matter what the source of the depolarizing stimulus, the response is potentiated in the presence of ACh.

M channels are blocked by Ba^{2+}, presumably as a result of a direct action on the channel (Constanti *et al.*, 1981). If the ACh response is mediated through M channels, it should be mimicked by Ba^{2+} application. Figure 12 shows that this

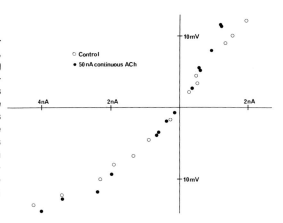

FIGURE 10. Current–voltage relations of the cell shown in Fig. 9, obtained by passing depolarizing and hyperpolarizing constant-current pulses of various amplitudes through the bridge circuit of the amplifier. Bridge balance was carefully controlled. A second curve was obtained during continuous application of 50 nA ACh, which caused potentiation of the response to ionophoretic aspartate but did not cause discharge. (From ffrench-Mullen et al., 1983.)

was indeed the case when Ba^{2+} was applied by ionophoresis in the region of the basal dendrites.

M channels also occur coupled to other transmitter receptors, such as those for lutenizing hormone-releasing hormone (Adams and Brown, 1980) and angiotensin II (Brown et al., 1980). Thus, even though our results show that there are no ACh receptors on apical dendrites, these dendrites have M channels coupled to some other receptor. To test this we applied Ba^{2+} ionophoretically on the apical

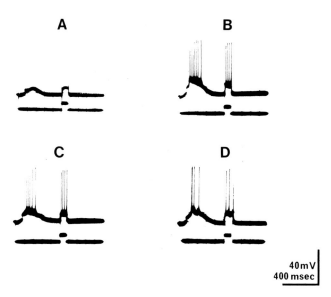

FIGURE 11. ACh potentiation of aspartate responses and of a depolarizing current pulse. The neuron had a resting potential of -72 mV. The upper record in each pair shows the voltage shifts recorded in response to ionophoretic application of 20 nA aspartate (left) and to a depolarizing current pulse of 1.1 nA (right). The lower trace is a current monitor. (A) Control, followed by ionophoretic application of ACh at 200 nA for 5 sec to the basal dendrites. (B, C, D) Responses to the same stimuli after 10, 20, and 40 sec, respectively. (From ffrench-Mullen et al., 1983.)

BASAL DENDRITE

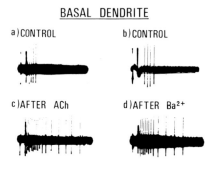

a)CONTROL   b)CONTROL

c)AFTER ACh   d)AFTER Ba²⁺

APICAL DENDRITE

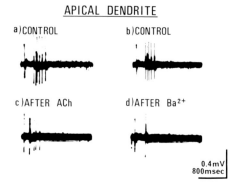

a)CONTROL   b)CONTROL

c)AFTER ACh   d)AFTER Ba²⁺

0.4mV
800msec

FIGURE 12. Effects of Ba^{2+} and ACh on basal and apical dendrites. The ionophoretic electrode for basal dendrites was at the cut surface; the electrode for the apical dendrites was at a 350-μm depth. The controls (a and b) are the response to 200-msec application of 50 and 30 nA aspartate, respectively, in basal and apical dendrites. ACh or Ba^{2+} was applied at 100 and 300 nA respectively, for 5 sec at each site, and traces (c) and (d) were taken 15 sec later. (From ffrench-Mullen *et al.*, 1983.)

dendrites. Neither ACh nor Ba^{2+} augmented the response to aspartate there, and Ba^{2+} actually depressed that response for reasons not understood (Fig. 12). Thus it is unlikely that there are M channels on apical dendrites associated with any type of receptor.

The existence of M channels in these neurons has recently been confirmed by voltage-clamp experiments (Constanti and Galvan, 1983). Thus the ACh receptors and their associated ion channel in this system are similar to those found elsewhere (Kelly *et al.*, 1979; Krnjević, 1981) but differ in being of restricted location.

4. DISCUSSION

4.1. Multiple Effects of a Single Transmitter on One Cell

The major conclusions from these studies are that (1) synaptic inputs and neurotransmitter receptors may be segregated to particular parts of a neuron and (2) a single transmitter may be used for totally different functions on different parts of the same single neuron, sometimes acting through different postsynaptic mechanisms. Although support for these conclusions comes from relatively few preparations, there is reason to believe that these are general principles of neuronal organization.

Until 15 years ago Dale's Principle, as enunciated by Eccles (1957), was a law of neurobiology. This principle stated that a neuron could make and release only a single transmitter and that the transmitter could have only one effect on postsynaptic neurons. Work done principally with invertebrate preparations showed that the latter postulate was not true. Kandel *et al.* (1967) found five interneurons in the abdominal ganglion of *Aplysia,* each of which mediated excitation of some and inhibition of other follower cells. Later Wachtel and Kandel (1967) and Gardner and Kandel (1972) showed that a single neuron could elicit a biphasic response on a postsynaptic neuron. There were differing rates of desensitization of the two components, such that the synapse was excitatory at low frequencies of stimulation but inhibitory at higher frequencies. Carew and Kandel (1976) studied a different *Aplysia* neuron that also caused a biphasic response. This response had two depolarizing phases, the first a conductance increase and the second a conductance decrease. These authors were able to ascribe different functions to the two phases: While the first phase had conventional effects, the second appeared to regulate the degree of electrotonic coupling between follower cells. Together these results show convincingly that a single presynaptic neuron, presumably releasing one transmitter, may have more than one action at a single site.

In vertebrate systems multiple responses to transmitters also exist. In sympathetic ganglia, for example, there are both nicotinic and muscarinic receptors, and some evidence indicates that they are selectively activated by different populations of afferents (Volle and Hancock, 1970). In parasympathetic ganglia ACh can cause both excitation and inhibition on the same neuron (Hartzell *et al.,* 1977). Bi- or triphasic responses to ionophoretic application of transmitters have been seen for ACh, histamine, serotonin, glutamate, and dopamine in invertebrates (Gerschenfeld, 1973) and to the catecholamines (Hosli *et al.,* 1971 ; Tebecis, 1970), GABA (Andersen *et al.,* 1980; Thalmann *et al.,* 1981), and ACh (Greene and Carpenter, 1981) in mammals. The existence of these varied ionic responses to most conventional transmitters is consistent with the hypothesis of Swann and Carpenter (1975) that transmitter receptors and ionophores are interchangeable.

4.2. Functional Relevance of Multiple Transmitter Actions

The possibility that these multiple effects of a single transmitter may reflect different functions of different parts of the neuron has not previously been considered. One exception is the biphasic GABA response seen in hippocampal neurons, for which Alger and Nicoll (1982) have proposed that the hyperpolarizing response is a result of functional synaptic receptors localized on the cell body, while the pharmacologically distinguishable depolarizing phase reflects a population of extrasynaptic receptors located on the dendrites.

Our observations support the premise that multiphasic responses may in at least some cases represent independent actions of the transmitter mediated by a spatial separation of responses. Receptors may be restricted to one portion of the cell, as in the prepyriform cortex, and when opposite polarity responses are present for one transmitter on a single cell, these may have distinct and independent locations. For the smooth muscle cell studied in culture, the biphasic response probably represents ionophoretic artifacts due to diffusion, rather than a spatial admixture of depolarizing and hyperpolarizing responses. How the cell maintains such clear demarcation remains to be investigated. If receptors may be segregated on a single neuron, what are the implications for transmitter-activated second messengers, such as cyclic AMP? A great variety of transmitters and peptides activate adenylate cyclase (Daly, 1976), often more than one on a single cell (Brunton *et al.*, 1977; Rimon *et al.*, 1978). If receptors are localized, different transmitters might use the same second messenger, such as cyclic AMP, and cause different cellular actions. Cyclic AMP is a small molecule and presumably diffuses easily in the cytoplasm, but if it is synthesized locally, the diffusion gradient is probably very steep due to rapid catalysis by phosphodiesterase. Thus, there is a real possibility that a cyclic AMP system in basal dendrites, whether activated by the same or a different transmitter, might regulate the activity of a different kinase and have quite different effects than a cyclic AMP system localized to apical dendrites.

While conventional transmitter responses that are due to non-voltage-dependent conductance increases may sometimes be asymmetrically distributed on neurons, it appears likely that transmitter actions that are more complex might have more significance when localized to particular portions of a neuron. M channels, shown in these studies to be located only on basal dendrites and/or cell bodies of prepyriform neurons, may have special actions by virtue of proximity to the axon hillock region. Other transmitter responses that cause a decreased membrane conductance would also be expected to be potentially important if so localized. Transmitters that either increase (McAfee *et al.*, 1981) voltage-dependent calcium currents, as well as transmitters that alter cyclic nucleotide levels, may also be of particular importance in this regard.

Although these considerations may mean that the single neuron is a more complex entity than the neurobiologist would desire, if such segregation of receptors and responses is indeed a general principal of neuronal organization, the neuron has a greater possibility of integration than often supposed. Perhaps this integration at a single cellular level is one reason why so many different neurotransmitters associated with so many different ionophores exist in the nervous system.

REFERENCES

Adams, P. R. and Brown, D. A., 1980, Luteinizing hormone-releasing factor and muscarinic agonists act on the same voltage-sensitive K^+ current in bullfrog sympathetic neurons, *Br. J. Pharmacol.* **68**:353–355.

Alger, B. E. and Nicoll, R. A., 1982, Pharmacological evidence for two kinds of GABA receptor on rat hippocampal pyramidal cells studied *in vitro*, *J. Physiol. (London)* **328**:125–141.

Andersen, P., Dingledine, R., Gjerstad, L., Langmoen, I. A., and Mosfeldt Laursen, A., 1980, Two different responses of hippocampal pyramidal cells to application of gamma-aminobutyric acid, *J. Physiol. (London)* **305**:279–296.

Brown, D. A. and Adams, P. R., 1980, Muscarinic suppression of a novel voltage-sensitive K^+ current in a vertebrate neurone, *Nature* **283**:673–676.

Brown, D. A., Constanti, A., and Marsh, S., 1980, Angiotensin mimics the action of muscarinic agonists on rat sympathetic neurones, *Brain Res.* **193**:614–619.

Brunton, L. L., Maguire, M. E., Anderson, H. J., and Gilman, A. G., 1977, Expression of genes for metabolism of cyclic adenosine 3':5'-monophosphate in somatic cells, *J. Biol. Chem.* **252**:1293–1302.

Carew, T. J. and Kandel, E. R., 1976, Two functional effects of decreased conductance EPSPS: Synaptic augmentation and increased electronic coupling, *Science* **192:**151–153.

Constanti, A. and Galvan, M., 1983, M-current in voltage clamped olfactory cortex neurones, *Neurosci. Lett.* **39:**65–70.

Constanti, A., Adams, P. R., and Brown, D. A., 1981, Why do barium ions imitate acetylcholine? *Brain Res.* **195:**403–420.

Daly, J. W., 1976, The nature of receptors regulating the formation of cyclic AMP in brain tissue, *Life Sci.* **18:**1349–1358.

Eccles, J. C., 1957, *The Physiology of Nerve Cells*, Oxford University Press, London.

ffrench-Mullen, J. M. H., Hori, N., Nakanishi, H., Slater, N. T., and Carpenter, D. O., 1983, Asymmetric distribution of acetylcholine receptors and M channels on prepyriform neurons, *Cell. Mol. Neurobiol.* **3:**163–181.

Gardner, D. and Kandel, E. R., 1972, Diphasic postsynaptic potentials: A chemical synapse capable of mediating conjoint excitation and inhibition, *Science* **158:**675–678.

Gerschenfeld, H. M., 1973, Chemical transmission in invertebrate central nervous systems and neuron-muscular junctions, *Physiol. Rev.* **53:**1–119.

Greene, R. W. and Carpenter, D. O., 1981, Biphasic responses to acetylcholine in mammalian reticulospinal neurons, *Cell. Mol. Neurobiol.* **1:**401–405.

Hartzell, C. H., Kuffler, S. W., Stickgold, R., and Yoshikami, D., 1977, Synaptic excitation and inhibition resulting from direct action of acetylcholine on two types of chemoreceptors on individual amphibian parasympathetic neurones, *J. Physiol. (London)* **271:**817–846.

Hori, N., Auker, C. R., Braitman, D. J., and Carpenter, D. O., 1982, Pharmacologic sensitivity of amino acid responses and synaptic activation of *in vitro* prepyriorm neurons, *J. Neurophysiol.* **48:**1289–1301.

Hösli, L., Tebécis, A. K., and Schonevetter, H. O., 1971, A comparison of the effects of monoamines on neurones of the bulbar reticular formation, *Brain Res.* **25:**357–370.

Kandel, E. R., Frazier, W. T., Waziri, R., and Coggeshall, R. E., 1967, Direct and common connections among identical neurons in *Aplysia, J. Neurophysiol.* **30:**1352–1376.

Kelly, J. S., Dodd, J., and Dingledine, R., 1979, Acetylcholine as an excitatory and inhibitory transmitter in the mammalian central nervous system, *Prog. Brain Res.* **49:**253–266.

Krnjević, K., 1981, Acetylcholine as modulator of amino-acid mediated synaptic transmission, in: *The Role of Peptides and Amino Acids as Neurotransmitters* (J. B. Lombardi and A. D. Kenney, eds.), A. R. Liss, New York, pp. 127–141.

McAfee, D. A., Henon, B. K., Horn, J. P., and Yarowsky, P., 1981, Calcium currents modulated by adrenergic receptors in sympathetic neurons, *Fed. Proc.* **40:**2246–2249.

Nelson, R., Lutzow, A., Kolb, H., and Guoras, P., 1975, Horizontal cells in cat retina with independent dendritic systems, *Science* **189:**137–139.

Rimon, G., Hanski, E., Braun, S., and Levitzki, A., 1978, Mode of coupling between hormone receptors and adenylate cyclase elucidated by modulation of membrane fluidity, *Nature* **276:**394–396.

Shepherd, G. M., 1979, *The Synaptic Organization of the Brain*, Oxford University Press, New York, pp. 289–307.

Sinback, C. N. and Shain, W., 1979, Electrophysiological properties of human oviduct smooth muscle cells in dissociated cell culture, *J. Cell. Physiol.* **98:**377–394.

Sinback, C. N., and Shain, W., 1980, Chemosensitivity of single smooth muscle cells to acetylcholine, noradrenaline and histamine *in vitro, J. Cell Physiol.* **102:**99–112.

Swann, J. W. and Carpenter, D. O., 1975, Organization of receptors for neurotransmitters on *Aplysia* neurons, *Nature* **258:**751–754.

Tebécis, A. K., 1970, Effects of monoamines and amino acids on medial geniculate neurones of the cat, *Neuropharmacology* **9:**381–390.

Thalmann, R. H., Peck, E. J., and Ayala, G. F., 1981, Biphasic response of hippocampal pyramidal neurons to GABA, *Neurosci. Lett.* **21:**319–324.

Volle, R. L. and Hancock, J. C., 1970, Transmission in sympathetic ganglia, *Fed. Proc.* **29:**1913–1918.

Wachtel, H. and Kandel, E. R., 1967, A direct synaptic connection mediating both excitation and inhibition, *Science* **158:**1206–1208.

IV

Biochemistry

26

Phosphorylation of Membrane Proteins in Excitable Cells and Changes in Membrane Properties

Experimental Paradigms and Interpretations, a Biochemist's View

TAMAS BARTFAI and BRITTA HEDLUND

1. INTRODUCTION

In 1969 Kuo and Greengard proposed that the diverse effects of signal substances that lead to increases in cyclic nucleotide levels are mediated via protein phosphorylation by the cyclic nucleotide-dependent (or activated) protein kinases (Kuo and Greengard, 1969). The role of protein phosphorylation in biological processes is now one of the fastest growing research areas, with several hundred reports monthly.

The role of protein phosphorylation in mediating or regulating the physiological response of nerve cells has recently been reviewed (Nestler and Greengard, 1983), indicating the widespread interest in the topic. Among the neuronal processes where involvement of protein phosphorylation has been shown are regulation of neurotransmitter biosynthesis (Haycock *et al.*, 1982), transport, release, neuronal growth and motility, and the conductance of specific neurotransmitter/voltage-dependent ion channels (cf. Nestler and Greengard, 1983; Greengard, 1978; Reuter, 1983).

This chapter will give a biochemist's assessment of the present experimental evidence and interpretation of the role of protein phosphorylation in regulation of ion conductances. Special reference will be made to the possibility that proteins phosphorylated at multiple sites may serve as the biochemical basis or correlate in processes such as conditioning.

TAMAS BARTFAI AND BRITTA HEDLUND ● Department of Biochemistry, Arrhenius Laboratory, University of Stockholm, S-106 91 Stockholm, Sweden.

2. EXTRACELLULAR SIGNALS AND SECOND MESSENGERS THAT REGULATE PROTEIN PHOSPHORYLATION IN NEURONS

The extracellular signals may include hormones (e.g., glucagon), neurotransmitters (e.g., noradrenaline, serotonin), or any signal, e.g., light quanta, sound, that can elicit at specific receptor sites a specific, graded or "all-or-none" change in the intracellular concentration of a "second messenger." The second messengers include $3'5'$-cyclic AMP (cAMP), $3'5'$-cyclic GMP (cGMP), and Ca^{2+}; the first two are assumed to act exclusively via activation of protein phosphorylation, whereas Ca^{2+} activates a large number of other proteins apart from the calcium-dependent protein kinases.

3. BIOCHEMICAL COMPONENTS AND REACTION MECHANISMS OF PROTEIN PHOSPHORYLATION IN NEURONS

Protein kinases represent a group of enzymes that transfers the terminal (-γ-) phosphate moiety of $5'$-ATP to serin or (less frequently) threonin group of proteins. The neuronal protein kinases that have been described until now comprise the cAMP-dependent protein kinases (Type I and II), cGMP-dependent protein kinase, four subtypes of the *calcium* (calmodulin)-activated protein-kinase, and a calcium-phosphatidylserine activated protein kinase (cf. Nestler and Greengard, 1983). Protein kinases catalyze a two-substrate reaction that leads to a covalent modification of the substrate protein, i.e., phosphorylation. One of the substrates, ATP, is kept at a rather steady ($\sim$ millimolar level) by several processes such as glycolysis and the Krebs or citric acid cycle. Thus the phosphorylation reaction proceeds as determined by the concentration of the active enzyme and by the concentration of the substrate proteins that are in their dephospho form at the moment. (Regulation of protein phosphorylation via changes in ATP has not been demonstrated and is unlikely to be of any importance, as the whole metabolic status of the cell must change before alterations of ATP concentration would significantly control the rate of protein phosphorylation.)

Covalent modification of proteins to alter their function is a commonly used regulatory mechanism in biology and represents a subclass of posttranslational modifications of proteins. (Peptide cleavage to turn chymotrypsinogen into the active chymotrypsin constitutes an example of the "irreversible" posttranslational modifications of proteins, whereas carboxymethylation (Kloog *et al.*, 1980), adenylation, or ribosylation of proteins represent other reversible posttranslational modifications of proteins, which are principally equivalent to protein phosphorylation although they are less widespread. In fact there is reason to believe that important regulatory proteins are targets of modification by several posttranslational changes, i.e., that phosphoproteins may also be substrates for carboxymethylation. Such an example is provided by the nicotinic acetylcholine receptor, which is phosphorylated at several distinct sites (cf. Huganir and Greengard, 1983), and also serves as substrate protein in a carboxymethylation reaction (Kloog et al., 1980).

3.1. Structure and Regulation of Protein Kinases

The cyclic AMP-dependent protein kinase is an oligomeric protein with two regulatory and two catalytic subunits. The latter are released in an active form from the tetramer when cAMP is bound to the regulatory subunits. Thus "the fully activated" cAMP-dependent protein kinase activity is expressed by the catalytic subunit of the oligomeric enzyme. Indeed, in microinjection experiments the dissociated catalytic subunit (which thus is not dependent on cAMP anymore for its activity) is used most often to mimic the effects of signals that lead to increases in cAMP levels. (See Section 5 for critique of this approach).

The calcium-dependent protein kinases are activated by calcium, which forms a complex with the ubiquitous, calcium-binding protein calmodulin while the Ca^{2+}/phosphatidylserine protein kinase is activated in the presence of this phospholipid. Thus, these protein kinases are active in the form of an oligomeric complex rather than in the form of a dissociated subunit.

The cGMP-dependent protein kinase has both the catalytic site and the cGMP binding domain located on the same polypeptide chain. Its activity is regulated by the reversible binding of cGMP to the regulatory site (Lincoln and Corbin, 1983).

3.2. Regulation of the Protein Kinase Activity

Most protein kinases show a basal activity in the absence of the second messenger. Increases in the second messenger concentration lead to a saturable increase in the rate of phosphorylation provided that the amount of substrate protein (and ATP) is not limiting.

The intracellular concentration of the ligands cAMP, cGMP, and Ca^{2+} is subject to increases upon activation of adenylate cyclase, or guanylate cyclase or opening the Ca^{2+} channels. The cAMP levels may rise from 10^{-8} to 10^{-4} M, the cGMP levels from 10^{-9} to 10^{-5} M, and the Ca^{2+} levels from 10^{-8} to 10^{-5} M upon appropriate stimuli with variation in different cell types. A number of intracellular processes act to reduce the increased intracellular levels of second messengers toward basal (unstimulated) level. Due to the activity of cyclic nucleotide phosphodiesterases (PDE) and Ca^{2+} sequestering processes, one cannot establish an activated steady state; rather the intracellular levels of cAMP, cGMP, and Ca^{2+} show a transient maximum shortly after stimulation. (The best approximation of a change in the steady-state level of the cyclic nucleotides is achieved by application of inhibitors of the phosphodiesterase or by a tonic activation of the cyclic nucleotide-generating enzymes (e.g., via cholera toxin) (Johnson and Bourne, 1977) or forskolin (Hudson and Fain, 1983), which activate adenylate cyclases, or by use of nitroso compounds, which activate the guanylate cyclases (DeRubertis and Craven, 1976). Penetrating analogues of cyclic nucleotides, e.g., mono- or dibutyryl cAMP, 8-Br cAMP, are more or less prone to act as substrates for the phospho-diesterases and therefore do not lead to establishment of a truly new steady-state of concentration of cyclic nucleotides (or their analogues).

3.3. Phosphoprotein Phosphatases

Although there is no doubt that repetitive signaling through protein phosphory-lation implies that the phosphorylated substrate proteins are eventually dephos-phorylated, there is very little known about protein phosphatases. In some *in vitro* experiments, protein phosphatase from heart (Osterieder *et al.*, 1982; Tsien, 1977) was used to dephosphorylate phosphoproteins before phosphorylation with [γ-^{32}P]-ATP. This procedure permits measurement of the total number of phosphorylation sites rather than of the portion of substrate proteins that are not in phosphorylated form at the moment [γ-^{32}P]-ATP is added.

3.4. Ion Channels as Direct (or Indirect) Substrates of Protein Kinases

The best characterized neuronal substrate for protein kinases is Synapsin I (Greengard, 1976; Kennedy and Greengard, 1981). In keeping with the theme of this volume, we shall focus on the effects of protein phosphorylation on K^+ con-ductances in *Hermissenda* (Alkon *et al.*, 1983) and K^+ and Ca^{2+} conductances in *Aplysia* (Kaczmarek *et al.*, 1980; Castelucci *et al.*, 1980; Kandel and Schwartz, 1982; Siegelbaum *et al.*, 1982) and on the effects of protein phosphorylation on the properties of the acetylcholine-regulated monovalent cation channel of the nico-tinic acetylcholine receptor from the electric organ of *Torpedo*.

4. MICROINJECTION EXPERIMENTS

4.1. In Vivo Approaches Using Whole Cells

Rationale: (1) If the external stimulus, dopamine, serotonin, etc., acts through activation of the adenylate cyclase with resulting increases in intracellular cAMP levels, then the extracellular stimulus can be mimicked by (a) extracellular appli-cation of penetrating cAMP analogues, (b) intracellular application of microinjected or iontophoresed cAMP, or (c) extracellular or intracellular application of inhibitors of cAMP-PDE. (2) If the increased cAMP levels bring about the response of the cell (e.g., change in ion conductance, discharge, etc.) by activation of the endog-enous cAMP-dependent protein kinase, then microinjection of the "activated" pro-tein kinase, i.e., that of the free, catalytic unit (C) should mimic the effect of the external stimulus or that of the increase in cAMP levels. (3) If phosphorylation of a certain protein by the catalytic unit of the cAMP-dependent protein kinase is not only a sufficient but also a necessary step evoking the response to the external stimulus, then one can prevent the response to this stimulus by microinjection of the inhibitor (Walsh inhibitor) of the cAMP-dependent protein kinase. (4) If activation of the protein phosphorylation influences the given conductance because the substrate of the protein kinase is the ion channel itself, then it should be possible by labeling the intracellular ATP store with [^{32}P]-phosphate to incorporate the radioactive [^{32}P]-(PO$_3$) group into the channel protein concomitant to the conductance change. If the channel protein can be identified by its size in gels or by its affinity for a specific drug/toxin, then direct evidence can be obtained that the labeled protein has also incorporated the [^{32}P]-PO$_3$ group.

Experiments according to paradigm 2 showed that in the photoreceptor cells of *Hermissenda* intracellular injection of the catalytic unit of cAMP-dependent protein kinase mimicks the effects of light in depressing the conductances of the early and late voltage-dependent K$^+$ channels (Alkon *et al.*, 1983). In identified neurons of *Aplysia* according to paradigms 1 and 2, it has been shown that the facilitating effect of serotonin on neurotransmitter release can be mimicked by cAMP, potentiated by phosphodiesterase inhibitors, or mimicked by injection of the catalytic subunit of the cAMP-dependent protein kinase, all leading to decreased conductance of a serotonin-regulated K$^+$ channel (Kaczmarek *et al.*, 1980; Castelucci *et al.*, 1980).

In the identified R15 neuron of *Aplysia*, Adams and Levitan (1982) showed that (cf. paradigm 1–3) the increased K$^+$ conductance elicited by serotonin can be fully blocked by injection of the protein kinase inhibitor, thus proving that the action of cAMP-dependent protein kinase is not only a sufficient but a necessary step in the serotonin-evoked change in K$^+$ conductance in this cell. Furthermore, the ATP stores of this cell were labeled by [^{32}P]-PO$_3$, and several phosphorylated proteins were identified by two-dimensional gel electrophoresis and subsequent autoradiography. One or several of these labeled proteins may represent a phosphorylated subunit of the K$^+$ channel or a protein that controls it.

4.2. In Vitro Approaches Using Purified Proteins

The purified ion channel protein is phosphorylated or dephosphorylated *in vitro* by protein kinases and phosphatases, incorporated into lyposomes or Black lipid membranes, and its conductance properties are studied. Such an approach may be possible in the case of the voltage-dependent sodium channel, where the identity of the purified protein was verified via its saxitoxin or tetrodotoxin or scorpion toxin binding ability and the subunit of the sodium channel was shown to incorporate 3–4 moles [^{32}P]-PO$_3$/mole saxitoxin binding activity when incubated with [^{32}P]-ATP and the catalytic unit of the cAMP-dependent protein kinase (Costa *et al.*, 1982).

Phosphorylation of the purified nicotinic acetylcholine receptor at two sites by the cAMP-dependent protein kinase was observed *in vitro* (cf. Huganir and Greengard, 1983, and references therein). In addition, the Ca^{2+}/phosphatidylserine-activated protein kinase can phosphorylate the nicotinic receptor (cf. Fig. 1).

Common target proteins for stimuli are phosphorylated at distinct sites as well as at common sites

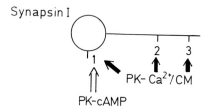

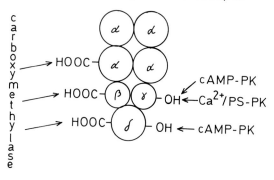

FIGURE 1. Schematic illustration of the multiple phosphorylation sites on two neuronal proteins.

5. INTERPRETATION AND CRITIQUE

The above-described experiments, together with many other examples of microinjection of cAMP and of the catalytic unit of the cAMP-dependent protein kinase, prove only that the given extracellular stimulus can be mimicked by the action of cAMP or the catalytic subunit of the protein kinase; thus, the net result of protein phosphorylation is similar to that of the extracellular stimulus mimicked. Whether or not the participation of the cAMP-dependent endogenous protein kinase is *necessary* the elicited response can only be established in experiments where the endogenous pool of cAMP and protein kinases are at work, but injection of the protein kinase inhibitor prevents the conductance change otherwise elicited by the extracellular stimulus (cf. Adams and Levitan, 1982).

5.1. Specificity Problems in Microinjection Experiments

Injection of cAMP raises cellular cAMP levels in all compartments of the cell with which the site of injection can be rapidly equilibrated, whereas the extracellular stimulus raises cAMP levels at the intracellular site where the receptor coupled adenylate cyclase catalytic unit resides: thus, physiologically, the cAMP gradient ranges from the membrane toward the cell interior, whereas in the injection experiment the cAMP concentration is highest at the tip of the electrode and lowest at the membrane. Since activation of the protein kinase occurs within a 2- to 10-fold increase in cAMP levels, this may lead to phosphorylation of a number of cytosolic proteins not normally phosphorylated on stimulation, which may only activate the membrane-bound protein kinases.

5.2. Cyclic Nucleotide Specificity

Cyclic GMP levels are generally 10-fold lower than cyclic AMP levels (cf. Greengard, 1976). Activation of cGMP-dependent kinases also occurs when the cGMP concentration is elevated 2- to 10-fold over basal level. The affinity of the cGMP-dependent protein kinase towards cGMP is only 10- to 50-fold higher than that for cAMP. Thus, microinjection of large amounts of cAMP that raise cAMP levels 10- to 20-fold is bound to lead to some activation of the cGMP-dependent protein kinases too.

Injection of phosphodiesterase inhibitors leads establishment of new "steady state" levels of cAMP (and of cGMP!), since we lack specific inhibitors of the hydrolysis of cAMP or cGPM.

5.3. Substrate Specificity of Protein Kinases

The substrate specificity of certain protein kinases is very high (e.g., phosphorylase kinase has only one substrate), whereas most of the protein kinases phosphorylate any available serine or threonine residue that occurs within the "right" sequence of amino acids. In particular one should be aware that although injection of the catalytic subunit of cGMP-dependent protein kinase seemingly circumvents the problem of cyclic nucleotide specificity, in high concentrations this protein can phosphorylate proteins that are normally substrates for the cGMP-dependent protein kinase (personal communication from P. Greengard).

5.4. Inhibitor Studies

Injection of material into neurons can inadvertantly, in a nonspecific way, change ion conductances; therefore, experimental controls with inactivated (preferably chemically inactivated with, e.g., 5'5' dithiobis benzoic acid) catalytic units of the cAMP-dependent protein kinase should also be tested, or protein kinase inhibitor and protein kinase should be injected together. The protein kinase inhibitor is rather stable but in 12–15 hr R-15 cells can degrade it (Adams and Levitan, 1982).

5.5. Phosphorylation State-Turnover of Phosphoprotein: An Ambiguity

In vivo phosphorylation of a protein is usually demonstrated by measuring the incorporation of $[^{32}P]$-PO_3 into proteins upon presentation of appropriate stimulus. This incorporation of $[^{32}P]$-PO_3 is difficult to interpret since it may mean a true increase in the portion of the given protein that is in this phosphorylated form; thus, the incorporation of $[^{32}P]$-PO_3 measures a change in the phosphorylation state of the protein brought about by the stimulus. Alternatively, the stimulus changes the turnover of the phosphate group on the protein. The activity of the phosphatase or protein kinase or of both may increase so that more sites are phosphorylated (and dephosphorylated) under the time lapse of the stimulus; thus, more $[^{32}P]$-PO_3 is incorporated, although the state of phosphorylation of the protein is not changed (cf. Rudolph *et al.*, 1978).

5.6. Convergent Stimuli Lead to Phosphorylation of Multiple Sites of Certain Key Proteins

Different stimuli reaching the postsynaptic cell within a well-defined time period (50–1000 μsec) may interact in bringing about the response of the cell. These interactions may take place (a) at the level of the plasma membrane, (b) in the cytosol, (c) at the level of individual proteins, or at any of these sites simultaneously.

(a) There are examples of neurotransmitters that activate adenylate cyclase, whereas others act to inhibit it. For example, noradrenaline stimulation of the adenylate cyclase in rabbit cardiac membranes is counteracted by occupancy of muscarinic acetylcholine receptors by agonists (Jakobs *et al.*, 1981). Thus, at the level of the plasma membrane noradrenaline and acetylcholine will interact to determine the resulting adenylate cyclase activity, the cellular cAMP level, and the phosphorylation state of several proteins.

(b) Simultaneous stimuli to activate adenylate cyclase will be summated in the cytosol, as the cAMP molecules generated in, e.g., response to noradrenaline or PGE, are indistinguishable; the cAMP concentration will determine the activity of the cAMP-dependent protein kinase.

(c) Convergent stimuli may interact at the level of individual phosphoproteins (Fig. 1).

Several examples of multiple phosphorylation sites on proteins involved in nervous function have been reported. Arbitrarily, we chose to discuss phosphorylation of a neuronal phosphoprotein Synapsin I (Greengard, 1976; Nestler and Greengard, 1983) and that of the nicotinic acetylcholine receptor.

Both of these proteins can be phosphorylated in a cAMP-dependent and in a Ca^{2+}-dependent manner; thus, different classes of stimuli leading to changes in cAMP or Ca^{2+} concentrations can converge on a common target protein and alter its function simultaneously.

Synapsin I, a neuronal phosphoprotein, can be phosphorylated on up to three sites; site 1 can either be phosphorylated by Ca^{2+}/calmodulin-dependent protein kinase or by cAMP-dependent protein kinase, whereas sites 2 and 3 are phosphorylated by a second Ca^{2+}/calmodulin-dependent protein kinase (Huttner and Greengard, 1979; Kennedy and Greengard, 1981) (Fig. 1).

The nicotinic receptor also serves as substrate of carboxymethylation, permitting an additional degree of freedom of regulation by another class of stimuli, leading to activation of carboxymethylation enzymes (Kloog *et al.*, 1980).

These arbitrarily chosen examples may indicate that phosphoproteins could provide "molecular substrates" for converging stimuli participating in higher forms of associative processes such as conditioning.

ACKNOWLEDGMENTS. This study was supported from grants from the Swedish Medical Research Council and the National Institute of Health, Bethesda, Maryland.

REFERENCES

Adams, W. B. and Levitan, I. B., 1982, Intracellular injection of protein kinase inhibitor blocks the serotonin-induced increase in K^+ conductance in *Aplysia* neuron R15, *Proc. Natl. Acad. Sci. USA*, **79**:3877–3880.

Alkon, D. L., Acosta-Urquidi, J., Olds, J., Kuzma, G., and Neary, J. T., 1983, Protein kinase injection reduces voltage-dependent potassium currents, *Science* **219**:303–306.

Castelucci, V. F., Kandel, E. R., Schwartz, J. H., Wilson, F. D., Nairn, A.C., and Greengard, P., 1980, Intracellular injection of catalytic subunit of cyclic AMP dependent protein kinase stimulate facilitation of transmitter release underlying behavioral sensitization in Aplysia, *Proc. Natl. Acad. Sci. USA*, **77**:7492–7496.

Costa, M. R., Casnellie, J. E., and Caterall, W. A., 1982, Selective phosphorylation of the alpha subunit of the sodium channel by cAMP-dependent protein kinase, *J. Biol Chem.* **257**:7918–7921.

DeRubertis, F. and Craven, P., 1976, Calcium independent modulation of cyclic GMP and activation of guanylate cyclases by nitrosamines, *Science* **193**:897–899.

Greengard, P., 1976, Possible role for cyclic nucleotides and phosphorylated membrane proteins in postsynaptic actions of neurotransmitters, *Nature* **260**:101–108.

Greengard, P., 1978, Phopshorylated proteins as physiological effectors, *Science* **199**:146–152.

Haycock, J. W., Bennett, W. F., George, R. J., and Waymore, P., 1982, Multiple site phosphorylation of tyrosine hydroxylase. Differential regulation in situ by 8-bromo-cAMP and acetylcholine, *J. Biol. Chem.* **257**:13699–13703.

Hudson, T. H. and Fain, J. N., 1983, Forskolin-activated adenylate cyclase, *J. Biol. Chem.* **258**:9755–9761.

Huganir, R. L. and Greengard, P., 1983, cAMP-dependent protein kinase phosphorylates the nicotinic acetycholine receptor, *Proc. Natl. Acad. Sci. USA*, **80**:1130–1134.

Huttner, W. B. and Greengard, P., 1979, Multiple phosphorylation sites in Protein I and their differential regulation by cyclic AMP and calcium, *Proc. Natl. Acad. Sci. USA*, **76**:5402–5406.

Jakobs, K. H., Aktories, K., and Schultz, G., 1981, Inhibition of adenylate cyclase by hormones and neurotransmitters, in: *Advances in Cyclic Nucleotide Research*, Vol. 14 (J. E. Dumont, P. Greengard, and A. G. Robison, eds.), Raven Press, New York, pp. 173–186.

Johnson, G. L. and Bourne, H. R., 1977, Influence of choleratoxin on the regulation of adenylate cyclase by GTP, *Biochem. Biophys. Res. Commun.* **78**:792–798.

Kaczmarek, L., Jennings, K. R., Strumwasser, F., Nairn, A. C., Walter, U., Wilson, F. D., and Greengard, P., 1980, Microinjection of catalytic subunit of cyclic AMP-dependent protein kinase enhances calcium action potentials of bag cell neurons in cell culture, *Proc. Natl. Acad. Sci. USA* **77**:7487–7491.

Kandel, E. R. and Schwartz, J. H., 1982, Molecular biology of learning: Modulation of transmitter release, *Science* **218**:433–443.

Kennedy, M. B. and Greengard, P., 1981, Two calcium/calmodulin-dependent protein kinases, which are highly concentrated in the brain: Phosphorylate Protein I at distinct sites, *Proc. Natl. Acad. Sci. USA* **78**:1293–1297.

Kloog, Y., Flynn, D., Hoffman, A. R., and Axelrod, J., 1980, Enzymatic carboxymethylation of the nicotinic acetylcholine receptor, *Biochem. Biophys. Res. Commun.* **97**:1474–1480.

Kuo, J. F. and Greengard, P., 1969, Cyclic nucleotide dependent protein kinases. IV. *Proc. Natl. Acad. Sci. USA* **64**:1349–1355.

Lincoln, T. M. and Corbin, J. D., 1983, Characterization and Biological Role of the cGMP-dependent protein kinase, in: *Advances in Cyclic Nucleotide Research,* Vol. 15 (P. Greengard and A. G. Robison, eds.), Raven Press, New York, pp. 139–203.

Nestler, E. J. and Greengard, P., 1983, Protein phosphorylation in the brain, *Nature* **305**:583–588.

Osterieder, W., Brum, G., Heschler, J., and Trautwein, W., 1982, Injection of subunits of cyclic AMP-dependent protein kinase into cardiac myocytes modulates Ca^{2+} current, *Nature* **298**:576–578.

Reuter, H., 1983, Calcium channel modulation by neurotransmitters, enzymes and drugs, *Nature* **301**:569–574.

Rudolph, S. A., Beam, K. G., and Greengard, P., 1978, Studies on protein phosphorylation in relation to hormonal control of ion transport in intact cells, in: *Membrane Transport Processes,* Vol. 1 (J. F. Hoffman, ed.), Raven Press, New York, pp. 107–123.

Siegelbaum, S. A., Camardo, J. S., and Kandel, E. R., 1982, Serotonin and cyclic AMP close single K^+ channels in *Aplysia* sensory neurons, *Nature* **299**:413–417.

Tsien, R. W., 1977, Cyclic AMP and contractile activity in heart, *Adv. Cycl. Nucleotide Res.* **8**:363–420.

27

Calcium- and Calmodulin-Dependent Protein Kinase:

Role in Memory

MARY LOU VALLANO, JAMES R. GOLDENRING, and ROBERT J. DELORENZO

1. INTRODUCTION

The molecular mechanisms that underlie learning and memory have intrigued investigators for over a decade. When formulating a model for memory, an interdisciplinary approach must be utilized. The specific brain regions that mediate information processing, storage, and retrieval should be identified and their role in each of these steps elucidated. Clearly, many different brain nuclei interact cooperatively in these processes, and a wide variety of experimental models for memory have been developed. Excellent reviews on the neuropsychology of memory (Squire, 1982) and possible biochemical correlates (Thompson *et al.*, 1983) are available.

At the cellular level, the site where a stable morphological and/or biochemical alteration has been produced should be identified and analyzed. After several years of intensive research utilizing both invertebrate (for reviews, see Alkon, 1980; Kandel, 1981) and mammalian systems (for reviews, see Eccles, 1983; Lynch and Baudry, 1984) as models for memory, the synapse has been targeted as the site that demonstrates plasticity. Ultimately, a successful model for memory must link the behavioral changes with the cellular changes that occur in the central nervous system.

The goal of this chapter is to review some of the evidence for synaptic involvement in mammalian memory and to suggest possible biochemical mechanisms

MARY LOU VALLANO, JAMES R. GOLDENRING, and ROBERT J. DELORENZO
● Department of Neurology, Yale University School of Medicine, New Haven, Connecticut 06510.
Present address for M. L. V.: Department of Pharmacology, State University of New York, Upstate Medical Center, Syracuse, New York 13210.

that contribute to this process. Particular emphasis will be placed upon the role of a calcium- and calmodulin-dependent protein kinase, since this area of research is a major focus of our laboratory.

1.1. Long-Term Potentiation as a Model for Memory

Substantial progress has been made using the phenomenon of "long-term potentiation" (LTP) in constructing a model for memory (Lynch and Baudry, 1984). LTP is a long-lasting synaptic facilitation in the postsynaptic target neuron that follows brief trains of high-frequency, repetitive stimulation of any one of several afferent pathways supplying the nucleus. It begins after a latency of 10–20 sec, peaks in minutes (Bliss and Gardner-Medwin, 1973), and persists for several days (Bliss and Lomo, 1973). Most of the available information on LTP has been obtained using animals with chronically implanted electrodes in the hippocampus, since the monosynaptic connections between the presynaptic afferent neurons and the postsynaptic target cells are readily available for analysis. The *in vitro* hippocampal slice preparation was developed as a means to circumvent the difficulties associated with *in vivo* experiments, while preserving the lamellar structure of the nucleus (for review, see Andersen, 1981). It offers the additional advantage of changing the extracellular neuronal environment, so that the effects of various chemical compounds on the development of LTP can be examined.

LTP has also been demonstrated in cerebral cortical slices (Lee, 1983), indicating that it may serve as a useful model for memory in both hippocampus and cerebral cortex. These two regions are primary loci for information storage and retrieval (Lynch and Baudry, 1984).

1.2. Postsynaptic Localization for LTP

The region that mediates the development of LTP is the synaptic complex where presynaptic neurons communicate with the dendritic spines of the postsynaptic neuron. In at least one of these pathways the excitatory amino acid, glutamate, appears to be the neurotransmitter released from the presynaptic neuron (Dunwiddie *et al.*, 1978). Specific blockade of postsynaptic glutamate receptors with 2-amino-4-phosphono-butyric acid inhibits LTP formation during stimulation of the afferent pathway (Dunwiddie *et al.*, 1978). Moreover, injection of EGTA into the postsynaptic target cells prevents LTP development (Lynch *et al.*, 1983). These experiments argue strongly in favor of a postsynaptic localization for LTP.

The salient features that relate to the functional and morphological changes that correlate with the appearance of LTP are well documented. First, extracellular calcium is necessary for initiation of LTP (Dunwiddie *et al.*, 1978; Dunwiddie and Lynch, 1979). Injection of EGTA, a calcium chelator, into the postsynaptic target cell inhibits the induction of LTP (Lynch *et al.*, 1983). The observation that calcium is not required once LTP is fully established suggests that calcium triggers a series of processes that induce and maintain LTP. Second, a role for calmodulin, the calcium binding protein, was suggested by studies in which trifluoperazine, a calmodulin inhibitor, blocked the appearance of LTP in hippocampus (Finn *et al.*,

1980). Third, an increase in the number of postsynaptic receptors for glutamate correlates with the development of LTP (Lynch and Baudry, 1984). An increase in the number of receptors may increase the efficacy of synaptic transmission and represent a stable modification in the activated dendritic spine. Thus, the postsynaptic events that mediate glutamate receptor insertion and/or uncovering of cryptic receptors present in the membrane are important. Fourth, a change in the dendritic ultrastructure (Lee *et al.*, 1980; Fifkova *et al.*, 1982), which may relate to the increase in protein synthesis and possible delivery of protein up the activated dendrites via the microtubular transport system, is observed.

A model that places primary emphasis on events occurring in the postsynaptic target cell, but also accounts for the data that favors a presynaptic role, has been formulated (Eccles, 1983). According to this model, calcium enters the activated dendrities of the postsynaptic neuron via voltage-sensitive calcium channels. Calcium then binds to calmodulin, thereby triggering a sequence of events that induce LTP. Eccles (1983) conjectures that activation of a calmodulin-dependent protein kinase in the postsynaptic density (PSD) modifies the function of various PSD proteins by phosphorylation and ultimately results in insertion of additional glutamate receptors in the postsynaptic membrane. The increased number of glutamate receptors in the postsynaptic membrane induces a secondary increase in glutamate release from presynaptic neuron by a trophic action across the synaptic cleft. Other proposed actions of calcium and calmodulin are acceleration of protein transport up the activated dendrites into the spines and induction of protein synthesis in dendritic polyribosomes and the nucleus. According to this model, calmodulin acts as a second messenger system in the development of LTP in the postsynaptic neuron by regulating PSD function, microtubule function, and protein synthesis. Thus, as a first step in testing the validity of this model, the calmodulin-dependent enzyme systems that mediate these effects must be identified and characterized.

2. CALMODULIN AS A SECOND MESSENGER SYSTEM IN NEURONS

The pioneering work of Katz and Miledi (1969, 1970) and Douglas (1968) established that calcium entry into the nerve terminal is required for neurotransmitter release. This information, coupled with the fact that calmodulin modulates the effects of calcium on several enzyme systems (Cheung, 1980; Klee *et al.*, 1980), prompted our laboratory to examine the possible role of calmodulin as a second messenger in synaptic function. These studies demonstrated that calmodulin is present in the synaptic terminal (DeLorenzo, 1980) and plays an important role in synaptic protein phosphorylation and depolorization-dependent synaptic processes (for review, see DeLorenzo *et al.*, 1982). A key event is the activation of an endogenous calcium/calmodulin-dependent protein kinase that phosphorylates several synaptic cytoskeletal proteins and alters their function. Therefore, we proceeded to isolate, biochemically characterize, and examine the effects of this calmodulin-dependent kinase on cytoskeletal function.

2.1 Isolation and Characterization of Calmodulin-Dependent Protein Kinase from Brain

Several laboratories have isolated and characterized calmodulin-dependent protein kinases from mammalian brain (Fukunaga *et al.*, 1982; Goldenring *et al.*, 1983; Bennett *et al.*, 1983; McGuinness *et al.*, 1983; Yamauchi and Fujisawa, 1983a; Schulman, 1984). These enzymes are remarkably similar, if not identical, although different substrates were utilized to follow their distribution during the purification procedures. They have been designated Type II calmodulin-dependent protein kinases.

Our laboratory has characterized a calmodulin-dependent protein kinase from rat brain cytosol that phosphorylates cytoskeletal proteins as major substrates, including microtubule-associated protein 2 (MAP 2), tubulin (Goldenring *et al.*, 1983), and neurofilament proteins (Vallano *et al.*, 1984). The enzyme is a 600,000-dalton complex containing two calmodulin-binding proteins of 52,000 and 63,000 daltons, designated as rho (ρ) and sigma (σ), respectively. The subunit isoelectric points are near neutrality and both the rho and the sigma subunits demonstrate calmodulin-dependent autophosphorylation. Rho subunits represent a larger proportion of the holoenzyme complex than sigma subunits. Figure 1 shows the two-dimensional isoelectric focusing/SDS–PAGE autoradiographs of calmodulin-dependent autophosphorylation and [^{125}I]-calmodulin binding to rho and sigma.

The calmodulin-dependent kinase activity previously identified as a second messenger system in synaptosomes (Burke and DeLorenzo, 1981), synaptic vesicles (Burke and DeLorenzo, 1982a), and synaptic cytosol (Burke and Lorenzo, 1982b) is identical to the purified cytosolic kinase on the basis of substrate specificities, enzyme subunit molecular weights, isoelectric points, and subcellular localization. While the cytosolic brain calmodulin-dependent kinase exhibits a broad range of substrate specificities, cytoskeletal proteins appear to be important. Thus, this multifunctional kinase may mediate the effects of calcium on cytoskeletal systems in the cell.

3. THE POSTSYNAPTIC DENSITY (PSD)

The PSD is an electron-dense, disc-shaped structure of variable thickness attached to the cytoplasmic face of the postsynaptic membrane at the synaptic junction (for review, see Matus, 1981). Based upon morphology and localization in the brain, two types of PSD have been described. Type I is thicker and typically found in regions thought to mediate excitatory responses, whereas the type II PSD may be localized to inhibitory synapses, i.e., cerebellum (Grab *et al.*, 1980). The PSD is closely associated with cytoplasmic microtubules that appear to course through it (Westrum and Gray, 1977). Due to its unique location, investigators have suggested that the PSD plays a central role in synaptic processing. With regard to development of LTP, the PSD may serve as a cytoskeletal framework for insertion of glutamate receptors and/or other important transmembrane proteins into the

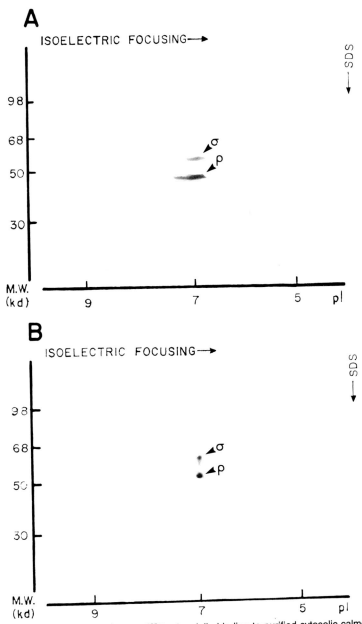

FIGURE 1. Autophosphorylation and [125I]-calmodulin binding to purified cytosolic calmodulin-dependent kinase. (A) Purified kinase was phosphorylated under standard conditions in the presence of calcium and calmodulin and resolved on two-dimensional isoelectric focusing/SDS–PAGE. (B) Purified kinase was resolved on isoelectric focusing/SDS–PAGE and assayed for [125I]-calmodulin binding proteins as described by Goldenring et al. (1983). Gels were subsequently dried and exposed to X-ray film. The autoradiographs are shown.

postsynaptic membrane. Long-lasting alterations in synaptic processing may be mediated by calcium-dependent modifications of postsynaptic cytoskeletal proteins.

3.1. Cytoskeletal Proteins in the PSD

The postsynaptic density is a highly insoluble cytoplasmic structure that can be isolated from synaptic membrane preparations by sequential detergent extractions (Cotman *et al.*, 1974; Cohen *et al.*, 1977). The PSD contains several cytoskeletal elements, including MAP 2, tubulin, and actin. They also contain calmodulin and several calmodulin-binding proteins. Tubulin is only a minor intrinsic component of the insoluble matrix, and the amount of tubulin isolated with the PSD is directly proportional to *post-mortem* preparation time (Carlin *et al.*, 1982). The source of additional tubulin is not known but may be provided by depolymerization of the microtubules that are closely associated with the PSD.

In addition to actin (Kelly and Cotman, 1978), the isolated PSD also contains the calmodulin-binding, actin-binding protein, fodrin (Carlin *et al.*, 1983). Fodrin is a ubiquitous cellular protein located just beneath the synaptic membrane and may serve as an anchor between the PSD and synaptic membrane proteins (Levine and Willard, 1981; Branton *et al.*, 1982).

3.2. Enzyme Activities in the PSD

Two types of phosphodiesterase activity have been described in the PSD, one of which is calmodulin-dependent (Grab *et al.*, 1981). The PSD also contains an intrinsic cyclic AMP-dependent kinase activity that phosphorylates synapsin I as a major substrate (Ueda *et al.*, 1979; Ng and Matus, 1979). Until recently, synapsin I was thought to be endogenous to the PSD, but this association was shown to be artifactual (DeCamilli *et al.*, 1983) due to the "sticky" nature of the PSD (Matus *et al.*, 1980). As a consequence, the function of cyclic AMP-dependent kinase in the PSD remains obscure.

The major protein component of the cerebral cortical PSD is a 52,000-dalton protein that comprises up to 50% of the PSD protein (Kelly and Cotman, 1978). The major postsynaptic density protein (mPSDp) is the major substrate for an endogenous calmodulin-dependent kinase, and is also the major calmodulin-binding protein in the isolated PSD (Grab *et al.*, 1981). Recently our laboratory (Goldenring *et al.*, 1984) and two other laboratories (Kennedy *et al.*, 1983; Kelly *et al.*, 1984) have demonstrated that the mPSDp is a subunit of the endogenous PSD calmodulin-dependent kinase and appears to be identical to the 52,000-dalton subunit of a Type II cytosolic calmodulin-dependent kinase. The isolated PSD also contains a 63,000-dalton calmodulin-binding protein, which is homologous to the 63,000-dalton subunit of the cytosolic calmodulin-dependent kinase. Figure 2 shows the protein patterns, autoradiographs for protein phosphorylation, and autoradiographs for [125I]-calmodulin binding from one-dimensional SDS–PAGE of the purified Type II calmodulin-dependent kinase (TACK) and PSD fractions from cerebral cortex. When the rho and sigma subunits of TACK were compared with the mPSDp and PSD 63,000-dalton protein by two-dimensional tryptic peptide mapping, the maps shown

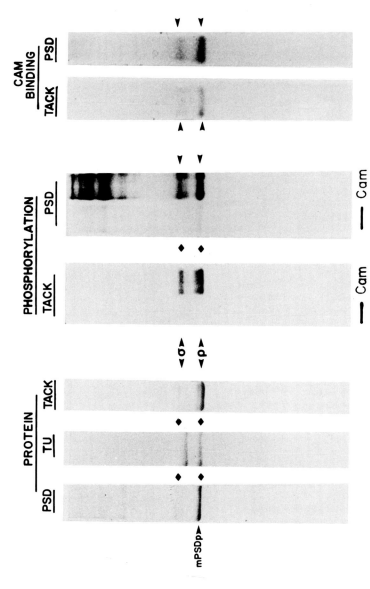

FIGURE 2. Autophosphorylation and [¹²⁵I]-calmodulin binding to calmodulin-dependent kinase in postsynaptic densities. Purified cytosolic calmodulin-dependent kinase (TACK) and PSDs were prepared and assayed for calmodulin-dependent autophosphorylation or [¹²⁵I]-calmodulin-binding proteins. The positions of the rho (ρ) and sigma (σ) enzyme subunits are depicted. Autophosphorylation of the enzyme and other PSD proteins were observed only when calmodulin (Cam) was present in the incubation medium (refer to bottom of appropriate gel lanes). The protein pattern of alpha and beta tubulin (Tu) is shown for comparison with TACK. (Reprinted from Goldenring et al., 1984.)

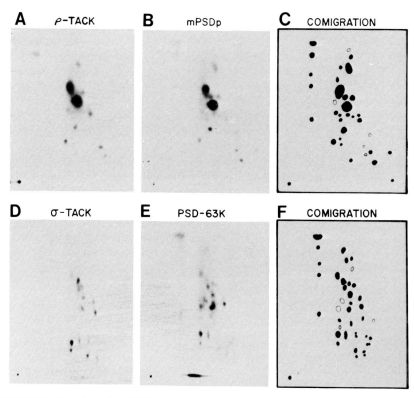

FIGURE 3. Two-dimensional [^{125}I]-tryptic peptide maps of purified calmodulin-dependent kinase and kinase endogenous to PSDs. Autoradiographic exposures of the two-dimensional tryptic peptide maps of: (A) rho (ρ) and (D) sigma (σ) subunits of the purified cytosolic calmodulin-dependent kinase (TACK); (B) the major PSD protein; and (E) the 63,000-dalton PSD protein. Electrophoresis was from left to right, and chromatography was from bottom to top. The schematic composites obtained from comigration of A + B are shown in (C), and D + E are shown in (F). The comigrating fragments are represented by black spots. (Reprinted from Goldenring *et al.*, 1984.)

in Fig. 3 were obtained. These results suggest that a Type II calmodulin-dependent kinase that is identical or closely related to the previously purified cytosolic kinase, is a major component of the insoluble PSD matrix in the cerebral cortex. It should be noted that mPSDp is present in small quantities in the cerebellar PSD (Flanagan *et al.*, 1982). This difference in protein composition may be reflected in the different morphologies of cerebellar and cerebral PSDs. Recent evidence indicates that the cerebellum may contain an altered form of calmodulin-dependent kinase where the 63,000-dalton enzyme subunit represents a larger proportion of the holoenzyme complex compared to the 52,000-dalton subunit (Miller and Kennedy, 1984; McGuinness *et al.*, 1984). Whether the cerebellar and cerebral kinases function differently in synaptic neurotransmission remains to be determined.

3.3. Role of Calmodulin-Dependent Kinase in PSD Function

The postsynaptic dendritic spine contains a filamentous trabecular network (Gulley and Reese, 1981). Alterations in dendritic spine structure have been implicated in the development of LTP (Lee *et al.*, 1980; Fifkova *et al.*, 1982). Lynch and Baudry (1984) have suggested that activation of a calcium-dependent proteinase degrades fodrin and results in glutamate receptor insertion into the synaptic membrane, indicating that changes in cytoskeletal proteins may produce changes in membrane protein composition.

Phosphorylation of PSD proteins or autophosphorylation of the endogenous calmodulin-dependent kinase may also be a major mechanism of cytoskeletal protein modification. Significantly, the distribution of calmodulin-dependent protein kinase in neurons parallels the distribution of glutamate binding sites (Nestler *et al.*, 1984). In addition, changes in the amount of mPSDp in the PSD correlates well with the demonstration of plasticity in cerebral synapses (Guldner and Ingham, 1979; Vrensen and Nunes Cardozo, 1981; Rostas *et al.*, 1984). Activation of the calmodulin-dependent kinase in the PSD may provide a biochemical mechanism for a rapid and stable response to calcium influx in the postsynaptic neuron.

4. CALMODULIN-DEPENDENT REGULATION OF MICROTUBULE FUNCTION

Microtubules play an integral role in several dynamic intracellular processes, including neuroplasmic transport. Therefore, the endogenous factors that rapidly modulate microtubule function are of interest. Successful repolymerization of tubulin *in vitro* was initially achieved in buffer containing sufficient EGTA to chelate free calcium ions (Weisenberg, 1972), suggesting that calcium reduces microtubule stability. Micromolar amounts of calcium induce microtubule depolymerization when calmodulin, ATP, and calmodulin-dependent kinase are added (Yamauchi and Fujisawa, 1983b). *In vitro* evidence indicates that calmodulin-dependent phosphorylation of MAP 2 mediates this effect (Yamamoto *et al.*, 1983). Microtubules contain calmodulin-binding proteins (Sobue *et al.*, 1981), and calmodulin has been shown to localize on specific populations of microtubules (Wood *et al.*, 1980). Moreover, calcium induces microtubule disassembly in cultured cells in a calmodulin-dependent manner (Schliwa, 1980; Keith *et al.*, 1983). These results indicate that calmodulin-regulated enzyme systems are associated with microtubules and may play a role in controlling microtubule dynamics.

4.1. Identification of Calmodulin-Dependent Kinase in Microtubules

A calmodulin-dependent kinase has recently been identified in cold-stable microtubules, a subpopulation of microtubules that are resistant to cold-temperature-induced depolymerization (Job *et al.*, 1983; Larson *et al.*, 1984). This calmodulin-dependent kinase is identical to the previously purified cytosolic enzyme with respect to subunit composition, isoelectric points, calmodulin-binding properties, substrate specificity, and kinetic properties (Larson *et al.*, 1985). Figure 4 compares the one-

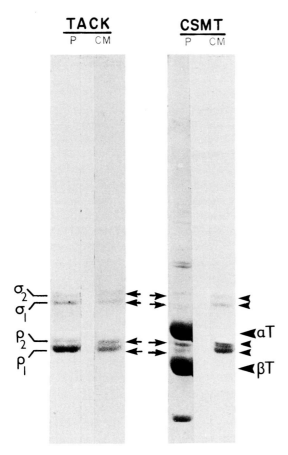

FIGURE 4. [^{125}I]-calmodulin-binding proteins in cold-stable microtubules. Purified calmodulin-dependent kinase (TACK) and cold-stable microtubules (CSMT) were assayed for protein staining (P) and [^{125}I]-calmodulin-binding proteins (CM) and resolved on high resolution SDS–PAGE as described by Goldenring *et al.* (1983). The rho and sigma subunit doublets of TACK are desginated, and the location of alpha (αT) and beta (βT) tubulin and the enzyme subunits in CSMT are indicated by arrowheads. (Reprinted from Larson *et al.*, 1985.)

dimensional high resolution SDS–PAGE autoradiographs of [^{125}I]-calmodulin binding to purified rho and sigma subunits and the enzyme subunits that are endogenous to microtubule preparations. Using this separation technique, the rho and sigma subunits of the enzyme can be resolved into calmodulin-binding doublets as described by Goldenring *et al.* (1983). These results demonstrate that the major 52,000- to 63,000-dalton calmodulin-binding proteins in cold-stable microtubules comigrate with the subunits of cytosolic kinase and can be separated from alpha and beta tubulin.

We have recently demonstrated that a high molecular weight fraction (>15 million) that is enriched for both neurofilament proteins and the calmodulin-dependent kinase can be isolated from microtubule preparations (Vallano *et al.*, 1985a,b). The calmodulin-dependent kinase was separated from a cAMP-dependent kinase that is endogenous to microtubules by gel filtration chromatography (Vallano *et al.*, 1985b). MAP 2 is a major substrate for both kinases and the two enzymes phosphorylate several distinct sites on the MAP 2 molecule (Goldenring *et al.*, 1985). An antibody against the calmodulin-dependent kinase specifically labels cytoskeletal elements in neurons (Vallano *et al.*, 1985a). These studies show that a Type II calcium/calmodulin-dependent kinase is specifically associated with the cytoskeleton, and phosphorylates cytoskeletal proteins with a high-specific activity. We have suggested that the calmodulin-dependent kinase may be a cross-bridging protein between microtubules and neurofilaments, and that calmodulin-dependent phosphorylation of MAP 2, or other cytoskeletal proteins may regulate the interaction between these structures.

4.2. Role of Calmodulin-Dependent Kinase in Microtubule Function

Evidence suggests that calcium and calmodulin accelerate axoplasmic protein transport by the axonal microtubule system (Iqbal and Ochs, 1980). By analogy, calcium and calmodulin may be involved in protein transport along the microtubules in the activated dendritic spine during the development of LTP. A possible mechanism for calmodulin-dependent kinase regulation of protein transport is sequential phosphorylation and detachment of MAP 2 from the surface of microtubules, permitting unidirectional protein transport. An excellent review concerned with asymmetry of cytoskeletal protein cross-bridges and directionality of transport vectors is available (Ellisman and Porter, 1983). The precise manner in which calmodulin-dependent kinase regulates microtubule dynamics and neuroplasmic transport remains to be determined.

5. SUMMARY

A Type II calmodulin-dependent kinase has been identified and biochemically characterized in PSD and microtubule preparations. In addition, a calmodulin-dependent protein kinase that exhibits a broad range of substrate specificities has recently been described in neuronal nuclei (Sahyoun *et al.*, 1984). The high level of enzyme activity suggests a role for this kinase in regulating neuronal nuclear function. The development of LTP in the postsynaptic target neuron is dependent upon calcium-mediated events and is accompanied by alterations in the postsynaptic membrane and underlying PSD, neuroplasmic transport up the activated dendrites, and protein synthesis (Eccles, 1983; Lynch and Baudry, 1984). A calmodulin-dependent protein kinase that phosphorylates cytoskeletal proteins as its major substrates is present in these regions and appears to play a pivotal role in mediating the effects of calcium at the synapse. Further investigations in this area should prove valuable in elucidating the role of the calmodulin-dependent kinase in the development and maintenance of LTP.

REFERENCES

Alkon, D. L., 1980, Cellular analysis of a gastropod (Hermissenda crassicornis) model of associative learning, *Biol. Bull.* **159**:505–560.

Andersen, P., 1981, Brain slices—a neurobiological tool of increasing usefulness, *Trends Neurosci.* **4**:53–56.

Bennett, M. K., Erondu, N. E., and Kennedy, M. B., 1983, Purification and characterization of a calmodulin-dependent protein kinase that is highly concentrated in brain, *J. Biol. Chem.* **258**:12735–12744.

Bliss, T. V. P. and Gardner-Medwin, A. R., 1973, Long-lasting potentiation of synaptic transmission in the dentate area of the unanaesthetized rabbit following stimulation of the perforant path, *J. Physiol. (London)* **232**:357–374.

Bliss, T. V. P. and Lomo, T., 1973, Long-lasting potentiation of synaptic transmission in the dentate area of the anaesthetized rabbit following stimulation of the perforant path, *J. Physiol. (London)* **232**:331–356.

Branton, D., Cohen, C. M., and Tyler, J., 1981, Interaction of cytoskeletal proteins on the human erythrocyte membrane, *Cell* **24**:24–32.

Burke, B. E. and DeLorenzo, R. J., 1981, Ca^{2+} and calmodulin-stimulated endogenous phosphorylation of neurotubulin, *Proc. Natl. Acad. Sci. USA* **78**:991–995.

Burke, B. E. and DeLorenzo, R. J., 1982a, Ca^{2+} and calmodulin-dependent phosphorylation of endogenous synaptic vesicle tubulin by a vesicle-bound calmodulin kinase system, *J. Neurochem.* **38**:1205–1218.

Burke, B. E. and DeLorenzo, R. J., 1982b, Ca^{2+} and calmodulin-regulated endogenous tubulin kinase activity in presynaptic nerve terminal preparations, *Brain Res.* **236**:393–415.

Carlin, R. K., Grab, D. J., and Siekevitz, P., 1982, Postmortem accumulation of tubulin in postsynaptic density preparations, *J. Neurochem.* **38**:94–100.

Carlin, R. K., Bartelt, D. C., and Siekevitz, P., 1983, Identification of fodrin as a major calmodulin-binding protein in postsynaptic density preparations, *J. Cell Biol.* **96**:443–448.

Cheung, W. Y., 1980, Calmodulin plays a pivotol role in cellular regulation, *Science* **207**:19–27.

Cohen, R. S., Blomberg, F., Berzins, K., and Siekevitz, P., 1977, The structure of the postsynaptic densities isolated from dog cerebral cortex. I. Overall morphology and protein composition, *J. Cell Biol.* **74**:181–203.

Cotman, C. W., Banker, G., Churchill, L., and Taylor, D., 1974, Isolation of postsynaptic densities from rat brain, *J. Cell Biol.* **63**:441–455.

DeCamilli, P., Harris, S. M., Jr., Huttner, W. B., and Greengard, P., 1983, Synapsin I (Protein I), a nerve terminal-specific phosphoprotein. II. Its specific association with synaptic vesicles demonstrated by immunocytochemistry in agarose-embedded synaptosomes, *J. Cell Biol.* **96**:1355–1373.

DeLorenzo, R. J., 1980, Role of calmodulin in neurotransmitter release and synaptic function, *Ann. N.Y. Acad. Sci.* **356**:92–109.

DeLorenzo, R. J., Gonzalez, B., Goldenring, J., Bowling, A., and Jacobson, R., 1982, Ca^{2+}-calmodulin tubulin kinase system and its role in mediating the Ca^{2+} signal in brain, in: *Progress in Brain Research,* Volume 56 (W. H. Gispen and A. Routtenberg, eds.), Elsevier Biomedical Press, Amsterdam, pp. 255–286.

Douglas, W. W., 1968, Stimulus-secretion coupling: The concept and clues from chromaffin and other cells, *Br. Pharmacol.* **34**:451–474.

Dunwiddie, T. V. and Lynch, G., 1979, The relationship between extracellular calcium concentrations and the induction of long-term potentiation, *Brain Res.* **169**:103–110.

Dunwiddie, T. V., Madison, D., and Lynch, G., 1978, Synaptic transmission is required for initiation of long-term potentiation, *Brain Res.* **150**:413–417.

Eccles, J. C., 1983, Calcium in long-term potentiation as a model for memory, *Neuroscience* **10**:1071–1081.

Ellisman, M. H. and Porter, K. R., 1983, Introduction to the cytoskeleton, in: *Neurofilaments* (C. A. Marotta, ed.), University of Minnesota Press, Minneapolis, pp. 3–26.

Fifkova, E., Anderson, C. L., Young, J. J., and van Harreveld, A., 1982, Effect of anisomycin on stimulation-induced changes in dendritic spines of dentate granule cells, *J. Neurocytol.* **11**:183–210.

Finn, R. C., Browning, M., and Lynch, G., 1980, Trifluoperazine inhibits hippocampal long-term potentiation and the phosphorylation of a 40,000 dalton protein, *Neurosci. Lett.* **19**:103–108.

Flanagan, S. D., Yost, B., and Crawford, G., 1982, Putative 51,000-Mr protein marker for postsynaptic densities is virtually absent in cerebellum, *J. Cell Biol.* **94**:743–748.

Fukunaga, K., Yamamoto, H., Matsui, K., Higashu, K., and Miyamoto, E., 1982, Purification and characterization of a Ca^{2+}-calmodulin-dependent protein kinase from rat brain, *J. Neurochem.* **39**:1607–1617.

Glenney, J. R., Glenney, P., and Weber, K., 1982, Erythroid spectrin, brain fodrin, and intestinal brush border proteins (TW-260/240) are related to molecules containing a common calmodulin-binding subunit bound to a variant cell type-specific subunit, *Proc. Natl. Acad. Sci. USA* **79**:4002–4005.

Goldenring, J. R., Mcguire, J. S., Jr., and DeLorenzo, R. J., 1984, Identification of the major post-synaptic density protein as homologous with the major calmodulin-binding subunit of a calmodulin-dependent protein kinase, *J. Neurochem.* **42**:1077–1084.

Goldenring, J. R., Gonzalez, B., McGuire, J. S., Jr., and DeLorenzo, R. J., 1983, Purification and characterization of a calmodulin-dependent kinase from rat brain cytosol able to phosphorylate tubulin and microtubule-associated proteins, *J. Biol. Chem.* **258**:12632–12640.

Goldenring, J. R., Vallano, M. L., and DeLorenzo, R. J., 1985, Phosphorylation of microtubule associated protein 2 at distinct sites by calmodulin-dependent and cyclic-AMP-Dependent kinase, *J. Neurochem.* (in press).

Grab, D. J., Carlin, R. K., and Siekevitz, P., 1980, The presence and functions of calmodulin in the postsynaptic density, *Ann. N.Y. Acad. Sci.* **356**:55–72.

Grab, D. J., Carlin, R. K., and Siekevitz, P., 1981, Presence of calmodulin in the postsynaptic density II. Presence of calmodulin-activatable protein kinase activity, *J. Cell Biol.* **89**:440–448.

Guldner, F. A. and Ingham, C. A., 1979, Plasticity in synaptic appositions of optic nerve afferents under different lighting conditions, *Neurosci. Lett.* **14**:235–240.

Gulley, R. L. and Reese, T. S., 1981, Cytoskeletal organization of the postsynaptic complex, *J. Cell Biol.* **91**:298–302.

Iqbal, Z. and Ochs, S., 1980, Calmodulin in mammalian nerve, *J. Neurobiol.* **11**:311–318.

Job, D., Rauch, C. T., Fischer, C. H., and Margolis, R. L., 1983, Regulation of microtubule cold stability by calmodulin-dependent and independent phosphorylation, *Proc. Natl. Acad. Sci., U.S.A.* **80**:3894–3898.

Kandel, E. R., 1981, Calcium and the control of synaptic strength by learning, *Nature* **293**:697–700.

Katz, B. and Miledi, R., 1969, Spontaneous and evoked activity of motor nerve endings in calcium Ringer, *J. Physiol. (London)* **203**:689–706.

Katz, B. and Miledi, R., 1970, Further study of the role of calcium in synaptic transmission, *J. Physiol. (London)* **207**:789–801.

Keith, C., DiPaola, M., Maxfield, F. R., and Shelanski, M. L., 1983, Microinjection of calcium-calmodulin causes a localized depolymerization of microtubules, *J. Cell Biol.* **97**:1918–1924.

Kelly, P. T. and Cotman, C. W., 1978, Synaptic protein: characterization of tubulin and actin and identification of a distinct postsynaptic density polypeptide, *J. Cell Biol.* **79**:173–183.

Kelly, P. T., McGuinness, T. L., and Greengard, P., 1984, Evidence that the major postsynaptic density protein is a component of a Ca^{2+}/calmodulin-dependent protein kinase, *Proc. Natl. Acad. Sci. U.S.A.* **81**:945–949.

Kennedy, M. B., Bennett, M. K., and Erondu, N. E., 1983, Biochemical and immunochemical evidence that the "major postsynaptic density protein" is a subunit of a calmodulin-dependent protein kinase, *Proc. Natl. Acad. Sci. USA.* **80::**7357–7361.

Klee, C. B., Crouch, T. H., and Richman, P. G., 1980, Calmodulin, *Annu. Rev. Biochem.* **49**:489–515.

Larson, R. E., Goldenring, J. R., Vallano, M. L., and DeLorenzo, R. J., 1985, Identification of endogenous calmodulin-dependent kinase and calmodulin binding proteins in cold-stable microtubule preparations from rat brain, *J. Neurochem.*, **44**:1566–1574.

Lee, K. S., 1983, Sustained modification of neuronal activity in the hippocampus and cerebral cortex, in: *Molecular, Cellular and Behavioral Neurobiology of the Hippocampus* (W. Seifert, ed.), Academic Press, New York, pp. 265–272.

Lee, K. S., Schottler, F., Oliver, M., and Lynch, G., 1980, Brief bursts of high-frequency stimulation produce two types of structural changes in rat hippocampus, *J. Neurophysiol.* **44**:247–258.

Levine, J. and Willard, M., 1981, Fodrin: Axonally transported polypeptides associated with the internal periphery of many cell types, *J. Cell Biol.* **90**:631–643.

Lynch, G. and Baudry, M., 1984, The biochemistry of memory: A new and specific hypothesis, *Science* **224**:1057–1063.

Lynch, G., Larson, J., Kelso, S., Barrionuevo, G., and Schottler, F., 1983, Intracellular injections of EGTA block induction of hippocampal long-term potentiation, *Nature (London)* **305**:719–721.

Matus, A., 1981, The postsynaptic density, *Trends Neurosci.* **4**:51–53.

Matus, A., Pehling, G., Ackermann, M., and Maeder, J., 1980, Brain postsynaptic densities: Their relationship to glial and neuronal filaments, *J. Cell Biol.* **87**:346–359.

McGuinness, T. L., Lai, Y., and Greengard, P., 1984, Multiple forms of calcium/calmodulin-dependent protein kinase II in rat brain, *Soc. Neurosci. Abstr.* **10**:919.

McGuinness, R. L., Lai, Y., Greengard, P., Woodgett, J. R., and Cohen, P., 1983, A multifunctional calmodulin-dependent protein kinase, *FEBS Lett.* **163**:329–334.

Miller, S. G. and Kennedy, M. B., 1984, Purification and characterization of distinct cerebellar form of brain "Type II" Ca^{2+}-calmodulin-dependent protein kinase, *Soc. Neurosci. Abstr.* **10**:544.

Nestler, E. J., Walaas, S. I., and Greengard, P., 1984, Neuronal phosphoproteins: Physiological and clinical implications, *Science* **225**:1357–1364.

Ng, M. and Matus, A., 1979, Protein phosphorylation in isolated plasma membranes and postsynaptic junctional structures from brain synapses, *Neuroscience* **4**:169–180.

Rostas, J. A. P., Brent, V. A., and Guldner, F. H., 1984, The maturation of post-synaptic densities in chicken forebrain, *Neurosci. Lett.* **45**:297–304.

Sahyoun, N., Levine, H., III, Bronson, D., and Cuatrecasas, P., 1984, Ca^{2+}-calmodulin-dependent protein kinase in neuronal nuclei, *J. Biol. Chem.* **259**:9341–9344.

Schliwa, M., 1980, Pharmacological evidence for an involvement of calmodulin in calcium-induced microtubule disassembly in lysed tissue culture cells, in: *Microtubules and Microtubule Inhibitors 1980* (M. DeBrabander and J. DeMey, eds.), Elsevier/North Holland, Amsterdam, New York, Oxford, pp. 57–70.

Schulman, H., 1984, Phosphorylation of microtubule-associated proteins by a calcium/calmodulin-dependent protein kinase, *J. Cell Biol.* **99**:11–19.

Sobue, K., Fujita, M., Muramoto, Y., and Kakiuchi, S., 1981, The calmodulin-binding protein in microtubules is tau factor, *FEBS. Lett.* **132**:137–140.

Squire, L. R., 1982, The neuropsychology of human memory, *Annu. Rev. Neurosci.* **5**:241–273.

Thompson, R. F., Berger, T. W., and Madden, J. IV, 1983, Cellular processes of learning and memory in the mammalian CNS, *Annu. Rev. Neurosci.* **6**:447–491.

Ueda, T., Greengard, P., Berzins, K., Cohen, R. S., Blomberg, F., Grab, D. J., and Siekevitz, P., 1979, Subcellular distribution in cerebral cortex of two proteins phosphorylated by a cAMP-dependent protein kinase, *J. Cell Biol.* **83**:308–319.

Vallano, M. L., Goldenring, J. R., Buckholz, T. M., and DeLorenzo, R. J., 1984, Isolation and characterization of a neurofilament-associated calmodulin kinase from microtubule preparations, *Soc Neurosci. Abstr.* **10**:545.

Vallano, M. L., Goldenring, J. R., Lasher, R. S., and DeLorenzo, R. J., 1985a, Association of calcium/calmodulin-dependent kinase with cytoskeletal preparations: phosphorylation of tubulin, neurofilament and microtubule-associated proteins. *Ann. NY Acad. Sci. in press.*

Vallano, M. L., Goldenring, J. R., Buckholz, T. M., Larson, R. E., and DeLorenzo, R. J., 1985b, Separation of endogenous calmodulin- and cAMP-dependent kinases from microtubule preparations, *Proc. Natl. Acad. Sci. USA* **82**:3202–3206.

Vrensen, G. and Nunes Cardozo, J., 1981, Changes in size and shape of synaptic connections after visual training: An ultrastructural approach to synaptic plasticity, *Brain Res.* **218**:79–97.

Weisenberg, R. C., 1972, Microtubule formation in vitro in solutions containing low calcium concentrations, *Science* **177**:1104–1105.

Westrum, L. E. and Gray, E. G., 1977, Microtubules associated with postsynaptic thickening, *J. Neurocytol.* **6**:505–518.

Wood, J. G., Wallace, R. W., Whitaker, J. N., and Cheung, W. Y., 1980, Immunocytochemical localization of calmodulin and a heat-labile calmodulin binding protein in basal ganglia of mouse brain, *J. Cell Biol.* **84**:66–76.

Yamamoto, H., Fukunaga, K., Tanaka, E., and Miyamoto, E., 1983, Ca^{2+}- and calmodulin-dependent phosphorylation of microtubule-associated protein 2 and τ factor, and inhibition of microtubule assembly, *J. Neurochem.* **41**:1119–1125.

Yamauchi, T. and Fujisawa, H., 1983a, Purification and characterization of the brain calmodulin-dependent protein kinase (Kinase II), which is involved in the activation of tryptophan-5-mono-oxygenase, *Eur. J. Biochem.* **132**:15–21.

Yamauchi, T. and Fujisawa, H., 1983b, Disassembly of microtubules by the action of calmodulin-dependent protein kinase (Kinase II) which occurs only in the brain tissues, *Biochem. Biophys. Res. Commun.* **110**:287–291.

28

Regulation of Neuronal Activity by Protein Phosphorylation

JOSÉ R. LEMOS, WILLIAM B. ADAMS,
ILSE NOVAK-HOFER, JACK A. BENSON,
and IRWIN B. LEVITAN

1. INTRODUCTION

During the last 30 years a great deal of progress has been made in our understanding of how neurotransmitters can regulate the activity of excitable cells. Much of our knowledge has come from studies on the vertebrate neuromuscular junction, in part because the preparation is easily accessible for experimental manipulation, but perhaps more importantly because a series of brilliant investigators have made it the focus of their highly imaginative studies. The resulting body of work has given us a detailed molecular picture of the nicotinic acetylcholine receptor/channel as a single macromolecular complex that can both bind acetylcholine and mediate the transport of ions across the plasma membrane. The opening of the channel (and the transport of ions) is rapid in onset after the binding of acetylcholine to the receptor and is rapidly reversible when the receptor is no longer occupied by the agonist; that is, the change in the activity of the ion channel is dependent on the continued occupation of a closely associated receptor by an agonist.

Longer-lasting modulation of ion channels by neurotransmitters is difficult to explain in terms of the scheme described above. Although it is conceivable that in some instances occupancy of receptor by agonist might persist for prolonged periods, there are examples of physiological responses that outlast the initial stimulus by

JOSÉ R. LEMOS, WILLIAM B. ADAMS, ILSE NOVAK-HOFER, JACK A. BENSON, and IRWIN B. LEVITAN ● Friedrich Miescher-Institut, CH-4002 Basel, Switzerland. *Present address* for J. R. L.: Worcester Foundation for Experimental Biology, Shrewsbury, Massachusetts 01545. *Present address* for W. B. A.: Biozentrum, University of Basel, CH-4056 Basel, Switzerland. *Present address* for J. A. B.: Ciba-Geigy AG, Entomology Basic Research, CH 4002 Basel, Switzerland. *Present address* for I. B. L.: Graduate Department of Biochemistry, Brandeis University, Waltham, Massachusetts 02254.

many seconds, minutes, or even hours. It has been convenient to think of such long-lasting changes in terms of a scheme such as that described in Fig. 1: here the changes in ion channel properties are not dependent on the continued occupation of the receptor by the transmitter, but rather result from some long-lasting metabolic modification (for example, phosphorylation) of the channel. This scheme suggests that the receptor and channel need not necessarily be intimately associated in a

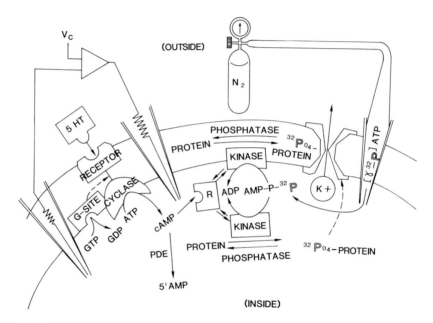

FIGURE 1. Schematic drawing outlining the hypothesized sequence of events underlying the response of neuron R15 to 5HT and the experimental paradigm used to measure single cell phosphorylation. When 5HT binds to its receptor on the plasma membrane of neuron R15, it activates the membrane-bound enzyme adenylate cyclase (cyclase) by displacing GDP from the GTP-binding protein (G-site) and allowing GTP to bind. This leads to the production of 3'5' adenosine monophosphate (cAMP) from ATP by the cyclase. This elevation in intracellular cAMP leads to the activation of either membrane-bound or cytosolic cAMP-dependent protein kinases by binding to the regulatory (R) subunit of the protein kinase and releasing the catalytic subunit (Kinase). These kinases can then phosphorylate specific proteins (protein), either in the membrane or cytosol, by transferring the terminal (γ) phosphate (P) from ATP to the protein. This reaction can be monitored by pressure injecting, using nitrogen (N_2) gas, γ-labeled ATP (AMP-P-^{32}P) into the cell via a microelectrode. The resulting phosphoproteins ($^{32}PO_4$-protein) can be resolved using two-dimensional polyacrylamide gel electrophoresis followed by auto-radiography (see Fig. 9), and they may regulate, either directly or via intermediaries (shown by dashed line), the conductance of the anomalously rectifying potassium (K^+) channel. The activity of this channel can be monitored by placing two microelectrodes into the cell and voltage clamping during the experiment. The process is reversed by enzymes (phosphatase), which remove the phosphate from the phosphoproteins and by phosphodiesterases (PDE) which hydrolyze cAMP to 5'AMP. Outside and inside refer to the extracellular and intracellular space, respectively, of Aplysia neuron R15.

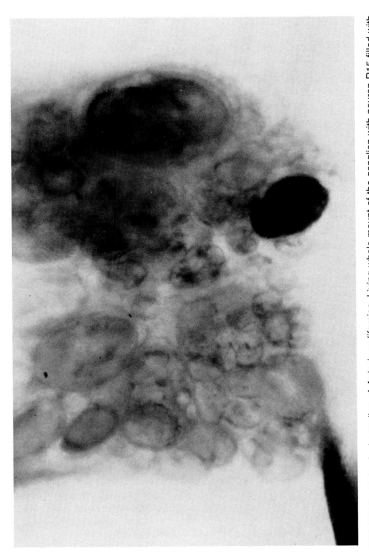

FIGURE 2. Abdominal ganglion of *Aplysia californica*. Living whole-mount of the ganglion with neuron R15 filled with the vital dye Fast Green. All the results discussed in this paper deal with this large (>250 μm diameter), identified cell. The branchial nerve can be seen entering the ganglion from the lower right.

single macromolecular complex but may communicate via some intracellular second messenger that is produced upon occupancy of the receptor by agonist. The second messenger sets in motion a series of steps, culminating in some covalent modification of the channel that alters its activity, and the functional changes persist until the covalent modification has been reversed (again this may require a series of steps).

The large size and ready identifiability of many molluscan neurons makes them particularly convenient for combined biochemical and electrophysiological studies on individual nerve cells. A number of laboratories have taken advantage of these favorable properties to investigate the role of intracellular second messengers in neurotransmitter actions and have implicated cAMP in the effects of serotonin (5HT) on several different molluscan neurons (Klein *et al.*, 1982; Drummond *et al.*, 1980a; Deterre *et al.*, 1981). Our studies have focused on the identified neuron R15 in the abdominal ganglion (see Fig. 2) of the marine mollusk *Aplysia californica*. R15 is an endogenous burster; it exhibits a pattern of spontaneous activity consisting of bursts of action potentials separated by interburst hyperpolarizations (Fig. 3). We have found that 5HT causes R15 to hyperpolarize and stop bursting (Fig. 3). This is also true if dopamine (DA), another putative neurotransmitter, is applied to R15 (Ascher, 1972). Both these responses are prolonged ones and long outlast the initial stimulus (application of the neurotransmitter). Furthermore, stimulation of the branchial nerve of the abdominal ganglion leads to a long-lasting hyperpolarization of neuron R15 (Fig. 4). In this chapter we review our current understanding of the molecular mechanisms underlying such long-lasting responses in this nerve cell.

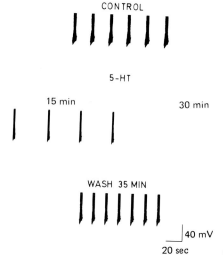

FIGURE 3. Voltage response of R15 to 5HT. The normal rhythmic activity of this neuron is a series of action potentials (burst) separated by an interburst hyperpolarization. When the abdominal ganglion is perfused with 1 μM 5HT, there is first a decrease in burst rate and an increase in the depth of the interburst hyperpolarization, and after about 20–30 min the cell becomes silent with its voltage stable near −80 mV. These effects normally reverse within 30 min after removal of 5HT. The effects of 100 μM dopamine (DA) on the activity of R15 are very similar. (Modified from Drummond *et al.*, 1980a.)

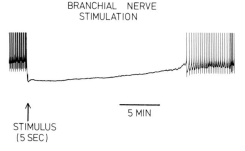

FIGURE 4. Long-lasting synaptic response of R15. If the branchial nerve is stimulated at 2 Hz for 5 sec, then R15 becomes hyperpolarized and bursting activity is inhibited. This response can last for several hours before the cell returns to rhythmic bursting.

2. RESULTS AND DISCUSSION

2.1. Mechanism of 5HT Response

We have studied the mechanism underlying the hyperpolarization of R15 by 5HT using voltage clamp techniques. The membrane potential was swept between -120 and -40 mV ($dV/dt = 4$mV/s) and the total membrane current was mea-

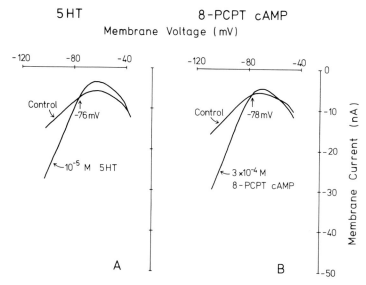

FIGURE 5. Effect of 5HT and cyclic AMP on R15. The membrane potential was swept between -120 and -40 mV ($dV/dt = 4$ mV/s), and the total membrane current was measured in nanoamperes (nA). (A) Normal response to 5HT. Current–voltage (I–V) characteristics of normal R15 (Control) and increase in conductance evoked by 10 μM 5HT. Note the reversal at -76 mV, near the K^+ equilibrium potential (E_K) for this neuron. (B) I–V characteristics of control R15 and increase in conductance elicited by a nonhydrolyzable analog of cAMP, 8-PCPT cAMP, at a concentration of 300 μM. Again note reversal near E_K. (Modified from Drummond et al., 1980a.)

sured. This rate of change is slow compared to the time constant of the cell's membrane but rapid compared to the response to 5HT. A plot of the membrane potential versus the total membrane current (Fig. 5A) yields a steady-state current–voltage (I–V) relationship. The slope of such an I–V relationship is the resistance (or conductance) of the cell membrane. Note that in this neuron there is a linear positive resistance region from -120 to -80 mV, a rectifying region above -80 mV, and a negative resistance region between about -60 and -40 mV.

If the abdominal ganglion is perfused with 5 μM 5HT, there is an increase in conductance that reverses direction (compared to the resting conductance) at around -80 mV (Fig. 5A), which is the equilibrium potential for K^+ (E_K) in this cell (Benson and Levitan, 1983). This reversal at E_K suggests that 5HT increases a K^+ conductance. To test this further the external K^+ concentration was changed and the cell's response to 5HT was examined. The results (Fig. 6) indicate that the current elicited by 5HT reversed at the theoretical E_K for each external K^+ concentration tested. This was not true for any other external ion. Furthermore, this 5HT-evoked current was not blocked by any of the normal K^+ channel blockers, e.g., TEA or 4AP, but was blocked by Cs^+, Rb^+, and Ba^{2+} (Benson and Levitan,

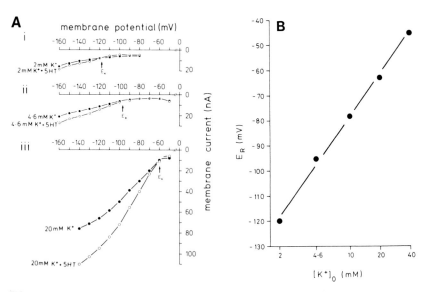

FIGURE 6. Identification of the conductance increased by 5HT. Effect of changing external potassium ($[K^+]_o$) on the resting and 5HT-evoked currents. (A) I–V curves measured at different $[K^+]_o$. The arrows indicate the theoretical E_K for each $[K^+]_o$ as calculated from the Nernst equation. Resting current (●), current evoked by μM 5HT (○). (B) E_r (reversal potential) plotted against log $[K^+]_o$. Line fitted by eye. Labeling as in Fig. 5. (Modified from Benson and Levitan, 1983.)

1983). These pharmacological treatments and the pronounced inward rectification indicate that the 5HT-evoked current is an anomalously rectifying K^+ conductance.

2.2. Intracellular Messenger

Perfusion of the ganglion with 8-parachlorophenylthio (8PCPT) or 8-benzylthio (8Bt) cAMP mimics the response to 5HT (Fig. 5B). These derivatives are resistant to hydrolysis by phosphodiesterases (Meyer and Miller, 1974) and are potent activators of *Aplysia* protein kinase (Levitan and Norman, 1980). The same response is elicited when the cAMP derivatives are injected directly into R15 (Levitan and Drummond, 1980), indicating that they act directly on this cell rather than on some pre-synaptic or non-neuronal element. It appears that cAMP affects the same K^+ channel as does 5HT, since the conductance increases evoked by saturating concentrations of the two are not additive (Drummond *et al.*, 1980a).

The above, together with a series of biochemical and pharmacological experiments, meet all of the criteria (Greengard, 1976) necessary to establish that cAMP mediates this response to serotonin: phosphodiesterase inhibitors, such as RO 20-1724, enhance the response to low concentrations of 5HT (Drummond *et al.*, 1980a); serotonin causes cAMP to accumulate within cell R15 (Levitan and Drummond, 1980); 5HT stimulates adenylate cyclase activity in membranes prepared from R15 somata (Levitan, 1978); and the serotonin receptors mediating adenylate cyclase stimulation and R15 hyperpolarization are pharmacologically very similar (Drummond *et al.*, 1980b).

2.3. Is Adenylate Cyclase Stimulation Necessary?

R15 is hyperpolarized following intracellular injection of the GTP analog guanylylimidodiphosphate (GppNHp), which stimulates adenylate cyclase and causes cAMP to accumulate within the cell (Treistman and Levitan, 1976). Treistman (1981) has found that this response is also mediated by an increase in K^+ conductance. GDPβS, a slowly hydrolyzable analog of GDP (Eckstein *et al.*, 1979), is a specific inhibitor of adenylate cyclase (Cassel *et al.*, 1979). At micromolar concentrations this GDP analog inhibits the stimulation of adenylate cyclase by 5HT in membranes prepared from *Aplysia* nervous system (Lemos and Levitan, 1984). If GDPβS is injected by pressure into a voltage-clamped R15 (see Fig. 1) to a final intracellular concentration of 10^{-6} M, then the increase in K^+ conductance normally elicited by 5HT (Fig. 7A) is blocked (Fig. 7B). The cell can recover from the GDPβS block (Fig. 7C), presumably after this GDP analog has been broken down. Dopamine, on the other hand, can still hyperpolarize R15 in the presence of the inhibitor, confirming that its response is not mediated by cAMP (Drummond *et al.*, 1980a). Furthermore, derivatives of cAMP can still evoke an increase in K^+ conductance in GDPβS-injected cells, pinpointing the block of the 5HT response at the adenylate cyclase (Lemos and Levitan, 1984). Thus the stimulation of adenylate cyclase is a *necessary* step in the activation of the anomalously rectifying K^+ conductance by serotonin in this cell.

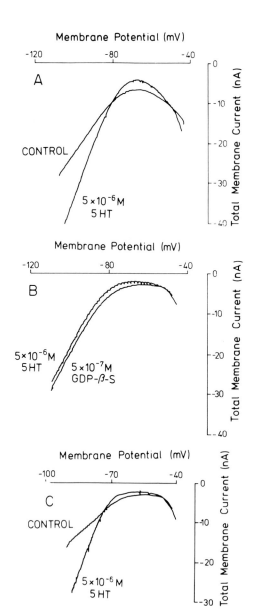

FIGURE 7. Effect of GDPβS on 5HT response. (A) Normal response to 5HT in cell R15. Steady-state I–V curves from an uninjected neuron before (Control) and 20 min after perfusion of 5 μM 5HT. Notice the reversal at about −80 mV. (B) The same cell after intraneuronal injection of 0.5 μM GDPβS. GDPβS had no direct effect on the I–V characteristics of this cell (compare control and GDPβS I–V curves), but blocked completely the cell's response to 5HT (compare to A). GDPβS is a nonphosphorylatable and slowly hydrolyzed analog of GDP that inhibits adenylate cyclase. (C) After 24 hr the cell is able to respond normally to 5HT, indicating breakdown of GDPβS. Labeling as in Fig. 5. (Reproduced from Lemos and Levitan, 1984.)

2.4. Is Protein Phosphorylation Involved in the 5HT Response?

Protein kinase inhibitor (PKI) is a 10,000-dalton protein that binds with high affinity to the active catalytic subunit of cAMP-dependent protein kinase and inhibits its activity (Walsh *et al.*, 1971). We have found that PKI purified to homogeneity from rabbit skeletal muscle (Demaille *et al.*, 1977) is a potent inhibitor of cAMP-dependent protein kinase from *Aplysia* (Adams and Levitan, 1982). When PKI is pressure-injected, via a microelectrode, directly into neuron R15 (see Fig. 1), the increase in K$^+$ conductance normally elicited by 5HT (Fig. 8A) is completely blocked (Fig. 8B). To test the selectivity of this inhibition by PKI, R15's response to dopamine was examined. As shown in Fig. 8C, dopamine causes a decrease in voltage-dependent inward current (Wilson and Wachtel, 1978). A comparison of Figs. 8C and D demonstrates that PKI injection does not affect this dopamine response. Furthermore, the cell's response to cAMP analogs is also blocked by PKI (Lemos and Adams, unpublished observations). Thus the blocking of the neurotransmitter effect appears to be produced specifically by PKI and is selective for

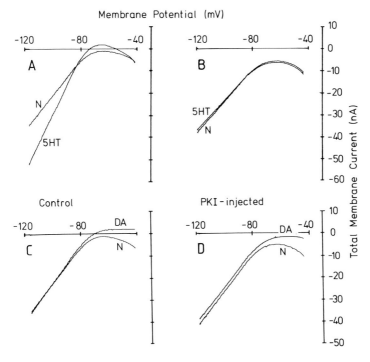

FIGURE 8. Protein kinase inhibitor (PKI) effects on R15. (A) Normal R15 response to 5μM 5HT. (B) After intraneuronal injection of PKI, the same concentration of 5HT elicits no increase in K$^+$ conductance. (C) Normal response of R15 to 100 μM DA. Note the decrease in inward current as compared to control (N). (D) The cell still responds normally to DA after injection of PKI. Labeling as in Fig. 5. (Modified from Adams and Levitan, 1982.)

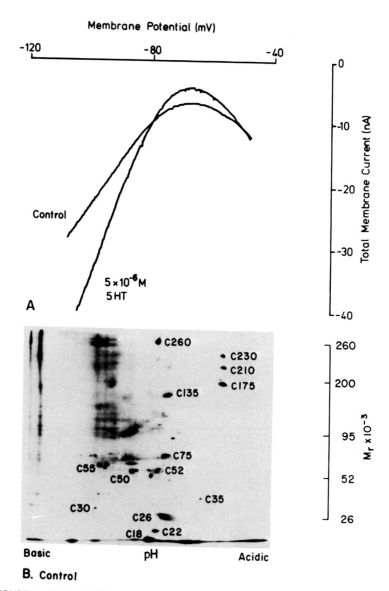

FIGURE 9. Effect of 5HT on protein phosphorylation in R15. (A) Current–voltage (I–V) relationship of normal (Control) R15 (A), and the increase in conductance evoked by perfusion for
20 min with 5 μM 5HT. This cell had been injected with [γ-32P]ATP 30 min prior to treatment
with 5HT. Labeling as in Fig. 5. (B) Protein phosphorylation pattern from a control R15, which
had been perfused with normal *Aplysia* medium for 50 min after injection with [γ-32P]ATP, then
frozen. Autoradiograph of a two-dimensional gel electrophoretic separation of phosphoproteins.
The numbers on the right side of the gel are apparent molecular weights (M_r) × 10^−3 daltons
and the acidic and basic extremes of the isoelectric focusing dimension are marked at the

the 5HT-induced, cAMP-mediated increase in K^+ conductance (Adams and Levitan, 1982). We therefore conclude that cAMP-dependent protein phosphorylation is involved in the regulation of electrical activity in neuron R15.

2.5. Proteins Phosphorylated in a Single Neuron

Having implicated protein phosphorylation in the control of K^+ conductance in R15, it is important to identify the phosphoproteins that may be invovlved in this regulation. Previous attempts to measure protein phosphorylation in individual nerve cells have involved incubating ganglia with ^{32}P-labeled inorganic phosphate, followed by isolation of individual nerve cell somata and analysis of radioactive phosphoproteins (Levitan et al., 1974; Jennings et al., 1982; Paris et al., 1981; Neary and Alkon, 1983). Although this approach has provided useful information, it suffers from several disadvantages. First, the cell body can never be isolated totally free of glia and portions of neighboring cell bodies, which will contribute to the labeling pattern, and, secondly, the neuropil processes of the cell, which are the sites at which most or perhaps all synaptic contacts occur (Frazier et al., 1967), are not sampled by this procedure. To circumvent these problems we have developed methods to inject $[\gamma\text{-}^{32}P]ATP$ directly into R15 (Lemos et al., 1982), in amounts

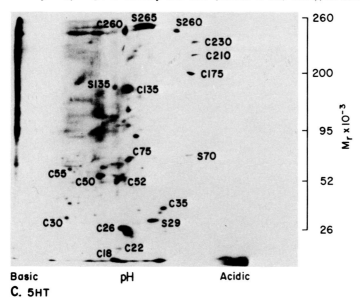

bottom. Some of the phosphoproteins present in control cells are marked with a C and their apparent molecular weight $\times\ 10^{-3}$. (C) Effect of 5HT on protein phosphorylation pattern of R15. This cell was injected with $[\gamma\text{-}^{32}P]ATP$ 30 min prior to perfusion with 5 μM 5HT and then frozen after an additional 20 min when the conductance changes were maximal (see A). Autoradiograph of a two-dimensional gel electrophoretic separation of phosphoproteins. Labeling as in (B), except that phosphoproteins present only in 5HT-treated cells are labeled with an S and their apparent molecular weight $\times\ 10^{-3}$. (Modified from Lemo et al., 1984.)

sufficient to label phosphoproteins (see Fig. 1). We have confirmed, by autora-diography of sections of the abdominal ganglion, that all the radioactivity remains within neuron R15 following such injections (Lemos *et al.*, 1985). Thus, we can process the entire abdominal ganglion, including the neuropil region, for gel elec-trophoresis with the confidence that any radioactive phosphoproteins we observe originate within R15. It is important to remember that the physiological properties of the cell are monitored with intracellular microelectrodes (Fig. 1) throughout the labeling period, so changes in the phosphoprotein labeling pattern may be related to changes in membrane conductance (Fig. 9A). In addition, voltage clamping assures that phosphorylation changes result directly from the effects of the neuro-transmitter, rather than indirectly from changes in the cell's spontaneous activity induced by the transmitter.

The injection protocol has been carefully worked out in order to minimize any damage or modification of normal neuronal function. In particular possible metabolic effects have been minimized by injecting less than 1% of the endogenous ATP levels in R15. Extraction of the acid-soluble counts from the ganglion after such injections indictes that at least 85% of the radioactivity injected is still in the form of [γ-^{32}P]ATP. The incorporated radioactivity is mainly in phosphoproteins and not RNA or phospholipids, although analysis of synaptically stimulated R15's does reveal some changes in phospholipid metabolism (Lemos and Drummond, unpub-lished observations). Furthermore, by using [γ-^{32}P]ATP of high (>5000 Ci/mmol) specific activity we are able to keep our injection volumes to less than 5% of the soma volume. This protocol has minimized any injection artifacts and results in no perceptible alteration of the I–V characteristics of the injected neuron (compare Figs. 5A and 9A).

2.5.1. Protein Phosphorylation Pattern in R15

Proteins phosphorylated within a single identified neuron during a 50-min labeling period were separated by two-dimensional gel electrophoresis. Fig. 9B shows that, in a control R15 perfused with normal *Aplysia* medium for 50 min after injection with [γ-^{32}P]ATP, more than 70 phosphoproteins can be detected. It is important to note that most of these are not major proteins in neuron R15 (or the abdominal ganglion) and thus this phosphorylation pattern does not merely reflect labeling of major substrates in the cell. Some of the phosphoproteins that are detectable in control cells are designated by a C followed by their molecular weight $\times$ 10^{-3}.

2.5.2. Serotonin Effects on Protein Phosphorylation

Concomitant with the K$^+$ conductance increase, 5HT alters the amount of ^{32}P incorporated into at least a dozen proteins (Fig. 9C and Table I). Five phospho-proteins are detected only after perfusion of the abdominal ganglion with 5HT. These 5HT-dependent phosphoproteins are indicated in Fig. 9C by the letter S followed by their molecular weight $\times$ 10^{-3} and by double arrows in Table I. In addition to causing the appearance of the 5HT-dependent phosphoproteins, serotonin

TABLE I. Summary of the Effects of Various Pharmacological Probes and Kinetic Manipulations on Phosphoproteins from Neuron R15[a]

Phosphoproteins	5HT	DA	cAMP	5HT + μM GDPβS	[high] DA	5HT Pre-gK$^+$	Branchial nerve stimulation	
							5HT-like	DA-like
S265	↑↑	—	0	—	—	—	—	—
C260	—	—	0	—	—	—	—	—
S260	↑↑	—	0	↑↑	↑↑	↑↑	↑↑	—
C230	↓	↓	↓	—	—	—	—	—
S135	↑↑	↑↑	—	↑↑	—	↑↑	—	↑
D135	—	↑↑	—	↑↑	↑↑	—	↑↑	↑↑
C135	↑	—	↑	↑	—	—	—	—
C75	—	—	—	—	—	—	—	—
*S70	↑↑	—	↑↑	—	↑↑	←	←	—
D69	—	↓↓	—	—	↓↓	—	↓↓	↓↓
C55	↓	—	↑	—	↑	—	—	↑
C52	↑	↓	—	—	—	—	↓	—
C35	↑	↑	↑	↑	—	—	—	—
C30	↑	↓	↑	—	—	—	↑	—
*S29	↑↑	—	↑↑	—	↑↑	←	↑↑	—
C26	↑	—	↑	↑	↑	↑	—	—
C22	↓	↓	↑	↓	↓	↓	—	↓

[a] A single upward arrow indicates an increase and a downward arrow a decrease in phosphorylation. Double arrows indicate the appearance or disappearance of phosphoproteins as a result of serotonin (5HT), dopamine (DA; normal and high concentrations), guanosine 5'-O-(2-thiodiphosphate) (GDPβS), branchial nerve stimuation (DA- or 5HT-like), or cAMP treatment. A single horizontal arrow indicates that the phosphoprotein appears to be partially shifted towards its final position. 0 indicates phosphoproteins that did not enter gel. * indicates phosphoproteins that could not be dissociated from the 5HT-induced increase in K$^+$ conductance (gK$^+$). (Modified from Lemos *et al.*, 1984, 1985.)

also stimulates the phosphorylation of five proteins that can be observed in control cells, C135, C52, C35, C30, and the doublet C26; and it inhibits the phosphorylation of three others, C230, C55, and C22 (Table I).

2.5.3. Dopamine Effects on Protein Phosphorylation

Dopamine, another putative neurotransmitter, does not affect the conductance of the anomalously rectifying K$^+$ channel when it is bath-applied at concentrations less than or equal to 100 μM (Fig. 8C; Adams *et al.*, 1980) but it can affect the phosphorylation pattern of R15 (Fig. 10C; Lemos *et al.*, 1984). Several phosphoproteins already observable in control cells are affected by dopamine (Table I), and there are at least two dopamine-dependent phosphoproteins (labeled with a D and their molecular weights × 10^{-3}): D135, which is observed only in the presence of dopamine; and D69, whose phosphorylation is very strongly inhibited by dopamine. Note that the 5HT-dependent phosphoproteins (with the exception of S135) are not detected in the presence of 100 μM dopamine (Fig. 8C). On the other hand, at higher concentrations dopamine can not only bind to 5HT receptors (Drummond *et al.*, 1980b) and cause an increase in cAMP (Bernier *et al.*, 1982), it can also

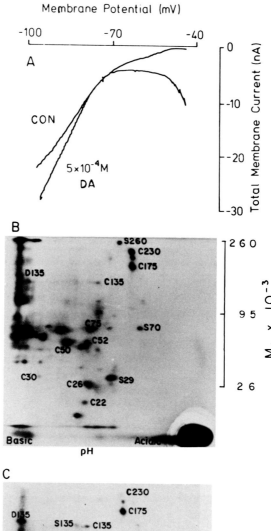

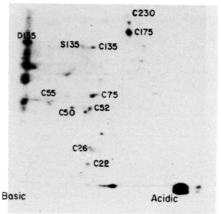

elicit an increase in K^+ conductance (together with the normal decrease in inward current: Fig. 10A). If one examines the phosphorylation pattern of a cell treated with 500 μM dopamine, one can see a combination of 5HT and dopamine effects (Fig. 10B). Note especially the appearance of the 5HT-dependent phosphoproteins S260, S70, and S29.

2.5.4. Synaptic Stimulation: Effects on Protein Phosphorylation

When the branchial nerve is stimulated with a train of 20 pulses at a rate of 2 Hz, there is a dual synaptic effect on R15: a fast, small depolarization after a short delay (milliseconds) and a long-lasting hyperpolarization after a delay of seconds (Fig. 4; Parnas *et al.*, 1974). There are two separate conductance changes underlying the long-lasting hyperpolarization, identical to those produced by the putative neurotransmitters dopamine and 5HT (Fig. 11A; Adams *et al.*, 1980). Concomitant with these conductance changes are alterations in the pattern of protein phosphorylation in R15 (Fig. 11B); in fact, the effects of synaptic stimulation on protein phosphorylation are different depending on the balance of the conductance changes elicited by branchial nerve stimulation. When the dopaminelike conductance changes are large compared with the 5HT-like changes (Lemos *et al.*, 1984), the protein phosphorylation pattern resembles a dopamine phosphorylation response (Table I; Lemos *et al.*, 1984). Furthermore, when the 5HT-like conductance change is at least as large as the dopaminelike changes (Fig. 11A), there is a further stimulation in the phosphorylation pattern with the appearance of S260, S70 and S29 (but not S265: Fig. 11B; Table I). In fact the latter type of synaptic response is very similar, both in conductance and phosphoprotein pattern, to the response to high concentrations of dopamine (compare Figs. 10 and 11). Thus, 5HT-like synaptic conductance changes are accompanied by changes in phosphorylation similar to those elicited by bath application of 5HT, whereas the phosphorylation pattern during dopaminelike synaptic action resembles that produced by bath-applied dopamine.

◄——

FIGURE 10. Dopamine effects on protein phosphorylation in neuron R15. (A) Current–voltage relationship of a normal (control) R15, and the combined decrease in voltage-dependent inward current and increase in the anomalously rectifying K^+ current evoked by perfusion for 20 min with a high concentration (500 μM) of dopamine (DA). Cell had been injected with [γ-^{32}P]ATP 30 min prior to treatment with DA. Labeling as in Fig 5. (B) Effects of 500 μM DA on protein phosphorylation pattern of R15. Same protocol as in Fig. 9C except that instead of 5HT, 500 μM DA was perfused during the last 20 min of the labeling period (the cell's conductance change is shown in A). Autoradiograph of a two-dimensional gel electrophoretic separation of phosphoproteins. Labeling as in Fig. 9C, except that those changes dependent on DA are labeled with a D and their apparent molecular weight × 10^{-3}. (C) Effects of 100 μM DA on protein phosphorylation pattern of R15. Same protocol as in (B), except that a lower concentration (100 μM) of DA was perfused during the last 20 min prior to freezing, resulting only in a decrease in inward current (see Fig. 8C). Autoradiograph of a two-dimensional gel electrophoretic separation of phosphoproteins. Labeling as in (B), but note the absence of high-molecular-weight phosphoproteins. (Modified from Lemos *et al.*, 1985.)

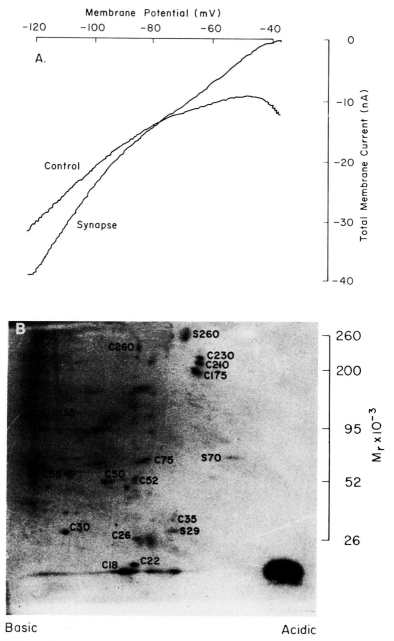

FIGURE 11. Effect of branchial nerve stimulation on protein phosphorylation pattern of R15.
(A) I–V relationship of R15 before (Control) and 3 min after stimulation of the branchial nerve
with 20 pulses at a frequency of 2 Hz (Synapse). Note the large increase in the slope of the
I–V curve at membrane potentials more negative than -80 mV, the K^+ equilibrium potential
for R15. This indicates an increase in K^+ conductance, which is accompanied by a decrease

2.6. Phosphoproteins Associated with the Increase in the Anomalously Rectifying K$^+$ Conductance

Table I summarizes the findings on the effects of 5HT, cAMP, synaptic action, and dopamine on the phosphorylation pattern of neuron R15. We have focused attention on those phosphoproteins that show the largest and most consistent changes in response to 5HT. In order to determine whether any of these phosphoproteins is involved in the regulation of the K$^+$ channel, we have utilized a variety of agents to probe specific sites in the sequence of events hypothesized to occur in neuron R15 as a result of 5HT application (see Fig. 1).

2.6.1. Receptor

The alteration in phosphoprotein pattern is receptor mediated, since whenever the receptor specific for 5HT is occupied by an agonist, the same changes in phosphoprotein pattern are seen (Figs. 9C, 10B). In the rare instances when treatment with 5HT does *not* evoke an increase in K$^+$ conductance, there is a concomitant lack of alteration in the phosphoprotein pattern of R15. When a different receptor is occupied, by 100 μM dopamine for example, and a different conductance response elicited (see Fig. 8C), a different phosphorylation pattern resulted (Fig. 10C). Changes that can be dissociated from the K$^+$ conductance increase would appear to be poor candidates for the regulation of the anomalously rectifying K$^+$ channel.

Whenever an agent (agonist, partial agonist, dopamine, etc.) that interacts with the 5HT receptor elicits an increase in the inwardly rectifying K$^+$ conductance in R15, it also evokes the appearance of the 5HT-dependent phosphoproteins. When 5HT itself, or dopamine, does not elicit this increase in the anomalously rectifying current, the above phosphorylation changes do *not* appear (Lemos *et al.*, 1985). Thus, the appearance of the 5HT-dependent phosphoproteins (with the exception of S135) and the increase in K$^+$ conductance seem to be closely associated.

2.6.2. Intracellular Messenger

Intraneuronal injection or perfusion with an analog of cAMP, 8BtcAMP, mimics some, but not all, of the changes in phosphoprotein pattern elicited by 5HT (Lemos *et al.*, 1983; Novak-Hofer *et al.*, 1985). Since stimulation of adenylate cyclase (Lemos and Levitan, 1984) and the subsequent elevation of cAMP levels (Drummond *et al.*, 1980a) are necessary for the increase in K$^+$ conductance to be elicited by 5HT, it would appear that only those phosphoproteins that respond *both* to 5HT and cAMP (see Table I) can be involved in the regulation of the anomalously

---

in inward current at less negative voltages. Labeling as in Fig. 5. (B) Autoradiograph of a two-dimensional gel electrophoretic separation of phosphoproteins from an R15 that had shown the response to synaptic stimulation in part A. Cell had been injected with [γ-^{32}P]ATP 30 min prior to synaptic stimulation, and was frozen 3 min after stimulation. Labeling as in Figs. 9 and 10. (Modified from Lemos *et al.*, 1984.)

rectifying K$^+$ channel. Another way to examine to role of cAMP is by using the adenylate cyclase modulators GDPβS and GppNHp. At high concentrations (millimolar intracellularly) GDPβS and GppNHp can potentiate or mimic the response to 5HT, both in terms of the increase in K$^+$ conductance (Lemos and Levitan, 1984) and the changes in phosphoprotein pattern (Fig. 12A). In contrast, low concentrations (micromolar intracellularly) of GDPβS completely block the conductance increase and many of the phosphorylation changes normally elicited by 5HT (Figs. 7B and 12B). It is significant that some of the changes in pattern are *not* blocked, i.e., S260, C135, S135, C35, C26, and C22, thus effectively dissociating these phosphoproteins from the increase in K$^+$ conductance (see Table I).

2.6.3. Protein Kinases

cAMP-dependent protein phosphorylation is a necessary step in the regulation of K$^+$ conductance by 5HT in neuron R15. Furthermore, catalytic subunit, the active component of cAMP-dependent protein kinases, can phosphorylate most of the same proteins *in vitro* as can 5HT *in vivo* (Novak-Hofer *et al.*, 1985). Some experiments involving dual injection of PKI and [γ-^{32}P]ATP result in a total inhibition of both the phosphoprotein pattern changes and the K$^+$ conductance response to 5HT in R15 (data not shown), but the results were variable from one experiment to another. Since these experiments are technically very difficult and did not reveal any new insights as to which phosphoprotein is responsible for channel regulation, they were not pursued further.

2.6.4. Potassium Channel

It seemed possible that the changes in phosphoprotein pattern seen in response to 5HT treatment could merely be the result of changes in intracellular K$^+$ concentration, especially since K$^+$ changes can alter protein kinase activity (Novak-Hofer and Lemos, unpublished). Experiments that effectively blocked such changes in K$^+$ concentrations, either by holding the cell at E_K or using Cs$^+$ to block the anomalous rectifier, revealed that net K$^+$ movement was not necessary to see the

---

▶

FIGURE 12. Effects of GDPβS on protein phorphorylation pattern in neuron R15. (A) Effect of mM GDPβS on protein phosphorylation in R15. The neuron was first injected with GDPβS until a final intracellular concentration of 10^{-3} M was achieved, then with [γ-^{32}P]ATP. Thirty minutes later the cell was perfused with 10^{-8} M 5HT. Under these conditions the cell responded with an increase in K$^+$ conductance similar to that seen with 5 μM 5HT in the absence of GDPβS (Lemos and Levitan, 1984). After 20 min the ganglion was frozen and processed for gel electrophoresis. Autoradiograph of a two-dimensional gel electrophoretic separation of phosphoproteins. Labeling as in Fig. 9C, except for the lack of higher-molecular-weight phosphoproteins. (B) Effect of μM GDPβS on protein phosphorylation in R15. Same protocol as in (A), except that the final intracellular concentration of GDPβS was 10^{-6} M and the concentration of 5HT was 5 μM. Under these conditons 5HT cannot evoke any increase in K$^+$ conductance (see Fig. 7B). Autoradiograph of a two-dimensional gel electrophoretic separation of phosphoproteins. Labeling as in (A). (Modified from Lemos *et al.*, 1985.)

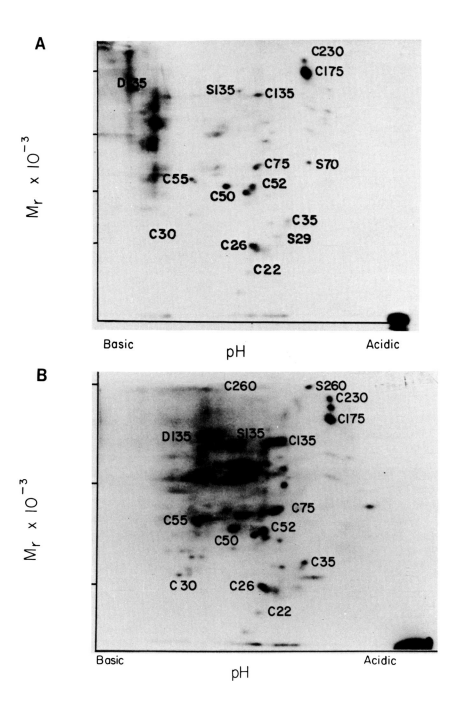

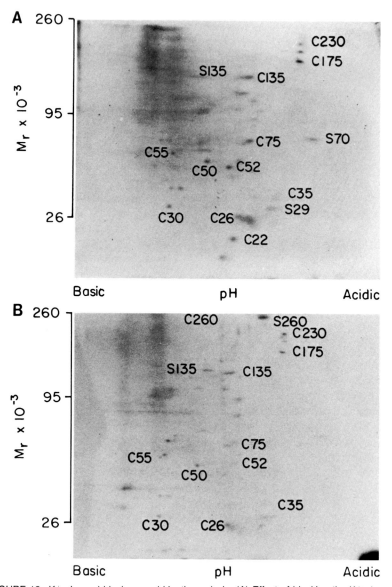

FIGURE 13. K$^+$ channel blockers and kinetic analysis. (A) Effect of blocking the K$^+$ channel on protein phosphorylation. Same protocol as in Fig. 9C except that 10 mM Cs$^+$ was present extracellulary during the entire labeling period. This concentration of Cs$^+$ is sufficient to block the anomalously rectifying K$^+$ channel (Benson and Levitan, 1983), and, as a result, 5HT elicited no increase in current in this cell. Autoradiograph of a two-dimensional gel electrophoretic

changes in phosphoprotein pattern (Fig. 13A). If it were possible to block access to the channel, by use of large molecules acting intracellularly, it might be possible to identify specific phosphoproteins as either constituents of the channel or regulatory proteins closely associated with it. Unfortunately *no* such intracellular blockers specific to this K^+ channel are presently available.

2.6.5. Kinetics of the Response

One would expect that phosphoprotein changes involved in the regulation of channel properties must necessarily accompany the change in K^+ conductance. Although for technical reasons it is difficult to do a rigorous kinetic analysis of the phosphorylation response, experiments designed to answer this question reveal that the phosphoproteins S265, S70, and S29 are most closely associated, in time, with the increase in K^+ conductance (Fig. 13B and Table I).

2.6.6. Localization

It also seems possible that important phosphoprotein changes might occur in synaptic regions of the cell. However, no differences between somata and neuropil were observed in terms of phosphoprotein pattern response to 5HT. This could be due to the application of 5HT by bath perfusion, which would allow occupancy of 5HT receptors on both the soma and neuropil of R15. Also, as elegantly shown by Siegelbaum *et al.*, (1982), cAMP would be able to affect K^+ channels throughout the cell (as is its function as a second messenger), even though its production might be restricted to a discrete site.

Although it might be thought that membrane phosphoproteins are more likely candidates for channel regulatory components, the only 5HT-dependent phosphoprotein found associated with the membrane, at least *in vitro*, is S70 (Lemos *et al.*, 1985). There is no *a priori* reason, however, to limit such regulatory proteins to either a membrane or cytosolic localization. It is even conceivable that the relevant phosphoprotein(s) is not the last or even near the last component in the cascade of events leading from occupancy of the receptor by 5HT to the gating of the anomalously rectifying K^+ channel. Single channel recording of this channel from R15

---

separation of phosphoproteins. Labeling as in Fig. 9C, except for the absence of high-molecular-weight phosphoproteins. (B) Early kinetics of the protein phosphorylation response to 5HT in R15. This cell was injected with [γ-^{32}P]ATP and after 50 min was perfused with 5 μM 5HT for 3 min and then frozen. The K^+ conductance had not yet increased at that time. Autoradiograph of a two-dimensional gel electrophoretic separation of phosphoproteins. Labeling as in Fig. 9C. (Modified from Lemos *et al.*, 1985.)

could help determine whether the channel or its constituents are phosphorylated directly.

If one examines Fig. 9B, or any such control pattern, carefully, it is possible to discern a phosphoprotein of 29,000 daltons, which is found to the right (more acidic) of the 5HT-dependent phosphoprotein S29 (Fig. 9C). More interestingly, when one phosphoprotein is present the other is absent. The same can be said for the S70 phosphoprotein. It is as if these two phosphoproteins are shifting in response to 5HT, but without knowing the identity of these two phosphoproteins it is hard to test this. The shift is of rather large magnitude, especially in the case of S70, and is in the "wrong" direction expected for a protein that is shifted as a result of an increase in negative charges due to phosphorylation. Note also that Fig. 13B reveals that just after (~3 min) treatment with 5HT and *before* a discernible increase in K^+ conductance, S29 and S70 are found at intermediate positions between the control 29,000 and 70,000 dalton phosphoproteins, respectively, and a phosphorylation pattern from an R15 showing a maximal response to 5HT (see Fig. 9C). It is precisely these two phosphoproteins that appear to be the best candidates (see asterisks in Table I) for involvement in the K^+ conductance response to 5HT. Using the probes and manipulations available to us, we were *never* able to dissociate the appearance of these phosphoproteins from the increase in conductance of the anomalously rectifying K^+ channel in *Aplysia* neuron R15.

3. CONCLUSIONS

1. The putative neurotransmitters serotonin and dopamine and stimulation of the branchial nerve all cause a long-lasting hyperpolarization of neuron R15.

2. Serotonin increases the conductance of the anomalously rectifying K^+ current, while dopamine decreases an inward current. The synpatic response is mediated by a combination of the two neurotransmitters' conductance effects.

3. Stimulation of adenylate cyclase is a necessary step in the activation of the K^+ conductance by serotonin. cAMP is the intracellular messenger mediating R15's response to serotonin but not to dopamine.

4. Stimulation of cAMP-dependent protein kinase is necessary for the serotonin response in R15 to occur. Thus protein phosphorylation plays a role in the regulation of the anomalously rectifying K^+ channel in this cell.

5. We have developed a technique for measuring *in vivo* protein phosphorylation in a single cell in order to identify phosphoproteins that might be involved in regulation of neuronal activity.

6. Serotonin changes the phosphorylation of more than a dozen proteins in R15, and five phosphoproteins are seen only after application of 5HT. Dopamine elicits a different phosphoprotein pattern response in R15.

7. Serotonin-like synaptic conductance changes are accompanied by changes in phosphorylation similar to those elicited by bath application of 5HT, whereas the phosphorylation pattern during dopamine-like synaptic action resembles that produced by bath-applied dopamine.

8. Using the pharmacological probes and manipulations available to us, it was possible to dissociate the appearance of all but two of the serotonin-affected phosphoproteins from the increase in K^+ conductance elicited by 5HT. These two phosphoproteins, S70 and S29, may be involved in the regulation of the anomalously rectifying K^+ conductance in *Aplysia* cell R15.

REFERENCES

Adams, W. B. and Levitan, I. B., 1982, Intracellular injection of protein kinase inhibitor blocks the serotonin-induced increase in K^+ conductance in *Aplysia* neuron R15, *Proc. Natl. Acad. Sci. USA* **79:**3877–3880.

Adams, W. B., Parnas, I., and Levitan, I. B., 1980, Mechanism of long-lasting synaptic inhibition in *Aplysia* neuron R15, *J. Neurophysiol.* **44:**1148–1160.

Ascher, P., 1972, Inhibitory and excitatory effects of dopamine on *Aplysia* neurons, *J. Physiol. (London)* **225:**173–209.

Benson, J. A. and Levitan, I. B., 1983, Serotonin increases an anomalously rectifying K^+ current in the *Aplysia* neuron R15, *Proc. Natl. Acad. Sci. USA* **80:**3522–3525.

Bernier, L., Castellucci, V., Kendel, E., and Schwartz, J. H., 1982, Facilitatory transmitter causes a selective and prolonged increase in cAMP in sensory neurons mediating the gill and siphon withdrawal reflex in *Aplysia*, *J. Neurosci.* **2:**1682–1691.

Cassel, D., Eckstein, F., Lowe, M., and Selinger, Z., 1979, Determination of the turn-off reaction for the hormone-activated adenylate cyclase, *J. Biol. Chem.* **254:**9835–9838.

Demaille, J., Peters, K., and Fischer, E., 1977, Isolation and properties of the rabbit skeletal muscle protein inhibitor of cAMP-dependent protein kinases, *Biochemistry* **16:**3080–3086.

Deterre, P., Paupardin-Tritsch, D., Bockaert, J., and Gerschenfeld, H. M., 1981, Role of cAMP in the serotonin-evoked slow inward current in snail neurons, *Nature (London)* **290:**783–785.

Drummond, A., Benson, J., and Levitan, I. B., 1980a, Serotonin-induced hyperpolarization of an identified *Aplysia* neuron is mediated by cyclic AMP, *Proc. Natl. Acad. Sci. USA* **77:**5013–5017.

Drummond, A., Bucher, F., and Levitan, I. B., 1980b, Distribution of serotonin and dopamine receptors in *Aplysia* tissues: analysis by ^{3}H-LSD binding and adenylate cyclase stimulation, *Brain Res.* **184:**163–177.

Eckstein, F., Cassel, D., Lefkowitz, H., Lowe, M., and Selinger, Z., 1979, Guanosine 5′-O-(2-thiodiphosphate): an inhibitor of adenylate cyclase stimulation by guanine nucleotides and fluoride ions, *J. Biol. Chem.* **254:**9829–9834.

Frazier, W., Kandel, E., Kupfermann, I., Waziri, R., and Coggeshall, R., 1967, Morphological and functional properties of identified neurons in the abdominal ganglion of *Aplysia californica*, *J. Neurophysiol.* **30:**1288–1351.

Greengard, P., 1976, Possible role of cyclic nucleotides and phosphorylated membrane proteins in postsynaptic actions of neurotransmitters, *Nature* **260:**101–108.

Jennings, K., Kaczmarek, L., Hewick, R., Dreyer, W., and Strumwasser, F., 1982, Protein phosphorylation during afterdischarge in peptidergic neurons of *Aplysia*, *J. Neurosci.* **2:**158–168.

Klein, M., Camardo, J., and Kandel, E., 1982, Serotonin modulates a specific $K+$ current in the sensory neurons that show presynaptic facilitation in *Aplysia*, *Proc. Natl. Acad. Sci. USA* **79:**5713–5717.

Lemos, J. R. and Levitan, I. B., 1984, Intracellular injection of guanyl nucleotides alters the serotonin-induced increase in potassium conductance in *Aplysia* neuron R15, *J. Gen. Physiol.* **83:**269–285.

Lemos, J. R., Novak-Hofer, I., and Levitan, I. B., 1982, Serotonin alters the phosphorylation of specific proteins inside a single living nerve cell, *Nature (London)* **298:**64–65.

Lemos, J. R., Novak-Hofer, I., and Levitan, I. B., 1984, Synaptic stimulation alters protein phosphorylation *in vivo* in a single *Aplysia* neuron, *Proc. Natl. Acad. Sci., USA* **81:**3233–3237.

Lemos, J. R., Novak-Hofer, I., and Levitan, I. B., 1985, Phosphoproteins associated with the regulation of a specific potassium channel in the identified *Aplysia* neuron R15, *J. Biol. Chem.* **260:**3207–3214.

Levitan, I. B., 1978, Adenylate cyclase in isolated *Helix* and *Aplysia* neuronal cell bodies: stimulation by serotonin and peptide-containing extract, *Brain Res.* **154:**404–408.

Levitan, I. B., and Drummond, A. H., 1980, Neuronal serotonin receptors and cAMP: biochemical, pharmacological and electrophsiological analysis, in: *Neurotransmitters and their Receptors* (U. Littauer, Y. Dudai, I. Silman, V. Teichberg, and Z. Vogel, eds.), John Wiley and Sons, London, pp. 163–176.

Levitan, I. B. and Norman, J., 1980, Different effects of cAMP and cGMP derivatives on the activity of an identified neuron: Biochemical and electrophysiological analysis, *Brain Res.* **187:**415–429.

Levitan, I. B., Madsen, C., and Barondes, S., 1974, Cyclic AMP and amine effects on phosphorylation of specific protein in abdominal ganglion of *Aplysia californica;* localization and kinetic analysis, *J. Neurobiol.* **5:**511–525.

Meyer, R. B. and Miller, J. P., 1974, Analogs of cyclic AMP and cyclic GMP: general methods of synthesis and the relationship of structure to enzymatic activity, *Life Sci.* **14:**1019–1040.

Neary, J. T. and Alkon, D. L., 1983, Protein phosphorylation/dephosphorylation and the transient, voltage-dependent potassium conductance in *Hermissenda crassicornis, J. Biol. Chem.* **258:**8979–8993.

Novak-Hofer, I., Lemos, J. R., Villermain, M., and Levitan, I. B., 1985, Calcium and cyclic nucleotide dependent protein kinases and their substrates in the *Aplysia* nervous system, *J. Neurosci.* **5:**151–159.

Paris, C., Castellucci, V., Kandel, E., and Schwartz, J. H., 1981, Protein phosphorylation, presynaptic facilitation, and behavioral sensitization in *Aplysia, Cold Spring Harbor Conf. Cell Prolif.* **8:**1361–1375.

Parnas, I., Armstrong, D., and Strumwasser, F., 1974, Prolonged excitatory and inhibitory synaptic modulation of a bursting pacemaker neuron, *J. Neurophysiol.* **37:**594–608.

Siegelbaum, S., Camardo, J., and Kandel, E., 1982, Serotonin and cAMP close single K^+ channels in *Aplysia* sensory neurons, *Nature (London)* **299:**413–417.

Treistman, S., 1981, Effect of adenosine 3′,5′-monophosphate on neuronal pacemaker activity: a voltage clamp analysis, *Science* **211:**59–61.

Treistman, S. and Levitan, I. B., 1976, Intraneuronal guanylylimidodiphosphate injection mimics long-term synaptic hyperpolarization, *Proc. Natl. Acad. Sci. USA* **73:**4689–4692.

Walsh, D. A., Ashby, C. D., Gonzales, C., Calkins, D., Fischer, E. H., and Drebs, E. G., 1971, Purification and characterization of a protein inhibitor of cAMP-dependent kinases, *J. Biol. Chem.* **246:**1977–1985.

Wilson, W. A. and Wachtel, H., 1978, Prolonged inhibition in burst firing neurons: synaptic inactivation of the slow regenerative inward current, *Science* **202:**772–775.

29

The Control of Long-Lasting Changes in Membrane Excitability by Protein Phosphorylation in Peptidergic Neurons

L. K. KACZMAREK

1. INTRODUCTION

Nerve cells are remarkably heterogeneous in their electrical properties. In the absence of synaptic input, neurons may show no spontaneous activity or may generate a variety of forms of endogenous pacing and bursting activities. This heterogeneity results from differences in the complement of ionic currents that each cell possesses (Koester and Byrne, 1980). In addition to the currents that determine the pattern of spontaneous and stimulated firing activity, the ionic currents that generate action potentials vary in their nature and distribution, giving rise to differences in the height, width, and cellular location of action potentials evoked in different types of neurons. In simple, experimentally tractable nervous systems, such as those provided by invertebrates, it has, in some cases, been possible to link the endogenous pattern of activity of a neuron to characteristics of specific behaviors. More importantly, it has been possible to demonstrate that stimulation may produce profound changes in the endogenous electrical properties of neurons, leading to changes in the behaviors that are controlled by these neurons (Byrne *et al.*, Chapter 3, this volume; Klein and Kandel, 1980; DeVlieger *et al.*, 1980; Strumwasser *et al.*, 1981; Gillette and Gillette, 1983). Evidence from a variety of laboratories has recently made it clear that changes in the phosphorylation state of proteins may play a central

L. K. KACZMAREK ● Departments of Pharmacology and Physiology, Yale University School of Medicine, New Haven, Connecticut 06510.

role in transformations of the electrical properties of neurons (Kaczmarek *et al.*, 1980; Castellucci *et al.*, 1980; Adams and Levitan, 1982; DePeyer *et al.*, 1982; Castellucci *et al.*, 1982; Alkon *et al.*, 1983).

The nervous system is particularly rich in protein kinases, enzymes that catalyze the phosphorylation of proteins. Much biochemical work has focused on characterizing kinases whose activity is controlled by second messenger substances, such as cyclic nucleotides, and intracellular calcium ions, whose concentrations change during neuronal activity (Rubin and Rosen, 1975; Nestler and Greengard, 1984). The stimulation of a neuron may activate these enzymes and bring about the phosphorylation of specific substrate proteins within the cells. This may in turn alter aspects of that cell's activity. Neuronal processes that may be altered by protein phosphorylation include energy metabolism, protein synthesis, neurotransmitter synthesis, and neurotransmitter release, as well as changes in the electrical properties of neuronal membranes (for a review see Nestler and Greengard, 1984).

This chapter describes the use of the bag cell neurons of *Aplysia* as a model system in which to investigate the role of protein phosphorylation in the control of electrical excitability. In response to brief electrical stimulation these neurons undergo a series of long-lasting transformations of their electrical properties. These, in turn, trigger and control egg-laying behavior. The first part of the chapter deals with the role of cyclic AMP-dependent protein phophorylation in the enhancement of calcium action potentials and the onset of repetitive discharge that leads to the release of neuroactive peptides from the bag cell neurons. The second part discusses the role of elevated intracellular calcium ions in the control of a subsequent transformation of the cells' properties and describes the major forms of kinases that are activated by calcium ions in these neurons.

2. AFTERDISCHARGE AND REFRACTORINESS IN THE BAG CELL NEURONS

The abdominal ganglion of *Aplysia* contains two clusters of peptidergic neurons, each situated at the base of one of the pleuroabdominal connective nerves that connect the abdominal ganglion to the head ganglia. Each cluster contains 200–400 relatively large (40–100 μm) neurons termed "bag cell neurons." The clusters are anatomically isolated from other neurons of the ganglion and the processes of the bag cell neurons extend down into the remainder of the ganglion and also travel a short distance (5–10 mm) along the pleuroabdominal connectives (Kaczmarek *et al.*, 1979; Chiu and Strumwasser, 1981).

When penetrated by a microelectrode, the bag cell neurons show no spontaneous activity. A brief stimulus train to the pleuroabdominal connective nerve (5–20 V, 2.5 msec, 1–6 Hz for 5–15 sec), however, generates a train of action potentials in the cells (Fig. 1), which is followed by a long-lasting depolarization and the onset of spontaneous discharge (Kupfermann and Kandel, 1970; Dudek and Blankenship, 1977; Kaczmarek *et al.*, 1978). This afterdischarge lasts for a mean duration of 30 min and is associated with a profound enhancement of the height

AFTERDISCHARGE

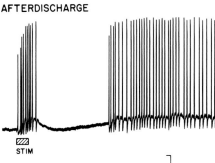

FIGURE 1. The upper part of the figure shows an intracellular recording from a bag cell neuron at the onset of an afterdis-charge triggered by brief stimulation of the pleuroabdominal connective nerve (2.5 msec, 20 V pulses, 1.67 Hz, five pulses). The lower half of the figure shows the response of the same cell to stimulation at the same frequency and intensity during the refractory period (2.5 msec, 20 V, 1.67 Hz, eight pulses). In the refractory state, stimulation fails to produce an afterdis-charge. (Kaczmarek and Kauer, 1983.)

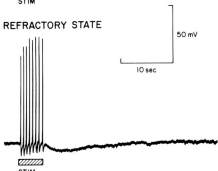

REFRACTORY STATE

and width of bag cell action potentials (Fig. 2) (Kaczmarek *et al.*, 1982). During stimulation and during the afterdischarge all neurons in a cluster fire in synchrony. This is believed to be due to the presence of numerous gap junctions on the processes of the cells, which result in all of the neurons within a cluster being electrically coupled during the afterdischarge (Blankenship and Haskins, 1979; Kaczmarek *et al.*, 1979). The afterdischarge in the bag cell neurons may also be initiated by peptides from the reproductive tract (Heller *et al.*, 1980) and serves to trigger the release of several neuroactive bag cell peptides the initiate egg-laying behavior (Kupfermann, 1970; Arch *et al.*, 1976; Chiu *et al.*, 1979; Dudek *et al.*, 1979; Stuart *et al.*, 1980; Scheller *et al.*, 1983; Rothman *et al.*, 1983).

After the end of the discharge, stimulation of the pleuroabdominal connectives generally fails to induce a second afterdischarge (Fig. 1) or succeeds in triggering only short discharges of low firing frequency. This period of refractoriness lasts for several hours, outlasting the sequence of stereotyped behaviors that is caused by the released bag cell peptides. The ability to stimulate full length afterdischarges is recovered after about 18 hr.

3. ELECTROPHYSIOLOGICAL EFFECTS OF CYCLIC AMP

Evidence indicates that the onset of an afterdischarge is intimately linked to an increase in intracellular cyclic AMP levels. The levels of cyclic AMP in a bag cell cluster increase during the first 2 min after stimulation of the pleuroabdominal

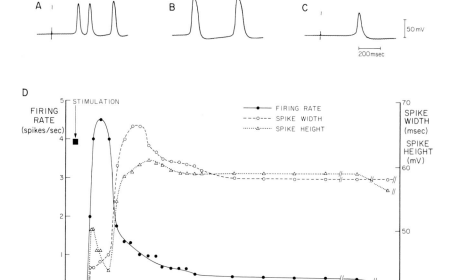

FIGURE 2. Traces (A), (B), and (C) show intracellularly recorded bag cell action potentials. Trace (A) shows spikes evolved by extracellular stimulation of a pleuroabdominal connective nerve at the onset of an afterdischarge. Trace (B) shows enhanced action potentials 10 min after the onset of afterdischarge. Trace (C) shows an action potential evoked after the end of the afterdischarge. The lower part of the figure (D) shows a plot of the firing rate, spike width, and spike height during a bag cell afterdischarge triggered by extracellular stimulation (20 V, 2.5 msec, 1 Hz, 10 sec) of a pleuroabdominal connective nerve. (Kaczmarek et al., 1982.)

connectives (Kaczmarek et al., 1978). An afterdischarge that resembles an electrically stimulated afterdischarge in all general aspects may be induced by extracellular application of a variety of membrane-permeant cyclic AMP analogues as well as by the adenylate cyclase activator, forskolin (Kaczmarek et al., 1978; Strumwasser et al., 1982). The duration of an afterdischarge may also be increased by phosphodiesterase inhibitors, which prevent the catabolism of cyclic nucleotides.

Because the bag cell neurons comprise an electrically coupled network of cells within the abdominal ganglion, their electrical properties are more readily assessed in isolated cultured neurons than in the intact clusters. The electrical effects of cyclic AMP analogues in isolated bag cell neurons qualitatively resemble those of the cells within intact clusters and include a marked enhancement of the height and width of action potentials and the onset of subthreshold oscillations in membrane potential that may drive repetitive firing (Kaczmarek and Strumwasser, 1981a). Cyclic AMP analogues and the cyclase activator forskolin also produce significant increases in input resistance in the cells.

Voltage clamp studies, using a two-microelectrode voltage clamp, have shown that the major effects of cyclic AMP are on potassium currents. Cyclic AMP analogues diminish both the delayed potassium currents and the early transient potassium current (I_A) and induce a region of negative slope resistance in the steady-state current voltage relations near the resting potential (Kaczmarek and Strumwasser, 1981b, 1984). No effect has been observed on the major inward currents. J. Strong has also demonstrated that elevation of cyclic AMP levels using forskolin causes similar effects in internally dialyzed isolated bag cell neurons, including the net diminution of I_A through an increase in its rate of inactivation (Fig. 3) (Strong, 1983).

4. CYCLIC AMP-DEPENDENT PROTEIN PHOSPHORYLATION

To test whether the electrophysiological effects of cyclic AMP could be duplicated by direct phosphorylation of substrate proteins, the injection of the catalytic subunit of the cyclic AMP-dependent protein kinase from bovine heart was carried out into bag cell neurons.

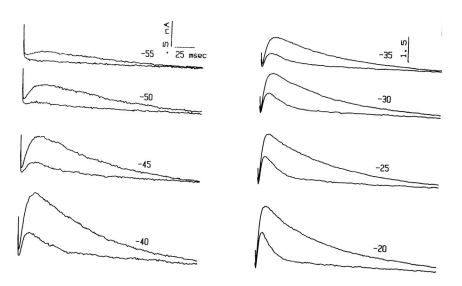

FIGURE 3. The effect of elevated cyclic AMP levels on the form of the early transient potassium current, I_A. Currents shown are those during 220-msec pulses to the indicated potential, after a 450-msec prepulse to -90 mV. The smaller current in each pair is that recorded 20 min after the addition of the adenylate cyclase activator forskolin (100 μM) with the phosphodiesterase inhibitor Ro20-1724. There is a change of scale between the left and right panels. (From Strong, 1983.)

Cyclic AMP-dependent protein kinase is a tetrameric enzyme consisting of two catalytic subunits and two regulatory subunits (Rubin and Rosen, 1975; Nestler and Greengard, 1984). On the binding of cyclic AMP to the regulatory subunits the tetramer dissociates and frees the catalytic subunits. The free catalytic subunits transfer phosphate from ATP to serine and threonine residues on substrate proteins. There exist two or more forms of the cyclic AMP-dependent enzyme, which differ in the nature and locations of their regulatory subunits. The catalytic subunits, however, appear to be the same, or very similar, in each of the forms of the enzyme and to have been well conserved throughout evolution. Thus catalytic subunit that is prepared from beef heart is capable, in an *in vitro* assay, of enhancing the phosphorylation of a large number of bag cell proteins (Kaczmarek *et al.*, 1980).

As is shown in Fig. 4, the injection of the catalytic subunit of the cyclic AMP-dependent protein kinase into the cultured neurons enhances their action potentials in a manner similar to that observed with elevations of cyclic AMP. The catalytic

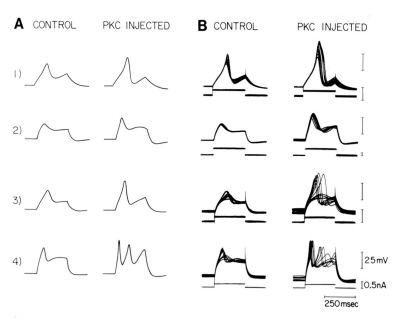

FIGURE 4. The effect of intracellular injection of the catalytic subunit of cyclic AMP-dependent protein kinase (PKC) on the action potentials of bag cell neurons in cell culture (A). The control column shows tracings of the first action potential evoked by a train of depolarizing current pulses prior to injection of PKC in four different cells. The second column shows the response of the cells to the same current pulses after injection. (B) Superimposed oscilloscope tracings of the response to multiple depolarizing current stimuli at a frequency of 0.83/sec before and after injection of PKC, for the same four cells as in (A). Lower traces show the applied transmembrane current. The solutions at the electrode tips contained PKC (0.5–1.13 mg/ml), 2-mercaptoethanol (10–15 mM), and 0.3 M K phosphate (cells 1 and 3), 0.3 M Na phosphate (cell 2), or 0.3 M KCl (cell 4). (From Kaczmarek *et al.*, 1980.)

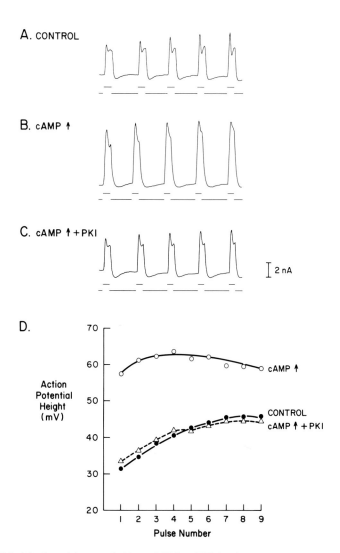

FIGURE 5. Injection of the protein kinase inhibitor (PKI) into isolated bag cell neurons antagonizes the enhancement of action potentials by elevated cyclic AMP levels. (A) shows control action potentials evoked by five consecutive depolarizing current pulses. (B) shows the response of the cell to the same depolarizing current pulses after exposure to 50 μM forskolin, 1 mM theophylline. Subsequent intracellular injection of PKI restores the height and width of action potentials towards control values (C). The lower part of the figure (D) plots the successive height of action potentials in a train of nine depolarizing current pulses applied at a frequency of 1.25 Hz. The graph shows heights before, and 15 min after, treatment with forskolin-theophylline and 10 min after a subsequent injection of PKI. The electrode tip contained 3.6 mg/ml PKI in 0.6 M KCl, 1 mM Tris-HCl, pH 7.8). (From L. K. Kaczmarek, A. C. Nairn, and P. Greengard, unpublished.)

subunit also produces an increase in input resistance and the onset of subthreshold oscillations in membrane potential (Kaczmarek *et al.*, 1980). These data are consistent therefore with the notion that the electrical effects of elevated cyclic AMP levels in these cells are mediated by the phosphorylation of proteins that are substrates for the cyclic AMP-dependent protein kinase.

Further evidence for the role of this enzyme in mediating the electrical effects of cyclic AMP comes from experiments in which a specific protein inhibitor was injected into these cells. Protein kinase inhibitor (PKI) is a protein isolated from rabbit skeletal muscle, which is able to bind to free catalytic subunit and to prevent its catalytic activity (Ashby and Walsh, 1972). We have found that, after the enhancement of action potentials by forskolin, the injection of this protein into bag cell neurons may diminish both their height and width towards control values (Fig.

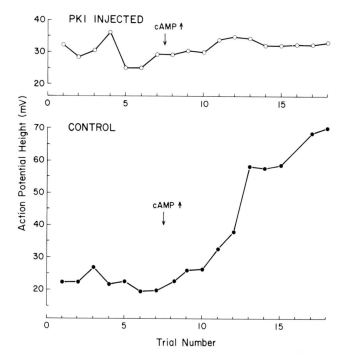

FIGURE 6. Prior injection of PKI into an isolated bag cell neuron prevents the enhancement of action potentials by elevated cyclic AMP levels (A). The graphs show the height of the first action potential evoked by a train of depolarizing current pulses. Successive trains of pulses (trials) were delivered at approximately 3-min intervals. The cell in the upper graph (A) had been injected with PKI by applying pressure to the inside of the microelectrode, which contained 3.6 mg/ml PKI in 0.6 M KCl, 1 mM Tris-HCl at pH 7.8. Exposure of the cells to 50 μM forskolin, 1 mM theophylline (cAMP) fails to produce enhancement of action potentials. The lower graph shows the control response for a cell injected with the carrier medium alone. (From L. K. Kaczmarek, A. C. Nairn, and P. Greengard, unpublished.)

5). Moreover, prior injection of the protein inhibitor prevents the electrical effects of a subsequent elevation of cyclic AMP with forskolin (Fig. 6).

5. CHANGES IN PHOSPHORYLATION STATE OF PROTEINS DURING AN AFTERDISCHARGE

The changes in the potassium currents that give rise to the altered electrical properties of bag cell neurons in response to cyclic AMP, or to its kinase, must be related to changes in the phosphorylation state of specific bag cell proteins. Alterations in the phosphorylation state of bag cell proteins have been investigated by radiolabeling intact clusters of cells with $Na_2H^{32}PO_4$ or by labeling phosphoproteins in homogenates of the bag cell neurons with $[\gamma\text{-}^{32}p]APT$ (Jennings et al., 1982). The phosphorylation state of at least two proteins, BCI and BCII, is enhanced during the bag cell afterdischarge. The time course of changes in phosphorylation state for these two proteins, however, appears to be slightly different. BCI showed enhanced phosphorylation within at least 2 min of the onset of an afterdischarge. Towards the end of an afterdischarge (20 min after stimulation) the phosphorylation state of BCI is not significantly different from control. No increase in the phosphorylation state of BCII was noted 2 min after the onset of afterdischarge, however, while a very significant increase was seen at 20 min (Jennings et al., 1982). Our preliminary evidence indicates that the phosphorylation state of BCII may remain elevated after the end of discharge (unpublished results).

The apparent molecular weight of BCI on SDS–polyacrylamide gels is 33,000, while that of BCII is 22,000. We have determined that these two proteins are the major substrates for the endogenous cyclic AMP-dependent protein kinase in the bag cell neurons (Fig. 7). BCI is found throughout the *Aplysia* nervous system. BCII, on the other hand, appears to be specific to, or highly enriched in, membrane preparations from the bag cell neurons. By electrophoretically eluting the protein band corresponding to BCII from an SDS gel, it was possible to obtain an amino acid composition for this protein and, by gas phase microsequencing, to obtain a partial sequence over 23 amino acid residues at the N-terminus (Fig. 8A) (Jennings et al., 1982). We have taken advantage of this information to generate antisera against part of this sequence. A synthetic sequence (Fig. 8B), which includes residues 3–9 of the N-terminal sequence, was conjugated to thyroglobulin and used as an immunogen. Antisera that recognize this short peptide sequence were generated. As is shown in Fig. 9, immunohistochemical staining of whole-mounts of abdominal ganglia demonstrate that the antisera recognize a determinant in the bag cell neurons but not in the remainder of the ganglion. Interestingly, the N-terminal sequence of BCII, has subsequently also been found in the precursor to the bag cell neurosecretory peptides (Scheller et al., 1983) suggesting that perhaps BCII is derived from this percursor.

Although BCI and BCII are the major substrates whose phosphorylation state changes with afterdischarge, we do not as yet know whether these proteins are

Bag Cells

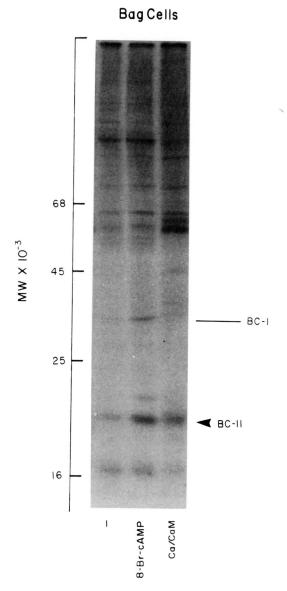

FIGURE 7. An autoradiogram showing the phosphorylation of endogenous substrate proteins in homogenates of bag cell neurons of *Aplysia* in the presence of 8-Br-cAMP or calcium plus calmodulin. Phosphorylation reactions were carried out in the presence of γ-^{32}P-ATP with either 1.5 mM EGTA (—), with 20 μM 8-Bromo-cAMP plus 1 mM Isobutylmethylxanthine (8-Br-cAMP), or with 1.0 mM calcium plus 10 μg/ml calmodulin (Ca/CaM). Radiolabeled phosphorylated proteins were subjected to SDS–PAGE and autoradiography. (DeRiemer *et al.*, 1984.)

A

(   )-(   )- | Val - His - Gly - Lys - Asn - Phe - Ala | - (Arg)

(positions: 5 above Gly; 10 above Arg)

- Asn - (Arg) - Ala - Val - Lys - (   ) - (   ) - (   ) - (   ) - Phe

(positions: 15 above Lys; 20 above Phe)

- Val - Val - (Leu) . . . .

B

Tyr - Gly - | Val - His - Gly - Lys - Asn - Phe - Ala |

(position: 5 above Gly)

FIGURE 8. (A) Partial N-terminal amino acid sequence of the protein band corresponding to the bag cell specific phosphoprotein BCII. (B) The amino acid sequence of a synthetic peptide containing residues 3–9 of the protein in (A). This synthetic peptide was used to prepare a bag cell-specific antisera. (From S. A. DeRiemer, J. Casnellie, P. Greengard, and L. K. Kaczmarek, unpublished.)

directly related to the changes in electrical properties or to some other aspect of the cells' response to cyclic AMP.

6. LONG-LASTING EFFECTS OF CALCIUM ENTRY IN THE BAG CELL NEURONS

As described above, the action potentials of the bag cell neurons are enhanced during a bag cell afterdischarge. Because calcium ions are a major carrier of inward current in these cells (Acosta-Urquidi, 1979; Kaczmarek et al., 1980), this results in an enhanced flux of calcium into the cells and brings about the secretion of the bag cell peptides. There is also evidence that calcium entry during the afterdischarge contributes substantially to the prolonged refractory period that follows an after-discharge.

In media that contain no extracellular calcium ions, afterdischarges may still be induced if a potassium channel blocking agent, such as tetraethylammoniun ions (TEA), is present in the medium (Kaczmarek et al., 1982). Such afterdischarges are short (1–2 min) and of high firing frequency (3–6 Hz). They resemble the early high-frequency phase of an afterdischarge in normal media. Interestingly, these afterdischarges in calcium-deficient media show no subsequent refractory period and may be triggered as many as 20 times in a cluster without attenuation (Fig. 10). Conversely, in a TEA- and calcium-containing extracellular medium lacking sodium ions, a single long afterdischarge is immediately followed by a prolonged refractory period (Fig. 10).

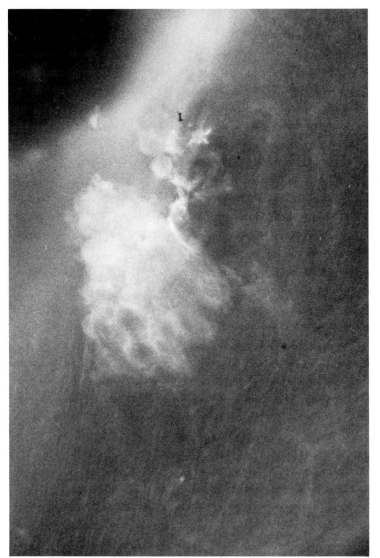

FIGURE 9. Immunocytochemical staining of a whole mount of an *Aplysia* abdominal ganglion, using antisera against the synthetic peptide of Fig. 8. The bag cell cluster in the center of the photograph is uniquely stained. The body of the abdominal ganglia is to the left and a pleuroabdominal connective nerve emerges to the right of the bag cell cluster.

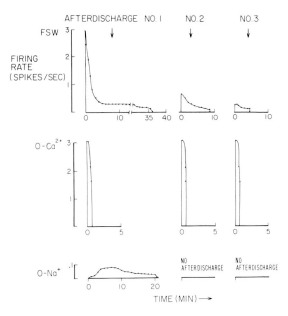

FIGURE 10. Refractoriness following bag cell afterdischarge in media of differing ionic composition. Firing rate of bag cells following brief stimulation of a pleuroabdominal connective nerve is plotted in all graphs. Afterdischarge No. 1 indicates the first afterdischarge that was triggered while No. 2 and No. 3 show successive responses to stimulation after the end of the first afterdischarge. The top row (FSW) shows responses in a normal seawater medium. The second row (O-Ca^{2+}) shows responses in a medium that contains 0.5 mM Ca^{2+} and 20 mM Co^{2+} in place of the normal calcium concentration and 100 mM TEA. The bottom row (O-Na$^+$) shows responses in a medium of normal calcium concentration (11 mM) but with sodium replaced by Tris-HCl (460 mM, pH 7.8) and with 100 mM TEA. (From Kaczmarek *et al.*, 1980.)

These results suggested that calcium entry during an afterdischarge may provide the intracellular signal for the onset of the refractory period. This hypothesis was tested further using the divalent cationophore X537A. The exposure of bag cell clusters to X537A in calcium-containing media does not trigger any electrical activity in the cells but does lead to the secretion of peptides. A concentration of 2.5–5.0 μM ionophore for a period of 20 min leads to an amount of radiolabeled peptide release from bag cell clusters that is quantitatively similar to that obtained on electrical stimulation of a bag cell afterdischarge (Kaczmarek and Kauer, 1983). Exposure to X537A at the same concentrations in calcium-containing media also induces a refractory state in the bag cell neurons (Fig. 11). The refractory state that is induced by the ionophore is pharmacologically and physiologically very similar to that induced by an afterdischarge, and recovery also takes place over 16–20 hr.

The nature of the change that is induced by calcium ions in bag cell neurons to prevent or attenuate the afterdischarge is not, as yet, known. Clues may be obtained, however, from studies with the cultured cells. Concentrations of ionophore that produce a refractory state have little effect on most of the electrical properties

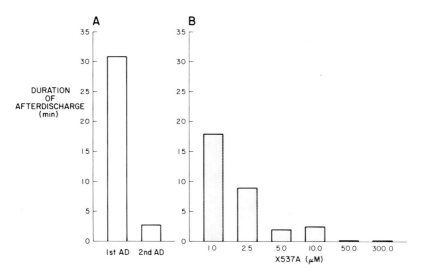

FIGURE 11. Histograms showing mean durations of afterdischarges before and after refractoriness induced either by a prior afterdischarge or by exposure to the cationophore X537A. (A) shows the mean duration of a first afterdischarge (1st AD) in a normal medium and the mean duration of discharges induced by subsequent stimulation (2nd AD) within 1 hr of the end of the first afterdischarge. (B) shows the effect of a 2-min exposure to different concentrations of X537A on the duration of a first afterdischarge. Exposure to an ionophore concentration of 2.5–5.0 μM produces a diminution in duration of afterdischarge that is similar to that produced by a prior afterdischarge. Kaczmarek and Kauer (1983).

of the cells. In particular, no significant effects are seen on the action potentials or input resistance of the cells nor on the ability of elevated cyclic AMP concentrations to alter these parameters. After exposure to the adenylate cyclase activator, forskolin, however, certain cultured bag cell neurons generate a cumulative depolarization in response to repetitive intracellular stimulation (Kaczmarek and Kauer, 1983). This depolarization is similar to the cumulative depolarization that is seen with stimulation of an afterdischarge in intact clusters of cells (see Fig. 1) and is abolished, or severely attenuated, by the ionophore. As the cumulative depolarization in intact clusters of cells is also attenuated in the refractory period, it is likely that the loss of this depolarizing response plays a major role in the onset on the refractory period.

7. CALCIUM-DEPENDENT KINASES IN THE NERVOUS SYSTEM OF *APLYSIA*

The finding that calcium produces prolonged changes in the electrical properties of neurons raises the possibility that the effects of calcium, like those of cyclic AMP, are mediated by changes in the phosphorylation state of specific proteins. The addition of calcium, or calcium with calmodulin, to homogenates of *Aplysia* nervous system stimulates protein phosphorylation (Novak-Hofer and Levitan, 1983). In contrast to cyclic AMP-dependent protein kinase, however, there are a variety of calcium-dependent kinases that differ in their catalytic activities and, therefore, in their ability to phosphorylate different substrates (Nestler and Greengard, 1984). We have, therefore, investigated the nature of the calcium-dependent protein kinases that are present in the nervous system of *Aplysia* and, in particular, in the bag cell neurons. We have determined that there are at least two calcium/calmodulin-de-

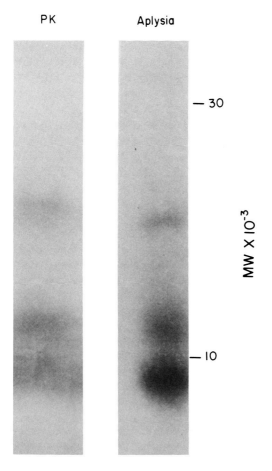

FIGURE 12. A comparison of the one-dimensional phosphopeptide map of the M_r 51,000 substrate for Ca/CaM-PK found in the *Aplysia* nervous system with that of purified mammalian calmodulin kinase II (PK). The M_r 51,000 substrates in the two preparations were labeled using γ-^{32}P-ATP separated by SDS-PAGE, and subjected to one-dimensional peptide mapping, and autoradiography (From DeReimer *et al.,* 1984.)

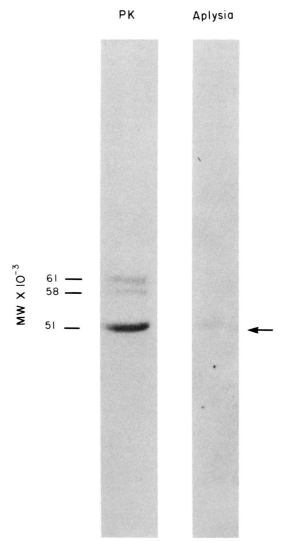

FIGURE 13. An immunoblot that demonstrates the cross-reactivity of M$_r$ 51,000 protein from *Aplysia* CNS ganglia with a monoclonal antibody to mammalian calmodulin kinase II. Partially purified calmodulin kinase II (PK; 20 μg) and *Aplysia* CNS ganglia homogenate (*Aplysia;* 100 μg) were transferred to nitrocellulose paper after separation of proteins by gel electrophoresis. Transfers were incubated with the monoclonal antibody, washed and then incubated in [^{125}I]-goat anti-mouse Ig's. The immunoreactive proteins were visualized by autoradiography (From DeRiemer *et al.,* 1984.)

pendent kinases (DeRiemer *et al.*, 1982, 1984), as well as a calcium-phospholipid-dependent protein kinase (DeRiemer *et al.*, 1983).

The major form of calcium/calmodulin-dependent protein kinase in the nervous system of *Aplysia* appears to be homologous to the mammalian enzyme calmodulin kinase II. As can be seen in Fig. 7, the major substrate for calcium/calmodulin-dependent phosphorylation in the bag cell neurons is a protein of apparent molecular weight 51,000. The proteolytic fragments generated from this protein in the *Aplysia* nervous system are very similar to those of a purified autophosphorylated component of calmodulin kinase II (Fig. 12). The M_r 51,000 protein is the major calmodulin binding protein in the *Aplysia* nervous system and is bound by a monoclonal antibody directed against mammalian calmodulin kinase II (Fig. 13). In addition, the substrate specificity of the major form of calcium/calmodulin kinase in the *Aplysia* nervous system matches that of the mammalian enzyme (DeRiemer *et al.*, 1982, 1984).

Interestingly, among the protein substrates for calcium/calmodulin-dependent phosphorylation is the bag cell-specific phosphoprotein BCII, whose phosphorylation state changes during a bag cell afterdischarge (Fig. 7). The phosphorylation state of BCI is, however, not affected by calcium ions. It is likely that the sensitivity of the phosphorylation state of BCII to changes in internal calcium concentrations accounts for the delayed and prolonged change in the phosphorylation state of BCII during an afterdischarge (see above).

8. CONCLUSIONS

The available evidence presents a strong case for the control of potassium channels in the bag cell neurons through the phosphorylation of proteins by a cyclic AMP-dependent protein kinase. It is not yet clear whether the substrate proteins that control these channels will turn out to be the membrane channels themselves or other proteins that regulate such channels. The characterization of such substrates and their role in the transformation of the electrical properties of neurons, as well as other aspects of long-lasting responses of neurons, therefore provides a fruitful area for future research.

Calcium entry into neurons may also produce long-lasting effects on their electrical properties, which may be accompanied by changes in protein phosphorylation that are regulated by calcium-dependent kinases. At present, the pharmacological specificity of drugs that affect calcium- and calmodulin-dependent processes does not permit one to unambiguously assign a role to calcium-dependent phosphorylation in the control of specific electrical events in neurons such as the bag cell neurons. The detailed characterization of which enzymes are activated by calcium, combined with techniques such as intracellular injection, may, however, cast more light on calcium-dependent transformations of the electrical properties of neurons that underlie long-lasting behavioral responses.

REFERENCES

Acosta-Urquidi, J. and Dudek, F. E., 1979, Soma spike of neuroendocrine bag cells of *Aplysia californica, Soc. Neurosci. Abstr.* **5:**239.

Adams, W. B. and Levitan, I. B., 1982, Intracellular injection of protein kinase inhibitor blocks the serotonin induced increase in K^+ conductance in *Aplysia* neuron R15, *Proc. Natl. Acad. Sci. USA* **79:**3877–3880.

Alkon, D. L., Acosta-Urquidi, J., Olds, J., Kuzma, G., and Neary, J., 1983, Protein kinase injection reduces voltage dependent potassium currents, *Science* **219:**303–306.

Arch, S., Earley, P., and Smock, T., 1976, Biochemical isolation and physiological identification of the egg laying hormone in *Aplysia californica, J. Gen. Physiol* **68:**197–210.

Ashby, C. D. and Walsh, D. A., 1972, Characterization of the interaction of a protein inhibitor with adenosine $3'$–$5'$ monophosphate dependent protein kinases, *J. Biol. Chem.* **247:**6637–6642.

Blankenship, J. E. and Haskins, J. T., 1979, Electrotonic coupling among neuroendocrine cells in *Aplysia, J. Neurophysiol.* **42:**347–355.

Castellucci, V. F., Kandel, E. R., Schwartz, J. H., Wilson, F., Nairn, A. C., and Greengard, P., 1980, Intracellular injection of the catalytic subunit of cyclic AMP-dependent protein kinase simulates facilitation of transmitter release underlying behavioural sensitization in *Aplysia, Proc. Natl. Acad. Sci. USA* **77:**7492–7496.

Castellucci, V. F., Nairn, A., Greengard, P., Schwartz, J. H., and Kandel, E. R., 1982, Inhibitor of adenosine $3'$-$5'$ monophosphate-dependent protein kinase blocks presynaptic facilitation in *Aplysia, J. Neurosci.* **2:**1673–1681.

Chiu, A. Y. and Strumwasser, F., 1981, An immunohistochemical study of the neuropeptidergic bag cells of *Aplysia, J. Neurosci.* **1:**812–826.

Chiu, A. Y., Hunkapiller, M. W. Heller, E., Stuart, D. K., Hood, L. E., and Strumwasser, F., 1979, Purification and primary structure of neuroactive egg-laying hormone of *Aplysia californica, Proc. Nat. Acad. Sci. USA* **76:**6656–6660.

DePeyer, J. E., Cachelin, A. B., Levitan, I. B., and Reuter, H., 1982, Ca^{2+}-activated K^+ conductance in internally perfused snail neurons is enhanced by protein phosphorylation, *Proc. Natl. Acad. Sci. USA* **79:**4207–4211.

DeRiemer, S. A., Kaczmarek, L. K., and Greengard, P., 1982, Calcium/calmodulin-dependent protein phosphorylation in *Aplysia* neurons, *Soc. Neurosci. Abstr.* **8:**565.

DeRiemer, S. A., Kaczmarek, L. K., Albert, K. A., and Greengard, P., 1983, Calcium/phospholipid-dependent protein phosphorylation in *Aplysia* neurons, *Soc. Neurosci. Abstr.* **9:**77.

DeRiemer, S. A., Kaczmarek, L. K., Lai, Y., McGuinness, T. L., and Greengard, P., 1984, Calcium/calmodulin-dependent protein phosphorylation in the nervous system of *Aplysia, J. Neurosci.* **4:**1618–1625.

DeVlieger, T. A., Kits, K. S., TerMaat, A., and Lodder, J. C., 1980, Morphology and electrophysiology of the ovulation hormone producing neuro-endocrine cells of the freshwater snail *Lymnea stagnalis, J. Exp. Biol.* **84:**259–271.

Dudek, F. E. and Blankenship, J. E., 1977, Neuroendocrine cells of *Aplysia brasiliana.* I. Bag cell action potentials and afterdischarge, *J. Neurophysiol.* **40:**1301–1311.

Dudek, F. E., Cobbs, J. S., and Pinsker, H. M., 1979, Bag cell electrical activity underlying spontaneous egg laying in freely behaving *Aplysia brasiliana, J. Neurophysiol.* **42:**804–817.

Gillette, M. V. and Gillette, R., 1983, Bursting neurons command consummatory feeding behaviour and coordinated visceral receptivity in the predatory mollusc *Pleurobranchaea, J. Neurosci.* **9:**1791–1806.

Heller, E., Kaczmarek, L. K., Hunkapiller, N. W., Hood, L. E., and Strumwasser, F., 1980, Purification and primary structure of two neuroactive peptides that cause bag cell afterdischarge and egg-laying in *Aplysia, Proc. Nat. Acad. Sci. USA* **77:**2328–2332.

Jennings, K. R., Kaczmarek, L. K., Hewick, R. M., Dreyer, W. J., and Strumwasser, F., 1982, Protein phosphorylation during afterdischarge in peptidergic neurons of *Aplysia, J. Neurosci.* **2:**158–168.

Kaczmarek, L. K. and Kauer, J., 1983, Calcium entry causes a prolonged refractory period in peptidergic neurons of *Aplysia*, *J. Neurosci.* **3**:2230–2239.

Kaczmarek, L. K. and Strumwasser, F., 1981a, The expression of long-lasting afterdischarge by isolated *Aplysia* bag cell neurons, *J. Neurosci.* **1**:626–634.

Kaczmarek, L. K. and Strumwasser, F., 1981b, Net outward currents of bag cell neurons are diminished by a cAMP analogue, *Soc. Neurosci. Abstr.* **7**:932.

Kaczmarek, L. K. and Strumwasser, F., 1984, A voltage-clamp analysis of current underlying cyclic AMP-induced membrane modulation in isolated peptidergic neurons of *Aplysia*, *J. Neurophysiol.* **52**:340–349.

Kaczmarek, L. K., Jennings, K., and Strumwasser, F., 1978, Neurotransmitter modulation, phosphodiesterase inhibitor effects, and cAMP correlates of afterdischarge in peptidergic neurites, *Proc. Nat. Acad. Sci. USA* **75**:5200–5204.

Kaczmarek, L. K., Finbow, M., Revel, J. P., and Strumwasser, F., 1979, The morphology and coupling of *Aplysia* bag cells within the abdominal ganglion and in cell culture, *J. Neurobiol.* **10**:535–550.

Kaczmarek, L. K., Jennings, K. R., Strumwasser, F., Nairn, A. C., Walter, U., Wilson, F. D., and Greengard, P., 1980, Microinjection of catalytic subunit of cyclic AMP-dependent protein kinase enhances calcium action potentials of bag cell neurons in cell culture, *Proc. Nat. Acad. Sci. USA* **77**:7487–7491.

Kaczmarek, L. K., Jennings, K. R., and Strumwasser, F., 1982, An early sodium and a late calcium phase in the afterdischarge of peptide secreting neurons of *Aplysia*, *Brain Res.* **238**:105–115.

Klein, M. and Kandel, E. R., 1980, Mechanism of calcium current modulation underlying presynaptic facilitation and behavioural sensitization in *Aplysia*, *Proc. Nat. Acad. Sci. USA* **77**:6912–6916.

Koester, J. and Byrne, J. H. (eds.), 1980, *Molluscan Nerve Cells: From Biophysics to Behavior*, Cold Spring Harbor Reports in the Neurosciences, Volume I, Cold Spring Harbor Laboratory, Cold Spring Harbor.

Kupfermann, I., 1970, Stimulation of egg laying by extracts of neuroendocrine cells (bag cells) of abdominal ganglion of *Aplysia*, *J. Neurophysiol.* **33**:877–881.

Kupfermann, I. and Kandel, E. R., 1970, Electrophysiological properties and functional interconnections of two symmetrical neurosecretory clusters (bag cells) in abdominal ganglion of *Aplysia*, *J. Neurophysiol.* **33**:865–876.

Nestler, E. and Greengard, P., 1984, *Protein Phosphorylation and Neuronal function*, John Wiley and Sons, New York.

Novak-Hofer, I. and Levitan, I. B., 1983, Ca^{++}/calmodulin-regulated protein phosphorylation in the *Aplysia* nervous system, *J. Neurosci.* **3**:473–481.

Rothman, B. S., Mayeri, E., Brown, R. O., Yuan, P., and Shively, J., 1983, Primary structure and neuronal effects of α-bag cell peptide, a second candidate neurotransmitter encoded by a single gene in bag cell neurons of *Aplysia*, *Proc. Natl. Acad. Sci. USA* **80**:5733–5757.

Rubin, C. S. and Rosen, O. M., 1975, Protein phosphorylation, *Ann. Rev. Biochem.* **44**:831–887.

Scheller, R. H., Jackson, J. F., McAllister, L. B. Rothman, B. S., Mayeri, E., and Axel, R., 1983, A single gene encodes multiple neuropeptides mediating a stereotyped behaviour, *Cell* **32**:7–22.

Strong, J., 1983, Modulation of A-current kinetics in bag cell neurons of *Aplysia*, Ph.D. Thesis, Yale University.

Strumwasser, F., Kaczmarek, L. K., Jennings, K. R., and Chiu, A. Y., 1981, Studies of a model peptidergic neuronal system, the bag cells of *Aplysia*, in: *Neurosecretion—Molecules, Cells, Systems* (D. S. Farner and K. Lederis, eds.), Plenum Press, New York, pp. 249–268.

Strumwasser, F., Kaczmarek, L. K., and Jennings, K. R., 1982, Intracellular modulation of membrane channels by cyclic AMP-mediated protein phosphorylation in peptidergic neurons of *Aplysia*, *Fed. Proc.* **41**:2933–2939.

Stuart, D. K., Chiu, A. Y., and Strumwasser, F., 1980, Neurosecretion of egg-laying hormone and other peptides from electrically active bag cell neurons of *Aplysia*, *J. Neurophysiol.* **43**:488–498.

30

Protein Phosphorylation, K^+ Conductances, and Associative Learning in *Hermissenda*

JOSEPH T. NEARY

1. INTRODUCTION

Research in our laboratory is directed toward investigations of the biochemical and biophysical processes that underlie associative learning in the nudibranch mollusc, *Hermissenda crassicornis*. Our studies to date suggest that two of these processes are protein phosphorylation and K^+ conductance(s) (Neary *et al.*, 1981; Alkon *et al.*, 1982a), and recently we have been investigating the possible relationships between K^+ conductances and protein phosphorylation. A number of studies in a variety of preparations have shown that several types of K^+ conductances can be altered by intracellular injection of protein kinases, enzymes that catalyze protein phosphorylation, and by a protein inhibitor of phosphorylation (Castellucci *et al.*, 1980; Kaczmarek *et al.*, 1980; Levitan and Adams, 1981; DePeyer *et al.*, 1982; Adams and Levitan, 1982; Strumwasser *et al.*, 1982; Castellucci *et al.*, 1982; Alkon *et al.*, 1983a; Acosta-Urquidi *et al.*, 1984a,b). In addition, agents that block K^+ conductance can also affect protein phosphorylation (Neary and Alkon, 1983). Some of the questions that arise from these studies include: (1) what proteins are phosphorylated by the injected kinases? (2) are the modified phosphoproteins part of functional K^+ channels? (3) what are the biochemical mechanisms that are involved in the modification of K^+ channels by protein phosphorylation and channel blockers, i.e., activation and/or inhibition of protein kinases, phosphatases, and regulatory proteins? and (4) are the phosphoproteins that are altered following associative learning identical to those that are phosphorylated by the injected protein kinases? This chapter presents a summary of our studies on the relationships between protein

JOSEPH T. NEARY • Section on Neural Systems, Laboratory of Biophysics, National Institute of Neurological and Communicative Disorders and Stroke, National Institutes of Health at the Marine Biological Laboratory, Woods Hole, Massachusetts 02543.

phosphorylation, K^+ conductances, and associative learning in *Hermissenda* and describes some recent directions of our work designed to address the above-mentioned questions.

2. ASSOCIATIVE LEARNING AND PROTEIN PHOSPHORYLATION

The presentation of paired, but not random or unpaired, light and rotation leads to a significant change in the phototactic behavior of *Hermissenda* (Crow and Alkon, 1978). It has subsequently been shown that several electrophysiological properties of photoreceptors from animals receiving paired light and rotation are altered following conditioning (Crow and Alkon, 1980; West *et al.*, 1982; Alkon *et al.*, 1982a). In order to extend these studies to the molecular level, we initiated a series of biochemical studies using eyes* from trained (paired) and control (ran-

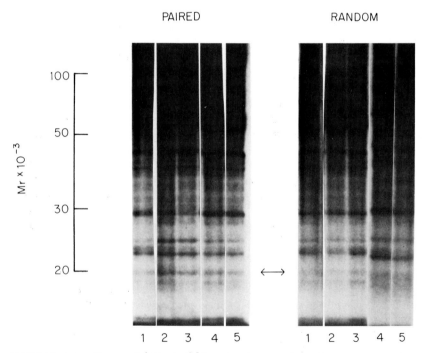

FIGURE 1. Autoradiogram of SDS–electrophoresis gels comparing endogenous protein phosphorylation in eyes of *Hermissenda* presented with paired or random light and rotation. Each lane represents an eye sample from a single animal. (From Neary *et al.*, 1981.)

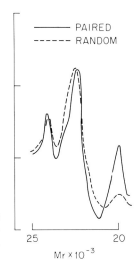

FIGURE 2. Densitometric scans of the 25,000–20,000 M_r region of autoradiograms of eye samples obtained from animals receiving paired (solid line; Fig. 1, lane 4) or random (dashed line; Fig. 1, lane 1) light and rotation. (From Neary *et al.*, 1981.)

dom, unpaired and naive) animals (Neary *et al.*, 1981). The first biochemical process chosen for study was protein phosphorylation (Neary, 1984). Animals were trained for three days (50 trials/day; Crow and Alkon, 1978), circumesophageal nervous systems (CNS) were dissected 2–3 hr after testing on the last day of training, a time period well within the range where associative effects of paired light and rotation are expressed (Crow, 1983). After dissection, CNS were incubated in artificial sea water (ASW) for 30 min prior to labeling for 2 hr in ASW containing glucose and ^{32}Pi. Following labeling, the eyes were dissected and lysed, and phosphoproteins were detected by SDS gel electrophoresis (Laemmli, 1970) and autoradiography (for experimental details, see Neary *et al.*, 1981). As compared to naive groups, a significant increase in ^{32}P incorporation in a 20,000 M_r phosphoprotein band (20K PP) was observed in eyes of animals whose phototactic behavior had been modified by paired light and rotation (Figs. 1 and 2), but not in control groups that had received random or unpaired stimuli and whose phototactic behavior was not significantly modified (Crow, 1983). No significant changes were found in ten other phosphoprotein bands that were present in all animals studied (Table I). Since the eye of *Hermissenda* consists of only five photoreceptors, a lens, and a few pigment and epithelial cells, this study demonstrated that a biochemical change that is correlated with associative learning could be localized to a few cells within a nervous system.

* Eyes were chosen as the preparation to investigate possible biochemical correlates of associative learning because electrophysiological correlates have been found in photoreceptors and because it has not been possible to dissect and isolate photoreceptors routinely from *Hermissenda*. The eye of *Hermissenda* is a relatively simple structure, which contains five photoreceptors, a lens, and a few pigment and epithelial cells.

Table I. Effect of Paired, Random, and Unpaired Stimulation on ^{32}P Incorporation in Specific Phosphoprotein Bands in *Hermissenda* Eyes[a]

Phosphoprotein band (M_r)	Ratio of experimental/untreated (mean ± S.E.M.)		
	Paired (N = 16)	Random (N = 12)	Unpaired (N = 5)
72,000	0.83 ± 0.08	1.05 ± 0.23	1.30 ± 0.38
55,000	1.02 ± 0.04	1.04 ± 0.09	0.88 ± 0.07
44,000	0.88 ± 0.12	1.35 ± 0.10	1.04 ± 0.44
42,000	1.27 ± 0.14	1.18 ± 0.08	1.08 ± 0.13
38,000	1.11 ± 0.07	0.87 ± 0.10	1.23 ± 0.14
34,000	1.55 ± 0.21	1.22 ± 0.20	1.56 ± 0.32
31,000	1.12 ± 0.14	1.23 ± 0.18	0.91 ± 0.16
29,000	0.89 ± 0.11	1.24 ± 0.17	1.15 ; ± pm 0.41
24,000	1.12 ± 0.17	0.90 ± 0.15	1.10 ; ± pm 0.18
22,000	1.04 ± 0.10	1.16 ± 0.14	0.76 ; ± pm 0.07
20,000	2.16 ± 0.28[b]	1.13 ± 0.10	1.18 ± ± 0.14

[a] For experimental details, see Neary *et al.*, 1981.
[b] $F_{2,30} = 6.49$; $P < 0.01$.

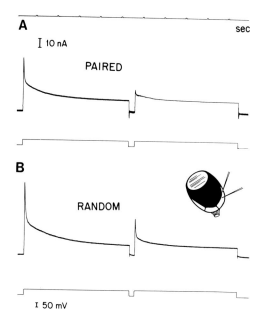

FIGURE 3. Outward K$^+$ currents from type B photoreceptors of animals receiving paired or random light and rotation. Initial peaks are the early, rapidly inactivating K$^+$ current (I_A). (From Alkon *et al.*, 1982a.)

3. MODIFICATION OF K⁺ CURRENTS BY ASSOCIATIVE LEARNING AND BY PROTEIN KINASES

Several electrophysiological properties of type B photoreceptors are altered following conditioning; these include an increase in spontaneous spike frequency, an increase in input resistance, an increase in the tail of the generator potential following a light step (long-lasting depolarization, LLD), and a tonic, light-evoked membrane depolarization (Crow and Alkon, 1980; West *et al.*, 1982). These changes are consistent with a decrease in K⁺ conductance(s), and a voltage clamp study of type B photoreceptors from conditioned animals showed a decrease in the early, transient K⁺ current (Fig. 3; Alkon *et al.*, 1982a). In addition, it has been suggested that other changes may also occur following conditioning (Alkon, 1982–1983; Crow, 1982, 1983), one of which may be a reduction in late K⁺ current(s) (Farley and Alkon, 1983, Forman *et al.*, 1984).

Because several studies in invertebrate neurons (e.g., Kaczmarek *et al.*, 1980; Castellucci *et al.*, 1980) had shown that intracellular injection of the catalytic subunit of cAMP-dependent protein kinase (cAMPdPK) could increase spike broadening and increase input resistance (changes which are consistent with a decrease in K⁺ current) and because we had established a correlation between protein phosphorylation and associative learning in *Hermissenda* eyes, we initiated a series of experiments designed to determine if intracellular injection of protein kinases into *Hermissenda* type B photoreceptors would mimic the effects of conditioning on the electrophysiological properties of the type B photoreceptors. In our first study, we injected the catalytic subunit (PKC) of cAMPdPK purified from bovine heart* into type B photoreceptors and found that it did in fact mimic the effects of conditioning; i.e, PKC injection led to an increase in input resistance and an increase in the tail of the generator potential after a light step (Alkon *et al.*, 1983a). In addition, voltage-clamp studies showed that PKC injection leads to decreases in early and late K⁺ currents (Alkon *et al.*, 1983a). The effect of the injected PKC was greater on the late K⁺ current(s), I_B†, than on I_A (Fig. 4).

The ability of the bovine heart PKC to phosphorylate *Hermissenda* CNS proteins has been measured and compared to the proteins that are phosphorylated by endogenous cAMPdPK (i.e., activated by addition of cAMP). Preliminary studies (Neary *et al.*, 1984) indicate that PKC phosphorylates at least 20 protein bands in *Hermissenda* CNS homogenates and that 19 of these bands co-migrate with the protein bands that are phosphorylated by *Hermissenda* cAMPdPK, thereby suggesting that bovine heart PKC phosphorylates proteins in *Hermissenda* that are similar to those phosphorylated by endogenous cAMPdPK.

* Our early experiments were done with a commercially obtained bovine heart PKC (Sigma P2645), while later experiments were conducted with a highly purified PKC, which was a generous gift from Dr. E. G. Krebs and associates.

† Under the conditions employed in the study of Alkon *et al.* (1983a), I_B consists of two components, a partially activated, voltage-dependent late K⁺ current (delayed rectifier) and partially inactivated, Ca^{2+}-dependent K⁺ current (Acosta-Urquidi *et al.*, 1984a).

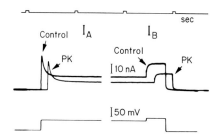

FIGURE 4. Reduction of K^+ currents in type B photoreceptors by intracellular injection of the catalytic subunit (PK) of cAMPdPK. (From Alkon et al., 1983a.)

Many of the observed changes which occur with conditioning appear to be related to a rise in intracellular Ca^{2+} (see Alkon, Chapter 1, in this volume). For example, light and voltage-dependent depolarization of type B photoreceptors is accompanied by a rise in intracellular Ca^{2+} (Connor and Alkon, 1984). Following offset of stimulus, the Ca^{2+} signal returns to baseline with a time course roughly parallel to that of LLD (Connor and Alkon, 1982). In addition, an increase in intracellular Ca^{2+} increases I_A inactivation (Alkon et al., 1982b). Because one of the means by which Ca^{2+} can regulate protein phosphorylation is via Ca^{2+}/calmodulin dependent protein kinases (Ca^{2+}/CaMdPK), we conducted our second study on the effects of protein kinases on K^+ currents by using phosphorylase kinase, a type of Ca^{2+}/CaMdPK that was suggested to us by Dr. Howard Rasmussen. We found that intracellular injection of phosphorylase kinase* into type B photoreceptors also mimicked the effects of conditioning; i.e., phosphorylase kinase injection into type B photoreceptors led to an increase in input resistance and an increase in the tail of the generator potential following light steps (Acosta-Urquidi et al., 1982, 1984a). In voltage clamp studies it was found that phosphorylase kinase also reduced I_A and I_B; under the conditions employed, the phosphorylase kinase induced effects were greater on I_A than on I_B (Fig. 5). In addition, the effects of phosphorylase kinase were Ca^{2+} dependent; i.e., the effects on input resistance and the generator potential following a light step were diminished in Ca^{2+}-free ASW, and the effects on the K^+ currents required an influx of Ca^{2+} that was obtained by pairing light and depolarization.

In addition to its effects on K^+ currents in photoreceptors, phosphorylase kinase also reduced K^+ currents in giant identifiable Hermissenda neurons; in particular, phosphorylase kinase potentiates the Ca^{2+}-mediated inactivation of I_A (Acosta-Urquidi et al., 1983). Although phosphorylase kinase is capable of modifying the activity of K^+ currents and of phosphorylating endogenous proteins in Hermissenda nervous system homogenates, we do not imply that endogenous phos-

---

* As in the PKC studies, both commercial (Sigma) and highly purified phosphorylase kinase (E.G. Krebs) were employed. Sigma preparations of phosphorylase kinase (P-2014) with lot numbers of 42F-9550 and 71F9610 and specific activities of 130 to 170 units per mg protein were effective in altering input resistance, LLD, and K^+ currents in our initial studies, but a later Sigma preparation (lot number 23F-9590) was only marginally effective in altering spike widths in giant neurons and was only 4% as active (on a protein basis) as previous lots of phosphorylase kinase when assayed for its ability to phosphorylate phosphorylase b (J. Stulman and J.T. Neary, unpublished observations).

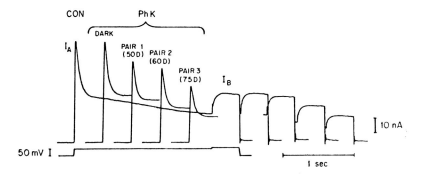

FIGURE 5. Reduction of K^+ currents in type B photoreceptors by intracellular injection of phosphorylase kinase (PhK), a type of $Ca^+/AAMdPK$. Con: control, before injection of phosphorylase kinase. Pair refers to pairings of light and depolarization (D, mV). Records of I_B on right are from the same experiment as on the left and are displaced for purposes of comparison. From Acosta-Urquidi *et al.* (1984a).

phorylase kinase is the main catalytic agent that alters K^+ currents. Phosphorylase kinase was used as a model for Ca^{2+}/CaM-regulated protein phosphorylation because of the wealth of information that is available about its properties and because of the difficulty in obtaining neuronal $Ca^{++}/CaMdPK$ in a stable form. Recently, however, DeLorenzo, Goldering, and colleagues have supplied us with a purified, relatively stable calmodulin kinase type II from rat brain. Iontophoresis of this enzyme into *Hermissenda* giant neurons (Acosta-Urquidi *et al.*, 1984b) and photoreceptors (M. Sakakibara , D. L. Alkon, R. DeLorenzo, J. R. Goldenring, J. T. Neary, and E. Heldman, unpublished observations) also leads to reductions in early and late K^+ currents although its effects appear to be more complex than phosphorylase kinase.

These studies indicate that both Ca^{2+}- and cAMP-regulated protein kinases can modify both early and late K^+ currents in *Hermissenda* neurons. cAMPdPK has a greater effect on late K^+ currents whereas $Ca^{2+}/CaMdPK$ has a greater effect on the early K^+ current, and it is tempting to speculate that the two types of protein kinases have preferential substrate specificity for distinct types of K^+ channels (or channel-associated proteins). In terms of regulation of channel function, interactive effects of cAMP and Ca^{2+} are also possible because both cAMPdPK and $Ca^{2+}/CaMdPK$ can modify the same type of K^+ current. Evidence for phosphorylation of different sites on the same protein by cAMPdPK and $Ca^{2+}/CaMdPK$ have been found in several systems (see review by Cohen, 1982), and multiple site phosphorylation could serve as a convergence point for the flow of information from two different second messenger systems (e.g., see Rasmussen, 1981). Alternatively, interactive regulatory effects of cAMP and Ca^{2+} on different proteins are also conceivable. For example, cAMP-mediated phosphorylation could activate a $Ca^{2+}/CaMdPK$, as in the case of phosphorylase kinase in skeletal muscle (Walsh *et al.*, 1971; Cohen, 1973). Finally it should be noted that activators of $Ca^{2+}/$ phospholipid-dependent protein kinase, in combination with a Ca^{2+} load (stimulated by light and depolarization), produce reductions in photoreceptor early and late K^+

currents which last longer than those obtained with either treatment alone (D. L. Alkon, J. T. Neary, S. Naito, D. Coulter, M. Kubota, and H. Rasmussen, unpublished observations). It is clear that, because of the complexities of cAMP and Ca^{2+} interactions, further studies in *Hermissenda* are needed in order to define the role of cAMP- and Ca^{2+}-stimulated phosphorylation in modulating the activities of the early and late K^+ channels.

4. PROTEIN PHOSPHORYLATION IN A SINGLE, IDENTIFIABLE NEURON IN *HERMISSENDA*

One of the important questions raised by the experiments described in the preceding section concerns the nature of the proteins that are phosphorylated by the injected Ca^{2+}/CaMdPK and cAMPdPK. In order to investigate this question, we have begun to study protein phosphorylation in a single, identifiable neuron in *Hermissenda* (Neary *et al.*, 1983). Such an approach allows for combined electrophysiological and biochemical studies in the same cell. The cell selected for study is located in the left pedal ganglion, has a diameter of 150–200 μm, and is designated LP-1 (Jerussi and Alkon, 1981). LP-1 may serve as a model cell for investigating biochemical processes that underlie associative learning and that are related to ionic conductances because LP-1 contains a voltage-dependent I_A that exhibits Ca^{2+}-mediated inactivation (Acosta-Urquidi *et al.*, 1983) and that is similar to that previously observed to change in *Hermissenda* type B photoreceptors following conditioning (Alkon *et al.*, 1982a).

The protocol for labeling phosphoproteins in LP-1 involves incubation of the ganglia in ^{32}Pi (in order to generate $[^{32}P]$-ATP and ^{32}P-labeled phosphoproteins by normal cellular metabolism) and dissection of LP-1 following freeze substitution in propylene glycol. This method is similar to that employed by Levitan *et al.* (1974) for single cell studies in *Aplysia*. However, because large dissected neurons in *Aplysia* are contaminated by glial membranes (Levitan *et al.*, 1983), Levitan and co-workers developed a technique for pressure injection of $[\gamma-^{32}P]$-ATP to study single cell protein phosphorylation without dissecting the cell (Lemos *et al.*, 1982). Thus, an advantage of this method is the ability to label and analyze the cell body and axon of interest without dissecting the cell, provided, of course, that the isotope is not transported to neighboring cells. The latter point deserves careful attention and needs to be investigated for individual preparations. No leakage has been observed from the R15 cell of *Aplysia* abdominal ganglion (Lemos *et al.*, 1982) but it appears that $[\gamma-^{32}P]$-ATP can be transported across neuronal membranes in squid (Pant *et al.*, 1979) and in *Hermissenda* (J.T. Neary, unpublished observations). Disadvantages of the pressure injection method include (1) the possible production of radiolytic-induced isotope contaminants due to the need for a highly concentrated, high-energy isotope in the injection electrode and (2) the limitation on the extent of *in vivo* labeling by the volume of isotope that can be injected without damaging the cell.

In our LP-1 studies, it has not been necessary to use the pressure injection technique because histological examination of dissected LP-1 cells revealed minimal contamination by glial cells or connective tissue. In addition, at this point in our studies, we are interested in a combined electrophysiological and biochemical analysis of the soma region of neurons. Although during conditioning of *Hermissenda* by paired light and rotation, the flow of information must be via synaptic communication between photoreceptors and statocysts, electrophysiological changes following conditioning have been found in cell bodies (e.g., Alkon *et al.*, 1982a). The techniques used in our LP-1 studies allow for ^{32}P-phosphoprotein labeling via bath-applied ^{32}Pi and for cell body separation from the neuropil region by dissection.

Prior to investigating the effects of injected protein kinases on labeled phosphoproteins in LP-1, we have carried out a series of experiments to optimize the conditions of labeling, freeze-substitution, and dissection. We have modified the freeze-substitution methods of Giller and Schwartz (1971), Ono and McCaman (1979), and Bernier *et al.* (1982) find that treatment of CNS with 60% propylene glycol at -12 to $-18°C$ for 45 min gives consistent fixation and yields a recovery of at least 90% of the protein content of LP-1. Time course labeling studies indicate that synthesis of ^{32}P proteins and lipids reach a plateau in 8–12 hr. ^{32}P proteins and lipids from a single cell can be detected by autoradiography of SDS electrophoresis gels and thin layer chromatograms after 2- to 4-day exposures using intensification techniques (Laskey and Mills, 1977; Neary *et al.*, 1981). Based on these findings, we are now conducting parallel biophysical and biochemical experiments in ^{32}P-labeled LP-1 neurons in order to determine which proteins are phosphorylated by the injected protein kinases.

5. PROTEIN PHOSPHORYLATION AND BLOCKADE OF I_A CHANNELS

A second approach for an investigation of the relationship between protein phosphorylation and ionic conductances involves the use of channel blockers that can preferentially block specific ionic currents. In molluscan neurons, 4-aminopyridine (4-AP) preferentially blocks I_A (Thompson, 1977, 1982; Byrne *et al.*, 1979). We applied 4-AP to *Hermissenda* CNS that were previously labeled with ^{32}Pi and found a marked reduction ($\geq 85\%$; Fig. 6) of ^{32}P incorporation in a 25,000 M_r phosphoprotein band (25K PP) in both eyes and ganglia (Neary and Alkon, 1983). This effect occurred in a concentration range of 4-AP (1–10 mM, see Fig. 7) and over a time course similar to those required to block I_A by 4-AP when the presence of the sheath surrounding the ganglia is taken into consideration. As shown in Fig. 8, the effect of 4-AP is reversible; removal of 4-AP leads to an increase in ^{32}P incorporation in 25K PP and also in a 23,000 M_r phosphoprotein band.

The effect of 4-AP on the level of ^{32}P in 25K PP does not appear to be the result of a 4-AP induced increase in impulse activity that can occur during 4-AP treatment (for review, see Thesleff, 1980). Neurons in the eye were isolated from the site of initiation of impulse activity and synaptic inputs by a lesion that was made in the optic tract between the eye and optic ganglion (Alkon, 1979). Eyes

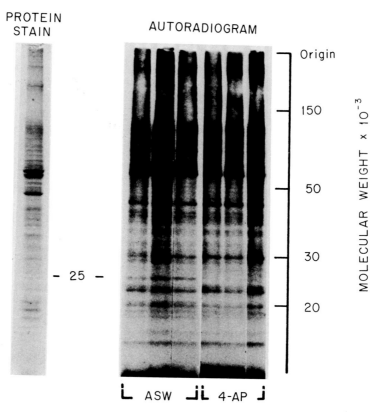

FIGURE 6. Reduction in level of ^{32}P incorporation in 25K PP by 4-AP. Three different samples from controls (ASW) and 4-AP experiments are shown to indicate sample to sample variations in the relative intensities of the phosphoprotein bands. The 4-AP induced decrease in ^{32}P incorporation in 25K PP can be observed in all 4-AP treated samples. (From Neary and Alkon 1983.)

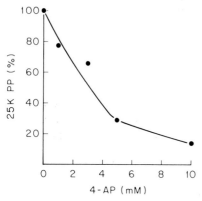

FIGURE 7. Effect of 4-AP concentration on the level of ^{32}P incorporation in 25K PP. (From Neary and Alkon, 1983.)

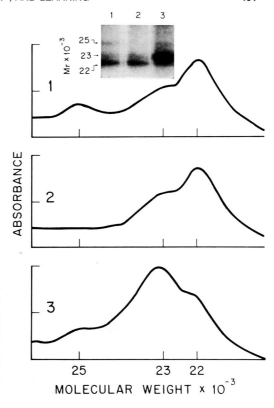

FIGURE 8. Reversibility of 4-AP effect on 25K PP. Autoradiograms (inset) and densitometric scans are from experiments in which ^{32}P-labeled CNS were incubated (1) in ASW alone, (2) in 10 mM 4-AP for 30 min, or (3) in ASW (30 min) following a 30-min incubation in 10 mM 4-AP. (From Neary and Alkon, 1983.)

from the lesioned preparations still exhibited the 4-AP effect on protein phosphorylation, suggesting that the 4-AP effect on 25K PP cannot be explained by an indirect effect of 4-AP on impulse activity.

As shown in Fig. 9, reduction of I_A by another means, sustained depolarization in high external K^+, also leads to a reduction in ^{32}P incorporation in 25K PP (Neary and Alkon, 1983). However, agents that block other types of K^+ currents in *Hermissenda* do not appear to affect ^{32}P incorporation in 25K PP. Neither Ba^{2+}, which blocks the delayed K^+ current (Alkon *et al.*, 1982b), nor Ni^{2+}, which blocks the Ca^{2+} current and the Ca^{2+}-dependent K^+ current (Alkon, 1979), have a significant effect on the level of phosphorylation in 25K PP (Fig. 9). However, the possibility of an effect of Ca^{2+} channel blockers on 25K PP remains open because the level of Ni^{2+} used in these experiments (1 mM) does not appear to give complete block of the Ca^{2+} current.

The mechanism(s) which underlies the effect of 4-AP and high external K^+ on protein phosphorylation are not known. Further studies are needed to determine the identity of 25K PP, whether or not it is a component of the transient K^+ channel, and the mechanism that leads to the observed change in protein phosphorylation. It is also not known if or how this change is related to the protein kinase-induced modification in I_A (see section on modification of K^+ currents by associative learning

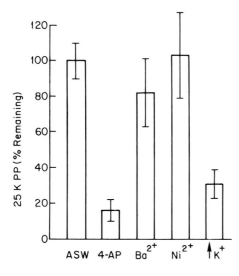

FIGURE 9. Effect of K^+ channel blocking agents and membrane depolarization on the level of ^{32}P incorporation in 25K PP. (From Neary and Alkon, 1983.)

and by protein kinases). One possibility is that the phosphorylation initiated by the injection of the protein kinases leads to activation of a protein phosphatase (Hemmings *et al.*, 1981; Yang *et al.*, 1981), which in turn leads to the reduction in ^{32}P incorporation in 25K PP. Another possibility is that an open K^+ channel may be related to the titration of a specific number of phosphorylation sites on the channel protein or a channel-associated protein, whereas a closed channel may contain too many or too few phosphorylated sites, in a manner analogous to the formation of an active antigen–antibody complex. In this case, multisite phosphorylation, as induced by protein kinases, or multisite dephosphorylation, as induced by channel blockers such as 4-AP, could both be related to a reduction in the activity of the K^+ channel.

Another question concerns the manner in which 4-AP acts to alter protein phoshorylation and affect K^+ channel formation. The effect of 4-AP on protein phosphorylation, if it is related to I_A activity, suggests that the mechanism of action of 4-AP involves more than simply plugging channel pores. One possibility is that the mechanism of action may be analogous to the interaction between hormones or neurotransmitters and membrane protein receptors in which ligand binding to the receptor leads to activation of enzyme systems that regulate phosphorylation. For example, 4-AP binding to I_A channel complexes may lead to activation of kinase/phosphatase systems that alters phosphorylation of integral or peripheral membrane proteins which in turn affect channel activity. Alternatively (or in conjunction with this), Ca^{2+} mobilization (via influx or release from internal stores) may be stimulated by 4-AP and the increased cytosolic Ca^{2+} may activate the kinase or phosphatase that regulates the level of phosphorylation of 25K PP. For example, Gainer and associates have shown that the 4-AP effect on phosphorylation in squid synaptosomes is Ca^{2+} dependent (Pant *et al.*, 1984). The preliminary studies described in the following section are designed to address some of these questions and possibilities.

6. ACTIVATION OF ENDOGENOUS PROTEIN KINASES BY cAMP AND Ca^{2+}

In order to begin to investigate the regulation of phosphorylation of the proteins that appear to be related to associative learning and K$^+$ conductance, we have begun to study the activation of endogenous protein kinases by cAMP, Ca^{2+}, calmodulin, and lipids. The experimental protocol involves adding [γ-^{32}P]-ATP to a homogenate of *Hermissenda* ganglia in the presence of Mg^{2+} and one or a combination of the second messengers incubating for various time periods, stopping the reaction with "SDS stop solution" and boiling for 2 min, separating the proteins by SDS–gel electrophoresis, and visualizing the labeled phosphoproteins by auto-radiography (Neary *et al.*, 1984, 1985). Preliminary results indicate that *Hermissenda* CNS contain endogenous Ca^{2+}/CaMdPK, cAMPdPK and Ca^{2+}/phospholipid-dependent protein kinases that phosphorylate both similar and different proteins. For example, it appears that some proteins are phosphorylated exclusively by cAMPdPK or by Ca^{2+}/CaMdPK, whereas other proteins can be phosphorylated exclusively by both types of kinases. As mentioned previously, phosphorylation of one protein by both cAMPdPK and Ca^{2+}/CaMdPK has been widely reported and may serve as a convergence point for the interaction between the two intracellular communication systems (see reviews by Rasmussen, 1981, and Cohen, 1982). Phosphorylation of the same protein by both kinases in *Hermissenda* is consistent with our experiments with injected kinases in which I$_A$ and I$_B$ are modified by both Ca^{2+}/CaMdPK and cAMPdPK. In addition to the presence of Ca^{2+}/CaMdPK and cAMPdPK, *Hermissenda* ganglia also appear to contain Ca^{2+}-dependent phosphatases that are particularly active in dephosphorylating proteins in the 20,000 to 30,000 Mr range and that are activated at higher Ca^{2+} concentrations than those which activate Ca^{2+}/CaMdPK. It is possible that an initial increase in intracellular Ca^{2+} may stimulate phosphorylation, while a further increase in Ca^{2+} may trigger dephosphorylation. The effects of Ca^{2+} on phosphorylation and dephosphorylation, as regulated by a difference in Ca^{2+} levels, may be related to the activity the Ca^{2+}-dependent K$^+$ current in *Hermissenda* photoreceptors, which is both activated and inactivated by Ca^{2+} (Alkon *et al.*, 1983b).

Our preliminary experiments indicate that the 25K PP which is affected by agents that reduce I$_A$ and the 20 KPP which is increased following acquisition can be phosphorylated by both Ca^{2+}-dependent protein kinase(s) and caMPdPK. However, 2-dimensional gel electrophoresis (O'Farrell, 1975; Neary, 1984) and tryptic peptide maps (Cleveland *et al.*, 1977) are needed to confirm these preliminary observations concerning the comparison of protein bands from *in vivo* labeling (^{32}Pi incubation of whole cell preparations) with *in vitro* labeling of studies ([γ-^{32}P]-ATP incubation of cell-free homogenates).

7. CONCLUDING REMARKS

The evidence obtained to date supports the hypothesis that protein phosphorylation is one of the biochemical processes that plays a role in K^+ conductances and in associative learning in *Hermissenda*. However, the nature of the relationships between protein phosphorylation, ionic conductances, and associative learning are not well understood, and the detailed biochemical mechanisms regulating phosphorylation of the 20K PP and 25K PP proteins and the identification of these proteins remain to be determined. Furthermore, it is important to keep in mind the fact that Ca^{2+} and cAMP are involved in many cellular processes, some of which include the regulation of proteins involved in activation of carbohydrate metabolism for energy requirements, in neurotransmitter and protein biosynthesis, and in intracellular movement via the cytoskeletal matrix. Studies on the subcellular localization and identification of proteins and the availability of antibodies to the proteins of interest will aid in determining how the phosphoproteins under investigation are related to ionic conductances and associative learning. Ultimately, it will be necessary to obtain purified components of K^+ channels in phosphorylated and dephosphorylated forms and to reconstitute these purified proteins in artificial membranes to see if K^+ flux is altered by changes in the phosphorylation state of the purified components. Although some interesting and suggesting observations have been made, it is clear that much work needs to be done in order to achieve our long-range goals of understanding how a biochemical mechanism such as protein phosphorylation can modify ionic conductances and how an organism can utilize biophysical and biochemical processes to alter its behavior.

ACKNOWLEDGMENTS. I am grateful to my colleagues Juan Acosta-Urquidi, Dan Alkon, Terry Crow, Susan DeRiemer, Hal Gainer, June Harrigan, Len Kaczmarek, Paul Kandel, Alan Kuzirian, Greg Kuzma, Shigetaka Naito, Jim Olds, Howard Rasmussen, Manabu Sakakibara, James Stulman, and Leslie Tengelsen for their contributions to the work described here. I also thank Jeanne Kuzirian for secretarial support.

REFERENCES

Acosta-Urquidi, J., Neary, J. T., and Alkon, D. L., 1982, Ca^{2+}-dependent protein kinase regulation of $K^+(V)$ currents: A possible biochemical step in associative learning of *Hermissenda, Soc. Neurosci. Abstr.* **8:**825.

Acosta-Urquidi, J., Alkon, D. L., Connor, J. A., and Neary, J. T., 1983, Intracellular injection of a Ca^{++}-dependent protein kinase amplifies Ca^{++}-mediated inactivation of a transient K^+ current (I_A) in *Hermissenda* giant neurons, *Soc. Neurosci. Abstr.* **9:**501.

Acosta-Urquidi, J., Alkon, D. L., and Neary, J. T., 1984a, Ca^{++} dependent protein kinase injection in a photoreceptor mimics biophysical effects of associative learning, *Science* **224:**1254–1257.

Acosta-Urquidi, J., Neary, J. T., Goldenring, J. R., Alkon, D., L., and DeLorenzo, R. J., 1984b, Modulation of I_{Ca} and late K currents by intrasomatic injection of Ca-calmodulin dependent protein kinase in *Hermissenda* giant neurons, *Soc. Neurosci. Abstr.* **10:**1129.

Adams, W. B. and Levitan, I. B., 1982, Intracellullar injection of protein kinase inhibitor blocks the seroton-induced increase in K^+ conductance in *Aplysia* neuron R15, *Proc. Natl. Acad. Sci. USA* **79:**3877–3880.

Alkon, D. L., 1979, Voltage-dependent calcium and potassium ion conductances: A contingency mechanism for an associative learning model, *Science* **205:**810–816.

Alkon, D. L., 1982–1983, Regenerative change of voltage-dependent Ca^{2+} and K^+ currents encode a learned stimulus association, *J. Physiol. (Paris)* **78:**700–706.

Alkon, D. L., Lederhendler, I., and Shoukimas, J. J., 1982a, Primary changes of membrane currents during retention of associative learning, *Science* **215:**693–695.

Alkon, D. L., Shoukimas, J. J., and Heldman, E., 1982b, Calcium-mediated decrease of a voltage-dependent K^+ current, *Biophys. J.* **40:**245–250.

Alkon, D. L, Acosta-Urquidi, J., Olds, J., Kuzma, G., and Neary, J. T., 1983a, Protein kinase injection reduces voltage-dependent potassium currents, *Science* **219:**303–306.

Alkon, D. L., Farley, J., Hay, B., and Shoukimas, J. J., 1983b, Inactivation of Ca^{++}-dependent K^+ current can occur without significant Ca^{2+} current inactivation, *Soc. Neurosci. Abstr.* **9:**1188.

Bernier, L., Castellucci, V. F., Kandel, E. R., and Schwartz, J. H., 1982, Facilitatory transmitter causes a selective and prolonged increase in adenosine $3':5'$-monophosphate in sensory neurons mediating the gill and siphon withdrawal reflex in *Aplysia, J. Neurosci.* **2:**1682–1691.

Byrne, J. H., Shapiro, E., Dieringer, N., and Koester, J., 1979, Biophysical mechanisms contributing to inking behavior in *Aplysia, J. Neurophysiol.* **42:**1233–1250.

Castellucci, V. F., Kandel, E. R., Schwartz, J. H., Wilson, F. D., Nairn, A. C., and Greengard, P., 1980, Intracellular injection of the catalytic subunit of cyclic AMP-dependent protein kinase simulates facilitation of transmitter release underlying behavioral sensitization in *Aplysia, Proc. Natl. Acad. Sci. USA* **77:**7492–7496.

Castellucci, V. F., Nairn, A., Greengard, P., Schwartz, J. H., and Kandel, E. R., 1982, Inhibitor of adenoisine $3':5'$-monophosphate-dependent protein kinase blocks presynaptic facilitation in *Aplysia, J. Neurosci.* **2:**1673–1681.

Cleveland, D. W., Fischer, S. G., Kirschner, M. W., and Laemmli, U. K., 1977, Peptide mapping by limited proteolysis in sodium dodecyl sulfate and analysis by gel electrophoresis, *J. Biol. Chem.* **252:**1102–1106.

Cohen, P., 1973, The subunit structure of rabbit-skeletal muscle phosphorylase kinase, and the molecular basis of its activation reactions, *Eur. J. Biochem.* **34:**1–14.

Cohen, P., 1982, The role of protein phosphorylation in neural and hormonal control of cellular activity, *Nature* **296:**613–620.

Connor, J. and Alkon, D. L., 1982, Light-induced changes of intracellular Ca^{2+} in *Hermissenda* photoreceptors measured with arsenazo III, *Soc. Neurosci. Abstr.* **8:**944.

Connor, J. and Alkon, D. L., 1984, Light- and voltage-dependent increases of calcium ion concentration in molluscan photoreceptors, *J. Neurophysiol.* **51:**745–752.

Crow, T., 1982, Sensory neuronal correlates of associative learning in *Hermissenda, Soc. Neurosci. Abstr.* **8:**824.

Crow, T., 1983, Conditioned modification of locomotion in *Hermissenda crassicornis:* Analysis of time-dependent associative and non-associative components, *J. Neurosci.* **3:**2621–2628.

Crow, T. J. and Alkon, D. L., 1978, Retention of an associative behavioral change in *Hermissenda, Science* **201:**1239–1241.

Crow, T. J. and Alkon, D. L., 1980, Associative behavioral modification in *Hermissenda:* Cellular correlates, *Science* **209:**412–414.

DePeyer, J. E., Cachelin, A. B., Levitan, I. B., and Reuter, H., 1982, Ca^{++}-activated K^+ conductance in internally perfused snail neurons is enhanced by protein phosphorylation, *Proc. Natl. Acad. Sci. USA* **79:**4207–4211.

Farley, J. and Alkon, D. L., 1983, Changes in *Hermissenda* type B photoreceptors involving a voltage-dependent Ca^{++} current and a Ca^{++}-dependent K^+ current during retention of associative learning. *Soc. Neurosci. Abstr.* **9:**167.

Forman, R., Alkon, D. L., Sakakibara, M., Harrigan, J., Lederhendler, I., and Farley, J., 1984, Changes in I_A and I_C but not in I_{Na} accompany retention of conditioned behavior in *Hermissenda, Soc. Neurosci. Abstr.* **10:**121.

Giller, E., Jr. and Schwartz, J. H., 1971, Choline acetyltransferase in identified neurons of abdominal ganglion of *Aplysia californica, J. Neurophysiol.* **34:**93–107.

Hemmings, B. A., Yellowlees, D., Kernohan, J. C., and Cohen, P., 1981, Purification of glycogen synthase kinase 3 from rabbit skeletal muscle. Copurification with the activating factor (F_A) of the (Mg-ATP) dependent protein phosphatase, *Eur. J. Biochem.* **119**:443–451.

Jerussi, T. P. and Alkon, D. L., 1981, Ocular and extraocular responses of identifiable neurons in pedal ganglia of *Hermissenda crassicornis*, *J. Neurophysiol.* **46**:659–671.

Kaczmarek, L. K., Jennings, K. R., Strumwasser, F., Nairn, A. C., Walter, U., Wilson, F. D., and Greengard, P., 1980, Microinjection of catalytic subunit of cyclic AMP-dependent protein kinase enhances calcium action potentials of bag cell neurons in cell culture, *Proc. Natl. Acad. Sci. USA* **77**:7487–7491.

Laemmli, U. K., 1970, Cleavage of structural proteins during the assembly of the head of bacteriophage T$_4$, *Nature* **227**:680–685.

Laskey, R. A. and Mills, A. D., 1977, Enhanced autoradiographic detection of ^{32}P and ^{125}I using intensifiying screens and hypersensitized film, *FEBS Lett.* **82**:314–316.

Lemos, J. R., Novak-Hofer, I., and Levitan, I. B., 1982, Serotonin alters the phosphorylation of specific proteins inside a single living nerve cell, *Nature*, **298**:64–65.

Levitan, I. B. and Adams, W. B., 1981, Cyclic AMP modulation of a specific ion channel in an identified nerve cell: Possible role for protein phosphorylation, *Adv. Cyclic Nucleotide Res.* **14**:647–653.

Levitan, I. B., Madsen, C. J., and Barondes, S. H., 1974, cAMP and amine effects on phosphorylation of specific proteins in abdominal ganglion of *Aplysia californica;* localization and kinetic analysis, *J. Neurobiol.* **5**:511–525.

Levitan, I. B., Adams, W. B., Lemos, J. R., and Novak-Hofer, I., 1983, A role for protein phosphorylation in the regulation of electrical activity of an identified nerve cell, *Progress in Brain Res.* **58**:71–76.

Neary, J. T., 1984, Biochemical correlates of associative learning: Protein phosphorylation in *Hermissenda crassicornis,* a nudibranch mollusc, in *Primary Neural Substrates of Learning and Behavioral Change* (D. L. Alkon and J. Farley, eds.), Cambridge University Press, New York pp. 325–336.

Neary, J. T. and Alkon, D. L., 1983, Protein phosphorylation/dephosphorylation and the transient, voltage-dependent potassium conductance in *Hermissenda crassicornis*, *J. Biol. Chem.* **258**:8979–8983.

Neary, J. T., Crow, T. and Alkon, D. L., 1981, Change in a specific phosphoprotein band following associative learning in *Hermissenda*, *Nature* **293**:658–660.

Neary, J. T., Acosta-Urquidi, J., Tengelsen, L. A., Kuzirian, A. M., and Alkon, D. L., 1983, Protein phosphorylation in a single identifiable molluscan neuron, *Soc. Neurosci. Abstr.* **9**:301.

Neary, J. T., DeRiemer, S. A., Kaczmarek, L. K., and Alkon, D. L., 1984, Ca^{2+} and cyclic AMP regulation of protein phosphorylation in the *Hermissenda* nervous system, *Soc. Neurosci. Abstr.* **10**:805.

Neary, J. T., Naito, S., and Alkon, D. L., 1985, Ca^{++}-activated phospholipid dependent protein kinase (C-kinase) activity in the *Hermissenda* nervous system, *Soc. Neurosci. Abstr.* in press.

O'Farrell, P. H., 1975, High resolution two-dimensional electrophoresis of proteins, *J. Biol. Chem.* **250**:4007–4021.

Ono, J. K. and McCaman, R. E., 1979, Measurement of endogenous transmitter levels after intracellular recording, *Brain Res.* **165**:156–160.

Pant, H. C., Terakawa, S., Yoshioka, T., Tasaki, I., and Gainer, H., 1979, Evidence for the utilization of extracellular [γ-^{32}P]ATP for the phosphorylation of intracellular proteins in the squid giant axon, *Biochim. Biophys. Acta* **582**:107–114.

Pant, H. C., Gallant, P. E., Cohen, R., Neary, J. T., and Gainer, H., 1983, Calcium-dependent 4-aminopyridine stimulation of protein phosphorylation in squid optic lobe synaptosomes, *Cell Mol. Neurobiol.* **3**:223–238.

Rasmussen, H., 1981, *Calcium and cAMP as Synarchic Messengers*, Wiley, New York.

Strumwasser, F., Kaczmarek, L. K., and Jennings, K. R., 1982, Intracellular modulation of membrane channels by cyclic AMP-mediated protein phosphorylation in peptidergic neurons of *Aplysia*, *Fed. Proc.* **41**:2933–2939.

Thesleff, S., 1980, Aminopyridines and synaptic transmission, *Neuroscience* **5**:1413–1419.

Thompson, S. H., 1977, Three pharmacologically distinct potassium channels in molluscan neurones, *J. Physiol. (London)* **265**:465–488.

Thompson, S. H., 1982, Aminopyridine block of transient potassium current, *J. Gen. Physiol.* **80:**1–18.

Walsh, D. A., Perkins, J. P., Brostrom, C. O., Ho, E. S., and Krebs, E. G., 1971, Catalysis of the phosphorylase kinase activation reaction, *J. Biol. Chem.* **246:**1968–1976.

West, A., Barnes, E., and Alkon, D. L., 1982, Primary changes of voltage responses during retention of associative learning, *J. Neurophysiol.* **48:**1243–1255.

Yang, S.-D., Vandenheede, J. R., and Merlevede, W., 1981, Identification of inhibitor-2 as the ATP-Mg-dependent protein phosphatase modulator, *J. Biol. Chem.* **256:**10231–10234.

The Role of Brain Extracellular Proteins in Learning and Memory

VICTOR E. SHASHOUA

1. INTRODUCTION

In mammalian brain, the cellular and biochemical mechanisms of learning and memory have the capacity to store information for long periods, in man, this may be upwards of 50 years. How is this achieved? If we search the components of the CNS looking for molecules that can fulfill this criterion of long-term stability, we find that everything except the DNA is in a dynamic state. The average half-life of proteins ranges between 6 and 14 days (Lajtha and Toth, 1966); the RNA turnover can vary from 1.5 to 24 hr (Appel, 1967); lipids and carbohydrates are in a rapid state of flux (Bourre *et al.*, 1977). Essentially we find that there are no biochemical components present in the CNS, except the DNA, that have a lifetime stability comparable to that required for long-term memory. Since no evidence indicating DNA has been found as yet, it would seem therefore that only the structure and connectivity patterns of the CNS have features with sufficient stability for use in establishing a long-term memory. Such a concept, first proposed in 1893 by Tanzi, reduces the search for the biochemical correlates of memory to the identification of specific physiological, metabolic, and molecular components that can ultimately lead to permanent alterations of neural circuits. These may be processes common to all cells but specially adapted for the CNS, or they may be unique to the CNS requiring specific molecules (Shashoua, 1976). Whether one or both of these types are used, the processes must have the additional property of being controllable by individual cells or parts of cells within the CNS. Such considerations suggest that learning and memory functions require biochemical mechanisms that can be linked to geographic loci at the cellular and subcellular level.

In our laboratory (Shashoua, 1977b, 1979) we studied the effects of the acquisition of new behaviors on the pattern of brain protein synthesis. Using goldfish

VICTOR E. SHASHOUA ● Mailman Research Center, McLean Hospital, Harvard Medical School, Belmont, Massachusetts 02178.

and mice as experimental animals and double labeling techniques, we identified a class of glycoproteins whose turnover rate was enhanced after training. These macromolecules were found to be released into the brain extracellular space. Investigations of their chemical properties suggest that they may have a functional role in the modification of neural circuits (Shashoua, 1984).

2. INVESTIGATION OF PROTEIN CHANGES IN GOLDFISH BRAIN

2.1. Behavioral Experiment

Figure 1 illustrates the "vestibular-motor" conditioning paradigm (Shashoua, 1968) used for training goldfish. In the procedure, animals were trained to swim with floats sutured at their ventral midline at positions 1 mm caudal to the base of their pectoral fins. Each goldfish (7 g), initially suspended by the float in an upside-down position, adapts to the float through a series of reproducible stages until it can swim upright in a horizontal posture. This task, chosen to provide a maximal challenge to the nervous system, can be considered to involve vestibular, cerebellar,

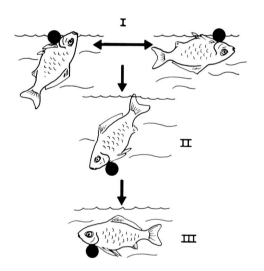

FIGURE 1. Vestibulomotor conditioning experiment: Diagram of principal stages in the sequences of adaptation of the goldfish to the float training procedure. The following table summarizes the stages and methods used for evaluating goldfish performance scores.

Stage	Behavior Score	Behavior during 30-sec observation period
I	0	Animal is upside down or fails three times to swim at 45°
I +	15%	Animal fails twice to maintain a 45° upright swimming posture
II −	30%	Animal fails once to maintain a 45° upright swimming posture
II	50%	Animal swims at a 45° angle
II +	65%	Animal swims at a 30–45° angle
III −	85%	Animal swims at a 15–30° angle
III	100%	Animal swims constantly in a horizontal posture

and lateral line systems in association with motor circuits that control swimming behavior. Thus, an animal readjusts practically all of its movements in order to swim upright, and presumably such radical changes in the swimming behavior would result in large biochemical changes within the nervous system. The training procedure requires 4–5 hr and is carried out by each animal at his own pace. This feature of the behavioral paradigm provides the advantage that there is no interference from the experimenter or the apparatus with the behavior of the animal. The performance of each animal is evaluated according to a fixed set of criteria (see Fig. 1) to obtain a general training score for groups of seven animals as a function of time. Figure 2 illustrates the time course of acquisition of the behavior for a group achieving a 100% training score (i.e., horizontal swimming posture in an upright position within 4 hr in trial 1). When the animals were tested with the same floats 3 days later (trial 2), the goldfish were able to swim in a horizontal posture within 5–10 min after the floats were attached, suggesting that there is a retention of the previous experience. Well-trained animals can recall the new swimming skill for at least 2 weeks. This behavioral paradigm was used in our initial experiments as a model system for looking for biochemical changes.

2.2. Specific Protein Changes Obtained after Training

The possibility that specific proteins might be required in some aspects of the mechanism of learning was investigated using the double-labeling procedure as the analytical method (Shashoua, 1976). Experimentally a group of seven animals was first trained for 4 hr; then the floats were removed; 1 hr later the trained group was labeled with [^{3}H]valine, while a group of seven untrained controls, in a separate tank, received injections of [^{14}C]valine. After a 1-hr incorporation time the animals were anesthetized by cooling, and the brains of the two groups were pooled together

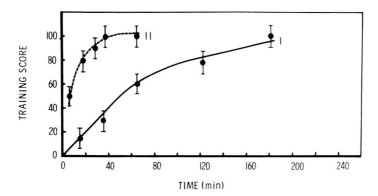

FIGURE 2. Performance scores during learning (I, day 1) and retention (II, day 4) trials for the goldfish. Seven animals were trained on day 1; then the floats were removed. In trial II on day 4, the same animals were tested with the same floats as on day 1.

and homogenized in isotonic sucrose. The homogenate was separated by ultracentrifugation (see Fig. 3) into the nuclear, cytoplasmic, synaptosomal, myelin, and mitochondrial subcellular fractions (Whittaker, 1959). Each of these fractions contained ^{3}H- and ^{14}C-labeled products derived from the trained and untrained controls, respectively. The products were then separated by SDS–gel electrophoresis (Laemmli, 1970) as a function of molecular weight to give the results shown in Fig. 4. Analysis of the isotope ratios as a function of migration distance showed that three proteins bands (α, β, and γ), associated with only one subcellular fraction (cytoplasmic), were labeled to a greater extent in the trained than in the control animals (see Table I). No double-labeling ratio changes were found for the membrane, nuclear, myelin, or mitochondrial fractions. Reversal of the label gave the

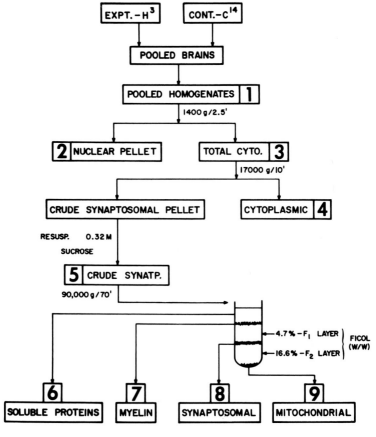

FIGURE 3. Subcellular fractionation procedure for analysis of double-labeling experiments. After training, seven goldfish received intracerebral injections of labeled [^{3}H]valine; an equal number of controls, in a separate tank, were labeled with [^{14}C]valine. The animals were labeled for 1 hr and anesthetized in ice for 10 min. The brains of the two groups were pooled and homogenized in 0.32 M sucrose and fractionated by centrifugation methods.

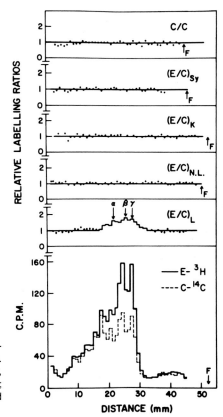

FIGURE 4. Gel electrophoresis data for labeled goldfish brain proteins. C/C, Control vs. control; (E/C), experimental vs. control; Sy, synaptosomal; K, kidney cytoplasmic fraction; L, N.L., and A.N.L., learning, nonlearning and active nonlearning, respectively.

same results. The average increases obtained for the ratio were 45%, 59%, and 72% for the proteins in the molecular weight range of 26–40K. It was surprising to find that no protein changes were obtained for the synaptosomal or the membrane fractions.

2.3. Control Experiments

The fact that enhanced labeling of specific proteins in goldfish brain occurs after training does not necessarily indicate that these proteins are correlated with the learning or memory aspects of the behavior (Shashoua, 1977b). Such changes might be the result of physiological stimulations, stress, or some other feature of the experiment. These possibilities were examined in several types of control experiments. It was found that in most training sessions some goldfish in each group did not learn the behavior. These were classified as two types: (1) passive nonlearners, which remained completely inactive in an upside-down position during the 4-hr training period and (2) active nonlearners, which would start the behavior at a given performance level and continue to swim actively at the same posture throughout the 4-hr period, without improving their score. A study of the pattern

Table I. Double-Labeling Data for Valine Incorporation
in the Brain Cytoplasmic Protein Fraction[a]

| | | Increase at bands (%) | | |
No.	Type	α	β	γ
1	E/C	60	80	100
2	E/C	60	78	100
3	E/C	41	47	91
4	E/C	37	44	43
5	E/C	22	26	31
6	E/C	35	30	40
7	E/C	15	20	30
8	E/C	17	25	18
Control Experiments				
9	PNL/C	0[b]	0	0
10	ANL/C	0	0	0
11	ANL/C	0	0	0
12	OG/C	0	0	0
13	OG/C	0	0	0

[a] Results are for gel electrophoresis data for incorporation of [³H]valine vs.
[¹⁴C]valine. In experiments 7 and 8, the trained goldfish received [¹⁴C]valine.
All other trained groups received [³H]valine. Each experiment compares seven
experimental with seven control goldfish. In experiments 12 and 13, the animals
are older goldfish (12 g). All others are younger animals (5–7 g). E/C, trained
vs. control; PNL/C, passive nonlearner vs. control; ANL/C, active nonlearner
vs. control; OG/C, older goldfish vs. control.
[b] 0, represents changes below the experimental error levels of ± 7%.

of labeling of both the active and the passive nonlearners in comparison with
untrained controls showed that there were no detectable protein changes in any of
the subcellular fractions of the goldfish brain. Figure 5 shows a typical result for
an active nonlearner group. This group, which started the training with an average
score of 29% and ended it 4 hr later with an average score of 33%, showed no
protein changes. Such data suggest that it is essential for the animals to acquire

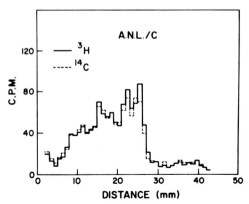

FIGURE 5. Comparison of the labeling
patterns of the ECF goldfish brain proteins from active nonlearners (A.N.L) with
untrained controls (C). The A.N.L. group
did not change their performance scores
during the 4-hr training period. They
continually swam throughout this time.
Both groups were labeled for 1 hr; [³H]
for the A.N.L. and [¹⁴C] for the C. Note
that the gel electrophoretic patterns for
the two groups are not significantly different in this double-labeling experiment.

some aspect of the behavior before any detectable protein changes can be observed. In addition, the active nonlearners became physically exhausted by their vigorous swimming during the 4-hr procedure; thus physical exercise or a general physiological stimulation per se is not sufficient to elicit the enhanced labeling of these specific proteins or any other proteins.

The possibility that stress was responsible for the protein changes was also investigated. Goldfish (1 year old or less) were found to learn the float training task and to recall the experience when tested 3 or even 11 days later. Older goldfish (12–15 g weight) learned the task at about the same rate as the young ones, but they could not recall the behavioral experience when tested 3 days later. Thus the younger goldfish appear to have both short- and long-term memory; i.e., they can learn the task and recall the behavior 3 days later. The older goldfish, however, appear to have short-term but not long-term memory, since they behave like naive animals when retested 3 days later. Double-labeling studies immediately after training showed that the younger animals had increased labeling in the α, β, and γ band region of the cytoplasmic fraction, whereas the older animals showed no protein changes. If stress were a determinant of the protein changes, then both the younger and older animals would be expected to show the changes. Presumably the effects of stress would be at a maximum during the acquisition phase of the behavior. The fact that no protein changes were obtained for the older goldfish, which could learn the task readily but not recall it, suggests that stress is not a major cause of the changes observed. However, one could argue that some other developmental factors such as the size and age of an animal might also be important in the sensitivity of the animal to stress, but this would not explain why older animals could not retain the behavior. These results raise the possibility that the metabolism of these proteins might have some relationship to the acquisition process of the new behavior.

2.4. Isolation and Purification of the β Protein

A combination of Sephadex gel chromatography and SDS preparative gel electrophoresis was used to isolate up to 1-mg quantities of the β protein from the total cytoplasmic fraction derived from 300 goldfish brains (Shashoua, 1977a). The purified protein was found to migrate as a single band on a variety of SDS gel electrophoretic systems. Analysis of its N-terminal amino acid end group showed the presence of a single group (serine), suggesting that the product contains a single polypeptide chain. Antisera raised in rabbits against the β antigen gave a single precipitin band when plated on Ouchterlony gels against the purified β protein or the total cytoplasmic fraction of goldfish brain. Amino acid analyses of the β protein (see Table II) showed it to have a high content of acidic amino acids (Schmidt and Shashoua, 1983). Its molecular weight is approximately 32–38K daltons. The γ protein was also purified and shown to be also acidic with a molecular weight in the range of 26–30K daltons. Immunochemical methods showed that both proteins were normal components of goldfish brain, suggesting that only their turnover rate was sensitive to training.

Table II. Amino Acid Compositions of Ependymins

Amino Acid	Ependymin β (mole %)	Ependymin γ (mole %)
Asx	8.9	9.2
Thr	5.8	6.3
Ser	8.9	9.2
Glx	13.1	12.5
Pro	5.5	6.3
Gly	10.0	10.8
Ala	6.2	6.3
Val	5.8	5.8
Cys	1.0	0.8
Met	0.7	0.4
Ile	3.4	3.3
Leu	7.2	7.5
Tyr	2.4	2.5
Phe	5.8	5.4
Orn	0.7	0.8
Lys	6.2	5.8
His	4.8	3.8
Arg	3.4	3.3
% acidic AA	22	21.7
% basic AA	15.1	13.7

[a] The data represent the mean from ten independent preparations.
[b] Tryptophan was not analyzed.

2.5. Neuroanatomical Localization of the β Protein

Immunohistochemical techniques of Coons (1968) and Hartman (1973) were used to investigate the neuroanatomical distribution of the β antigen in the brains of untrained goldfish. The protein was found to be present in the cytoplasm of specific cells and fibrous elements of the nervous system (see Fig. 6). A neuroanatomical map, generated from serial sections, established that the protein was localized in a system of cells (see Fig. 7) along the periventricular gray of the goldfish nervous system (Benowitz and Shashoua, 1977). The cells were most highly concentrated in the *zona ependyma* region of the goldfish brain, and we have proposed the name "ependymins" for the proteins. An immunohistochemical study of the localization of the γ protein also showed it to be distributed in a manner similar to that of the β protein (Dimino, unpublished data).

2.6. Amnestic Effects of Antisera to the Ependymins

There are several possibilities that can be proposed to explain how proteins such as the ependymins, whose metabolism is enhanced after the acquisition of a new pattern of behavior, may be involved in learning processes. One possibility is that the whole system of β and γ cells is activated by the training. In this case the ependymins would be merely markers for the specific neural circuits that are ac-

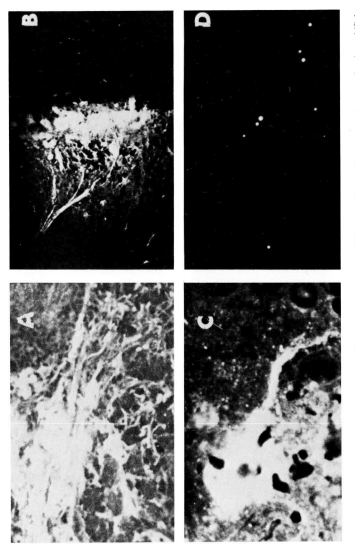

FIGURE 6. Immunohistofluorescence localization of the cells and fibers that contain the β and γ proteins in goldfish brain. (A) Regions in the ependymal zone below the optic tectum (150×). (B) Cells and fibers in the basal forebrain (150×). (C) A single cell in the dorsal tegmentum (1000×). (D) Preimmune serum control.

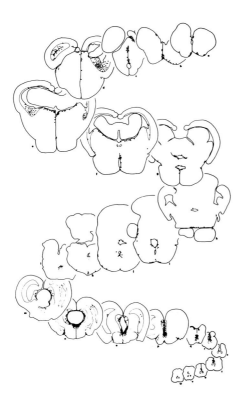

FIGURE 7. Localization of β protein cells in goldfish brain. Serial cross-sections are drawn at 400-μm intervals. Triangles show the locations of individual β ependymal cells.

tivated by the training and thus would have no direct functional role in the mechanism of long-term memory formation. Another possibility is that the ependymins might be directly participating in some aspect of the neural plasticity process. To test for this hypothesis we investigated the effect of antisera on the retention of training (Shashoua and Moore, 1978). The procedure was to train animals and then inject antisera to β and γ ependymins into the 4th ventricle of the brain. Control animals from the same group, trained at the same time, were injected with normal or pre-immune rabbit serum. The experiments were run blind. After 3 days the floats were reattached and the rate of reacquisition of the task was tested. Table III illustrates the results of such experiments. It was found that animals that received injections of antisera to the ependymins, either β or β + γ, could not recall the behavior, whereas those receiving pre-immune sera had good retention. Thus far, 500 animals have been tested by this procedure, and the results were highly statistically significant (see Table III).

There are several possible explanations for these observations. One is that the antisera might generate a toxic reaction and thus indirectly cause the amnestic behavior. As a control for this, the effects of injections of β and γ antisera prior to training were tested. Such injections at 30 min and 24 hr before training were found to have no influence on the rate of learning or the recall of the behavior. This indicates that neither acute nor delayed toxicity factors can be important in

TABLE III. Studies of the Effect of Ependymin Antisera on Behavior[a]

Expt. no.	Antisera	Time (hr)	Experimental		Control			T-test p-value
			No. of animals	Average retention score (%)	No. of animals	Average retention score (%)		
1	β	+8	28	36 ± 19	21	94 ± 7		<0.0025
2	β	+8, +20	21	25 ± 11	21	94 ± 16		<0.0005
3	β + γ	+8, +20	98	49 ± 21	97	92 ± 27		0.0005
4	β + γ	+48	15	28 ± 33	14	81 ± 27	<0.01	>0.05
5	β + γ	+72	13	70 ± 32	12	77 ± 37	<0.35	>1.3
Controls								
6	β + γ	−0.5	21	90 ± 13	21	92 ± 6	<0.45	>0.4
7	β + γ	−24	21	94 ± 11	21	120 ± 35	<0.2	>0.15
8	NS-6	+8	20	89 ± 39	20	20 ± 38	<0.48	>0.45
9	β + γ (antigen adsorbed)	+8, +20	12	82 ± 32	11	71 ± 24	<0.2	>0.15

[a] Experimental goldfish received injections, into the fourth brain ventricle, of antisera to either β or β + γ ependymins. Controls received preimmune sera at times specified before or after the initiation of the 5-hr training periods.

the observed amnestic effects of the antisera. Another possibility is that any anti-serum to any brain-specific protein might produce amnesia. To test for this, an antiserum to a brain-specific protein NS 6 (Chaffee and Schachner, 1978) was tested and found to have no effect. Also, antisera to the ependymins adsorbed with the β and γ antigens were found to have no effect on the rate of acquisition or the recall of behavior, suggesting that the specific IgG molecules directed against the β and γ ependymins may be important for the observed biological effects.

A study of the time course of the amnestic effects of the ependymin antisera indicated that there was a window of time, between 3 and 24 hr after training, during which injections of antisera were effective. Injections at 48 and 72 hr after training were found to produce no statistically significant amnestic effects. These observations suggest that learning may initiate a series of sequential biochemical events, which at some stage may require the participation of ependymins. Once completed (i.e., about 24 hr later), the process seems to be no longer vulnerable to attack by the antisera to the ependymins.

2.7. Evidence for Release of the β and γ Ependymins into the Brain Extracellular Fluid

Several types of experiments indicate that the ependymins are released from their site of synthesis into the extracellular space to become highly localized in the brain extracellular fluid (ECF). (1) Goldfish brain cerebrospinal fluid (CSF) and ECF, when plated against ependymin antisera, were found to give precipitin bands identical to those of the pure antigen in an Ouchterlony assay (Shashoua, 1979). (2) Quantitative measurements, using ^{125}I-labeled β ependymin in a radioimmu-noassay, showed that about 14% of the total proteins present in goldfish brain ECF fraction consist of ependymins (Schmidt and Shashoua, 1981). (3) Double-labeling studies (Shashoua, 1979) of the pattern of protein synthesis after training by isolation of the ECF fraction indicated that most of the enhanced labeling obtained after training was localized at the molecular weight position of the β and γ ependymin. In fact, in some experiments the total increased incorporation associated with the β and γ ependymins could be extracted with the ECF fraction, leaving marginal amounts in the cytoplasmic fraction. This suggests that the ependymins are syn-thesized in specific cells and rapidly released into the extracellular space after learning.

Additional proof that the β and γ ependymins are released into the ECF fraction was obtained by tissue culture experiments (Majocha *et al.,* 1982). *Zona ependyma* cells of goldfish brain were grown *in vitro* on polylysine-coated plates. Immuno-histochemical studies of the cultures (10–20 days old) showed that specific cells and fibers were stained with antisera to the ependymins (see Fig. 8). Analysis of the culture media by radioimmunoassay showed that the ependymins were released products. There was a progressive increase of ependymins in the media as a function of days in culture without any significant change in the amount present in the cells. In addition, labeling studies with [^{3}H]valine indicated that newly synthesized epen-dymins were rapidly released into the medium. These data support the hypothesis

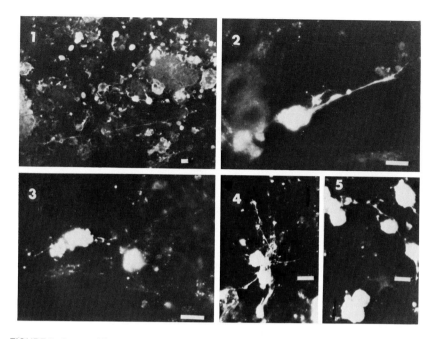

FIGURE 8. Immunohistochemical staining patterns of zona ependyma cultures with antisera to ependymins β and γ. The photographs show the fluorescent cells after 24 hr in culture (1), (2,3) after 5 days in cultures, and (4,5) after 10 days in culture. Note the presence of cells with multiple processes. The white bar coresponds to a length of 20 μm.

that these proteins are normally released into the extracellular space for a probable function at targets distant from the site of their synthesis.

3. STUDIES OF PROTEIN CHANGES IN MAMMALIAN BRAIN

Experiments using Balb-c mice as experimental animals and a self-return T-maze (Greene *et al.*, 1972) as the behavioral paradigm were carried out to find out if ependyminlike or other specific protein changes can be obtained in mammalian brain after learning. Thirsty animals were trained to find water in one arm of a T-maze. The mice were water deprived for 2 days prior to training. During this period each mouse was placed daily for 30 min in the maze with all doors open (see Fig. 9) to allow for the animal to become familiar with the apparatus. The orientation preference (left of right) for one arm of the maze was noted for each animal. It was surprising to find that even litter mates from a single strain of animals have a distribution of orientation preferences (Shashoua and Moore, 1980). Sixty percent had a right-arm preference, 30% had a left-arm preference, and about 10% of the mice had no specific behavioral preference. Figure 9 shows a diagram of the self-

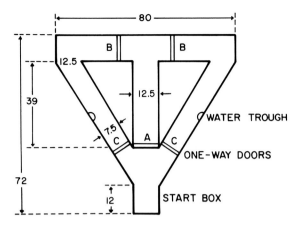

FIGURE 9. Diagram of the self-return T-maze apparatus. Thirsty mice are trained to find water in one arm of the T-maze. Doors A, B, and C are one-way clear plastic swinging gates that allow a mouse to pass through but not return. In each trial a mouse receives 8 μl of water in the water trough. Dimensions are in centimeters.

return T-maze. Doors A, B, and C are one-way clear plastic swinging gates that allow the mouse to pass one way into the maze but not to return through the same gate. In this paradigm, each animal learns at his own pace without interference by the experimenter or the apparatus. An animal trained to find water at his preferred orientation side shows no savings, whereas an animal trained to find water on the opposite side of his preference requires longer to acquire the criterion performance rate (85% correct for 30 consecutive trials) and recall the experience when tested 4 days later. After about 100 trials, in which an animal receives 8 μl of water in each trial, a mouse becomes satiated and his performance rate begins to decline. Following training in such a behavioral paradigm, the rate of valine incorporation was compared to that of an untrained litter mate in a double-labeling type of experiment (Shashoua and Moore, 1984). Table IV and Fig. 10 show the results of such experiments. Only the ECF and cytoplasmic fractions showed changes in double-labeling ratios at specific protein bands of the SDS electrophoretic gels. None were obtained for the nuclear, mitochondrial, synaptosomal, and membrane fractions. The cytoplasmic fraction had enhanced incorporation at a band position migrating at 68K. After 1 hr of labeling the predominant changes in the ECF fraction were at about 33K and 25.5K. At shorter times (30 min) the ECF fraction showed increases at 68K, 64K, 59K, 38K, 30K, and 19K (see Table II). These results are suggestive of the type of association products previously noted for the ependymins in goldfish brain.

Table IV also shows a number of control experiments in which no protein changes were obtained. These include animals trained to their preferred orientation side that show no retention and highly stressed animals. The stressed mice were obtained using three sequential sessions of training and testing of each water-

TABLE IV. Double-Labeling Studies with Valine: Balb C Mice[a]

Expt. no.	Label time (min)	E-isotope	Increase at molecular weight (%)					
			68,000	64,000	59,000	38,000	30,000	19,000
1	60	^{3}H	—	—	—	280	100	—
2	60	^{3}H	—	—	—	540	200	65
3	60	^{3}H	—	—	—	130	24	14
4	60	^{14}C	—	—	—	30	—	—
5	60	^{14}C	—	—	—	140	70	48
6	45	^{14}C	170	90	100	20	40	—
7	45	^{14}C	50	30	30	20	30	30

Controls

	Type	Result
5	E/C kidney	No changes[b]
8	C/C	No changes
9	Stress	No changes
10	Stress	No changes
11	P-Side/C	No changes
12	Thirsty/satiated	No changes

[a] Each experiment consists of two litter mates labeled with valine. A trained animal was matched to a control animal. The label was introduced I.P.; 1 mCi [^{3}H]valine and 100 μCi [^{14}C]valine were used. E, experimental; C, control; P-Side, trained to the preferred orientation. Experiments 1–7: all experimental animals were trained opposite to their preferred orientation.
[b] No change, represents changes below the experimental error levels of ±7%.

deprived animal to firmly fix its behavior to its preferred side. Next each mouse was water deprived for a fourth time and an attempt was made to switch its orientation to the opposite side. Some of the animals even after 180 trials could not be forced to reverse their preferred orientation. They clearly worked hard and were presumably highly frustrated and stressed by their unsuccessful attempts to find water. Such stressed animals (Expt. 9 and 10, Table IV) exhibited no protein changes for any brain subcellular fraction when tested against a control litter mate. Similar experiments comparing protein incorporation patterns for a thirsty vs. a satiated animal showed that the stress of being water deprived was not sufficient to cause any detectable protein labeling changes. Such results are consistent with the hypothesis that it is essential for an animal to acquire a new behavior before specific protein changes can be observed.

The data from the double-labeling experiments indicate that proteins with similar molecular weights and subcellular localization properties have an enhanced turnover rate in mammalian brain to that previously observed in goldfish brain. Thus, two completely different learning experiments in two separate species appear to cause similar protein changes in the brains of trained animals.

In attempts to further characterize these observations, two of the proteins (38K and 19K) that showed changes after training in mouse brain were isolated and purified by a combination of gel electrophoresis and Sephadex gel chromatography

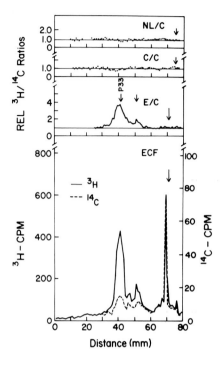

FIGURE 10. Electrophoretic migration properties of the extracellular fluid proteins of mouse brain. Balb c litter-mates are compared. A thirsty mouse was labeled I.P. with 1 mCi [³H]valine, at 3 hr after completion of training, and compared to an untrained control animal labeled with 100 μCi [¹⁴C]valine I.P. Incorporation was for 1 hr. Note enhanced incorporation at peaks 1 and 2 for E/C (experimental vs. control) and the findings that no changes are obtained for the ³H/¹⁴C label ratios for the control vs. control (C/C) and the nonlearning vs. control (NL/C).

(Shashoua and Moore, 1984). The purified products isolated from ECF preparation from 100 brains of Balb-c mice were characteried by one- and two-dimensional SDS gel electrophoresis as single migrating bands. In the absence of electrolytes both purified proteins were found to aggregate into insoluble products. These were then individually resuspended in 1% SDS and used to raise antisera in rabbits. The antisera raised against the 38K and 19K protein were found to have the same type of antigenic properties when tested by western blots against mouse ECF. Bands located at 68K, 38K, and 19K were stained, suggesting that common antigenic determinants are present in these ECF proteins.

The 38K Antiserum was used for immunohistochemical localization of the "ependyminlike" proteins in mouse brain. Figure 11 shows data for horizontal sections mapping the locus of immunoreactive sites (Shashoua and Moore, 1984). The staining appears to be concentrated in the thalamus, caudate, and hippocampus. In fact, every pyramidal cell of the hippocampus and dentate region had staining processes associated with its soma. The superficial cortical areas were generally devoid of straining areas, whereas some deeper cortical areas contained immunoreactive sites. These preliminary studies indicate that the proteins with "ependyminlike" properties exist in mouse brain and that they are localized in specific cells and regions.

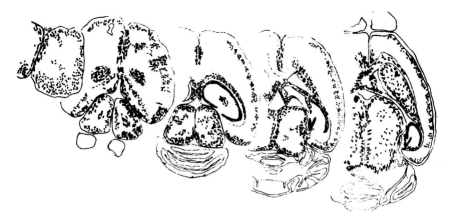

FIGURE 11. Localization of ependymin-immunoreactive sites in mouse brain. Serial horizontal sections (left to right) show staining regions for dorsal to ventral at various levels of the CNS. Note the cerebellum is unlabeled and that there is an intense labeling in the hippocampus, thalamus, caudate, and deep layers of the cortex.

4. INVESTIGATIONS OF THE MOLECULAR PROPERTIES OF EPENDYMINS

The above results illustrate that in two vertebrate species (goldfish and mice) the turnover rate of a class of brain extracellular proteins is enhanced after the animals learn two completely different types of behavior. The data suggest that the brain extracellular space may be an important communications channel in which ECF proteins might have a role in the neuroplasticity of the CNS. In attempts to find out how ECF proteins can participate in such a process we devised procedures for the isolation of the ECF proteins and investigated their properties, looking for molecular mechanisms that might be related to function.

4.1. Procedures for Isolation of Brain ECF Proteins

Goldfish brain is surrounded by a large external layer of fluid (Cserr and Ostrach, 1974) commonly referred to as the extradural fluid (EDF). This occupies most of the space in the cranial cavity and is reported to be different from CSF, the fluid within the ventricular spaces, and ECF, the fluid in the extracellular spaces of brain tissue. In attempts to investigate the nature and relationships of the proteins of these compartments, an extraction procedure was developed for the isolation of ECF (Shashoua, 1981) from perfused goldfish brains after washing off EDF and CSF. Incubation of the tissue in isotonic sucrose containing 1–4 mM Ca^{2+} at 0°C was found to result in the preferential leaching of ECF proteins without disruption of the integrity of the brain cells. The validity of this extraction procedure and its application to mammalian brain was established by kinetic studies and the fact that

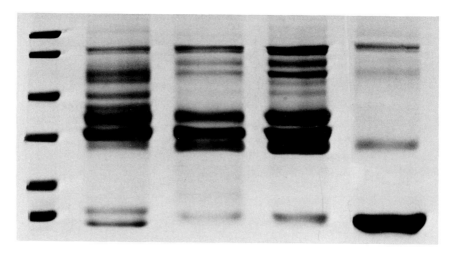

FIGURE 12. SDS-gel electrophoretic patterns comparing the components of ECF, CSF, and EDF. Note the similarity of the compositions of these three extracellular protein fractions and their distinct differences from goldfish serum proteins (SR). The standards (ST; top to bottom) correspond to the following molecular weights: 96K, 68K, 45K, 30K, 21K, and 14.5K.

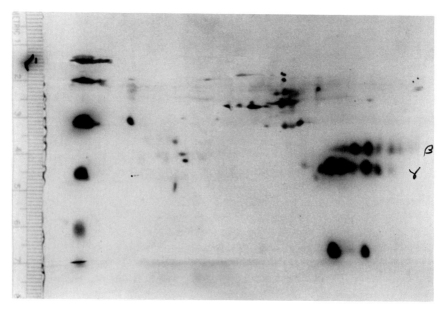

FIGURE 13. Two-dimensional gel electrophoretic pattern of goldfish ECF proteins. Note the microheterogeneity of the β and γ ependymin chains. ST, standards; same molecular weights as in Fig. 12.

cytoplasmic marker enzymes such as tyrosine hydroxylase (Hofstein *et al.*, 1983) and lactate dehydrogenase (Hesse *et al.*, 1984) were essentially absent from the extracts. Figures 12 and 13 show the one-dimensional and two-dimensional gel electrophoretic patterns of goldfish ECF proteins. The similarities of ECF to EDF and CSF are clearly evident in the one-dimensional gels. All three fluids contain a surprising collection of proteins with a wide range of molecular weights (10–100K). The prominent bands at 39K and 31K are the β and γ ependymins. In the two-dimensional gels (Fig. 13) the microheterogeneity of the bands at the positions of β and γ are clearly evident. Each chain appears to have five subtypes with isoelectric points in the pH range of 5.1 to 5.5.

4.2. Glycoprotein Nature of the Ependymins

The fact that the β and γ ependymins are released into the brain ECF raises the possibility that they may be glycoproteins. A study of the staining pattern of ECF proteins separated by SDS gel electrophoresis showed that a strong periodic-Schiffs (PAS) reaction (Clarke, 1967) occurred at the position of the β and γ ependymins, indicating their glycoprotein (Shashoua, 1982) nature. This was confirmed by analysis of hydrolysates of the purified β ependymin (J. Codington, private communication). Gas chromatographic data obtained by the method of Reinhold (1972) showed that the protein contains at least 5% carbohydrate with mannose galactose, *N*-acetylglucosamine and *N*-acetyl-neuraminic acid as the predominant components (see Table V).

4.3. Isolation of Goldfish Brain Ependymins in Their Native State

An affinity chromatographic method was developed for the isolation and purification of the ependymins in their native state. The procedure uses Con A-

Table V. Carbohydrate Analysis of Ependymins

Carbohydrate	Type G[a] (wt %)	Type M[b] (wt %)
Fucose	0.14	0.08
Xylose	0.16	0.05
Mannose	0.60	0.59
Galactose	1.21	0.94
Glucose	1.66	1.93
N-acetyl glucosamine	1.93	0.49
N-acetyl neuraminic acid	0.83	0.65
Total carbohydrate	5.6	4.7

[a] Type G = β + γ ependymins eluted from Con A sepharose with 0.1 M glucose.
[b] Type M = β + γ ependymins eluted from Con A sepharose with 0.1 M α-methyl mannoside.

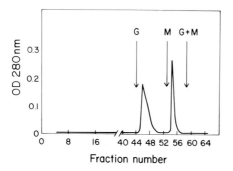

FIGURE 14. Elution of bound ependymins from an affinity chromatographic Sepharose-Con A column. Two fractions eluted with 0.1 M glucose (G), 0.1 M α-methylmannoside (M). These give the $(\beta + \gamma)_G$ and $(\beta + \gamma)_M$ fractions, respectively.

Sepharose as the lectin to bind the ependymins at room temperature. Figure 14 illustrates the procedures in which ECF extracts from 200–300 goldfish brains are used as the starting material. After binding to Con A, the unbound proteins are washed off with buffer prior to a sequential elution with 0.1 M glucose and 0.1 M α-methylmannoside. This yields two fractions, M and G, which, upon analysis by SDS gel electrophoresis (Schmidt and Shashoua, 1981) prior to heating in the presence of β-mercaptoethanol, indicates the presence of three closely migrating

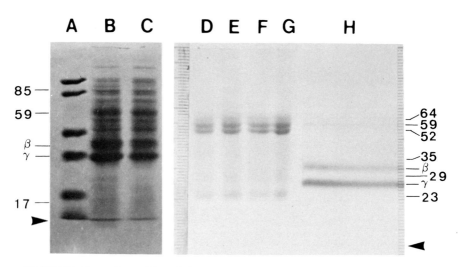

FIGURE 15. Comparison of the gel electrophoretic patterns of the native β and γ ependymin complex with that of the denatured products. (A) shows the molecular-weight markers: Phosphorylase B (94K), bovine serum albumin (68K), ovalbumin (45K), carbonic anhydrase (30K), soybean trypsin inhibitor (21K), and lysozyme (14.3K). (B) and (C) show the patterns for the separation of the total extracellular fluid proteins; the bands stained with Coomassie blue include ependymin β and γ and other constituents including P85, P59, and P17. (D–G) show the products as isolated by affinity chromatography. Note that three components are clearly visible at P64, P59, and P52. In H the same sample heated with β-mercaptoethanol dissociates into β and γ. The components P64, P59, and P52 correspond to molecular weights equivalent to β_2, $\beta\gamma$, and γ_2, respectively.

bands with molecular weights corresponding to β_2, $\beta\gamma$, and γ_2, respectively. However, if the samples were denatured by heating either in the presence of β-mer-
captoethanol or in a SDS-containing buffer alone, then only two bands migrating
at the positions of the β and γ were obtained in the gel electrophoretic patterns
(see Fig. 15). This suggests that the native protein is a complex dimer of two chains
that can dissociate to give β and γ. The M and G fractions appear to be subtypes
of the protein with differing carbohydrate compositions. As shown in Table V,
there is a significant difference in the N-acetylglucosamine and galactose levels
present in the M and G components, although they both appear to have the same
total carbohydrate content. These values must, however, be considered as minimal
amounts, since we do not know the extent of hydrolysis that may take place during
the isolation and purification of the glycoproteins.

4.4. Antigenic Properties of the Native and Denatured Ependymins

The antigenic properties of the native ependymins (β_2, $\beta\gamma$, and γ_2 complex)
were found to be substantially different from those of denatured single β or γ
polypeptide chains (Schmidt and Shashoua, 1981). Antisera raised against the purified denatured β polypeptide were at least 40 times more active towards β than the
native $\beta\gamma$ dimer. Moreover, the cytoplasmic and ECF fractions become more immunoreactive if they are heated for 5 min at 93°C, whereas the pure β and γ chains
exhibit no heat-induced antigenicity changes (see Table VI).

The β and γ polypeptide chains of the ependymins were found to have identical
immunoreactive sites (Schmidt and Shashoua, 1983). Investigations of protease
digests of the two proteins indicate that their peptide maps, with the exception of
one β-derived peptide, are identical, suggesting that γ may be derived from β chain.
[125]I-labeled β when incubated with ECF proteases yields labeled γ among its
breakdown products, whereas ^{125}I-labeled γ does not yield any labeled β. These
observations support the hypothesis that the ependymins are released into ECF as

TABLE VI. Increase in Antigenicity of Ependymins
After Heat Denaturation[a]

Sample	Percent antigenic reactivity relative to protein content	
	Before denaturation	After denaturation
Brain ECF	0.06 ± 0.1 (58)	14.2 ± 0.7 (59)
Brain cytoplasm	0.008 ± 0.001 (16)	4.6 ± 0.3 (25)
Ependymin	100 ± 12.4 (13)	96.2 ± 6.7 (5)
Ependymin	80 ± 16.9 (8)	70.6 ± 12.4 (3)
β_2 native dimer	9.2 ± 2.7 (8)	96.2 (1)
$\beta\gamma$ native dimer	12.8 ± 3.7 (8)	96.4 ± 4.8 (2)
γ_2 native dimer	4.6 ± 0.4 (4)	15.7 (1)

[a] The percent antigenic reactivity was measured by radioimmunoassay. Denaturation was achieved
by heating for 5 min at 100°C prior to the assay. All data are given with their S.E.M.;
number of determinations are shown in parentheses.

β_2 dimers, which may then be converted to $\beta\gamma$ and γ_2. The major antigenic sites of the dimers appear to be buried within the molecules. These sites only become available for reaction with antiserum raised against the denatured β or γ chains, after heating. Such results raise the possibility that association–dissociation phenomena might be important in functional properties of the molecules.

4.5. Aggregation Properties of ECF Proteins and Ependymins

The ependymins are highly soluble in aqueous media in the presence of physiological concentrations of electrolytes and calcium (2.5 mM in goldfish CSF). When calcium is removed from such solutions by dialysis at 4°C, the proteins spontaneously form insoluble aggregates (Shashoua, 1984). Similar changes occur, yielding fibrous products (see Fig. 16), when the calcium chelating agent ethylene-bis (oxyethylene-nitrilo) tetraacetate (EGTA) is added to ECF preparations from goldfish brain. The initiation and propagation of the polymerization reaction was found to require critical concentrations of EGTA and ECF proteins. The best results were obtained using freshly extracted ECF in which polymerization could be initiated by EGTA at pH 7.4 but not at pH 7.8. ECF samples stored for several days tended to lose their pH 7.4 polymerization properties, progressively requiring lower pH conditions for the initiation of the reaction. The most rapid polymerization occurred at pH values close to the isoelectric points (pH 5.1 to 5.5) of the ependymins.

Figure 17 illustrates a study of the kinetics of the polymerization process. Measurements of turbidity as a function of time indicate that the ECF proteins can aggregate even when less than the equivalent amount of EGTA required to chelate the Ca^{2+} present in solution is added (see Fig. 17A) to the medium. This suggests that the EGTA might be able to interact with the macromolecules more readily than with the Ca^{2+} in the solvent. In additional experiments, the rate of rise in turbidity initiated by EGTA was found to be inhibited by the addition of calcium ions (Fig. 17B). Moreover, such Ca^{2+}-blocked polymerizations could be re-initiated by adding another aliquot of EGTA. This observation suggests that calcium can inhibit the initiation and propagation steps of the polymerizations. The fibrous products once formed, however, could not be redissolved in most protein solvents, including boiling 1% SDS in 6 M urea and even trifluoroacetic acid. The fact that the ependymins are involved in the polymerization properties of ECF was established by immunohistochemical methods. Antisera to the ependymins were capable of staining the fibrous aggregates in the presence of goat serum and BSA, the reaction products being visualized by the standard horseradish peroxidase-goat antirabbit IgG method (Sternberger, 1979). The fibers were found to stain very heavily with the antisera to the ependymins but not with pre-immune sera.

These results suggest that the capacity to aggregate may be built into the molecular structure of the proteins. The fact that the aggregates are insoluble raises the possibility that covalent bonds may be formed during the polymerization process. One mechanism that could lead to insolubility is the formation of disulfide bonds between polypeptide chains using cysteine residues of the proteins. A conformational change in the native dimer cold be triggered by the removal of calcium from an allosteric site to initiate a process of molecular aggregation to the fibrous state.

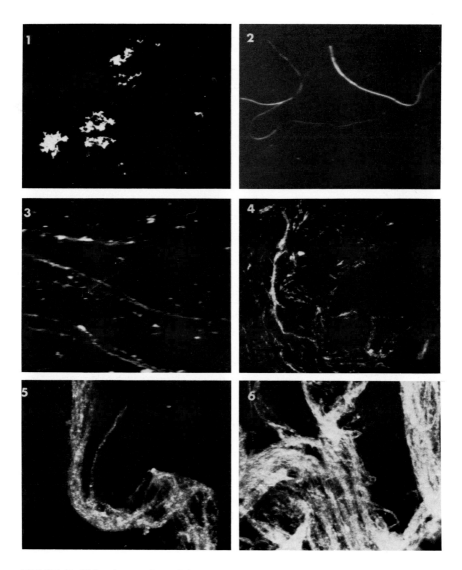

FIGURE 16. Light microscopic studies of the polymerization of ECF proteins. Panels 1–6 show dark-field photomicrographs. (1) shows typical aggregates (400× magnification) obtained by adding a large excess of EGTA (18 mM) to ECF solutions with 2.5 mM Ca^{2+}. Addition of low amounts of EGTA (2.1 mM) produce fibrous products at 5 min (panels 2 and 3) and 15 min (panel 4) (400× magnification). At 2 hr (panel 6) fiber bundles aggregate into matts in a parallel array (100× magnification).

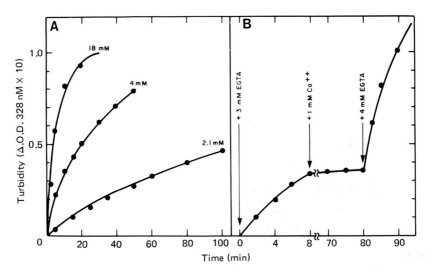

FIGURE 17. Studies of the kinetics of the polymerization of the ependymins. (A) shows the effect of adding increasing amounts of EGTA on the rate of increase in turbidity of ECF solutions (0.23 mg protein/μl + 2.5 mM Ca^{2+}) as a function of time. (B) illustrates the capacity of Ca^{2+} to block an ongoing polymerization initiated by 3 mM EGTA and that the Ca^{2+} inhibition effect can be overcome by further addition of EGTA at pH 6.3.

An alternative mechanism may involve the carbohydrate moieties of the glycoproteins. Such a hypothesis would account for the observed loss of polymerization properties in the ECF fraction after storage for several days at room temperature. Ependymins isolated from stored ECF samples tended to have a lower carbohydrate content than those prepared from freshly extracted ECF. Further studies are in progress to determine which of the above or other molecular mechanisms are responsible for the conversion of the highly soluble ependymins into insoluble aggregates.

5. INVESTIGATIONS OF THE FUNCTIONAL PROPERTIES OF THE EPENDYMINS

The above experiments demonstrate that the ependymins are a class of brain glycoproteins whose turnover rates are enhanced when goldfish or mice acquire a new pattern of behavior. The proteins are highly concentrated in the brain extracellular fluid and are released from cells located in the *zona ependyma* of goldfish brain. In the native state, the ependymins are soluble dimers derived from two acidic polypeptide chains that contain sulfhydryl and/or disulfide bonds and at least 5% covalently linked carbohydrates. *In vitro*, in the absence of Ca^{2+} ions, the proteins can rapidly polymerize to form insoluble aggregates. Is this property important for their *in vivo* functions?

5.1. Evidence for Aggregation of Ependymins in Hippocampal Slices

The fact that an aggregation of ECF proteins and the ependymins can take place in a test tube does not necessarily mean that the same phenomenon can occur in neural tissue and *in vivo*. In attempts to explore this question, two types of experiments were carried out using the rat hippocampal slice as a model system to look for a role for extracellular proteins. In the first series of experiments we studied the pattern of protein synthesis (Duffy *et al.*, 1979) after stimulation of monosynaptic pathways in the slice to obtain long-term potentiation (LTP) (Bliss and Lømo, 1973; Lynch and Schubert, 1980; Schwartzkroin and Wester, 1975; Teyler, 1980). Using double-labeling procedures we found that, after LTP, a slice released more labeled proteins (an average increase of 175%) into the extracellular medium than an unstimulated control. No protein changes after LTP were detected in other subcellular fractions or in a variety of control experiments including stimulation at low frequencies that produced no LTP. This observation suggests the possibility that during LTP, proteins present in the extracellular space may be preferentially used up in some process—perhaps the formation of ependymin aggregates. Thus the observed increased labeling of ECF proteins after LTP might be due to a homeostatic mechanism that is turned on to restore protein levels in the extracellular space. If such a phenomenon were to occur, then it should be possible to demonstrate the presence of aggregates in the extracellular space after LTP.

The second series of experiments with the hippocampal slice system were designed to look for the presence of polymerized ependymins after LTP, using immunohistochemical methods. The slices were first potentiated and then incubated for 24 hr at 4°C in an isotonic medium (Cragg, 1980), containing 2 mM Ca^{2+} in the presence of goat serum and BSA to leach out all soluble ECF proteins. This procedure was shown to be capable of removing ECF proteins from brain tissue (Shashoua, 1985). The slices were next incubated with the following reagents in sequence: rabbit antiependymin serum (1/200), followed by extensive washing in isotonic medium, fluorescent goat antirabbit IgG (1/200), and final washing in isotonic medium. Figure 18 shows the results of such an experiment. Both control (unpotentiated) and experimental slices showed fluorescent regions surrounding the pyramidal cells of the hippocampus and dentate gyrus. These are the cells that normally contain the proteins and release them into the extracellular space. In the potentiated slice, however, there was additional staining in the stratum radiatum (Shashoua and Hesse, 1985). This appeared as dots scattered throughout the zone. Presumably these are polymeric ependymin aggregates that might have been generated by LTP. No staining was observed using preimmune sera. These results suggest that the process of ECF aggregation can occur in a viable neural tissue.

5.2. Studies of the Effect of Training on Ependymin Aggregation

In attempts to find out whether the process of ependymin aggregation can occur *in vivo*, we carried out a series of experiments using the antisera to the ependymins to localize immunohistochemical staining sites in the brains of trained goldfish.

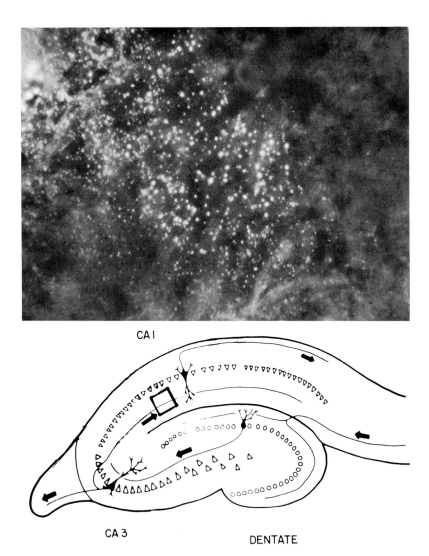

FIGURE 18. Effect of LTP on the pattern of staining hippocampal slices with antisera to mouse brain ependymins. The photograph shows a fluorescent staining region in the stratum radiatum. The dotlike appearance is localized at 1–2 mm away from the site of the stimulation (S) and abruptly stops as shown in the photograph. Unpotentiated slices show no such staining. Both control and potentiated slices show staining at the pyramidal cell layer of the dentate and hippocampus. There are cells (not pyramidal) that synthesize and release the ependymins into the extracellular space.

Following vestibulomotor conditioning, each animal received two injections, 24 hr apart, of anti-ependymin sera into the 4th ventricle of the brain. Such animals, when tested 3 days later, were found to have no recall of the training (Shashoua, 1985). In addition they appeared unable to relearn the task. They repeatedly attempted, but did not successfully improve in, learning the behavior. They could, however, learn another task (shock avoidance training). Thus we cannot assume that all learning abilities had been blocked by the antibody treatment. Is it possible that a temporary block of the specific sites in circuits that subserve the behavior occurs as a result of the prolonged exposure to the antibody? Such a specific blockade of behavior following a distinct lesioned site has recently been reported for the nictitating membrane response in rabbit brain (McCormick et al., 1982; Thompson et al., 1983). If the 3-day nonrelearning goldfish were retested 10 days later, then they behaved as naive animals, capable of learning the task within 4 hr. Presumably any antibody present at blocked sites in the brain was removed by proteolysis by this time. Figure 19 compares horizontal sections at the same anatomical level of a goldfish brain from a 3-day tested animal, which could not relearn, with a 10-day retested animal, which could relearn. The binding sites for the antibody were localized with fluorescent goat antirabbit IgG. It is clear that the 3-day nonrelearner has many staining regions, including some in brain areas that do not normally contain ependymin-synthesizing cells, whereas the 10-day animal has only a few sites that stain. So far, 10 and 9 animals of the 3- and 10-day goldfish, respectively, have been studied by this procedure. A consistent difference between the two groups was easily distinguishable in a double-blind experiment. If we assume that the high-molecular-weight IgG molecules do not enter the brain cells, then most of the staining sites have to be localized on external surfaces of cell membranes or in the extracellular space. Such a possibility would require the formation of ependymin polymers, since any products of antibody interaction with an excess of soluble antigen (i.e., the conditions present in ECF) would tend to be soluble and easily removable from the tissue during the staining procedure.

5.3. Ependymin Polymerization Hypothesis

The experiments described in this chapter suggest the following as a working hypothesis for the functional role of the ependymins in the CNS. The ependymins are normally present as β_2, $\beta\gamma$, and γ_2 dimers throughout the brain extracellular space as soluble molecules. During learning, at specific sites where a transient Ca^{2+} depletion of the ECF occurs, the soluble ependymins are rapidly converted to the insoluble fibrous state. This forms an extracellular matrix at the specific neuroanatomical sites where a subsequent modification of neural circuits has to occur. This could ultimately lead to the growth of preexisting synaptic areas or even the formation of new synapses, perhaps in a manner similar to previous findings in neural development (Bonner-Frazer and Cohen, 1980) and the regeneration of the neuromuscular junction (McMahon et al., 1980, Sanes, 1983). Thus the role of the ependymins in this hypothesis is to define the extracellular space in which the subsequent events leading to pre- and postsynaptic changes might take place. The protein is always ready to be fixed at the specific geographic site where a signal for its transformation (i.e., forming of an insoluble fibrous matrix) is generated.

The hypothesis essentially has three requirements: (1) the presence of a steady supply of the ependymins in the soluble form throughout the extracellular space, (2) a signal generation mechanism that distinguishes normal use from the type of novel use that may occur during learning, i.e., a process for removal of Ca^{2+} from the extracellular environment that is much larger during stimulation of converging imputs than during normal use of single pathways, and (3) that the ECF polymer initiation signal (the calcium-depletion process) should be rapid, localized at specific sites, and transient. In the goldfish the supply of the ependymins in the ECF seems to be well regulated (Shashoua, 1981). In the mammalian brain there is a rapid turnover of the protein with a half-life of 4 hr (Hesse *et al.*, 1984).

The possibility that the ependymin polymerization signal may involve transient

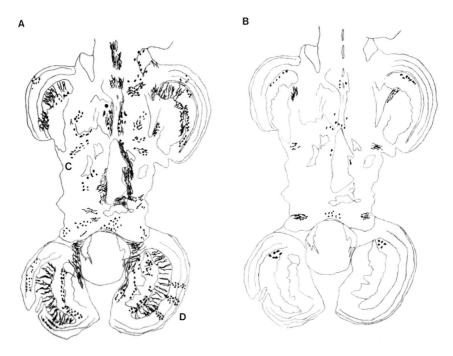

FIGURE 19. Immunohistochemical staining pattern of horizontal sections of brains of trained goldfish. (A) and (B) received two injections of ependymin antisera (24 hr apart) at 3 hr after completion of learning. (A) was stained at 3 days after learning, after noting the animal had no recall of the training and was incapable of relearning the task. (B) was stained at 10 days after the learning when the goldfish had no recall of the behavior but was capable of relearning. Note that the staining regions were plotted on an identical diagram for cross-sections of the brain. There is a marked difference in the fluorescent staining regions in (A) as compared to (B). The results are consistent with the hypothesis that the ependymin antisera can block crucial sites at which an extracellular matrix of insoluble ependymins was formed during learning. Photographs (C) and (D) show the type of punctate cell surface labeling obtained for the vestibular region and perimeter staining of the columnar array of cells in the vagal lobe in section A.

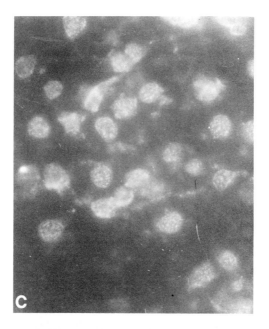

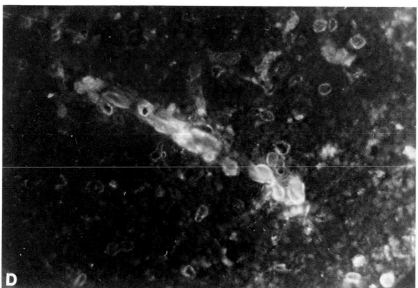

FIGURE 19. (*Continued*)

changes in the concentration of Ca^{2+} in the extracellular environment can be supported by previous experimental evidence in studies of associative learning in invertebrates and of long-term potentiation of hippocampal slices in mammalian brain. Alkon (1980) has demonstrated by direct measurements that the neurophysiological events depicting associative learning do result in a transient accumulation of calcium within the specific cells (Alkon, Chapter 1, this volume) that exhibit a long-lasting depolarization. Moreover, this increase, produced by a paired association of two inputs, is substantially greater than the transient calcium changes observed following stimulation of each of the same circuits as a single pathway (i.e., in an unpaired mode). The calcium changes are considered to arise from the opening of calcium channels to allow an influx of extracellular calcium. Similar changes have been postulated in learning in *Aplysia* (Carew *et al.*, 1981). Thus, in both systems a transient decrease in the level of calcium in the extracellular fluid would be expected. Direct measurements of the concentrations of Ca^{2+} in the extracellular space of mammalian CNS during stimulation indicate that transient decreases in Ca^{2+} levels can occur (Krnjevic *et al.*, 1982a; King and Somjen, 1981). In the rat hippocampus Krnjevic *et al.* (1982a,b) have observed decreases in extracellular calcium following stimulation *in vivo*. Stimulation of the fimbria at 10 Hz resulted in a Ca^{2+} decreases in the range of 0.1-0.75 mM in the vicinity of CA1 hippocampal pyramidal cell layer. Changes of a similar magnitude were observed in *in vitro* studies of the hippocampal slice (Krnjevic, Chapter 16, this volume). Such fluctuations in the calcium level are within the range that can cause the polymerization of ECF proteins. These data would tend to support the ependymin polymerization hypothesis. We clearly do not yet know if the hypothesis is valid. It is, however, a testable one and suggests a role for the proteins of the brain extracellular fluid in the neuroplasticity of the CNS. Thus the formation of an insoluble fibrous extracellular matrix may be one step in a complex series of events that can ultimately lead to the modification of the CNS after learning.

REFERENCES

Alkon, D. L., 1980, Cellular analysis of a gastropod (Hermissenda crassicornis) model of associative learning, *Biol. Bull.* **159**:505–560.

Appel, S. H., 1967, Turnover of brain messenger RNA, *Nature (London)* **213**:1253–1254.

Benowitz, L. I. and Shashoua, V. E., 1977, Localization of a brain protein metabolically linked with behavioral plasticity in the goldfish, *Brain Res.* **136**:227–242.

Bliss, T. V. P. and Lømo, T., 1973, Long-lasting potentiation of synaptic transmission in the dentate area of the anesthetized rabbit following stimulation of the perforant path, *J. Physiol. (London)* **232**:331–356.

Bonner-Frazer, M. and Cohen, A. M., 1980, Analysis of the neural Crest ventral pathway using injected tracer cells, *Dev. Biol.* **77**:130–141.

Bourre, J. M., Pollet, S., Paturneau-Jovas, M., and Baumann, N., 1977, Function and biosynthesis of lipids, *Adv. Exp. Med. Biol.* **83**:103–109.

Chaffee, J. and Schachner, M., 1978, A new cell-surface antigen of brain kidney and spermatozoa, *Dev. Biol.* **62**:173–184.

Carew, T. L., Walters, E. T., and Kandel, E. R., 1981, Associative learning in Aplysia: Cellular correlates supporting a conditioned fear hypothesis, *Science* **211**:501–504.

Clarke, J. T., 1967, Simplified "disc" (polyacrylamide gel) electrophoresis, *Ann. N. Y. Acad. Sci.* **121**:428–436.

Coons, A. H., 1968, Fluorescent antibody methods, in: *General Cytological Methods* (J. F. Danielle, ed.), Academic Press, New York, pp. 399–422.

Cragg, B., 1980, Preservation of extracellular space during fixation of the brain for electron microscopy, *Tissue Cell* **12**:63–72.

Cserr, H. F. and Ostrach, L. H., 1974, On the presence of subarachnoid fluid in the mudpuppy, Necturus maculosus, *Comp. Biochem. Physiol.* **48A**:145–151.

Duffy, C., Teyler, T. J., and Shashoua, V. E., 1981, Long-term potentiation in the hippocampal slice: Evidence for stimulated secretion of newly synthesized proteins, *Science* **212**:1145–1151.

Greene, E., Stauff, C., and Walters, J., 1972, Recovery of function with two-stage lesion of the fornix, *Exp. Neurol.* **37**:14–22.

Hartman, B. K., 1973, Immunofluorescence of dopamaine β-hydroxylase. Application of improved methodology to the localization of the peripheral and central noradrenergic nervous system, *J. Histochem. Cytochem.* **21**:312–332.

Hesse, G., Hofstein, R., and Shashoua, V. E., 1984, Protein release from hippocampus in vitro, *Brain Res.* **305**:61–66.

Hofstein, R., Hesse, G., and Shashoua, V. E., 1983, Protein of the extracellular fluid of mouse brain: Extraction and partial characterization, *J. Neurochem.* **40**:1448–1455.

King, G. L. and Somjen, G. G., 1981, Extracellular calcium and action potentials of soma and dendrites of hippocampal pyramidal cells, *Brain Res.* **226**:339–344.

Krnjević, K., Morris, M. E., and Reiffenstein, R. J., 1982a, Stimulation-evoked changes in extracellular K^+ and Ca^{2+} in pyramidal layers of the rat's hippocampus, *Can. J. Physiol. Pharmacol.* **60**:1643–1657.

Krnjević, K., Morris, M. E., Reiffenstein, R. J., and Ropert, N., 1982b, Depth distribution and mechanism of changes in extracellular K^+ and Ca^{2+} concentrations in the hippocampus, *Can. J. Physiol. Pharmacol.* **60**:1658–1671.

Lajtha, A. and Toth, J., 1966, Instability of cerebral proteins, *J. Biochem. Biophys. Res. Commun.* **23**:249–299.

Lynch, G. S. and Schubert, P., 1980, The use of in vitro brain slices for multidisciplinary studies of synaptic function, *Annu. Rev. Neurosci.* **3**:1–22.

Laemmli, U. K., 1970, Cleavage of structural proteins during the assembly of the head of bacteriophage T4, *Nature* **227**:680–685.

McCormick, D. A., Clark, G. A., Lavond, D. G., and Thompson, R. F., 1982, Initial localization of the memory trace for a basic form of learning, *Proc. Natl. Acad. Sci. USA* **79**:2731–2735.

McMahan, V. J., Edgington, D. R., and Kuffler, D. P., 1980, Factors that influence regeneration of the neuromuscular junction, *J. Expt. Biol.* **89**:31–38.

Majocha, R. E., Schmidt, R., and Shashoua, V. E., 1982, Cultures of zona ependyma cells of goldfish brain: An immunological study of the synthesis and release of ependymins, *J. Neurosci. Res.* **8**:331–342.

Reinhold, V. N., 1972, Gas-liquid chromatograpahic analysis of constituent carbohydrates in glycoproteins, in: *Methods of Enzymology*, Volume 25 (C. H. Hirs and S. N. Timasheff, eds.), Academic Press, New York, pp. 244–249.

Sanes, J. R., 1983, Roles of extracellular matrix in neural development, *Ann. Rev. Physiol.* **45**:581–600.

Schmidt, R. and Shashoua, V. E., 1981, A radioimunoassay for ependymins β and γ: Two goldfish brain proteins involved in behavioral plasticity, *J. Neurochem.* **36**:1368–1377.

Schmidt, R. and Shashoua, V. E., 1983, Structural and metabolic relationships between goldfish brain glycoproteins participating in functional plasticity of the central nervous system, *J. Neurochem.* **40**:652–660.

Schwartzkroin, P. A. and Wester, K., 1975, Long-lasting facilitation of a synaptic potential following tetanization in the *in vitro* hiippocampal slice, *Brain Res.* **89**:107–119.

Shashoua, V. E., 1968, RNA changes in goldfish brain during learning, *Nature (London)* **217**:238–240.

Shashoua, V. E., 1976, Brain metabolism and the acquisition of new behaviors. I. Evidence for specific changes in the pattern of protein synthesis, *Brain Res.* **111**:347–367.

Shashoua, V. E., 1977a, Brain metabolism and the acquisition of new behaviors. II. Immunological studies of the α, β and γ proteins of goldfish brain, *Brain Res.* **122**:113–124.

Shashoua, V. E., 1977b, Brain protein metabolism and the acquisition of new patterns of behavior, *Proc. Natl. Acad. Sci. USA* **74**:1743–1747.

Shashoua, V. E., 1979, Brain metabolism and the acquisition of new behaviors. III. Evidence for secretion of two proteins into the brain extracellular fluid after training, *Brain Res.* **166**:349–358.

Shashoua, V. E., 1981, Extracellular fluid proteins of goldfish brain: Studies of concentration and labeling patterns, *Neurochem. Res.* **6**(10):1129–1147.

Shashoua, V. E., 1982, Molecular and cell biological aspects of learning: Towards a theory of memory, *Adv. in Cell. Neurobiol.* **3**:97–141.

Shashoua, V. E., 1984, The role of extracellular glycoproteins in CNS plasticity: Calcium effects on polymerization, *Soc. Neurosci.* **10**:195.12.

Shashoua, V. E., 1985, The role of brain extracellular proteins in neuroplasticity and learning, *Cell. Molec. Neurobiol.* **5**:183–206.

Shashoua, V. E. and Hesse, G., 1985, Role of brain extracellular proteins in the mechanism of long-term potentiation in rat brain hippocampus, *Soc. Neurosci.* **11**:225.19.

Shashoua, V. E. and Moore, M. E., 1978, Effect of antisera to β and γ goldfish brain proteins on the retention of a newly acquired behavior, *Brain Res.* **148**:441–449.

Shashoua, V. E. and Moore, M. E., 1980, Enhanced labeling of ECF proteins in mouse brain after training, *Neurosci. Abstr.* **6**:290.4.

Shashoua, V. E. and Hesse, G., 1985, Role fo brain extracellular proteins in the mechanism of long-term potentiation in rat brain hippocampus, *Soc. Neurosci.* **11**:225.19.

Sternberger, L. A., 1979, *Immunocytochemistry*, J. Wiley & Sons, New York.

Tanzi, E., 1893, Nel'odierna istologia de sistema nervoso, *Riv. Sper. Freniatr. Med. Leg.* **19**: Alienazioni Ment. 419–472.

Teyler, T. J., Lewis, D., and Shashoua, V. E., 1981, Neurophysiological and biochemical properties of the goldfish optic tectum maintained in vitro, *Brain Res. Bull.* **7**:45–56.

Teyler, T. J., 1980, Brain slice preparation: Hippocampus, *Brain Res. Bull.* **5**:391–403.

Thompson, R. F., Berger, T. W., and Madden, J., IV, 1983, Cellular processes of learning and memory in the mammalian CNS, *Ann. Rev. Neuroscience* **6**:447–492.

Whittaker, V. P., 1959, The isolation and characterization of acetylcholine particles from brain, *Biochem. J.* **72**:694–706.

Index

Acetylcholine
  "M" channel and, 362
  receptors
    on basal and apical dendrites, 358, 360
    chloride channel conductance and changes
      in, 346
    facilitation of, 351
    phosphorylation of, 375, 377
Acetylcholinesterase, 341–355
  ACh-hydrolizing function of, 344–345
  inhibitors of, 342–343
Actin, 131, 388
Action potential, *see also* Membrane potential
  calcium, 283–289
  enhancement of, 428
Adenylate cyclase, neuronal response to
  serotonin and, 403
Afference memory, 119
Affinity chromatography, 477
γ-aminobutyric acid, IPSP alterations induced
  by, 231
Angiotensin II, receptors for, 365
Aplysia, 118, 261, 263, 400
  associative learning, 55–73
  bag cell neurons of, 422, 423, 424, 426, 427,
    431–434
  calcium inactivation of neuron of, 264, 265,
    268
Associative learning, *see also* Classical
    conditioning
  central neural pathways mediating, 85–93
  characteristics in *Hermissenda*, 3–17, 20–26
  depolarization and, 5–10, 36
  electrolyte currents and, 3–17, 47–49
  electrophysiological recording and, 3–17, 29,
    151
  evidence for, 4, 78
    in *Pleurobranchaea*, 83–84
  in insects, 110

Associative learning (*cont.*)
  model of, 65, 76
  potassium ion currents and, 3–17, 445–448
  protein phosphorylation and, 3–17, 442–443
  role of, 19
  sensory neuron and, 3–10, 67
  sites of, 5–10, 29–31
  test for, 83
Autoradiography, visualizing phosphoproteins
  by, 453
Avoidance conditioning, 76
Az III, monitoring intracellular free calcium ions
  with, 287

Backward conditioning, 155
Barium ions, 268
Brain
  gel electrophoresis for proteins in, 463
  metabolism, 239
  protein changes in mammalian, 471–474
  protein synthesis, 459
Brain stem, lesions, effect on conditioning, 213

Cadmium blockade, of calcium ion channels,
  275
Calcium, LTP and, 322
Calcium action potential, 135–136, 283–289
Calcium channel
  inactivation, 261–282
    computer simulations of, 274
    phases of, 266–267
Calcium ion(s)
  conditioning and intracellular, 13
  cytoplasmic buffering of free, 270, 271
  dyes sensitive to, 254
  flux into bag cells neurons, 431–434
  intracellular pH and, 265
  iontophoresis, 12
  membrane voltage and, 262–263

Calcium ion(s) (*cont.*)
 microinjection of, 12, 264
 modulation, 277
 protein phosphorylation and, 435
 red nucleus neurons and, 135
 regulatory function, 261
 role in learning, 12–15, 251–259
 sequestration, 255
 transmitter synthesis and influx of, 252
 Type B photoreceptor depolarization and,
  12–13
Calcium ion channels
 cadmium ion blockade of, 275
 cyclic nucleotides and, 375
 hydrogen ions and, 264
 inactivation, physiological significance of,
  277–278
Calcium ion current, mathematical model of,
  272
Calcium-phospholipid protein kinase, 436
Calmodulin
 protein kinase, 386
 role of, 385
Calmodulin/calcium dependent protein kinases,
  14–15, 435–436
Calmodulin kinase type II, vs. phosphorylase
  kinase, 447
Campbell's theorem, 342
Causal detection
 mechanisms of, 19–51
 systems, features of, 19
 within the visual vestibular system, 37–46
Causal relations, responding, 2
Central nervous system
 regeneration in, 187
 role of ependymin in, 485–488
Cerebellum, lesions, effect on conditioning, 213
Cerebral cortex, LTP in the, 384
Cerebral hemispheres, mnemonic interaction
  between and within, 223–231
Chicken, passive avoidance training in, 233–248
Chromatography, affinity, 477
Classical conditioning
 eye blink, 161–162
 Hermissenda, 1–2
 hypothalamic stimulation and, 151
 vs. operant conditioning, 120, 121
 red nucleus mediated, 127–139
Conditioned reflex, 158, 221–222
Conditioned responses
 cerebellar lesions and, 213
 motorneuron pool controlling, 197–208
Conditioning
 avoidance, 76, 80, 81, 82, 83
 backward, 82

Conditioning (*cont.*)
 classical, 1–2, 120, 121, *see also* Classical
  conditioning
 cyclic AMP and, 68–70
 discriminative, 162
 effects mimicked by phosphorylase kinase,
  446
 ependymin aggregation and, 483
 as a function of elevated intracellular calcium
  ions, 13
 operant, 120, 121, *see also* Operant
  conditioning
 phosphorylation and, 14
 rabbit, 16
 rapid, 157, 158–161, 162–163
 savings of, 80, 117
 trace, 213
 transfer of, 217
 "vestibular-motor," 460
Contingency learning, 25, 26, 37
Controlled stimulus, in food avoidance learning,
  80, 81, 82 83
Cortex, pyramidal cells of, 356, 357, 360
Cortical neurons
 input resistance of, 163, 291–305
 persistent changes in excitability, 162–163,
  291–305
Cortical pyramidal tract, 162, 292
Cortical unit
 activity,
  during rapid conditioning, 157
  hypothalamic stimulation and, 157
Corticorubral synaptic transmission, long-term
  potentiation of, 133–134
Cyclic AMP
 analog of, 413
 conditioning and, 68–70
 electrophysiological effects of, 423–425
 potassium ion channels and, 403
 potassium ion current and, 425
 protein kinase and effects of, 428
 protein phosphorylation and, 422, 425–429
 serotonin depolarization and, 63–64
Cycloheximide, neuronal firing and, 291
Cytoplasmic buffering, 270, 271

Dendritic spine, structure and function, 141–149
Dopamine, protein phosphorylation and, 409–411
Dorsal column section, 190–191, 191–192

Efference memory, 119
EGTA
 inactivation of calcium ions and, 264
 LTP and, 384
 steady state current and, 268

Electrolyte currents, associative learning and, 47
Electromyogram, 152
Electrophoresis, gel, 14
Energy metabolism, protein phosphorylation and, 422
Ependymin
  aggregation generated by LTP, 483
  aggregation properties of, 480–482, 483, 485
  amnesic effects of antisera to, 466, 468–470
  antigenic properties of, 479–480
  glycoprotein nature of, 477
  isolation of, 477–479
  molecular properties of, 475–482
  release into brain extracellular fluid, 470
  role in central nervous system, 485–488
EPSP: see Excitatory postsynaptic potential
Excitatory postsynaptic potential (EPSP)
  cerebral peduncular, 131
  corticorubral, 134
  dendritic, 130–131
  intracellular, 323
  morphological changes in dendritic spikes and alterations in, 130
  potentiation of, 321
  serotonin and, 59–62
  stimulus pairing and, 6
  in tail shock, 65, 66
  tetanization and, 321
Eye, retraction of, 197
Eye blink reflex
  rapid conditioning of, 151–165
  unconditioned, 156
Eyelid eye blink reflex, 221–222

Feeding behavior, avoidance conditioning of, 76
Fodrin, 388
Food avoidance learning, 76–84
  acquisition parameters for, 78
  cellular mechanisms underlying, 93–99, 100
  controlled stimulus in, 80, 81, 82, 83
  in vitro analysis of, 95–97
  selectivity in, 82–83
  uncontrolled stimulus in, 80, 82
Forskolin
  depolarizing effects, 62–63
  effect on action potential, 428
  input resistance and, 425

Gel electrophoresis, 14
  2-dimensional, 453
  for labeled brain proteins, 463
Glutamate, postsynaptic receptors for, 385
Glycoproteins, enhancement of turnover rate, 460

Hermissenda crassicornis, 3–17, 19–51, 441–457
  associative learning in, 1–2, 19
  memory in, 1–2, 19
Hippocampus
  calcium ion sequestration in, 255
  heterogenicity of spine structure in the, 147
  integrative firing in the, 315–317
  ionic conductance of pyramidal cells of the, 19, 313–314
  long-term potentiation and, 253, 319
  LTP in the, 384
  neuron firing patterns in the pyramidal cells of, 311–313
  spines and synaptic junctions in the, 145–146
Hydrogen ions, calcium ion channels and, 264
Hyperpolarization, 183
  posttetanic, 302
Hyperstriatum ventral, location of, 237
Hypothalmus
  associative conditioning and electrical stimulation of the, 151
  stimulation, 152
    cortical unit activity and, 157
    unconditioned eye blink response and, 156

Inhibitory postsynaptic potential (IPSP)
  hippocampal, 321
  intracellular, 323
Input resistance, 291, 293
  excitability and, 297
  measurement of changes in, 5–8, 293–294
  of motoneurons, 178
Insects, associative learning in, 110
Intermediate medial hyperstriatum ventrale, biochemical changes during PAT, 234, 237
Ion channels, neurotransmitter modulation of, 397
Ionic conductance
  protein phosphorylation and, 454
  in pyramidal cells, 313–314
Iontophoresis, 12
IPSP, see Inhibitory postsynaptic potential

Learning
  analog of, 76
  calcium ions and, 12–14, 251–259
  contingency, 25, 26, 57
  "passive" electrical interaction in, 254
  role of brain extracellular proteins in, 459–490
Limax, as model system of associative learning, 76
"Local enzyme" hypothesis, 333

Long-term facilitation (LTF), 334–336
  in isolated neuromuscular preparation, 336
Long-term potentiation (LTP), 252
  calcium and, 322
  EGTA and, 384
  ependymin aggregation generated by, 483
  glutamate postsynaptic receptors and the
    development of, 385
  hippocampal, 253, 319, 384
  homosynaptic, 334
  inhibition of, 384
  mechanisms underlying, 319–329
  memory and, 384
  at neuromuscular junctions, 331
  postsynaptic cell firing and, 322
  postsynaptic localization for, 384
  synaptic efficacy and, 320, 321
  trifluoperazine and, 384
Luteinizing hormone receptors, 365

MAP-2, 388, 392
"M" channel, 362, 363, 364
  coupled to other receptors, 365
  evidence for, 366
Membrane currents, 6–16
Membrane potential, *see also* Action potential
  calcium channel inactivation and, 275
  depolarization of, 283
  modulation of, 277
Membrane voltage, calcium ions and, 262–263
Memory
  age and, 465
  calcium and calmodulin-dependent protein
    kinase and, 383–396
  cellular events associated with, 3–19, 108
  defined, 107
  inhibition, following PAL, 239
  long-term, 465, 468
  LTP and, 384
  model for, 384
  protein kinase and, 383–396
  protozoan systems of, 119
  role of, 19
  role of brain extracellular proteins in,
    459–490
  short-term, 5–8, 465
    stores for, 119
  synaptic plasticity as neuronal basis for, 127
Microinjection experiments, 376–377
  specific problems in, 379
Microtubule, calmodulin-dependent regulation of
    function of, 391–393
Mnemonic interaction between cerebral
    hemispheres, 223–231

Mollusk, 3–17, 19–51, 441–457
  cellular mechanisms of causal detection in a,
    19–53
Motoneurons, 56, 57
  alpha, 167, 173, 177–180
  control of conditioned response via, 197–208
  input resistance, 178
  spinal, 255
Motor activity, sensory input in, 187–196
Motor cortex, organization of, 193

Neomycin, neuronal firing and, 291
Nervous system, as input/output information
    processor, 120
Neuron(s)
  bag cell, 422, 423, 424, 426, 427, 431–434
  cortical, 157, 291–305
  depolarization required to reach firing
    threshold of, 295
  firing of, 174, 291, 311–313
  increases in input resistance of, 163, 297
  modeling responses of, 307–310
  motor, 56, 57, 167, 173, 177–180, 197–208,
    255
  potentiation of activity of, 16
  protein phosphorylation and, 407–412, 422
  regions of specialization in, 355
  sensitization in, 58
  sensory, 56, 57, 67
Neurotransmitter
  release of, 422
  synthesis of, 422
Nictitating membrane, reflex arc, 197
Nucleotides, calcium ion channels and, 375

Olfactory tract, lateral fibers of, 356, 357, 358
Operant conditioning, vs associative
    conditioning, 120

Paracerebral neurons
  intracellular responses to food stimuli, 94
  role in feeding behavior, 89–93
Passive avoidance training (PAT), 233–248
Pavlovian conditioning, 19
  characteristics accompanying extinction of, 27
  model of, 3, 209–219
  of vertebrates, 4
pH, intracellular, 265
Pleurobranchaea, evidence for associative
    learning in, 83–84
Pleurobranchaea californica, 75–105
Phosphatase, phosphoprotein, 376
Phosphodiesterase inhibitors, increase in
    duration of after discharge by, 424

Phosphoprotein
  5HT-dependent, 417
  protocol for labeling, 448
  visualization by autoradiography, 453
Phosphorylase kinase
  vs. calmodulin kinase type II, 14–15, 447
  effects of conditioning mimicked by injection
    of, 14–15, 446
Phosphorylation
  calcium and calmodulin-dependent protein,
    7–15
  conditioning and, 14
Photoreceptors, Type B, role in conditioning, 4
Phototoxic behavior, suppression, 1–2, 20, 21,
    22, 23, 24, 25, 27, 39, 41, 47
Postsynaptic density (PSD), 386–391
  calmodulin-dependent kinase and function of,
    391
  cytoskeletal proteins in the, 388
  enzyme activities in the, 388, 390
Postsynaptic membrane, effects of glutamate and
    acetylcholine on properties of, 163
Posttetanic potentiation, 252
Posture, standing, neuronal mechanisms related
    to, 167–185
Potassium, persistent reductions in currents of,
    12
Potassium ion channels, 7–15
  cyclic AMP and, 403
  protein kinase activity and, 414
  serotonin and, 403
Potassium ion conductance, 136
  calcium-activated, 49
  cyclic AMP and, 425, 429
  phosphoproteins and, 413–414
  protein phosphorylation and, 407
  within visual vestibular system, 37–46
Prepulse inactivation, 49, 275
Protein
  beta, 465, 466, *see also* Ependymins
  changes in, in mammalian brain, 471–474
  half life of, 459
Protein kinase, 414
  abundance in nervous system, 422
  calcium-phospholipid dependent, 436
  calmodulin/calcium dependent kinase,
    435–436
  function of, 374
  inhibitor, 405
  isolation from brain, 386
  memory and, 383–396
  phospholipid-dependent, 447
  regulation of the activity of, 275–276
  role in mediating effects of cyclic AMP, 428

Protein kinase (*cont.*)
  structures for, 376, 379
  substrates for, 376, 379
Protein phosphatase, activation of, 452
Protein phosphorylation
  associative learning and, 442–443
  calcium and, 435
  changes during an after discharge, 429–431
  cyclic-AMP dependent, 422, 425–429
  dopamine and, 409–411
  energy metabolism and, 422
  ionic conductance, 454
  long-lasting changes in membrane excitability
    by, 421–439
  neuronal response to serotonin and, 422
  pattern of, 408
  potassium ion conductance and, 407
  protein synthesis and, 422
  in regulation of ion conductances, 373–382
  regulation of neuronal activity by, 397–419
  serotonin effects on, 408–409
  in a single neuron, 407–412
  synaptic stimulation and, 411–412
Protein synthesis
  passive avoidance training and, 234
  protein phosphorylation and, 422
Protozoa, species memories of instruction in,
    119
Purkinje cell, 221
  anatomy of, 356
  inhibition, 222
  spines of, 141, 142, 143, 144
Pyramidal cells
  ACh effects on, 360
  ionic conductance of, 313–314
  neuron firing patterns in, 311–313

Rabbit, conditioning of, 16
Rabbit nictitating membrane/eye blink
    conditioning, 212–217
Radioimmunoassay, 470
Rapid conditioning, 158–161
  cortical unit activity during, 157–158
  mechanisms of, 162–163
Red nucleus
  calcium ion-dependent potentials in neurons
    of, 135–136
  classical conditioning mediated by, 127–139
  lesions, effect on conditioning, 215
Reflex
  eye blink, 151–165
  tail withdrawal, 55–57
Renshaw cell, suppression of firing frequency
    of, 174

Resting potential, changes associated with
        increased excitability, 301–302
RNA
    synthesis, passive avoidance training and, 234
    turnover, 459

"savings of conditioning," 80, 117
SDS gel electrophoresis, 442, 443
Sensitization control cell SN3, 66, 67
Sensory cortex ablation, 189–190, 191–192
Sensory neurons, 1–19, 56, 57
    associative conditioning of, 67
    role in reflex action, 57
Serotonin, 118
    cyclic AMP and, 63–64
    depolarizing effects, 61
    EPSPs and, 59–62
    mechanism of neuronal response to, 401–402
    modulation of type B photoreceptor cell by,
        35
    potassium ion channels and, 403
    protein phosphorylation and, 408–409
    phosphoprotein and, 417
    receptor, 398, 413
Spinal motoneurons, calcium ion sequestration
        in, 255
Sprouting, 127–128
    corticorubral, 132
Steady state current, 268, 275
Stimulus
    presentation of, 152–153
    uncontrolled, uncontrolled stimulus
Stimulus pairing, 5–6, 8, 37, 39, 47
    excitatory postsynaptic potential and, 6
    in food avoidance conditioning, 77
    repeated, 6–7
    temporal relation for, 41
Supratrigeminal reticular formation, in transfer
        of conditioning, 217

Synapse
    changes in performance, 334
    neuroneuronal vs. neuromuscular junction,
        341
Synaptic function, segregation of, 355–369
Synaptic plasticity, 127
Synaptic potential, recording of, 337
Synaptic stimulation, protein phosphorylation
        and, 411–412

Tail shock, EPSP in, 65, 66
Tail withdrawal reflex, 55–57
    unconditioned stimulus and, 64
Tetanization, 322
    EPSP and, 321
    LTP-inducing, 324, 325, 326
Tetraethylammonium calcium ion action
        potential and, 286
Trace conditioning, 213
Trifluoperazine, LTP blockade with, 384
Tubulin, 388
Type A photoreceptor cell, 31
    depolarization, 5
Type B photoreceptor cell
    associative learning and depolarization of,
        5–8, 36
    depolarization of, 5
        cumulative, 5–8, 34
        response to light, 11
    hyperpolarization, 5
    intracellular calcium and depolarization of,
        12–13
    intracellular recordings from, 1–19, 29
    persistent increased excitability, 7–8
    role in conditioning, 4
    serotonin modulation of ionic currents in, 35
Uncontrolled stimulus
    in tail withdrawal reflex and, 64
    in food avoidance conditioning, 80, 82